ANNUAL REVIEW OF PHARMACOLOGY AND TOXICOLOGY

ANNUAL REVIEW OF PHARMACOLOGY AND TOXICOLOGY

HENRY W. ELLIOTT, *Editor*
California College of Medicine, University of California, Irvine

ROBERT GEORGE, *Associate Editor*
University of California School of Medicine, Los Angeles

RONALD OKUN, *Associate Editor*
California College of Medicine, University of California, Irvine

VOLUME 16

1976

ANNUAL REVIEWS INC.   4139 EL CAMINO WAY   PALO ALTO, CALIFORNIA 94306

ANNUAL REVIEWS INC.
Palo Alto, California, USA

International Standard Book Number: 0–8243–0416–0
Library of Congress Catalog Number: 61–5649

REPRINTS

The conspicuous number aligned in the margin with the title of each article in this
volume is a key for use in ordering reprints. Available reprints are priced at the
uniform rate of $1 each postpaid. The minimum acceptable reprint order is 10
reprints and/or $10.00, prepaid. A quantity discount is available.

PRINTED AND BOUND IN THE UNITED STATES OF AMERICA

PREFACE

Old friends of Annual Review of Pharmacology will have noticed by now that something new has been added—we start our fourth quinquennium as Annual Review of Pharmacology and Toxicology. While we have always recognized toxicology as an important area of pharmacology, there are many reasons for this special recognition in 1976. Perhaps the most important are increasing concern with the toxicology of nonmedical agents, the many toxicologists now in the field who were not trained primarily in classical pharmacology, and the proliferation of societies and regulatory agencies devoted to toxicology. We hope that the new title will help preserve the unity of the discipline. We are all concerned with the effects of chemicals (drugs) upon biological systems, and all chemicals can cause adverse effects (toxicity). No review is complete without some reference to toxicity, but it is not by accident that this volume contains nine reviews dealing predominantly with some aspect of toxicology. Some deal with toxicity related to therapeutics, others with accidental or industrial poisoning, and three with various methods for evaluation of pulmonary toxicity. These reviews emphasize both the scope of toxicology and its interdependence with other aspects of pharmacology.

We trust that old and new friends alike will be pleased with this and future volumes of Annual Review of Pharmacology and Toxicology and will join us in expressing here our thanks to our assistant editor Toni Haskell and our indexers Dorothy Read and Mary Glass.

THE EDITORIAL COMMITTEE

CONTENTS

ANNUAL REVIEWS INC. is a nonprofit corporation established to promote the advancement of the sciences. Beginning in 1932 with the *Annual Review of Biochemistry,* the Company has pursued as its principal function the publication of high quality, reasonably priced Annual Review volumes. The volumes are organized by Editors and Editorial Committees who invite qualified authors to contribute critical articles reviewing significant developments within each major discipline.

Annual Reviews Inc. is administered by a Board of Directors whose members serve without compensation.

Annual Reviews are published in the following sciences: Anthropology, Astronomy and Astrophysics, Biochemistry, Biophysics and Bioengineering, Earth and Planetary Sciences, Ecology and Systematics, Energy, Entomology, Fluid Mechanics, Genetics, Materials Science, Medicine, Microbiology, Nuclear Science, Pharmacology and Toxicology, Physical Chemistry, Physiology, Phytopathology, Plant Physiology, Psychology, and Sociology. In addition, two special volumes have been published by Annual Reviews Inc.: *History of Entomology* (1973) and *The Excitement and Fascination of Science* (1965).

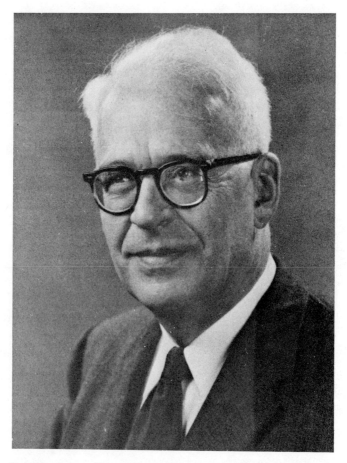

In 1959, when president of The American Society for Pharmacology and Experimental Therapeutics, and president-elect of The American Association for the Advancement of Science

Chauncey D. Leake

HOW I AM

❖6632

Chauncey D. Leake

University of California, San Francisco, California 94143

Although I am primarily a pharmacologist, I have a great diversity of related interests. This is natural. Pharmacology and toxicology are diverse disciplines, related to all the life sciences (including psychology and sociology); to the various clinical specialties of the expanding health professions; to agriculture, agronomy, ecology, forestry, oceanography, and even meteorology; to law, politics, and public policy, and to the arts and humanities, even to philosophy, especially the ethics, the logics, and the esthetics.

My entrance into pharmacology came by chance. During World War I, I was full of adolescent idealism to "save the world for democracy," and I was in service in March 1917. Universities were generous in those days: Princeton gave me a bachelor's degree (with a major in chemistry, biology, and philosophy), even though I missed half of the last semester of my senior year and did not turn in a thesis expected of me.

A top sergeant in a machine gun outfit training in Anniston, Alabama, I was transferred to the newly organized Chemical Warfare Service and sent to the Medical Defense Division, operating under Majors J. A. E. Eyster (1881–1955) and Walter J. Meek (1878–1963), in the physiology and pharmacology laboratories of the University of Wisconsin. The pharmacologist of the group was Arthur S. Loevenhart (1878–1929). He was in Washington. So was the biochemist, Harold C. Bradley (1878–1975).

Harold Bradley was a personnel officer for the Chemical Warfare Service, and it was he who spotted my chemistry-biology background. After the war, he taught me physiological chemistry, and we became close friends. His Madison home was a happy gathering place for his pupils. When he retired, he moved back to his father's home in Berkeley, California and became a leader in conservation. We enjoyed many pleasant evenings together at the Chit Chat Club meetings in San Francisco.

My job in the Chemical Warfare Service, in the basement of old Science Hall on the Madison Campus, was to study the effects of toxic war gases on the acid-base balance of blood. We used morphinized dogs. Samuel Amberg (1874–1966), who had come from the Mayo Clinic to work with us, and Walter Meek taught me well. We studied chlorine, chlorpicrin, mustard gas, and lewisite. When the war was over,

1

I was asked to stay on and run the necessary controls: what does morphine do to blood reaction in mammals?

In dogs, morphine causes first an increase in respiration, usually with vomiting, followed by respiratory depression, lassitude, and analgesia. I interpreted this as an initial decrease in cellular oxidative mechanisms in the medulla oblongata with subsequent increase of oxidative processes, in accordance with ideas expressed by Arthur Loevenhart and his pupil, Herbert Gasser (1888–1963). I showed that initial stimulation of the vomiting center by morphine is followed by depression, when vomiting cannot be induced either centrally by apomorphine or peripherally by stomach irritants. A ketosis develops after morphine, with a mild acidosis.

These findings (*J. Pharmacol.* 20:359–64, 1922; *Arch. Int. Pharmacodyn. Ther.* 27:221–27, 1922) suggested that it might be worthwhile to see what anesthetic agents do to blood reaction. So with my ever patient wife, Elizabeth, whom I was fortunate enough to marry in 1921, and with Alfred Koehler, a graduate student, we studied blood reaction in dogs under anesthesia with ether, chloroform, and nitrous oxide oxygen. We found an acidosis under ether and chloroform, with an initial alkalosis going into an acidosis under nitrous oxide and oxygen. The latter involves oxygen want if real anesthesia is to be obtained.

Meanwhile, Arno Luckhardt (1885–1957) in Chicago had introduced ethylene anesthesia. This has an advantage over nitrous oxide in that it can be successful with 15% oxygen (at sea level), instead of the 10% with nitrous oxide. Twelve percent is needed for satisfactory blood oxygenation. With Alrick Hertzman, I found that there is relatively little change in blood reaction with ethylene oxygen, and I thought this could be correlated with the generally superior clinical condition of patients under ethylene and oxygen.

This set me thinking about combining the chemical unsaturation of the carbon atoms in ethylene into the ether configuration. Long discussions were held on this, especially with my toxicology associate, Clarence Muehlberger (1896–1966). The compound in question, divinyl ether, was not in existence, but I determined to try to get it.

Meanwhile I had become engaged in many other search and research efforts. I reported a summary of our work on anesthesia and blood reaction at the Third Congress of Anesthetists in 1924 (*Br. J. Anaesth.* 2:1–20, 1924). With Frank G. Hall, I showed that alkalosis gives vascular constriction, while acidosis brings vascular relaxation. With Thomas K. Brown I found that infections, such as in experimental pneumonia, when there is respiratory involvement, are accompanied by an acidosis, due to an anoxic anoxemia.

With my wife, I became interested in blood regulation in anemias. Figuring that there might be some kind of a hormonal regulation, with red blood cell production geared to red cell destruction, we studied the effects of giving saline extracts of mammalian spleen and bone marrow to dogs. Stupidly we used healthy dogs, instead of trying to make them anemic. We found that spleen extracts give equivocal effects on erythrocyte counts, while bone marrow causes some increase. When we combined spleen and bone marrow we found a considerable rise in the red cell count. Liver, kidney, and heart extracts had no effect in our healthy dogs. So we introduced combined desiccated spleen and bone marrow for the treatment of secondary anemias. Clinically it seemed to be helpful. It had no effect in pernicious anemia. Years later, it seemed that spleen and bone marrow might give a kick to the reticuloendothelial system. My clinical balance was maintained by William S. Middleton, the sharp professor of medicine, who later became dean.

Those were busy years and happy ones, although we lived on a pittance. We canoed on Lake Mendota, picnicked on Picnic Point, and even got a secondhand auto for a trip to the East Coast. The university generously gave me a doctoral degree with publications in lieu of a thesis. My patient wife coached me in passing French in a qualifying exam. Walter Meek arranged for me to go to the Cleveland meeting of the Federated Societies in 1922, where Frederick Banting (1891–1941) thrilled us with his report on insulin. Meek got me into the American Physiology Society in 1923, but Torald Sollmann (1874–1962) kept me out of the Pharmacology Society until the following year, because as he said I was too young. Later he was a good friend.

I had become interested in historical and philosophical affairs, as a result of the stimulus of the William Snow Miller (1858–1939) seminar in medical history. One of my contributions was on the history of anesthesia (*Sci. Mon.* 20:304–28, 1925). This was later put into cadence, with a huge bibliographical chronology, and published by the University of Texas Press in 1947. I had written an account of Thomas Percival (1740–1804) and his misnamed "Medical Ethics" (*J. Am. Med. Assoc.* 81:366–71, 1923). This attracted the attention of Harvey Cushing (1869–1939), who asked me to come to Boston to present it there. He became one of my best friends and mentors. In 1927, this effort resulted in a book, *Percival's Medical Ethics,* which was published by Williams and Wilkins in Baltimore, under the direction of Charles C. Thomas, who later became his own distinguished publisher. This book fell flat as a mud pie. Amazingly, now, with much excitement over medical ethics, it is appearing in a second edition, nearly half a century after the first.

I became interested in William Harvey (1578–1657) and his great classic, *De Motu Cordis,* first issued in 1628. With coaxing from Charles Thomas, I undertook a new English translation to appear as a tercentennial tribute. Charles Thomas published it in fine format, and soon issued it in paperback, the first such in USA medical publishing. This has gone through five editions, the most recent in 1970. Harvey was probably the first to suggest giving drugs by injection into the blood circulation.

Meanwhile, Ralph Waters, the great anesthetist, came to Madison to develop anesthesia in the new Wisconsin General Hospital, the main clinical facility for the university. He came, in part, he said to have a chance to work with pharmacologists. He established a great residency training program in anesthesia, and we started a long work effort. In 1828, Henry Hill Hickman (1800–1830), in England, had used carbon dioxide as an anesthetic in dogs. No one had studied it since from that standpoint. Ralph Waters and I decided to try it out. We found that carbon dioxide, 30% with 70% oxygen, is indeed anesthetic, with no asphyxia involved. This we reported at the Seventh Congress of Anesthetists held at the University of Wisconsin in 1928, a century after Hickman.

Although I had started as a physiologist, Arthur Loevenhart persuaded me to move alone with him in pharmacology, and I soon was an associate professor, with major teaching responsibilities. In reality at Wisconsin, physiology, pharmacology, and physiological chemistry worked together. We had a joint weekly seminar in Arthur Loevenhart's pleasant laboratory; the large graduate student laboratory, under the calm, efficient eye of William Young, our English "diener," was a center of experimentation, with its big kymograph, and I had a convenient office-laboratory of 300 square feet, with a chemical bench and hood on one side, a microscope bench along the windows, and desks along the other side. I had graduate students with me: Peter K. Knoefel, later professor of pharmacology at the University of Louisville; George Wakerlin, later professor of physiology at Louisville and director of the American Heart Association, and Warren Stratman-Thomas, who worked so well on African sleeping sickness and its chemotherapy. The chemotherapy of trypanosomiasis was one of Arthur Loevenhart's major contributions.

From the way the four of us worked together in one office-lab came the idea for "The Student's Unit Medical Laboratory" (*J. Am. Med. Assoc.* 82:114–17, 1924). This attracted the interest of Abraham Flexner (1866–1959) and was the beginning of the now popular multidiscipline medical laboratories. Lathan Crandall, later director of research for Miles Laboratories, also worked with us on a broad study of the pharmacology of nitrites and nitrates, initiated by Arthur Loevenhart at the request of the DuPont interests to see whether or not it would be possible to get the headache out of dynamite. It is not, unless one has a nonnitroglycerine dynamite.

I was fortunate in having many keen colleagues at Wisconsin. K. K. Chen, who introduced ephedrine and later became research director for Eli Lilly, was one. Elmer Sevringhaus, who later was research director for Hoffman-LaRoche, was another. Another was Fred Jenner Hodges, later professor of radiology at the University of Michigan, and one of our greatest leaders in the field. We had some great graduate students: Samuel Lepkovsky, distinguished in vitamin nutrition and my colleague in Berkeley; Karl Link, who developed the coumarin anticoagulants, and Conrad Elvehjem (1901–1962), who isolated niacin, and later was president of the University of Wisconsin. These students came over from the College of Agriculture, where they had been trained by the vitamin pioneers, Edwin B. Hart (1874–1953) and Harry Steenbock (1886–1967).

When I arrived at the University of Wisconsin, I roomed with Edwin and Mrs. Fred, on Mendota Court, close to the lake with its swimming and boating. Edwin Fred was a kind mentor; he later became dean of the College of Agriculture and president of the university. He was a distinguished bacteriologist. My Wisconsin experiences have been a continuing inspiration to me.

In July 1927, I had a telegram from Carl L. A. Schmidt, professor of biochemistry at the University of California in Berkeley, asking me to come out in August for four months to teach pharmacology to the second-year medical students, then studying in Berkeley. Out we went, full of excitement, leaving the hot Midwest, and arriving in foggy, cool Berkeley, where the palms waved over fur-coated coeds. My office was in old Budd Hall, and the class met in the redwood Spreckles Laboratory where Jacques Loeb (1859–1924) had taught. The class was an alert one. I had time to do a bit of work on the effect of anesthetics on the osmotic resistance of erythrocytes. It was a stimulating atmosphere, with Karl F. Meyer (1884–1974) as professor of microbiology, and Herbert M. Evans (1882–1971), the neurotic discoverer of vitamin E, and pioneer on the estrus cycle and anterior pituitary hormones, as professor of anatomy.

The Medical School of the University of California was being reorganized, and President William Wallace Campbell (1862–1938), the great astronomer, asked me to come back in July 1928 as professor of pharmacology. We did so, but found that a laboratory had been provided on the top floor of the old medical school building in San Francisco. I had an office, and arranged a small laboratory under a mezzanine which was built for graduate students at the front of the large high general laboratory. It was a great place. With William Gilmore as an efficient "diener," we soon had the place humming.

Peter Knoefel came as a National Research Council fellow; Eric Reynolds (who later was president of the California Medical Society) lent us clinical guidance, and Hamilton H. Anderson, with Norman A. David and Anderson Peoples, worked with us while getting their medical degrees. Peter Knoefel and I began work on divinyl ether, which had been prepared for us, along with other unsaturated ethers, by Randolph Major at Princeton. Major later became director of research for Merck. With Mei-Yu Chen, a remarkably able worker, whom I had met at the Boston Physiology Congress, we found that divinyl ether has the anesthetic properties we had predicted for it. We had the good, practical help of Arthur E. Guedel of Los Angeles, who had been an associate of Ralph Waters. Our experimental study was summarized in 1933 (*J. Pharmacol.* 47:5–16), and the agent soon went into clinical use. But it is flammable, very powerful, and likely to injure livers if anesthesia with it is too long maintained.

We experimented with various halogenated hydrocarbons and both saturated and unsaturated ethers, but found nothing safe or useful. It remained for John Krantz, the keen pharmacologist at the University of Maryland, to study fluorinized compounds, which became available after World War II. These led to halothane, now a popular anesthetic, developed by my friend, Yule Bogue, of Imperial Chemical Industries.

K. F. Meyer, director of the Hooper Foundation for Medical Research, was interested in tropical medicine. He suggested that we study the chemotheraphy of amebiasis. This, we found, has about a 10% incidence in the USA, mostly as carriers. We got a dozen or so organic arsenical compounds from Lilly, and an equal number of halogenated hydroxyquinolines from Ciba, and started screening them. Hamilton Anderson handled the arsenicals, and Norman David the hydroxyquinolines.

First, Hamilton Anderson showed the unsatisfactory toxicity of emetine, the standard remedy for amebiasis. It injures heart muscle. Then, using natural amebic infestations in macaques, we found that 4-carbaminophenyl arsonic acid, called *carbarsone* for short, is only mildly effective, but safe. It also seems to have a general "tonic" effect. So we started using it clinically, after taking it ourselves, and finding that most of it is excreted within a day. Alfred Reed, a skilled clinician, directed clinical trials. Later, Hamilton Anderson, with his wife Jeanette, studied amebiasis and treated it successfully in many parts of the tropics in Africa, Latin America, and Asia. Herbert Johnstone (1903–1956) aided in much of this.

Quite as easy to show carbarsone better than stovarsol for amebiasis was it to show iodochlorhydroxyquinoline superior to iodohydroxyquinoline. Indeed, we found iodochlorhydroxyquinoline (Vioform ®) to be a useful intestinal antiseptic generally. Soon after Norman David introduced it for use in amebiasis, it was in wide use throughout the world for intestinal infections, and could be purchased by travelers over-the-counter, except in the USA. We noted no neurotoxic symptoms, as have been described, because our evidence showed it is not absorbed from the gut. A general review of our studies on the chemotherapy of amebiasis was prepared by me in 1932 (*J. Am. Med. Assoc.* 98:195–98). Norman David later became professor of pharmacology at the University of Oregon, Portland.

Our strategy in the amebiasis effort was simple: we eliminated many proposed remedies as ineffective, and concentrated on types of chemicals showing promise. We tried the same strategy in tackling the chemotherapy of leprosy, but soon abandoned the effort because we found the disease so hedged by politics and vested interests that clearly we were not welcome. We did, however, carefully study the characteristics of the organism, and used murine leprosy in test animals. George Emerson, a brilliant chemical biologist who came to us from Berkeley, devised the water-soluble chaulmoogryl-glycerophosphate for intravenous medication.

Meanwhile, Peter Knoefel studied acetals and aldehydes and added much stimulus to our efforts as he joined us each summer. Through K. F. Meyer, we brought over Myron Prinzmetal, later the distinguished cardiologist from Los Angeles, to work on "mussel poison." He persuaded us to offer a place for animal experimentation to Gordon Alles (1901–1963), a keen organic chemist from Los Angeles. Alles was trying to find a synthetic substitute for ephedrine, the price of which had gone sky-high, to use in treating asthma. Alles was supported by George Piness, the leading West Coast allergist from Los Angeles.

Alles was a most meticulous experimenter. He properly used molal solutions of the drugs he had made, thus being able to compare them in millimole doses on a strict molecular basis. He developed the amphetamines. I have told of his important work in the summary entitled *The Amphetamines* (Thomas, Springfield, Ill., 1958, 167 pp.).

Many graduate students came to work with us: Carroll Handley (1911–1958), later professor of pharmacology at Baylor Medical College in Houston; Benedict Abreu (1913–1965), later in charge of pharmacological research for Pitman-Moore in Indianapolis and professor of pharmacology at the University of Texas Medical Branch in Galveston; Nilkanth Phatek (1898–1971), a political refugee from Bombay and later professor of pharmacology at the University of Oregon Dental School; Michael Shimkin, keen administrator from Tomsk, who later became professor of medicine at Temple and professor of community medicine and oncology at the University of California at San Diego; James Morrison, later at Emory University, Atlanta; David Marsh (1919–1961), later director of research at McNeil Laboratories, Philadelphia; Jack Ferguson (1918–1959), later at the Medical College of Virginia, and E. Leong Way, later professor of pharmacology at the University of California in San Francisco, and famed for his studies on morphine derivatives.

Some of these students came from Berkeley as a result of a general course on pharmacology I offered there at the instigation of Carl L. A. Schmidt, others as a result of our cooperation with the School of Pharmacy in San Francisco. This had been reorganized by Carl Schmidt into a fine teaching and research institution, with a brilliant faculty, including the physical-chemist Troy Daniels, who later became dean; Robertson Pratt, microbiologist; John Eiler, biochemist; Warren Kumler, physical-chemist; and Louis Straight, spectrometrist. Michael Hrenoff helped develop mass spectrometry, and his brother, Arseny, was a devoted worker in our laboratory. We all worked rather closely together.

We had regular seminar sessions, which overflowed into the Crummer Room, and often for Sunday meetings in the Santa Cruz redwoods in a spot on the San Lorenzo River, which my wife and I developed for happy weekends. We had a large redwood circle with rustic benches around and a blackboard on a big tree. There, with our two sons, Chaunc and Wilson, we would entertain our friends and their families, and have vigorous scientific discussions. Arthur Guedel often came from Los Angeles, with friends, to debate metabolic effects under anesthesia. We tried out our proposed publications here, and then often reported them before the quarterly meetings of the West Coast section of the Society for Experimental Biology and Medicine. In these meetings we usually had sharp but pleasant debate with our colleagues from Stanford. Maurice Tainter, later the distinguished director of the Winthrop Laboratories, often joined us.

Maurice Tainter studied dinitrophenol as a stimulant of biological oxidation. We aided in studies on its toxicity. This suggested that we might use its respiratory-stimulating power to counteract the respiratory depression of morphine. So George Emerson easily made dinitrophenylmorphine, and it was well studied by Benedict Abreu, George Emerson, and Nilkanth Phatek. It is pain relieving without causing respiratory depression, and we had evidence that it might be less addictive than morphine. But bureaucratic red tape kept us from trying it clinically, except on ourselves.

By this time we had an arrangement with the Shell Development Company, under Clifford Williams, to test the toxicity of new organic chemicals and solvents, not only to protect the public but the workmen in the plant as well.

We had a heavy teaching load. We enjoyed it. I lectured to medical, dental, and pharmacy students jointly, but we split laboratory assignments. We offered a special course for nurses, and for collegiate students in Berkeley. We had postgraduate sessions. We made up our reference sources, and did not use texts. We tried to get our students to contribute. We were quite informal, and had the laboratory hung with pictures of the leading pharmacology contributors. Otto Guttentag, Charles Gurchot, and Salvatore Lucia added philosophical spice. Milton Silverman gave us helpful journalistic aid in writing. He got his degree from Stanford, but did the work for it (sugar synthesis under ultraviolet light) in our laboratory. He later became one of our best science writers, the author of *Magic in a Bottle* (Macmillan, New York, 1941, 332 pp.); *Alcoholic Beverages in Clinical Medicine* (Yearbook Medical Publishers, Chicago, 1966, 160 pp.); and with Philip Lee, *Pills, Profits and Politics* (University of California Press, Berkeley, 1974, 403 pp.).

My wife and I finally made the Grand Tour in 1938. We visited A. J. Clark (1885–1941) in Edinburgh, with his great collection of poisons brought together by T. R. Fraser (1841–1920). We stopped in Oxford for the meeting of the British Pharmacology Society, where I reported on dinitrophenylmorphine, and where we watched J. H. Burn and Edith Bulbring do some of their careful experimentation. We enjoyed meetings with A. V. Hill and Sir Henry Dale. In Ghent we had a marvelous visit with Corneel Heymans (1892–1968), with his fine institute, and in neat 18th Century Darmstadt, with the Mercks. We went to the Physiology Congress in Zurich, where we enjoyed a visit with Hans Fischer out on the lake, and where we met Arthur Stoll (1887–1971) contemplating one of the huge military murals of Ferdinand Hodler (1853–1918). We later became good friends with the Stolls, who had one of the greatest art collections anywhere. Stoll, a pupil of Richard Willstätter (1872–1942), the great chlorophyll chemist, worked brilliantly on digitalis glycosides and ergot alkaloids. He directed the great Sandoz drug company.

The Zurich Congress was exciting. We had an extemporaneous discussion on the status of pharmacology as a science. This became the subject of my address as retiring president of the American Association for the Advancement of Science in 1961. I try to get double duty out of ideas, if I can!

So we worked cheerfully along. Ross Hart and Elton McCawley came as graduate students. Taking up our observation that the allyl radical stimulates respiration, they made N-allylnormorphine, in an effort to get the pain-relieving properties of morphine without its respiratory depression. But it turned out to be a morphine antagonist. As "nalorphine" it was widely used to detect morphine or heroin addiction and to treat narcotic overdose, as suggested by Eddie Way, another brilliant graduate student.

In order not to use too much space in the professional journals, we started *University of California Publications in Pharmacology* in 1938. This assured us prompt publication through the University of California Press, and we could distribute as we wished. Here we published many of our toxicity studies on new solvents made by the Shell Development Company. Here Benedict Abreu and Nilkanth Phatak published their important studies on nitrofuran antiseptics. These later came to wide clinical use. We also made furan local anesthetics, but these had no particular advantage. We even tried a furan aspirin, but this came to grief: animal experiments showed its value and apparent low toxicity. But when I took it, it deposited on my bladder wall, and I had to be hospitalized to be cleaned out. We had not looked at the bladders of our animals in our routine postmortem examinations of sacrificed animals in our toxicity studies. Now we do.

We had contact with the great cyclotron radiation laboratory in Berkeley, through Joseph Hamilton (1907–1957), one of our clinical associates, who was interested in radioactive iodine for thyroid studies. This he prepared himself in the Berkeley laboratory, and somehow got exposed so that he developed leukemia. He succeeded in correlating the deposition of iodine in the thyroid with the histology of the gland. This publication of 1940 was reproduced by Lloyd Roth at the University of Chicago Symposium on *Autoradiography of Diffusible Substances* (Academic Press, New York, 1969). Another worker with us was Charles Pecher, a Belgian, who studied whole body autoradiography in mice with radioactive calcium and strontium. He used these substances clinically in osteoblastic bone tumors. When we were blown into World War II, he enlisted and was killed within a year.

With war upon us, we turned our attention to war gases, the use of which was threatened by the Japanese. I went up and down the West Coast talking to high school students (who were sensible, and could tell their elders) about simple protection against war gases: if exposure is suspected, breathe through a wet handkerchief or rag, using urine if no water is available; get out of the area, shed outer clothing, and as soon as possible get a thorough scrubbing with soap and water. I was not popular with official stuffed shirts who issued elaborate instructions for identification of the gases and the different ways to handle each one—as if the enemy would oblige by shelling over one gas alone. David Marsh and I prepared an article for clinicians, based on our direct experiments with mustard gas on our own arms, showing that sodium hypochlorite solutions or soap and water would protect one, if applied within ten minutes of exposure.

In the midst of all this, when I was getting a little respite at the glorious Bohemian Grove on the Russian River, in the summer of 1942, I got an urgent phone call asking me to come to Texas to clear up a messy administrative situation at the University of Texas Medical Branch in Galveston. I went down, met the regents, and we liked each other, especially Lutcher Stark of Orange, who noted calluses on my hands and said I'd do. It was easy enough to get the place in order, with an open door to my office, and with Sunday afternoon receptions which Elizabeth, my always efficient wife, arranged at our home for faculty, students, and townspeople. But this all left no time for pharmacology. Actually, when we admitted two classes a year, and increased the size of each to 120, as part of the war effort, I continued to teach.

The pharmacologist at Galveston, Wilfred Dawson, had killed himself in frustration over the administrative situation, and I had to try to take over. Pharmacology had its own building, a wooden one, but quite adequate, and we soon had a seminar going, as well as classes. Both students and clinicians seemed interested in a new point of view. We used no text but asked the students to submit a couple of term papers properly documented, and graded from excellent to poor. We started publication of a quarterly *Texas Reports on Biology and Medicine,* which soon attracted contributions from all over, since we sent it without charge to the libraries of medical institutions throughout the world. The response in exchange journals made our library the best in the Southwest. It was especially gratifying to get a generous response from Russia.

As soon as the war was over, we planned and built new hospital and laboratory facilities. We promoted Galveston as a health resort, and I traveled over the South and Midwest spreading the gospel of the rational use of drugs, and the ever widening scope of pharmacology. I had helped that energetic gynecologist, William Bertner, organize the great medical center in Houston, with wise leadership from Fred Elliott, dean of the University of Texas Dental Branch, and Lee Clark, the efficient director of the M. D. Anderson Tumor Clinic and Hospital. I helped Baylor Medical School get started in Houston, getting Anderson Peoples and Carroll Handley to take over pharmacology. We gave library and laboratory equipment and books to these new developments, and even lent personnel to help get them going. Then they got the money, and soon had a huge and flourishing center. We aided in the establishment of the University of Texas Medical School in Dallas and tried to promote one in San Antonio.

I was fortunate in persuading Charles Marc Pomerat (1905–1964) to join our staff in anatomy, which had been so well maintained by Donald Duncan. Pomerat was a brilliant cytologist and teacher, a fine artist and bon vivant. He got our students interested in etching and lithography and established as fine a tissue culture laboratory as could be found. His great contribution was to use time-lapse cinematography to record changes in tissue culture under different conditions. I worked with him on drug effects on cells in tissue culture, and reported with him on this work at a tissue culture symposium he arranged with the New York Academy of Sciences. His studies even inspired me to write a half dozen "Tissue Culture Cadences." His biobibliography appears in the June 1965, issue of *Texas Reports on Biology and Medicine,* with many of his drawings and watercolors.

Meanwhile I began serving on many national committees dealing with problems of alcohol and with various aspects of medical education. These were tiresome. Frank Fremont-Smith (1895–1973), director of the Macy Foundation, made a great success of arranging series of conference discussions. I was invited to join one on neuropharmacology, chaired by Harold Abramson. This met pleasantly in Princeton and gave me a chance to get back to that delightful place. Elizabeth and I spent several months on three occasions in Princeton, when I worked at the Institute for Advanced Study, under Robert Oppenheimer (1904–1967) whom I had known at Berkeley. I was preparing a translation and annotation of the Hearst Medical Papyrus, a drug formulary from Egypt about 1550 BC, which was a prized possession of the Anthropology Museum of the University of California, which was in San Francisco when I first went there. It had attracted my interest then, and it still does. My work resulted in the Logan Clendenning Lecture at the University of Kansas (*The Old Egyptian Medical Papyri,* University of Kansas Press, 1952, 111 pp.).

With George Emerson in charge of pharmacology, my effort therein turned to writing reviews. I prepared one on drugs acting on the central nervous system, including the hallucinogenic agents, and then a more pertinent clinically oriented one on an analysis of drugs used in allergy (*Texas Reports on Biology and Medicine* 9:322–40, 1951). Ever interested in training programs, I wrote on the training of professional pharmacologists, and also on the training of physicians for general practice. Disturbed by the McCarthy witch-hunting, I wrote on the ideals of science in relation to national security (*Texas Rep. Biol. Med.* 13:434–45, 1955), and was denied clearance to go to Ecuador to survey medical education there. But I also wrote on ideals for a community health library.

Political machinations began again in Texas. I should have been alerted when a new bunch of regents fired James Hart, a distinguished barrister, as president of the University after a year of helpful leadership. The big corporations, anxious to avoid severance taxes on natural resources, set up the Texas Research League (nonprofit, and thus tax-exempt) to advise state agencies on operating with efficiency and economy. The university was hard hit. Most of the administrators resigned, as did I. When Charles Doan, the brilliant hematologist, and dean of the Ohio State University Medical School, asked me to join his program, we packed up and left Galveston to settle in Columbus. It took a decade for the University of Texas to recover. Now under the inspiring leadership of Truman Blocker, the University of Texas Medical Branch is flourishing, with an Oceanographic institute and an institute for the Humanities in Medicine, both of which Charles Pomerat and I had dreamed about. Galveston also has a superb seaorama, with a great aquarium, and performing seals, dolphins, and whales. We had tried to get an aquarium going years before, but it was a flop.

At Columbus my main job was to try to organize a laboratory for pharmacology. This was not easy in a predominately clinical school. Fortunately, I had the interest of Bernard Marks, and he took hold in admirable style, building a splendid group of teachers and graduate students. He worked on cardiovascular drug problems, while I went back to the stimulant action of spleen-marrow on the reticular endothelial system. I thought that stimulation of red blood cell production might aid in counteracting the fatal anemia following whole-body radiation. I used hundreds of mice, but had only slight indication that spleen-marrow fed ad lib before radiation might be helpful. The evidence was too slight to publish.

Now there were too many meetings: Macy Foundation Conferences on Central Nervous System and Behavior, National Research Council on Problems of Alcohol, The National Medical Library, Physiology Congress in Buenos Aires, History of Medicine Congress in Athens and Cos, and meetings of pharmacologists and the too big sessions of the federated societies at Atlantic City. I was up to my neck with travel. But my wife topped it off with two trips around the world.

With me home in bed, I was nominated from the floor and made president of the American Society for Pharmacology and Experimental Therapeutics. Ben Abreu told me I'd better get over to Chicago. I did not get a warm reception from the "establishment," but we soon were humming along with news letters and *Pharmacological Reviews,* and I started *The Pharmacologist.* I became involved with the American Association for the Advancement of Science, and presently was its president. My historical interests appeared in my address on retiring: "The Status of Pharmacology as a Science" (*Science,* Dec. 29, 1961).

But even with growing preclinical strength at Columbus, there were difficulties. We had a fine seminar, cooperating with Arthur Tye in pharmacy, and with Eric Ogden (1903–1973) who had built a great department of physiology. A new administration began cutting. With Bernard Marks running pharmacology well, I thought it was time to quit. We enjoyed Columbus. We helped get the symphony rolling under Evan and Jean Whalon, and the Kit-Kat Club was a stimulus to me.

Robert Featherstone had come to San Francisco from Iowa to take charge of pharmacology after Hamilton Anderson retired. John Saunders had built a big laboratory building, and pharmacology had new quarters, with much stimulus for growth. Robert Featherstone (1914–1974) was interested in mechanisms of anesthesia, promoted student research and asked me to guide it. So out we came again to San Francisco, where my brother Russell, found an apartment with a view for us near the school. I was given an office in the dining room of an old house below the school, and assured that I'd soon have fine quarters. I'm still there.

Actually I'm having a good time and enjoying it. Occasionally I'm asked to lecture in pharmacology to nurses or pharmacists, and I get to pharmacology seminars once in a while. Mostly I'm busy in my book-crowded office, trying to write what I think is worthwhile. The ethical problems of medical practice have long interested me; now they are hot subjects of debate. I'm interested in how theories of ethics apply. There is vast confusion in ethical theory in organ transplants, for example, and human experimentation raises many questions. Even euthanasia is pharmacologically related.

Since I can do quite as I wish, I offer a no-credit course on the ethics, the logics, and the esthetics. It is fairly well attended, but not by the graduate students for whom it is designed. I think that persons holding the degree, doctor of philosophy, should know something about the subject. I also teach a no-credit course on the history and philosophy of the health professions, quite as I have done yearly for over fifty years. This course is well attended. I offer coffee and cookies as bait.

Thanks to Henry Elliott, my former colleague, and now handling both pharmacology and anesthesiology well at our Irvine campus, I was asked to write a review of reviews for *Annual Review of Pharmacology,* when Murray Luck's great series was expanded in 1960 to include pharmacology. Thanks to Henry Elliott again, I have written such a review each year since. It helps to keep me abreast of the rapidly expanding field of pharmacology and toxicology. My colleagues, Harold Hodge and Charles Hine, help with toxicology, and Eddie Way always helps, as does Vi Sutherland, with details of pharmacology.

James Dille, developing a keen pharmacology program for the University of Washington in Seattle, persuaded the West Coast pharmacologists to organize the Western Pharmacology Society. He guided it well for many years. After a decade, he turned it to me as secretary-treasurer, and I enjoyed preparing the meetings and the proceedings, until I got in trouble with a president who wanted to run things his way, so I quit and let him do so.

Meanwhile I traveled a lot. Under the auspices of our State Department (having somehow been cleared), I went to the Brussels Physiology Congress, where I put on an exhibit entitled *Some Founders of Physiology,* and then via Helsinki, to Leningrad. There I enjoyed the high morale of the devoted staff of S. V. Anichkov, and of the keen workers at the Institute for Experimental Medicine, with their high regard for Charles Darwin. In Moscow it was a joy to know P. K. Anokhin (1898–1974), director of the Sechenov Institute for Physiology, who later visited and stayed with us.

My regard for Frank Berger was always high. He had developed meprobamate as a mild tranquilizer. Thanks to him, and Charles Hoyt, we went to Japan, and had a great time in the pharmacology laboratories in Tokyo, Osaka, and Kyoto. It was a special pleasure to meet Professor Hiroshi Kumagai, and his colleague, Setsuro Ebashi, and to learn of their fine work on muscle contraction. With Frank Berger again, I had the joy of meeting Silvio Garattini at his fine Instituto Mario Negri in Milan, at a conference on anti-inflammatory drugs.

Elizabeth and I enjoyed visiting Arthur and Martha Stoll at their lovely art gallery villa at Vevey on Lake Geneva, and going to Spain for an exciting visit with Francisco Guerra, who had done so well for pharmacology in Mexico. Francisco Guerra had explored Mexican hallucinogenic drugs, and had written widely on Mayan drugs. His baronial holdings in Santillana-sur-Mar include the famed Altamira Caves. Guerra had raised a company to protect his village in the Spanish

Civil War, and after losing a leg in the fighting, had fled to Mexico, where he became professor of pharmacology at the National University.

My interest in what goes on in pharmacological and medical fields led me to put out a monthly mimeographed sheet, "Calling Attention To," for the benefit of my friends. At Galveston and Columbus this grew to over 1500 copies a month. The postage was too much on my return to California, so I restricted the effort to books, a list of which appears monthly in *Current Contents—Life Sciences.* This is one of the helpful publications of the Institute for Scientific Information in Philadelphia, started on a shoestring by my long-time friend, Eugene Garfield, and now a large and vigorous enterprise. I had worked with Garfield while trying to convert what was then the Armed Forces Medical Library into a truly national library of medicine.

My pharmacological interests may sometimes seem to be far afield. I was once president of the Sex Education Society in San Francisco back in depression days. We ran a birth-control clinic, and our effort later grew into the Planned Parenthood program. In 1940, the students in Berkeley petitioned the faculty for a sex education course. I was put in charge. I made it a non-credit affair, with emphasis on human relations. If interpersonal relations are in order, sex relations will usually be so too. It was a shock to find 2600 students showing up for the weekly illustrated lectures. World War II stopped this undertaking.

The Hastings College of the Law in San Francisco was made by Sam Snodgrass, its informal dean, into one of the best in USA, simply by asking retired deans and professors from other law schools to join his faculty. His 65 Club included some of the greatest law teachers in USA. He asked me to join, in order to teach medical jurisprudence. I knew no law, but I had had much experience as an expert witness, and I did know something about toxicological analysis. The course went well for several years, until Dean Snodgrass died and a new, more formal and pedantic dean took over. He didn't like my informal grading system of good, bad, or indifferent, since law schools grade to decimal points. So I quit. But I enjoyed the experience.

Stanley Jacob, at the University of Oregon Medical School, had found dimethyl-sulfoxide (DMSO) to be an excellent solvent and skin absorbable. He used it to dissolve steroids for local application in arthritis. On trying DMSO alone, as a control, he found it was effective. It tends to dissolve collagen and fibrous tissue. So he began using it in a variety of clinical conditions for which it was indicated, and ran smack into the new regulations of the Food and Drug Administration, of which he knew nothing. He was accused of violating practically all of them. I persuaded James Goddard, FDA Director, that Jacob was not criminally minded, and we arranged a big symposium on DMSO under the auspices of the New York Academy of Sciences (*Ann. NY Acad. Sci.* 141:1–671, 1967). Schering AG, under the keen direction of Gerhard Laudahn, arranged for a notable clinical conference on DMSO in Vienna (*Dimethyl-sulfoxyd: DMSO,* Salabruck, Berlin, 1966, 219 pp). In spite of countless handicaps, Stanley Jacob has persisted in the careful, patient accumulation of data, so that DMSO now has a chance again of helping people.

My Princeton classmate, Harry Hoyt, who developed the Carter-Wallace Company with Frank Berger in charge of drug research, asked me to join his board of directors. This I did, and I have learned much of the tough problems continually faced by drug companies in trying to develop new drugs. It is nothing like the way we did it during the depression. But the drugs we introduced, spleen-marrow, divinyl ether, carbarsone, Vioform®, the amphetamines, and nalorphine, are still useful drugs, when used appropriately and properly. We never made a penny from our work, except Gordon Alles from amphetamine, but we were well content to have enjoyed the effort.

Actually, we had quite a close association at the big, open lab in San Francisco where we all worked together. We called ourselves the Blakians, in reference to James Blake (1814–1893), the brilliant London physician who by 1846 had shown clear relationships between chemical constitution and biological action using inorganic salts. He showed that their biological activities permitted their arrangement into families having similar actions, and there is the outline of the periodic table, 20 years ahead of Dmitri Mendeleev (1834–1907). Blake got into trouble and came to St. Louis in 1847, and then came to California in the Gold Rush. He was professor of midwifery and diseases of women and children at the University of California Medical School when it was organized in 1873, and became president of the California Academy of Sciences. He retired to Middletown where he returned to his earlier pharmacological studies. The Blakians made frequent pilgrimages to his grave in the Middletown cemetery. When I gave an account of his career at the Aberdeen meeting of the British Association for the Advancement of Science, I found that the old scandal, whatever it was, precluded the possibility of publishing my account in England.

When it comes to writing, scientists are often no better than their secretaries. I've been fortunate in having fine secretaries, keen, efficient, dedicated, often with us in family affairs, and always helpful in arranging laboratory parties. At Wisconsin there was Irene Blake, and at California, Marjorie Williams, both of whom died too young. At Texas there was Isobel Aiklin, now Mrs. Clemens, who visits my wife each year at Chautauqua, and Mary Jane Steding. At Columbus there was Jane Nolan, and now back in San Francisco there is Mia Lydecker, who really works for Milton Silverman, but who helps me when she can. Here also is Aline Steward, who actually is secretary for the group in environmental health, which shares the old house with me. Mrs. Steward keeps my mail in order.

My historical interest resulted in a large manuscript on the history of pharmacology. This was prepared for Pergamon Press *Encyclopedia of Pharmacology.* But I ran into editorial blocks, so now it appears from C. C. Thomas, who was my first publisher anyway. Peter Knoefel, working on Felice Fontana (1730–1804), pioneer student of the toxicity of venoms, comes over from Firenze once in a while to work with us, and to run to see what we can find on Blake. So we keep rolling along. Even at the Bohemian Grove, where each summer is "the greatest men's party on earth," I get a chance to talk at the lakeside on alcoholic beverages, and other drugs. My chief joy there, however, is lighting the Concert-at-the-Lake, throwing 250 foot beams of colored lights on the redwoods behind the orchestra in coordination with the music. This I've done for 40 years. So this is how I am: still at it for the excitement, the knowledge, and the fun of pharmacology, and related matters.

GASTROINTESTINAL PHARMACOLOGY

❖6633

Thomas F. Burks
Department of Pharmacology, The University of Texas
Medical School at Houston, Houston, Texas 77025

Control of gastrointestinal function is accomplished by a diverse extrinsic autonomic innervation, a sophisticated intrinsic neural system, extramural humoral influences, and a plethora of hormones produced by the gastrointestinal organs themselves. Because drugs generally do not create new physiological or biochemical functions, they are useful only insofar as they modify ongoing processes. In the gastrointestinal tract, drugs modify mainly the various mechanisms that control secretion and motility. Unfortunately, often so little is known about the gastrointestinal tract that understanding of drug actions seems difficult or impossible and pharmacology is still presented in descriptive terms. While certainly the answers to the major problems in gastrointestinal pharmacology are not yet available, perhaps we can gain some satisfaction from the belief that at least the quality of the questions is improving.

GASTRIC SECRETION

Previous empirical approaches to the treatment of diseases in which decreased gastric acid secretion might offer benefit have been either ineffective because of inherent limitations in the drugs themselves or have been directed at the result, not the cause, of the disorder. The use of atropine, which is completely rational, is usually ineffective because of dosage limitations (1). We therefore rely heavily on neutralization of secreted acid; this approach completely ignores the control mechanisms involved in gastric secretion and in fact increases secretory stimuli (2).

The primary stimulus for gastric acid secretion is the gastrointestinal hormone, gastrin (3–6). Gastrin is present in the mucosa of the antrum of the stomach and, decreasing caudally, in the small intestine; it is also present in the pancreas (6). Gastrin occurs in several molecular forms. The forms isolated from antral mucosa are heptadecapeptides known as gastrins I and II (gastrin II differs from I only in

15

that the tyrosine residue in position 12 is sulfated), or frequently as the "little gastrins," with molecular weights of approximately 2,100. The principal molecular species of gastrin in the circulation, "big gastrin," has a molecular weight of approximately 7,000 (6). Big gastrin is a major component of gastrin extracted from intestinal mucosa. A third gastrin, delightfully called "big, big gastrin," has been isolated from serum and jejunal mucosa and has a molecular weight of approximately 20,000 (7). A "minigastrin" of 13 amino acid residues has also been identifed (3). A stimulating account of the discovery and identification of gastrin and other gastrointestinal hormones was published recently (3).

Stimuli for the release of gastrin include alkaline pH of the antral contents, mechanical distention of the antrum, neural acetylcholine, and the presence in the antrum of food, particularly proteins and amino acids (4). The acetylcholine released by vagal stimulation causes the release of antral gastrin and also has a direct stimulatory effect on the parietal cells. The negative feedback control that inhibits gastrin release is acid in the stomach antrum. The regulation of release of intestinal gastrin is less well understood (6).

Gastrin stimulates acid secretion by interacting with a gastrin receptor in the parietal cell. This receptor, but not receptors for acetylcholine or histamine, is blocked by secretin (8). Gastrin and other gastric secretagogues may stimulate acid secretion through activation of parietal cell adenylate cyclase with subsequent increases in intracellular cyclic adenosine monophosphate (cAMP). The arguments for and against a role of cAMP in gastric acid secretion are presented in the comprehensive review by Kimberg (9).

The logical points for pharmacological modification of gastric acid secretion are the control mechanisms for gastrin release, gastrin interaction with the parietal cell, and the events that lead to acid secretion subsequent to that interaction.

H_2 Receptor Blockers

The relative inability of conventional (H_1) antihistamines to block the gastric secretory and certain other effects of histamine is part of the treasured lore of pharmacology. In the belief that the non-H_1 effects of histamine represent actions on a second kind of histamine receptor, Black and his colleagues designed and tested hundreds of compounds for gastric antisecretory activity. The success of their effort (10) not only provided a valuable new class of pharmacological tools and potentially useful therapeutic agents, but also stands as a tribute to scientific perseverence and rational drug design. The gastric antisecretory actions of the H_2 receptor antagonists have recently been reviewed (11); only the significant studies that have appeared since that thorough review are discussed here.

Studies of H_2 receptor antagonists have focused on burimamide and metiamide. A third promising agent, cimetidine, was only recently described (12). The gastric antisecretory effects of burimamide and metiamide have been confirmed in animals and man (13–15). In addition to inhibition of acid secretion, burimamide and metiamide also reduce gastric mucosal blood flow. Since there is a close relation between acid secretion and gastric mucosal blood flow (16), the question arose whether the inhibition of histamine-induced acid secretion by the H_2 receptor antagonists could be due to inhibition of mucosal vasodilatation through an effect on vascular H_2 receptors (17). Studies in dogs with gastric fistulas and Heindenhain pouches demonstrated that while metiamide decreased mucosal blood flow, the ratio of aminopyrine concentration in the gastric juice and blood plasma was not changed by metiamide (18). This result indicated that the reduction in gastric mucosal blood flow was secondary to the inhibition of gastric secretion induced by metiamide. In anesthetized cats with acute gastric fistulas, burimamide and metiamide reduced acid secretion more than they reduced gastric mucosal blood flow (19, 20). Finally, metiamide was shown to inhibit stimulated acid secretion in isolated gastric mucosa of frog and isolated stomach of rat, preparations in which blood flow was not a consideration (17). It now appears, therefore, that the basic effect of the H_2 receptor antagonists on gastric acid secretion is exerted directly on the acid secretory mechanisms in the gastric mucosa. An additional contributory effect of reduced gastric mucosal blood flow, however, cannot yet be ruled out. Some portion of the gastric antisecretory effect of burimamide, but not metiamide, may be attributable to release of catecholamines (19).

In their original study of the antisecretory effects of burimamide, Black et al (10) found it to be effective against gastric acid secretion induced by histamine, pentagastrin, and feeding, but not against secretion induced by reflex or direct vagal stimulation. It is now apparent, however, that metiamide inhibits also the gastric acid secretion induced by vagal stimulation, bethanechol, and methacholine (14, 18, 21–25). Acid output induced by pentagastrin, bethanechol, methacholine, reflex vagal stimulation, feeding and caerulein, but not by histamine, is antagonized also by atropine (18, 24, 25). These data indicate an anticholinergic component of metiamide action, a nonspecific gastric antisecretory effect, or some complicated interaction of H_2 receptors with those for acetylcholine and gastrointestinal hormones. Both cholinergic and histaminergic links in the acid secretory responses to food, vagal stimulation, and gastrin-like gastrointestinal hormones could be postulated. The histamine receptor would be more proximal to the secretory mechanism than the cholinergic receptor, thus explaining the ability of metiamide to antagonize all the stimuli tested and the ability of atropine (in dogs and cats) to inhibit all but the histamine stimulus. Grossman & Konturek (25) have proposed a far more provocative hypothesis to account for the data. According to this hypothesis, the parietal cell has separate receptors for histamine, acetylcholine, and gastrin. Blockade of one receptor may change the properties of one or both of the other two receptors. For example, blockade of the histamine receptor by metiamide, or blockade of the acetylcholine receptor by atropine, would change the properties of the gastrin receptor so that stimulation by pentagastrin would be less effective. This interesting hypothesis is worthy of testing by appropriate pharmacological techniques. One result of the studies with atropine and metiamide, as pointed out by Grossman & Konturek (25), is the conclusion that it is not necessary for a drug to be an effective antagonist of histamine for it to inhibit acid secretion in response to a meal. The reason that atropine has relatively little practical therapeutic value in depressing gastric acid secretion in patients with duodenal ulcer is not because it does not have a broad enough spectrum of stimulants against which it is effective. It is therapeutically ineffective because it cannot be used in high enough doses to provide the desired degree of inhibition of acid secretion without intolerable side effects.

Prostaglandins

Despite their varied effects on the gastrointestinal tract, it is the actions of prostaglandins on gastric secretion where hope for therapeutic utility has largely focused. It has been known for several years that several prostaglandins (particularly E_1 and E_2) can inhibit gastric secretion (26). Studies in man were disappointing in that the natural prostaglandins exhibited no antisecretory activity when administered orally and produced undesirable side effects when administered intravenously. These effects of the prostaglandins have been reviewed extensively (27–30). The oral inactivity of the natural prostaglandins results from their breakdown by prostaglandin 15-hydroxydehydrogenase. Several prostaglandin analogs resistant to this enzyme have been developed (31). 15-Methyl-PGE$_2$-methyl ester (R and S isomers) and 16:16-dimethyl-PGE$_2$-methyl ester are active orally and are more potent than the natural prostaglandin E_2 (32). After intragastric administration in man, 15(S)-15-methyl-PGE$_2$-methyl ester, 16:16-dimethyl-PGE$_2$, and 16:16 dimethyl-PGE$_2$-methyl ester inhibited spontaneous and pentagastrin-induced gastric acid secretion (33, 34). When administered into the intestine, however, these compounds were considerably less effective than after intragastric administration (35). The 16:16 dimethyl-PGE$_2$ analogs were virtually inactive when given into any part of the human upper small bowel, yet 16:16 dimethyl-PGE$_2$ did inhibit dog Heidenhain pouch acid secretion following administration into the jejunum (32). The curious inactivity of the methyl prostaglandins after intraintestinal administration in man may indicate chemical instability in the intestinal environment or raises the possibility of a direct, local effect of these agents on the oxyntic glands. At high doses, the methyl prostaglandin derivatives can decrease stomach and intestinal motility (36). Three other synthetic prostaglandin analogs, 15-hydroxy-9-oxoprostanoic acid, 15-hydroxy-15-methyl-9-oxoprostanoic acid, and 15-hydroxy-15-methyl-9-oxoprostanoic acid methyl ester, inhibited gastric acid secretion when administered parenterally in rats, but the compound lacking a 15-methyl substitution was not effective when administered orally (37). The synthetic analogs of the prostaglandins may hold great promise as effective gastric antisecretory agents if they do not produce prostaglandin-like side effects, such as diarrhea, in further clinical trials.

Although there are differences in degree of inhibition, prostaglandin E_1 has a broad spectrum of inhibitory activity against several secretagogues, including carbachol, direct and reflex vagal stimulation, histamine, pentagastrin, and food (11). Since their antisecretory activity appears not to result from changes in mucosal blood flow (38), the prostaglandins may act by interfering with events that couple parietal cell stimulation to acid secretion. Prostaglandins could alter activity of adenylate cyclase or membrane permeability to ions, or act as feedback inhibitors (9, 11, 28). Whether or not prostaglandin derivatives will ever serve as useful therapeutic antisecretory agents, understanding their mechanism of action will represent a major advance in gastrointestinal pharmacology.

Gastrointestinal Hormones

Perhaps the most promising method for control of gastric secretion will occur as a result of advances in knowledge about the physiology and biochemistry of the endogenous gastrointestinal hormones. There are three generally recognized gastrointestinal hormones: gastrin, secretin, and cholecystokinin (CCK). There are also a number of what Grossman (39) has called "candidate hormones." The candidate hormones include chymodenin, gastric inhibitory peptide, motilin, vasoactive intestinal peptide, coherin, urogastrone, gastrone, bulbogastrone, duocrinin, enterocrinin, enterogastrone, enteroglucagon, incretin, and villikinin. The list could be extended by including potential hormones postulated on the basis of physiological evidence but for which chemical evidence is so far absent.

A great deal is known about the effects of the three established hormones on gastrointestinal function and on processes elsewhere in the body. Some of these effects are summarized in Table 1. In the table, no distinction is made between low-dose and high-dose effects of the hormones. The effects of gastrin on release of insulin and on intestinal contractions, for example, may be observed only with high doses and may not represent physiological actions (3). Since the gastrointestinal hormones exhibit such a variety of effects, there is frequent disagreement about "physiological" and "pharmacological" effects. One of the more interesting controversies concerns the potential role of gastrin in maintenance of tone in the lower esophageal sphincter (49–52).

The role of gastrin in acid secretion is reviewed above. CCK is a 33 amino acid polypeptide hormone that has been prepared in pure form from duodenal mucosa (44). The major stimulus for release of CCK is entry of peptides, amino acids, and especially fats into the small bowel. CCK shares many of the physiological properties of gastrin and can be considered a member of the gastrin family of hormones (3). In the rat and cat, CCK is a full agonist at parietal cell gastrin receptors and

Table 1 Effects of gastrointestinal hormones on selected functions of the gastrointestinal tract

	Gastrin	Cholecystokinin	Secretin
Secretion			
Gastric			
H+	increase (3)	partial agonist (3)	decrease (3, 48)
Pepsin	increase (3)	none (3)	increase (3, 48)
Intestine	increase (3)	increase (39)	increase (3)
Pancreas	increase (3)	increase (3)	increase (3)
Bile flow	increase (3)	increase (44)	increase (3)
Insulin release	increase (3)	increase (45)	increase (3, 45)
Motility			
Lower esophageal sphincter	contraction (3)	relaxation (46)	relaxation (3)
Gastric			
Contractions	increase (40)	decrease (44)	decrease (48)
Emptying	delayed (41)	delayed (44)	delayed (3, 48)
Intestinal contractions	increase (3, 4, 42)	increase (47)	decrease (3, 42, 47)
Gastrointestinal blood flow	increase (43)	increase (43)	increase (3, 48)

can stimulate gastric acid secretion as strongly as gastrin (3). In dog and man, CCK is a partial agonist; given alone it evokes only a small response and, given in conjunction, it inhibits the response to gastrin (3). Caerulein, a decapeptide, has physiological activity almost identical with the C-terminal octapeptide of CCK.

Secretin is a 27 amino acid polypeptide hormone present in high concentration in the upper portion of the small bowel (4). While products of fat and protein digestion may stimulate secretin release, the major stimulus for its release is the presence of hydrochloric acid within the proximal small bowel (4). Secretin induces the secretion of water and electrolytes by the pancreas. As the volume increases, so does the bicarbonate concentration. In addition to providing the alkaline pancreatic juice that neutralizes the acid gastric contents as they pass into the duodenum, secretin also inhibits the action of gastrin on the parietal cell, as mentioned above, and inhibits the release of gastrin from the stomach antrum (3).

Two candidate gastrointestinal hormones, gastric inhibitory peptide (GIP) and vasoactive intestinal peptide (VIP), share several actions of secretin and can be thought of as members of the secretin family (3). GIP is a 43 amino acid polypeptide obtained from duodenal mucosa (3, 53). GIP is effective in inhibiting gastric acid secretion stimulated by pentagastrin, histamine, and reflex vagal stimulation (53). VIP is a 28 amino acid polypeptide isolated from hog intestine (54). Although it shares some physiological actions with secretin, such as ability to inhibit both histamine- and pentagastrin-induced acid secretion, VIP also has properties unlike those of secretin. For example, VIP is a potent vasodilator and it inhibits gastric pepsin secretion (53). The hormonal role of VIP is in doubt because it is largely inactivated in passing through the liver (55). Other candidate gastrointestinal hormones capable of inhibiting gastric acid secretion have been postulated (39).

A recent arrival on the gastrointestinal hormone scene is growth hormone–release inhibitory hormone (GH–RIH) or somatostatin. It is a 14 amino acid polypeptide first isolated from hypothalamic nuclei but now known to be present in rat pancreas and stomach (56). Evidence to date indicates that GH–RIH inhibits release of growth hormone, thyroid-stimulating hormone, insulin, glucagon, and gastrin. In dogs, cats, and humans, GH–RIH inhibited gastric acid secretion in response to histamine, pentagastrin, and feeding (57, 58). The inhibitory effect was most pronounced with food-induced acid secretion and was least prominent against histamine. Although conclusions must await establishment of dose-response relationships, the efficacy against food-stimulated acid secretion could be due to a combined effect on release of gastrin and on the parietal cell.

Directions for the Future

It would appear that several means exist by which gastric acid secretion should be subject to modification by drugs. Endogenous substances, such as secretin and GH–RIH, are capable of inhibiting release of gastrin and thereby reducing the primary stimulus for acid secretion. Secretin, gastric inhibitory peptide, vasoactive intestinal peptide, GH–RIH, and H_2 receptor antagonists may decrease acid secretion by interference with the ability of gastrin and other secretagogues to interact effectively with their parietal cell receptors. Certain natural prostaglandins and their synthetic derivatives appear to decrease acid secretion by virtue of actions on secretory mechanisms that are distal to parietal cell receptor activation.

All three of these approaches to prevention of acid hypersecretion call for a greater investment by pharmacologists in analysis of the control mechanisms responsible for gastric secretion. The likely dividends may include highly selective and effective drugs for precise modulation of specific secretory events.

MOTILITY

The primary myogenic control of gastrointestinal motility results from the electrical slow waves generated in the longitudinal layer of smooth muscle. Neurogenic control is exerted primarily via the neurons of the myenteric plexus and determines whether spike potentials will be initiated by the depolarization phase of the slow waves. Spike potentials are associated with muscle contractions (59, 60). Excitatory stimuli, such as release of acetylcholine from myenteric nerves, raise the level of excitability of the muscle and promote spike bursts and contractions. The distribution in time and space of contractions is determined by the slow wave or control electrical activity (59). Propulsion of intestinal contents requires an aboral net pressure gradient (59) and results from the sum of many separate events. These events require neural, muscular, and temporal integration for proper regulation of flow. The integration occurs over long periods of time and across large distances. The dimensions differ considerably from the rapid events of the cardiac cycle or the short distances of the capillary.

Extrinsic Control

Neural control of gastrointestinal motility occurs primarily from the activity of the intrinsic nerves which are subject to modulation by the extrinsic innervation. Electrical stimulation of vagal or sympathetic nerves or local field stimulation can provoke both excitatory and inhibitory effects in the stomach and intestine (61–65). Signals over the extrinsic nerves originate in the central nervous system after appropriate afferent input. Perhaps the most striking example of extrinsic modulation of motility is the intestinal interdigestive myoelectric complex, first described by Szurszewski (66). The complex consists of distinct bands of electrical burst activity and segmenting contractions that migrate aborally in a cyclic fashion in fasted animals. Each band is approximately 25–35 cm long and requires 5–7 min (depending on part of intestine involved) to pass a point in the bowel. The bowel is quiet after passage of a complex; activity increases again as the subsequent complex develops. As one complex reaches the ileum, another develops in the duodenum (66). The complex is under extrinsic control, mediated probably over sympathetic nerves, since Thiry-Vella loops of bowel taken out of continuity still display the characteristic pattern at the appropriate time in the passage of the activity down the remainder of the small intestine (67). The interdigestive myoelectric complex has implications for drug studies of intestinal motility. Ideally, the effects of drugs on motility should be characterized in unanesthetized animals against defined backgrounds of fed or fasting motility patterns.

Presumptions of extrinsic control over specific motility patterns frequently are shown to be unfounded. Such may be the case with esophageal peristalsis. Because the peristaltic wave in the esophagus travels over a relatively long distance and requires several integrated events in the musculature of the esophagus and the lower esophageal sphincter, it was thought to represent an extrinsically controlled, preordained motility pattern (68). The idea of medullary control over the mechanical events of swallowing was based primarily on studies in dogs and other species whose esophagi are composed of striated muscle. Recent studies in the opossum, in which, like the human, the distal two thirds of the esophagus is composed of smooth muscle, refute the classical view of central control (69). These studies demonstrate that electrical stimulation of the distal end of the divided vagus nerve induced fully coordinated, propagated peristaltic contractions in the body of the esophagus. The results indicate that esophageal peristalsis is under the control of local intrinsic mechanisms rather than the central nervous system. In order to avoid cardiac responses to vagal stimulation, the animals in this experiment were treated with 0.1 mg/kg of atropine. This may indicate that the local control mechanisms are noncholinergic.

Intrinsic Control

The most familiar intrinsic neural reflex of the intestine is the peristaltic reflex. This reflex requires simultaneous ascending contraction and descending inhibition of the circular muscle (70). The neural basis for descending inhibition has been established by intracellular recordings from the myenteric plexus (63). In the cat colon, atropine can impair propulsion by selective blockade of the descending inhibition (71), which thus seems to contain muscarinic cholinergic receptor links. The descending inhibition associated with propulsion in the large intestine appears to involve a nonadrenergic inhibitory system (71).

Extracellular recordings from ganglion cells in cat small intestine myenteric and submucous plexuses before and after exposure to drugs suggested the presence of cholinergic excitatory neurons, tonic inhibitory neurons, and adrenergic fibers that synapse with nonadrenergic inhibitory neurons (72). Excitatory myenteric neural pathways with transmitters other than ACh or 5-hydroxytryptamine (5-HT) may exist (73). Tonic inhibition of gut circular muscle can be revealed by tetrodotoxin even during blockade of cholinergic and adrenergic receptors (74, 75). The hypothesis has been put forward that adenosine triphosphate or related nucleotides may be the transmitters released by the nonadrenergic inhibitory neurons (76).

Humoral Control

The gastrointestinal hormones deserve special attention as potential physiological modulators that are subject to pharmacological intervention. They may also be important as mediators of some indirect actions of existing gastrointestinal drugs. The actions of catecholamines on gastrointestinal motility have been reviewed previously (77).

In addition to its effects on gastric secretion, gastrin has effects on gastrointestinal motor activity. Gastrin can increase tone of the lower esophageal sphincter (78);

increase antral slow wave activity; increase force of antral contractions, yet delay gastric emptying (41); and, in relatively high doses, increase spike bursts and contractile activity of intestine (42). The effect of gastrin on tone of the lower esophageal sphincter is particularly noteworthy. Gastrin release during the gastric phase of digestion may help tighten the sphincter against esophageal reflux. Also, the role of antacids in treating esophageal reflux may be not only to neutralize acid, but to strengthen the sphincter by inducing the release of endogenous gastrin (79).

Secretin reduces gastric motility, delays gastric emptying, decreases intestinal motility, and causes relaxation of the lower esophageal sphincter (4, 42). As in the case of gastric acid secretion, secretin appears to be a competitive inhibitor of the stimulant effect of gastrin on the lower esophageal sphincter (78).

Cholecystokinin (CCK), caerulein, and the C-terminal octapeptide of CCK exhibit essentially identical diverse actions on gastrointestinal motility. Like secretin, CCK produces dose-related decreases in lower esophageal sphincter pressure (46). Upper small bowel activity in humans was stimulated by CCK and inhibited by secretin (47). The motility effects of the two hormones were mutually antagonistic, but too few dose levels were tested to allow conclusions about mechanisms. In isolated ileum of rabbit, caerulein increased spike bursts associated with contractions of the circular muscle (80). The effect of caerulein on spike bursts and muscle contraction was abolished by tetrodotoxin. When administered to mice, caerulein enhanced transit through the intestine, but delayed gastric emptying (81).

The mechanisms by which the gastrointestinal hormones produce their motility effects are not established, but progress in that direction is being made. The experiments of Lecchini & Gonella (80), for example, suggest that intrinsic nerves participate in motor responses to caerulein. This suggestion has been confirmed in other experiments. The guinea pig ileum contractor effects of CCK, CCK-octapeptide, caerulein, and pentagastrin were virtually abolished by tetrodotoxin (82). There seems to be a difference between the modes of CCK stimulation of intestine and gall bladder. Contractions of guinea pig ileum induced by purified CCK were blocked by low concentrations of atropine, but even at 500 times higher concentration, atropine failed to block CCK-induced contractions of gall bladder strips (83). CCK-induced contractions of guinea pig ileum were not blocked by hexamethonium. The contracting effect of CCK on gall bladder appears to be a direct effect, that on intestine an indirect effect. Vizi et al (84) examined the mechanism of stimulatory action of caerulein, CCK-octapeptide, gastrin, and pentagastrin on longitudinal muscle (with myenteric plexus) of guinea pig ileum. The contractor effects of all four peptides were blocked by atropine, tetrodotoxin, and morphine. The peptides were found to release acetylcholine, confirming the involvement of cholinergic nerves in the response. Norepinephrine, presumably by a presynaptic action, decreased responses to the peptides. This suggested that the neural pathway activated by the peptides contains ganglia, but the peptide effects were not blocked by hexamethonium. The intestinal effect of CCK and related peptides seems similar in some respects to those of 5-HT, which may act upon intramural cholinergic ganglia by activation of a receptor distinct from the nicotinic cholinergic receptor (85). This mechanism was subsequently confirmed in a model set of experiments (86). Guinea

pig ileum longitudinal muscle was stimulated by CCK-octapeptide, caerulein, nicotine, and dimethylphenylpiperazinium (DMPP). All four agents were found to
release acetylcholine, and their contractor effects were blocked by atropine. Nicotine
and DMPP contractions were blocked by hexamethonium; contractions induced by
CCK-octapeptide and caerulein were not. Participation of 5-HT in the responses to
the peptides was ruled out by 5-HT receptor desensitization experiments. Responses
to the peptides were prevented by ganglionic depolarization with large concentrations of nicotine. To demonstrate that the blocking effect of nicotine was due to
depolarization, the action of nicotine was prevented by prior administration of
hexamethonium. In the presence of hexamethonium and nicotine, CCK-octapeptide
exerted its usual effects. The author concludes from these experiments that parasympathetic ganglion cells in the myenteric plexus contain receptors for CCK and
related peptides. While this is certainly the most likely explanation, the experiments
do not rule out another mode of action involving ganglionic transmission but not
nicotinic cholinergic receptors.

Indirect evidence was presented recently that some intestinal effects of *cis*–fatty
acids could be due to release of CCK (87). The fatty acids, including *cis*-ricinoleic
acid, caused initial stimulation, then prolonged inhibition, of upper small bowel
motility. Intravenous CCK-octapeptide produced similar effects. The stimulatory
effects of ricinoleic acid (the active ingredient of castor oil) and CCK-octapeptide
were both blocked by atropine (because atropine alone inhibited motility, the inhibitory phase of ricinoleic acid or of CCK-octapeptide action could not be observed
after atropine). This report is almost surely the first of many that will implicate
gastrointestinal hormones as participants in responses to drugs.

Narcotic Drugs

The intestinal effects of narcotics have been studied primarily from two different
points of view: (*a*) as a model system to understand actions of narcotics in the
central nervous system and (*b*) as a means of improving understanding of gastrointestinal pharmacology and physiology with the aim of perfecting therapeutic
modalities in humans. The guinea pig ileum, for better or worse, has frequently been
the object of investigations intended for extrapolation to the central nervous system.
Morphine and related narcotic drugs decrease release of acetylcholine from guinea
pig lieum and thus decrease responses of the preparation to 5-HT and electrical field
stimulation (88). It would be easy to attribute the constipating effect of morphine
to a decrease in intestinal motility. In mammalian species other than the guinea pig,
however, morphine in fact increases intestinal contractile activity and, except sometimes in high doses (89), does not block responses to 5-HT (90, 91). The increase
in intestinal tone and motility induced by morphine retards propulsion through the
bowel (92), increases resistance to flow of bile through the choledochoduodenal
junction (93), and contributes to a delay in gastric emptying (89, 94).

The mechanisms by which morphine and related opiates produce their intestinal
effects are becoming clarified. In isolated segments of dog small intestine perfused
via the vasculature with a physiological salt solution (95), morphine and similar
narcotics produce tonic and phasic contractions essentially identical with those
recorded in situ. This demonstrates that the major component of morphine con-

tractile activity results from a direct effect on the intestine. The contractions produced by the opiates were associated with release of 5-HT (96). Narcotic-induced contractions and release of 5-HT were dose related, stereospecific (97), and blocked by naloxone (98). The stimulatory effects of narcotics in dog intestine appear to be due largely to mobilization of endogenous 5-HT (85). The 5-HT released by morphine stimulates intestinal smooth muscle directly and by activation of intramural cholinergic neural elements. Tetrodotoxin, atropine, methoxamine, and bufotenidine block the neural component of the response (85, 99–101). Although 5-HT does not stimulate nicotinic cholinergic receptors, the neural pathway acted upon by 5-HT contains ganglia (85, 102). Isoproterenol, prostaglandin E_1, and theophylline selectively inhibit intestinal responses to 5-HT and morphine (99, 101). This observation led to a proposal that the direct component of 5-HT action on intestinal smooth muscle results from interference with cAMP tonic inhibition.

The 5-HT hypothesis of morphine action on the dog intestine does not explain why morphine is constipating and 5-HT generally is not. The intestinal pressure gradient required for aboral flow through the gut results primarily from the gradient of circular muscle contractions at frequencies determined by electrical slow wave activity (59, 60, 103). Yet morphine, 5-HT, and cholinergic drugs produce grossly similar spike bursts and circular muscle contractions (104, 105). Close examination, however, often reveals slightly different patterns of circular and markedly different patterns of longitudinal muscle contractions induced by morphine and bethanecol (85, 105, 106). The interactions between longitudinal and circular muscle layers are still controversial (107–109), but differential drug effects on the two muscle layers could account for some of their different effects on intestinal flow. Only the intestinal stimulatory effect of morphine may be due to 5-HT release, and even this hypothesis should be questioned if a treatment blocks the intestinal stimulatory effect of 5-HT without reducing responses to morphine.

The inhibitory effect of opiates on guinea pig ileum results from inhibition of release of acetylcholine. Nicotine-, caerulein-, pentagastrin-, and 5-HT-induced increases in neuronal firing rate in myenteric plexus of guinea pig ileum were blocked by morphine (110, 111). The site of action of morphine appears to be on the postganglionic nerve fibers that secrete acetylcholine toward the muscle (112, 113). Indomethacin also can inhibit twitches in electrically stimulated guinea pig ileum. Ehrenpreis et al (114) have postulated that morphine and indomethacin interfere with an essential prostaglandin link in secretion of acetylcholine from intramural postganglionic nerve fibers. According to this theory, indomethacin inhibits prostaglandin synthesis, and morphine acts as a prostaglandin antagonist at a neural receptor. Evidence has been presented, however, that the indomethacin inhibition of contractions results from indirect effects (disinhibition) on intramural inhibitory adrenergic nerves (115). Morphine does not alter release of norepinephrine from guinea pig ileum myenteric plexus (116).

Tolerance to Narcotics

Tolerance to the intestinal effects of morphine and related opiates has been demonstrated often in guinea pig ileum (117–121). The mechanism by which tolerance to morphine develops in guinea pig ileum has been pursued in a series of related investigations (120, 121). These investigations were based on the knowledge that opiates decrease acetylcholine release from electrically stimulated guinea pig ileum (88, 122) as well as the striking similarity of potency rank order of several opiates in this preparation as compared to their central narcotic agonist and antagonist activity (123). Goldstein & Schulz (121) prepared myenteric plexus–longitudinal muscle strips from control guinea pigs or animals that had been implanted subcutaneously with 300 mg of morphine base. Contractions of the strips were induced by supramaximal electrical field stimulation at a frequency of 0.1 Hz. Strips taken from the morphine-implanted animals were less sensitive than control strips to the depressant effects of morphine added to the bath. Tolerance was observed within 24 hr after morphine pellet implantation and became maximal 3–6 days after implantation. Maximum twitch tension and contractile responses to acetylcholine were not altered by tolerance to morphine. Interestingly, the depressant effects of epinephrine, isoproterenol, and dopamine were reduced considerably in strips from morphine-tolerant animals. A parallel study by the same authors (120) indicated that ileal strips from morphine-tolerant animals are supersensitive to the contracting effects of 5-HT. The authors proposed that tolerance to morphine results from an increase in the number or intrinsic sensitivity of 5-HT receptors. While this interpretation would account simultaneously for tolerance to morphine and catecholamines, a 5-HT link in ileal responses to field stimulation has not been demonstrated. Moreover, continuous interruption of neural activity, such as treatment with ganglion-blocking drugs, can cause supersensitivity in guinea pig ileum (124). The proposal by Schulz & Goldstein (120), however, is strengthened by the specificity of the supersensitivity to 5-HT during morphine tolerance. Van Neuten & Lal (125) found that ileal segments from morphine-tolerant guinea pigs were more sensitive (larger contractions with lower intensities of stimulation) to coaxial stimulation than strips from control animals. Interpretation of this observation is difficult because the experiments involved submaximal stimulation; the effect of morphine treatment could have been to decrease stimulus threshold in the intramural excitatory nerves.

In contrast to the above studies, Shoham & Weinstock (126) observed enhancement of responses of guinea pig ileum to acetylcholine during acute tolerance produced by addition of morphine to the bath fluid for 90 min. The increased sensitivity to acetylcholine was accompanied by a diminished effect of morphine on twitch height (contractions induced by supramaximal field stimulation). During the acute tolerance to morphine, there was no change in the ability of morphine to inhibit release of acetylcholine. It thus appeared that morphine had altered the smooth muscle acetylcholine receptors to cause supersensitivity. The acute tolerance to morphine in this case, and the enhanced responsiveness to acetylcholine, may in fact be due to the anticholinesterase property of morphine. After the twitch of coaxially stimulated guinea pig ileum was depressed by low concentrations of morphine, both dextrorphan and levorphanol were effective in restoration of the contractions (127). Dextrorphan and levorphanol differ considerably in narcotic agonist potency, but were about equally active as cholinesterase inhibitors in homogenates of the test preparation. Also, physostigmine in low concentrations restored the twitch that had been depressed by morphine. Acute tolerance of the guinea pig ileum to morphine cannot be explained in terms of the proposed negative feedback neural inhibitory control of acetylcholine release (128), because the effect of morphine on acetylcholine release is undiminished during acute tolerance (126). The same consideration would argue against an inhibitory effect of morphine on a neural acetylcholine uptake site (129).

Tolerance to morphine has been demonstrated also in the small intestine of dog (130), in which morphine is stimulatory and, acting presumably through release of 5-HT, increases release of acetylcholine (85). Tolerance to the stimulatory effect of morphine in situ and in vitro was not associated with significant changes in dose-response curves for 5-HT or for bethanechol. The results indicated that in the dog, at least, intestinal tolerance to morphine does not occur as a consequence of changes in transmitter receptor sensitivity. Similar conclusions were prompted by a study of acute tolerance to opiates in dog intestine (98). Perfusion of intestinal segments with morphine nearly abolished responses to intraarterial bolus doses of morphine, but did not decrease responses to bethanechol, DMPP, or 5-HT. Levorphanol and morphine showed cross-tolerance; responses to morphine (but not responses to bethanechol, DMPP, or 5-HT) were blocked by naloxone. 5-HT receptor desensitization did not alter responses to bethanechol or DMPP, but caused a considerable reduction in responses to morphine. While the specific mechanisms of acute and chronic tolerance of the dog intestine to morphine may be quite different, both kinds of experiments indicate that tolerance reflects events at the opiate receptor or on 5-HT release, not events at 5-HT or cholinergic receptors.

ANTIDIARRHEAL AND CATHARTIC DRUGS

Selectivity of drug action is a principal goal in pharmacology. The opiates are our most effective antidiarrheal drugs, but their actions are not limited to the gastrointestinal tract. It may, however, be possible to separate the intestinal and the central effects of the opiates. Promising agents such as loperamide demonstrate significant antidiarrheal activity in animals and man without notable central actions (131–135). Behavioral tests in rats trained to discriminate between fentanyl and saline indicated that fentanyl, morphine, codeine, and diphenoxylate produced narcotic cues, but loperamide was completely inactive in this test (135). Bass and his colleagues (136) subjected a novel indoline derivative, coded Cl-750, to rigorous pharmacological testing. Cl-750 was shown to have minimal central narcotic agonist activity, but produced narcotic-like constipation in rats and monkeys. The gastrointestinal motor effects of the compound were similar to those produced by morphine. Unlike morphine, however, its actions were only partially antagonized even by high concentrations of naloxone. It was not established whether the naloxone-insensitive actions of Cl-750 contribute to its constipating effects. If the intestinal and central opiate receptors are identical, selective opiate actions on the intestine can be achieved only by preventing entry of the opiate drug into the central nervous system. It is quite important, therefore, that all new antidiarrheal agents be tested in the absence and presence of naloxone to determine whether their constipating effects are blocked by naloxone. If they are blocked, the intestinal effect can be attributed to interaction with a conventional opiate receptor.

The constipating actions of narcotics can occur as a troublesome side effect of analgesic or narcotic addict maintenance therapy. Coadministration of cyproheptadine, a 5-HT antagonist, decreased the spasmogenic effect of methadone in dog intestine (137). Cyproheptadine also diminished the antipropulsive effect of methadone in mice, but did not alter the lethal dose of methadone.

Although little or no experimental evidence exists, "irritant" cathartics have been generally thought to stimulate intestinal smooth muscle. Stewart et al (138) performed a careful study of the effects of castor oil and magnesium sulfate on dog gastrointestinal contractile activity in vivo. Circular muscle activity, measured with extraluminal strain gages, was characterized during fed motility patterns and after twenty hours of fasting in the unanesthetized animals. Both laxative agents produced diarrhea when administered during the fasted state, but only mild laxation when administered after food. Both cathartics decreased motility, particularly in the ileum, especially when given during the interdigestive period. This interesting study provides support for the contention that increased circular muscle activity is obstructive and that some optimal decrease in activity might be associated with increased flow (136, 139). It is also noteworthy that castor oil and a saline cathartic, magnesium sulfate, had similar effects on both motility and absorption of water from the intestine (138).

Literature Cited

1. Ivey, K. J. 1975. *Gastroenterology* 68: 154–66
2. Feurle, G. E. 1975. *Gastroenterology* 68:1–7
3. Gregory, R. A. 1974. *J. Physiol. London* 241:1–32
4. Katz, J. 1973. *Med. Clin. North Am.* 57:893–905
5. Lin, T. M. 1974. *Med. Clin. North Am.* 58:1247–75
6. McGuigan, J. E. 1973. *Gastroenterology* 64:497–501
7. Yalow, R. S., Berson, S. A. 1972. *Biochem. Biophys. Res. Commun.* 48: 391–95
8. Johnson, L. R., Grossman, M. I. 1971. *Gastroenterology* 60:120–44
9. Kimberg, D. V. 1974. *Gastroenterology* 67:1023–64
10. Black, J. W., Duncan, W. A. M., Durant, G. J., Ganellin, C. R., Parsons, E. M. 1972. *Nature London* 236:385–90
11. Bass, P. 1974. *Adv. Drug Res.* 8:205–328
12. Brimblecombe, R. W., Duncan, W. A. M., Durant, G. J., Ganellin, C. R., Parsons, M. E., Black, J. W. 1975. *Br. J. Pharmacol.* 53:435–36P
13. Hirschowitz, B. I. 1974. *Am. J. Dig. Dis.* 19:811–17
14. Konturek, S. J., Biernat, J., Oleksy, J. 1974. *Am. J. Dig. Dis.* 19:609–16
15. Mainardi, M., Maxwell, V., Sturdevant, R. A. L., Isenberg, J. I. 1974. *N. Engl. J. Med.* 291:373–76
16. Main, I. H. M., Whittle, B. J. R. 1973. *Br. J. Pharmacol.* 49:534–42
17. Wan, B. Y. C., Assem, E.-L. K., Schild, H. O. 1974. *Eur. J. Pharmacol.* 29: 83–88
18. Konturek, S. J., Tasler, J., Obtulowicz, W., Rehfeld, J. F. 1974. *Gastroenterology* 66:982–86
19. Albinus, M., Sewing, K.-F. 1974. *Arch. Pharmacol.* 285:337–54
20. Albinus, M., Sewing, K.-F. 1974. *Experientia* 30:1435–37
21. Carter, D. C., Forrest, J. A. H., Werner, M., Heading, R. C., Park, J., Shearman, D. J. C. 1974. *Br. Med. J.* 3:554–56
22. Kowalewski, K., Kolodej, A. 1974. *Pharmacology* 11:207–12
23. Lundell, L. 1975. *J. Physiol. London* 244:365–83
24. Konturek, S. J., Demitrescu, T., Radecki, T. 1974. *Am. J. Dig. Dis.* 19:999–1006

25. Grossman, M. I., Konturek, S. J. 1974. *Gastroenterology* 66:517–21
26. Robert, A., Nezamis, J. E., Phillips, J. P. 1967. *Am. J. Dig. Dis.* 12:1073–76
27. Wilson, D. E. 1972. *Prostaglandins* 1:281–93
28. Weeks, J. R. 1972. *Ann. Rev. Pharmacol.* 12:317–36
29. Wilson, D. E. 1974. *Arch. Int. Med.* 133:112–18
30. Robert, A. 1974. *Prostaglandins* 6: 523–32
31. Weeks, J. R., DuCharme, D. W., Magee, W. E., Miller, W. L. 1973. *J. Pharmacol. Exp. Ther.* 186:67–74
32. Robert, A., Magerlein, B. J. 1973. *Adv. Biosci.* 9:247–53
33. Nylander, B., Anderson, S. 1974. *Scand. J. Gastroenterol.* 9:751–58
34. Nylander, B., Anderson, S. 1975. *Scand. J. Gastroenterol.* 10:217–20
35. Nylander, B., Anderson, S. 1974. *Scand. J. Gastroenterol.* 9:759–62
36. Nylander, B., Anderson, S. 1975. *Scand. J. Gastroenterol.* 10:91–95
37. Lippman, W. 1973. *Experientia* 29: 990–91
38. Jacobson, E. D. 1970. *Proc. Soc. Exp. Biol. Med.* 133:516–19
39. Grossman, M. I. 1974. *Gastroenterology* 67:730–55
40. Thompson, J. C. 1973. *Int. Encycl. Pharmacol. Ther.*, Sect. 39(A). 1: 261–86
41. Cooke, A. R., Chvasta, T. E., Weisbrodt, N. W. 1972. *Am. J. Physiol.* 223:934–38
42. Waterfall, W. E., Duthie, H. L., Brown, B. H. 1973. *Gut* 14:689–96
43. Fasth, S., Filipsson, S., Hultin, L., Martinson, J. 1973. *Experientia* 29:982–84
44. Jorpes, E., Mutt, V. 1973. *Int. Encycl. Pharmacol. Ther.*, Sect. 39(A). 2: 383–98
45. Creutzfeldt, W., Feurle, G., Ketterer, H. 1970. *New Engl. J. Med.* 282: 1139–41
46. Resin, H., Stern, D. H., Sturdevant, R. A. L., Isenberg, J. I. 1973. *Gastroenterology* 64:946–49
47. Gutiérrez, J. G., Chey, W. Y., Dinoso, V. P. 1974. *Gastroenterology* 67:35–41
48. Mutt, V., Jorpes, E. 1973. *Int. Encycl. Pharmacol. Ther.*, Sect. 39(A). 2: 361–81
49. Grossman, M. I. 1973. *Gastroenterology* 65:994
50. Cohen, S. 1974. *Gastroenterology* 66:479–80
51. Davidson, J. S. 1974. *Gastroenterology* 67:558–59
52. Dodds, W. J., Hogan, W. J., Miller, W. N., Barreras, R. F., Arndorfer, R. C., Stef, J. J. 1975. *Am. J. Dig. Dis.* 20:201–7
53. Brown, J. C. 1974. *Gastroenterology* 67:733–34
54. Said, S. I. 1974. *Gastroenterology* 67:735–37
55. Said, S. I. 1973. *Fed. Proc.* 32:1972–76
56. Arimura, A., Sato, H., DuPont, A., Nishi, N., Schally, A. V. 1975. *Fed. Proc.* 34:273 (Abstr.)
57. Barros D'Sa, A. A. J., Bloom, S. R., Baron, J. H. 1975. *Lancet* 1:886–87
58. Gomez-Pan, A., Reed, J. D., Albinus, M., Hall, R., Besser, G. M., Coy, D. H., Kastin, A. J., Schally, A. V. 1975. *Lancet* 1:888–90
59. Daniel, E. E. 1973. *Int. Encycl. Pharmacol. Ther.* Sect. 39(A). 2:457–545
60. Bortoff, A. 1969. *New Engl. J. Med.* 280:1335–37
61. Sarna, S. K., Daniel, E. E. 1975. *Gastroenterology* 68:301–8
62. Abrahamsson, H. 1973. *Acta Physiol. Scand. Suppl.* 390:1–38
63. Hirst, G. D. S., McKirdy, H. C. 1974. *J. Physiol. London* 238:129–43
64. Tansey, M. F., Kendall, F. M., Murphy, J. J. 1972. *Surg. Gynecol. Obstet.* 135:763–68
65. Wood, J. D. 1975. *Physiol. Rev.* 55: 307–24
66. Szurszewski, J. H. 1969. *Am. J. Physiol.* 217:1757–63
67. Carlson, G. M., Bedi, B. S., Code, C. F. 1972. *Am. J. Physiol.* 222:1027–30
68. Ingelfinger, F. J. 1958. *Physiol. Rev.* 38:533–84
69. Mukhopadhyay, A. K., Weisbrodt, N. W. 1975. *Gastroenterology* 68:444–47
70. Frigo, G. M., Lecchini, S. 1970. *Br. J. Pharmacol.* 39:346–56
71. Crema, A., Frigo, G. M., Lecchini, S. 1970. *Br. J. Pharmacol.* 39:334–45
72. Ohkawa, H., Prosser, C. L. 1972. *Am. J. Physiol.* 222:1420–26
73. Bennett, A., Fleshler, B. 1971. *Am. J. Dig. Dis.* 16:550–51
74. Tonini, M., Lecchini, S., Frigo, G., Crema, A. 1974. *Eur. J. Pharmacol.* 29:236–40
75. Wood, J. D., Marsh, D. R. 1973. *J. Pharmacol. Exp. Ther.* 184:590–98
76. Burnstock, G. 1972. *Pharmacol. Rev.* 24:509–81
77. Daniel, E. E. 1969. *Ann. Rev. Physiol.* 31:203–26
78. Cohen, S., Lipshutz, W. 1971. *J. Clin. Invest.* 50:1241–47

79. Castell, D. O., Levine, S. M. 1971. *Ann. Intern. Med.* 74:223–27
80. Lecchini, S., Gonella, J. 1973. *J. Pharm. Pharmacol.* 25:261–62
81. Piccinelli, D., Ricciotti, F., Catalani, A., Sale, P. 1973. *Arch. Pharmacol.* 279:75–82
82. Yau, W. M., Makhlouf, G. M., Edwards, L. E., Farrar, J. T. 1974. *Can. J. Physiol. Pharmacol.* 52:298–303
83. Hedner, P., Persson, H., Rorsman, G. 1967. *Acta Physiol. Scand.* 70:250–54
84. Vizi, E. S., Bertaccini, G., Impicciatore, M., Knoll, J. 1972. *Eur. J. Pharmacol.* 17:175–78
85. Burks, T. F. 1973. *J. Pharmacol. Exp. Ther.* 185:530–39
86. Vizi, E. S. 1973. *Br. J. Pharmacol.* 47:765–77
87. Stewart, J. J., Bass, P. 1975. *Gastroenterology* 68:991 (Abstr.)
88. Schaumann, W. 1957. *Br. J. Pharmacol.* 12:115–18
89. Daniel, E. E. 1966. *Can. J. Physiol. Pharmacol.* 44:981–1019
90. Weinstock, M. 1971. *Narcotic Drugs— Biochemical Pharmacology*, ed. D. H. Clouet, 394–407. New York: Plenum
91. Pruitt, D. B., Grubb, M. N., Jaquette, D. L., Burks, T. F. 1974. *Eur. J. Pharmacol.* 26:298–305
92. Vaughan Williams, E. M., Streeten, D. H. P. 1950. *Br. J. Pharmacol.* 5:584–603
93. Persson, C. G. A. 1971. *Acta Pharmacol. Toxicol.* 30:321–29
94. Weisbrodt, N. W., Wiley, J. N., Overholt, B. F., Bass, P. 1969. *Gut* 10:543–48
95. Burks, T. F. 1974. *Proc. 4th Int. Symp. Gastrointest. Motility* 305–12. Vancouver: Mitchell
96. Burks, T. F., Long, J. P. 1967. *J. Pharmacol. Exp. Ther.* 156:267–76
97. Burks, T. F., Long, J. P. 1967. *J. Pharmacol. Exp. Ther.* 158:264–71
98. Burks, T. F., Grubb, M. N. 1974. *J. Pharmacol. Exp. Ther.* 191:518–26
99. Grubb, M. N., Burks, T. F. 1974. *J. Pharmacol. Exp. Ther.* 189:476–83
100. de Oliveira, L. F., Bretas, A. D. 1973. *Eur. J. Pharmacol.* 21:369–71
101. Grubb, M. N., Burks, T. F. 1975. *J. Pharmacol. Exp. Ther.* 193:884–91
102. de Oliveira, L. F., Bretas, A. D., Sollero, L. 1974. *Pharmacology* 12:7–11
103. Weisbrodt, N. W. 1974. *Am. J. Dig. Dis.* 19:93–99
104. Weinbeck, M., Christensen, J. 1971. *Gastroenterology* 61:470–78
105. Weinbeck, M. 1972. *Res. Exp. Med.* 158:280–87
106. Bass, P., Wiley, J. N. 1965. *Am. J. Physiol.* 208:908–13
107. Wood, J. D., Perkins, W. E. 1970. *Am. J. Physiol.* 218:762–68
108. Bortoff, A., Ghalib, E. 1972. *Am. J. Dig. Dis.* 17:317–25
109. Gonella, J. 1972. *Am. J. Dig. Dis.* 17:327–32
110. Sato, T., Takayanagi, I., Takagi, K. 1973. *Jpn. J. Pharmacol.* 23:665–71
111. Dingledine, R., Goldstein, A., Kendig, J. 1974. *Life Sci.* 14:2299–2309
112. North, R. A., Nishi, S. 1974. See Ref. 95, pp. 667–76
113. Waterfield, A. A., Kosterlitz, H. W. 1974. See Ref. 95, pp. 659–66
114. Ehrenpreis, S., Greenberg, J., Belman, S., 1973. *Nature London New Biol.* 245:280–82
115. Kadlec, O., Mašek, K., Šeferna, I. 1974. *Br. J. Pharmacol.* 51:565–70
116. Henderson, G., Hughes, J., Kosterlitz, H. W. 1975. *Br. J. Pharmacol.* 53:505–12
117. Mattila, M. 1962. *Acta Pharmacol. Toxicol.* 19:47–52
118. Takagi, K., Takayanagi, I., Irikura, T., Nishino, K., Ichinoseki, N., Shishido, K. 1965. *Arch. Int. Pharmacodyn. Ther.* 158:39–44
119. Haycock, V. K., Rees, J. M. H. 1973. *Agonist and Antagonist Actions of Narcotic Drugs*, ed. H. W. Kosterlitz et al, 235–39. Baltimore: University Park Press
120. Schulz, R., Goldstein, A. 1973. *Nature London* 244:168–70
121. Goldstein, A., Schulz, R. 1973. *Br. J. Pharmacol.* 48:655–66
122. Paton, W. D. M. 1957. *Br. J. Pharmacol.* 12:119–27
123. Gyang, E. A., Kosterlitz, H. W. 1966. *Br. J. Pharmacol.* 27:514–27
124. Fleming, W. W. 1968. *J. Pharmacol. Exp. Ther.* 162:277–85
125. Van Neuten, J. M., Lal, H. 1974. *Arch. Int. Pharmacodyn. Ther.* 208:378–82
126. Shoham, S., Weinstock, M. 1974. *Br. J. Pharmacol.* 52:597–603
127. Kosterlitz, H. W., Waterfield, A. A. 1975. *Br. J. Pharmacol.* 53:131–38
128. Kilbinger, H., Wagner, P. 1975. *Arch. Pharmacol.* 287:47–60
129. Carson, V. G., Jenden, D. J., Russell, R. W. 1973. *Toxicol. Appl. Pharmacol.* 26:39–48
130. Burks, T. F., Jaquette, D. L., Grubb, M. N. 1974. *Eur. J. Pharmacol.* 25:302–7

131. Niemegeers, C. J. E., Lenaerts, F. M., Janssen, P. A. J. 1974. *Arzneim. Forsch.* 24:1633–35
132. Niemegeers, C. J. E., Lenaerts, F. M., Janssen, P. A. J. 1974. *Arzneim. Forsch.* 24:1636–40
133. Schuermans, V., Van Lommel, R., Dom, J., Brugmans, J. 1974. *Arzneim. Forsch.* 24:1653–56
134. Van Neuten, J. M., Janssen, P. A. J., Fontaine, J. 1974. *Arzneim. Forsch.* 24:1641–44
135. Colpaert, F. C., Niemegeers, C. J. E., Lal, H., Janssen, P. A. J. 1975. *Life Sci.* 16:717–28
136. Bass, P., Kennedy, J. A., Wiley, J. N., Villarreal, J., Butler, D. E. 1973. *J. Pharmacol. Exp. Ther.* 186:183–98
137. Kennedy, D. K., Grubb, M. N., Burks, T. F. 1974. *Gastroenterology* 66:396–402
138. Stewart, J. J., Gaginella, T. S., Olsen, W. A., Bass, P. 1975. *J. Pharmacol. Exp. Ther.* 192:458–67
139. Dubois, A., Bremer, A. 1972. *Arch. Int. Pharmacodyn. Ther.* 198:162–72

THE PHARMACOLOGY OF THE PINEAL GLAND

✦6634

Kenneth P. Minneman[1] *and Richard J. Wurtman*
Laboratory of Neuroendocrine Regulation, Department of Nutrition and Food Science,
Massachusetts Institute of Technology, Cambridge, Massachusetts 02139

INTRODUCTION

Only recently have a sufficient number of publications been available to legitimize a review of the pharmacology of the mammalian pineal organ. Two decades ago Kitay & Altschule reviewed the world literature on pineal physiology, which comprises several thousand papers, and concluded only that removal of the pineal, or administration of pineal extracts, somehow affected pigmentation in lower vertebrates and gonadal function in mammals (1). As the studies described below demonstrate, much more information is now available concerning the pharmacology of the pineal. This review subdivides present knowledge into two areas: (*a*) the effects on mammals of administering pineal extracts or pure synthetic or natural pineal constituents and (*b*) the effects of drugs and hormones on the pineal itself.

As might be anticipated, the bulk of studies cited in both categories deals with the pineal hormone, melatonin. Melatonin was first isolated from bovine pineal extracts in 1958 by Lerner and his colleagues (2), who used as a marker the capacity of the hormone to aggregate the pigment granules in amphibian melanophores around the cell nucleus. Five years later, Wurtman et al (3) showed that melatonin affected a physiological function in mammals, that is, the size and secretion of the ovary, and subsequent studies have demonstrated that melatonin administration also modifies the growth, composition, and functional activities of numerous other organs. Only recently an assay was developed that allows quantification of the melatonin in human urine (4). The concentrations of the compound vary with a characteristic daily rhythm, peaking at night. The pineal's apparent role as the sole or major source of melatonin, the presence of melatonin in urine, and the demonstration that physiologic effects follow a pinealectomy or the administration of melatonin seem to justify labeling it a pineal hormone.

[1]Present address: Department of Pharmacology, University of Cambridge, Cambridge CB2 2QD, England.

33

Melatonin synthesis and pineal biosynthetic activity are generally controlled by the sympathetic nerves of this organ (5, 6). Therefore, it should not be surprising that drugs known to modify the synthesis, release, or metabolism of norepinephrine in peripheral organs also affect pineal function. Melatonin is itself a derivative of another biogenic amine, serotonin, whose metabolism and actions are also affected by numerous drugs. Indeed, the pineal has often provided an apt tool for examining monoaminergic mechanisms for pharmacologists not specifically concerned with its particular functional properties.

EFFECTS OF MAMMALIAN PINEAL EXTRACTS
ON GONADAL FUNCTION

The ability of mammalian pineal organ constituents to modify gonadal function has been recognized for at least four decades. Initial reports (7) were interpreted as showing that pineal extracts stimulated the gonads. However, O. Fischer (8), and then Engel (9), and E. Fischer (10) showed that the administration of pineal extracts to rats or mice slowed gonadal maturation (i.e. it delayed the spontaneous rupture of the vaginal membrane). In 1954, Kitay & Altschule (11) produced ovarian atrophy by giving young rats daily injections of a bovine pineal extract. This effect was confirmed in 1959 by Wurtman et al (12) who used a protein-free extract, and it was subsequently shown (13, 14) that pineal extracts, as well as media in which rat pineals have been incubated (15), can suppress the compensatory hypertrophy of the remaining ovary after unilateral gonadectomy.

In 1960, Fiske et al (16) demonstrated that maintaining rats in a continuously illuminated environment caused pineal weight to decrease. [It had been previously shown (17–19) that this treatment also caused persistence of estrous cytology in rat vaginal smears.] Suspecting that the ovarian effects of light might be related to an inhibition of the synthesis of an antigonadal factor in the pineal, Wurtman et al (20) in 1961, administered bovine pineal extracts to light-treated rats, and found that such extracts blocked the ovarian hypertrophy. In 1962, Ifft (21) provided further evidence that light suppresses the synthesis of antigonadal factors in the pineal by showing that treatment with pineal extracts interrupted the persistent vaginal estrus in light-treated animals. The ability of pineal extracts to block light-induced changes in ovarian function provided the experimental basis for the original evidence that melatonin was the—or at least one of the—antigonadal factor(s) in pineal extracts (3). Once this evidence was obtained, most investigators stopped using crude or partially purified pineal extracts to explore pineal function in favor of melatonin and other pure compounds that had been identified in these extracts.

In 1963, Reiss and his co-workers (22) reported that while pineal extracts decreased gonadal weight in mature animals, they stimulated gonad growth in immature mice, rats, and rabbits. (A similar age-dependence was observed in the effects of pineal extracts on pituitary and thyroid weights.) In 1961, Meyer et al (23) observed that the same bovine pineal extracts that reversed the persistent vaginal estrus caused by exposure to continuous illumination also corrected the spontaneous persistent estrus exhibited by "middle-aged" (18-month-old) rats.

Evidence has been adduced that a constituent of pineal extracts directly inhibits gonadal responses to gonadotropins. Thus, Soffer et al (24) in 1965, and Hipkin (25) in 1970, observed that the concurrent administration of pineal extracts suppressed the increase in uterine weight caused by giving human chorionic gonadotropin (HCG) to immature mice. Extracts of human pineals failed to modify this response to HCG (26). Davis (27), in 1971, noted that bovine pineal extracts potentiated the direct effects of another pituitary hormone, pitocin, on contractions of the perfused rat uterus.

Several investigators have prepared pineal extracts that allegedly lack melatonin and that produced antigonadal effects in rats and mice. Benson and his associates reported that (a) a "melatonin-free" extract, prepared by subjecting aqueous extracts of human pineals to centrifugation and ultrafiltration, partially blocked compensatory ovarian hypertrophy (28); (b) an aqueous extract of bovine pineals, allegedly containing only 0.0035 μg per dose of melatonin, caused as much inhibition of compensatory ovarian hypertrophy as 30 μg of melatonin in pure solution (29); (c) an isobutanol extract of pineals subjected to ultrafiltration also suppressed this phenomenon in 6- to 10-week-old mice to a greater extent than could be attributed to its melatonin content (30); and (d) aqueous extracts subjected to ultrafiltration decreased the postcastration rise in serum luteinizing hormone (LH) in rats (31). A similar suppression of compensatory ovarian hypertrophy was noted by Vaughan & Reiter (32) in 1972, and by Bensinger et al (33) in 1973, working in Reiter's laboratory. In contrast, Debeljuk (34) could find no effects of a melatonin-free pineal extract on the weight of the gonads, or on pituitary LH concentration. Studies reporting antigonadal effects of pineal homogenates that have been treated to remove their melatonin are certainly of some significance, if only because they encourage exploration for additional antigonadal pineal constituents, which might be hormones. However, their interpretation is complicated by a number of problems: (a) quantitation of the melatonin concentrations in the extracts, before and after organic extraction or other treatment, has been crude at best; and (b) it seems likely that the extraction procedure removes other substituents of the pineal homogenates in addition to melatonin, and contaminates the homogenates with small amounts of organic solvents which could modify biologic responses to authentic pineal constituents in test animals. Positive findings using such extracts have, so far, been obtained by only two laboratories.

Moszkowska and her co-workers have utilized Sephadex G-25 gel filtration to separate various peptide fractions from pineal extracts. When given to rats or added to brain cultures, their F3 fraction reportedly increases the concentrations of the releasing factor(s) for follicle-stimulating hormone (FSH) and LH in the hypothalamus (35). Its administration, or the administration of an ultrafiltrate (36), also decreases gonadal weight, presumably by suppressing the release of hypothalamic-releasing factors and, thereby, of pituitary gonadotropins (37). The addition of whole pineals to hypothalamus-adenohypophysis tissue culture also reportedly decreases LH content (38).

Pineal extracts have also been reported to inhibit adrenocortical function in rats (39) and electric-shock-induced seizures in cats (40). Their administration suppresses compensatory adrenal hypertrophy following unilateral adrenalectomy and decreases the thickness of the zona fasciculata and the plasma corticosterone concentration in intact animals (39, 41).

EFFECTS OF EXOGENOUS MELATONIN ON MAMMALS

Gonadal Function

In 1963, evidence was first presented that melatonin administration affected gonad function in experimental animals (3). It was shown that the injection of relatively low doses of the pineal compound (1 μg per day, subcutaneously) could slow the growth of a maturing rat ovary and decrease the incidence of estrous vaginal smears in animals exposed to continuous illumination. During the next few years, additional studies revealed that environmental light, acting via the eyes, brain, and sympathetic nervous system, decreases the activity of the pineal enzyme, hydroxyindole-O-methyltransferase (HIOMT), that catalyzes the terminal step in melatonin biosynthesis (5, 42). On the basis of these observations, a widely accepted theory of pineal function was formulated, according to which the mammalian pineal functions as a *neuroendocrine transducer,* synthesizing and secreting melatonin—and perhaps other methoxyindole hormones—in response to the release of norepinephrine from its sympathetic nerve terminals (6, 43, 44). The rate at which impulses traverse the pineal sympathetic nerves is, in turn, controlled inversely by environmental lighting: light acts indirectly to *decrease* impulse flow to the pineal, thereby slowing melatonin synthesis. Once released, melatonin acts on neuroendocrine centers in the brain to suppress the secretion of LH and to produce other effects, which are described below.

Numerous other investigators have subsequently examined the antigonadal effects of melatonin in rats and other mammals. In 1965, Moszkowska (45) confirmed that melatonin administration reduces ovarian weight and showed that its repeated administration also delayed vaginal opening. Chu et al (46), and then McIsaac et al (47), demonstrated that exogenous melatonin decreased the incidence of estrous vaginal smears in rats and mice exposed to normal lighting regimens, and thus probably interfered with ovulation. Collu et al (48) in 1971, and then Ying & Greep (49) in 1973, showed directly that it blocked spontaneous ovulation. Most recently, Thorpe & Herbert (50) demonstrated that melatonin administration causes premature termination of estrus in ferrets exposed to constant light. Melatonin inhibits the compensatory ovarian hypertrophy that follows unilateral oophorectomy in mice, when administered on the day of birth (51) or the day of surgery (52), but not when administered 40 hr after unilateral oophorectomy (53). It inhibits the increase in rat ovarian, but not uterine, weight caused by the administration of HCG (54, 55) and, in large doses, decreases the incidence of induced ovulations in immature mice treated with pregnant mares' serum gonadotropin (PMSG) (56–58). Mature monkeys given 10 mg melatonin per day for seven days exhibited anovulation and a shortened luteal phase (59).

Exogenous melatonin also inhibits the growth and functional activity of the male gonad: it causes testicular weight to regress in weasels (60), suppresses the light-induced increase in testicular (and ovarian) weight in rats (61), inhibits the testicular recrudescence in hamsters that normally follows exposure to a long photoperiod (62), decreases the weights of the rat seminal vesicle and ventral prostate (63–67), and lowers the concentration of testosterone in testicular venous blood (68). That melatonin may act directly on the testes, as well as indirectly, via the brain, is suggested by evidence that it suppresses testosterone synthesis in vitro (69) and that it accelerates testicular and prostatic regression in hypophysectomized animals (70). Melatonin may also indirectly affect testicular function by modifying the metabolism of testosterone in the liver and hypothalamus (71, 72).

It has also been reported (73, 74) that melatonin implanted subcutaneously in golden hamsters blocks the antigonadotropic effects of exposure to short periods of light, that is, the decreases in testicular and ovarian weight and in pituitary LH and prolactin levels. This observation has been taken as evidence that melatonin is not the antigonadotropic substance of the pineal body in golden hamsters. Unfortunately, no data on plasma melatonin levels were presented in this study; hence, it is not possible to rule out such alternative explanations for its paradoxical effects as the induction of melatonin-metabolizing enzymes by the constant high levels of this compound in the plasma.

The doses of melatonin reportedly needed to inhibit sexual maturation and spontaneous gonadal growth have generally been well under 1 mg/kg per day; those required to block spontaneous or hormone-induced ovulation are greater and probably vary according to when they are administered in relation to the Critical Period (49). It should be noted that Ebels & Prop in 1965 and DeProspo & Hurley in 1971 failed to detect any effect of melatonin or pineal extracts on the weight of the rat ovary (75–77), while Thieblot et al (78) in 1966, reported that large doses of melatonin stimulated gonadal growth and increased the luteinization of the ovaries. Melatonin also reportedly increases the synthesis of progesterone by perfused corpora lutea taken from humans on the twenty-first day of the menstrual cycle (79).

Pituitary Gland and Gonadotropin Secretion

Adams and his colleagues (80) reported in 1965 that doses of melatonin that delayed puberty and decreased ovarian weight also increased the content of LH in the pituitary. They interpreted this finding as suggesting that melatonin suppresses LH secretion. A number of investigators have subsequently used the increase in LH secretion following castration to amplify melatonin's effects on the pituitary. Thus, Clementi et al (81, 82), Fraschini et al (83, 84), and Debeljuk et al (85) reported that melatonin implants placed in particular brain regions—the median eminence and the "reticular area" of the brain stem—or injected daily for 33 days suppressed the postcastration rise in pituitary LH content. Melatonin's parallel suppression of the castration-induced rise in serum LH was observed by Roche et al (86) in 1970, and Fraschini et al (87) in 1971, but not by Talbot & Reiter (88) in 1973. Some investigators have observed melatonin-induced decreases in pituitary weight among untreated (89, 90), light-exposed (91), or castrated (85) rats; others (76) have failed to detect such changes. Melatonin administration has also been reported to decrease serum FSH (92), to block the preovulatory surge in serum LH (49), and to increase serum prolactin (93, 94). The pineal hormone may act by decreasing the synthesis or release of gonadotropin-releasing factors in the hypothalamus (35).

Other Glands

A decrease in thyroid weight following melatonin administration was described as early as 1963 by Baschieri and co-workers (95) and confirmed by Turner and associates (96, 97), who correlated it with a decrease in the pituitary concentration of thyroid-stimulating hormone (TSH). In doses of 10–150 μg per animal per day, melatonin also was found to decrease the uptake of ^{131}I by the thyroid (95, 98–100) and to decrease oxygen consumption (101). Using the rate at which ^{131}I disappears from the thyroid as an index, Turner and his associates have concluded that melatonin also slows the secretion of iodinated thyroid hormones (89, 102–104).

Some investigators have observed in vivo decreases in adrenal corticosterone production in rats given large doses of melatonin (50–200 μg/100 g body weight) (105). Others, using smaller doses, have failed to observe changes in either the synthesis of corticosterone or the plasma or pituitary levels of ACTH (1 μg/kg body weight) (106). Melatonin may decrease the formation of Δ^4-3-ketonic corticosteroids in vitro (107) and may suppress the compensatory adrenal hypertrophy that follows unilateral adrenalectomy (51, 108).

Melatonin reportedly suppresses the secretion of insulin in vitro from islets of Langerhans perfused with a glucose-containing medium (109), but does not affect basal insulin secretion (110).

While melatonin apparently does not affect its own synthesis—from ^{14}C-tryptophan in cultured rat pineals (111)—it does influence pineal metabolism in vivo. Thus, Fiske & Huppert (112) found that melatonin administration extinguished the daily rhythm in rat pineal serotonin content, and Cady & Dillman (113) reported that melatonin increased the uptake of thyroxine in bovine pineal slices. Pavel (114) observed a 50% decrease in the arginine-vasotocin content of the pineal, as well as a decrease in the antidiuretic activity of the cerebrospinal fluid following melatonin administration to cats.

High doses of melatonin (80 mg/kg) reportedly suppress the secretion of growth hormone (GH) (115, 116); this action may be related to the effect of melatonin on brain serotonin levels (117). It has also been reported that melatonin decreases the somatomedin-like activity of rat plasma (118). Gram quantities of melatonin also reduce the rise in plasma GH among humans made hypoglycemic with insulin (119). One report suggests that melatonin stimulates the synthesis of GH by the pituitary (120).

Effects on the Brain

That melatonin might directly influence the central nervous system was first suggested by the demonstrations that ^{3}H-melatonin passes freely from the bloodstream into the brain (121), and that melatonin implants placed within the median eminence or the brain stem "reticular formation," but not within the pituitary, could block the castration-induced rise in pituitary LH content (81, 83, 84). In 1968, Anton-Tay and his collaborators (117) demonstrated that the systemic administration of melatonin modified brain serotonin levels: the concentration of the neurotransmitter initially fell within the cerebral cortex, a brain region containing only the axons and terminals of serotoninergic neurons, while it rose within the brain stem, presumably reflecting changes within cell bodies. Increases in the serotonin content of particular brain regions after melatonin administration were also subsequently observed by Piezzi & Wurtman (122).

The mechanism responsible for melatonin's effects on brain serotonin remains to be characterized. It could represent direct hormonal action on processes occurring within serotoninergic neurons—e.g. the synthesis, storage, release, or intraneuronal metabolism of the amine—or, perhaps, a transsynaptic effect resulting from a primary action of other neurons. The observation (123) that melatonin administration also increases pyridoxal kinase activity in the rat brain would seem to suggest that the pineal hormone accelerates serotonin synthesis, if, as appears unlikely, decarboxylation is the rate-limiting step in this process. Melatonin could affect brain serotonin by acting peripherally to modify the plasma amino acid pattern and, thereby, brain tryptophan levels (124). Parenthetically, drugs and lesions that affect serotonin-containing brain neurons have, like melatonin administration, been found to affect the secretion of gonadotropins and growth hormone from the pituitary gland (125, 126). In a recent study, intraarterial injections of melatonin (250 μg/kg) were reported to increase brain dopamine and decrease brain norepinephrine in rats, while a lower dose (40 μg/kg), injected intracisternally, raised the levels of both monoamines (127). Effects of melatonin on brain neurotransmitter metabolism may be related to the behavioral effects discussed below.

Relatively low doses of melatonin (under 50 μg/kg per day, for five days) were found to enhance the incorporation of ^{3}H-leucine into brain proteins (128), especially within the hypothalamus (129). In contrast, much larger doses (1–3 mg/kg) were needed to change brain serotonin levels. The determination of whether a particular dose of melatonin is physiologic, i.e. that it presents its site of action with melatonin concentrations that might occur in untreated animals as a result of its endogenous secretion, is rendered impossible by the paucity of information about the locus and rate of melatonin secretion: it is not known whether the pineal hormone normally is secreted into the bloodstream or into the cerebrospinal fluid. If the latter, then a several hundredfold greater fraction of endogenous melatonin enters the brain than the fraction of exogenous melatonin injected systemically (130); hence a 1-mg dose would be physiologically equivalent to 2–5 μg secreted from the pineal organ. Moreover, until very recently (4), no quantitative data were available concerning even that small fraction (131) of endogenous melatonin that passes, unchanged, into the urine.

That melatonin acts directly on the brain is also suggested by numerous reports describing its effects on sleep and other forms of behavior. Melatonin has been shown to decrease both wheel-running activity in rats (132, 133) and the incidence of adventitious movements in mice receiving large doses of L-DOPA (134). [Its administration apparently failed to affect total activity in rats (135)]. It induces sedation, and sometimes sleep, in cats (136) and humans (137–139), potentiates hexobarbital sleeping time in mice (140), and causes electroencephalographic patterns consistent with sleep stages in cats (141). Its administration also reportedly blocks ouabain-induced seizures in rats (142).

Other Effects

In concentrations of 1.25–300 $\times$ 10^{-6} M, melatonin inhibits spontaneous contractions by the isolated, perfused duodenum (143) and uterus (144); higher concentrations also suppress pitocin-induced concentrations by perfused uterine horns (145). The induction of bronchoconstriction in serotonin-treated dogs can be inhibited by large doses (6 $\times$ 10^{-5} mol/kg) of melatonin (146).

Melatonin administration has been reported to decrease urinary estrogens in women with advanced breast cancer (147), but to increase the incidence of mammary adenocarcinomas among rats treated with 9,10-dimethyl-1,2-benzanthracene (148), as well as tumor growth in mice (149); implants of melatonin reportedly suppress bile production in rabbits (150). The hormone allegedly decreases blood glucose in rats (151, 152), increases the amount of brown adipose tissue present in hamsters (153), and is as effective as serotonin in raising cyclic GMP (3',5'-guanosine monophosphate) levels in human monocytes (154).

EFFECTS OF OTHER PINEAL CONSTITUENTS ON MAMMALS

Mammalian pineals can deaminate serotonin to form an aldehyde, which is then rapidly oxidized to 5-hydroxyindoleacetic acid (5-HIAA), or reduced to form 5-hydroxytryptophol; these compounds can then be O-methylated, yielding 5-methoxyindoleacetic acid (5-MIAA) or 5-methoxytryptophol (155). This latter methoxyindole has been reported to have biological activities similar to those of melatonin. Its administration, via implants or intraperitoneally (20 μg/day), decreases ovarian weight and the proportion of daily vaginal smears exhibiting estrous cytology (47), delays spontaneous vaginal opening (156), suppresses HCG-induced uterine weight gain (55), and decreases pituitary LH content (83); however, it reportedly fails to suppress the increases in pituitary and plasma LH levels resulting from castration (88). Very large doses of methoxytryptophol (300–700 mg/kg) also reportedly induce sleep in mice (157), while lower doses (100 μg) block compensatory adrenal hypertrophy following unilateral adrenalectomy (108). DeProspo & Hurley reported that the administration of 100 μg of 5-methoxytryptophol, but not of serotonin or 5-hydroxytryptophan, for 10 days increased adrenal weight (76).

In 1962, Milcu, Pavel & Neascu (158) identified an oxytocic principle in bovine pineal extracts; this compound was a peptide closely related to, but differing from, arginine vasopressin, lysine vasopressin, or oxytocin. A similar agent was found in pig pineals three years later (159). In 1966, synthetic arginine vasotocin was found to have biological activities and chromatographic properties similar to those of the pineal compound (160), and in 1970, Cheesman & Fariss (161) confirmed the structure of this pineal principle as 8-arginine vasotocin. Very low doses of this compound inhibit the compensatory ovarian hypertrophy that follows unilateral ovariectomy (162, 163), the stimulation of ovarian and uterine growth caused by PMSG (160), and the compensatory adrenal hypertrophy that follows unilateral adrenalectomy (164). The incubation of mouse pituitaries with arginine vasotocin decreases the levels of a gonad-stimulating constituent (165), while the administration of 1 μg of arginine vasotocin daily for three days reportedly decreases the weights of the ovary, testicle, and accessory sex organs in rats (166, 167). Crude extracts of ovine, bovine, and porcine pineals were recently found to contain high levels of gonadotropin-releasing hormones (168). Lipolytic peptides were found by Rudman et al (169) to increase the tissue responsiveness to lipolytic agents of pineal extracts from animals fasted for 48 hr.

EFFECTS OF DRUGS AND HORMONES ON THE MAMMALIAN PINEAL

The biosynthetic activity of the mammalian pineal is primarily controlled by the release of norepinephrine from its postganglionic sympathetic nerves. One major consequence of norepinephrine release is an acceleration in the synthesis of the biogenic amine, serotonin, and its derivative hormone, melatonin. Inasmuch as most of the drugs known to affect the mammalian pineal do so by acting either on noradrenergic synapses or at steps in the conversion of tryptophan to serotonin and melatonin, a brief description is provided of these synapses and of pineal indole biosynthesis.

Sympathetic Nervous Control of Pineal Indole Biosynthesis

The mammalian pineal organ receives most or all of its innervation via postganglionic sympathetic neurons, which originate in the superior cervical ganglia (170) and terminate near pineal parenchymal cells and blood vessels (171); the density of noradrenergic nerve terminals within the pineal is unusually great. Pineal sympathetic terminals contain relatively large quantities of serotonin (172) in addition to their "true" neurotransmitter, norepinephrine; this phenomenon probably reflects competition for norepinephrine storage sites between the catecholamine and serotonin molecules, which are present in very high concentrations within neighboring pineal parenchymal cells (173). Rat pineal "gliocyte" cells can concentrate another presumed neurotransmitter, aminobutyric acid (GABA), in vitro (174).

The effects of norepinephrine on pineal metabolism have been most thoroughly studied within a rat organ culture system in which individual rat pineals are incubated for up to 48 hr with synthetic media containing isotopically labeled tryptophan (175, 176). The pineals readily take up the tryptophan and convert it to protein (177) or to 5-hydroxy- and 5-methoxyindoles (111). Norepinephrine accelerates the syntheses of serotonin and melatonin in cultured pineals by a process involving β-adrenergic receptors (178, 179), and possibly, adenylate cyclase and cyclic AMP (3',5'-adenosine monophosphate). The evidence that cyclic AMP participates in the control of melatonin synthesis is threefold: (a) norepinephrine activates adenylate cyclase in pineal homogenates (180–186); (b) dibutyryl cyclic AMP, but not cyclic

AMP itself, accelerates melatonin synthesis from ^{14}C-tryptophan within cultured pineal organs (176, 178, 187–189); and (c) dibutyryl cyclic AMP was found in some studies (179, 190) to enhance the activity of serotonin-N-acetyltransferase—an enzyme involved in melatonin biosynthesis—when added to pineal organ cultures. This evidence is, of course, only indirect; at present there seems to be a paucity of plausible theories to explain just how cyclic AMP might control the enzymatic steps in melatonin biosynthesis.

The first step in melatonin biosynthesis involves the hydroxylation of tryptophan to form 5-hydroxytryptophan; this process is catalyzed by a tryptophan hydroxylase enzyme, which may differ from the tryptophan hydroxylase in the brain (191), and which is probably not saturated with its amino acid substrate in vivo (192). The 5-hydroxytryptophan is then converted to a serotonin (5-hydroxytryptamine) through the action of the pyridoxal-dependent enzyme, aromatic L-amino acid decarboxylase. Some of the serotonin formed is inactivated by oxidative deamination, which is catalyzed by monoamine oxidase, an enzyme present in both sympathetic terminals and parenchymal cells in the rat pineal (193). The remainder (and larger fraction) is converted first to N-acetylserotonin, through the action of serotonin-N-acetyltransferase (SNAT), and then to melatonin, through the action of hydroxyindole-O-methyltransferase, which catalyzes the transfer of a methyl group from S-adenosylmethionine.

The mammalian pineal synthesizes and contains relatively enormous amounts of serotonin (172, 194). During daylight hours the rat pineal probably stores most of this amine. With the onset of darkness, 80–90% of it is released and probably converted to melatonin, causing marked daily rhythms in the pineal concentrations of both serotonin (195) and melatonin (196). The onset of darkness, by activating the sympathetic nerves to the pineal (197), also causes major increases in the activities of SNAT and HIOMT, the two enzymes that catalyze the conversion of serotonin to melatonin (5, 198). Pineal sympathetic nerves can also be activated by stress, hypoglycemia (199), and, possibly, endogenous factors. Thus, some rhythmicity in melatonin biosynthesis appears to persist when animals are deprived of light-dark cycles by being placed in a continuously dark environment (200). [Weekly rhythms in melatonin synthesis may also exist (201).] Obviously, in examining the effects of any drug on pineal indole metabolism, great care should be taken to include adequate types of controls for the time-dependent changes that normally characterize melatonin biosynthesis.

Almost all of the melatonin synthesized by cultured pineal organs is found in the culture medium, and not within the pineal itself (202). This observation, plus the chemical structure of melatonin—a highly lipophilic compound that is uncharged at physiologic pH—suggests that melatonin secretion from the pineal, like corticosterone secretion from the adrenal cortex, is not an active process, but depends simply on the gradient between intracellular and extracellular melatonin concentrations. As lamented above, it is not presently known whether melatonin is secreted into the blood or into the cerebrospinal fluid. In any event, sympathetic stimulation, by accelerating melatonin biosynthesis, should also accelerate the secretion of the hormone.

Effects of Drugs on Pineal Indole Synthesis

SEROTONIN   The rate at which cultured rat pineals synthesize serotonin can be increased by adding 5-hydroxytryptophan to, or elevating the tryptophan concentration of, the medium (192, 202), although it has been reported that high tryptophan concentrations can inhibit total tryptophan hydroxylation in cultured pineal organs (203). L-norepinephrine lowers the serotonin content of cultured pineals, possibly by increasing the conversion of the indole to N-acetylserotonin (204); this effect is blocked by propranolol. Mescaline increases the conversion of ^{14}C-tryptophan to ^{14}C-serotonin by cultured pineals, an effect that is not mimicked by LSD or psilocybin (205).

In vivo, pineal serotonin levels are increased by injecting tryptophan (206–208) or 5-hydroxytryptophan (206), and decreased by p-chlorophenylalanine (pCPA) (208), an inhibitor of both tryptophan hydroxylase and catechol synthesis (209), or by RO4-4602 (210), an inhibitor of aromatic L-amino acid decarboxylase. The daily rhythm in pineal serotonin content is disrupted by giving rats reserpine or the monoamine oxidase inhibitor, β-phenylisopropylhydrazine (206, 211), but not by bretylium or guanethidine (206). As a result, pineal serotonin levels fail to decline nocturnally. N-methyl-3-piperidyl benzoate, an anticholinergic agent, exerts similar effects (212). The administration of norepinephrine, dopamine (207), or actinomycin D (211) blocks the daytime increase in pineal serotonin. Presumably, the catecholamines do so by accelerating the N-acetylation of the serotonin; the mechanism by which actinomycin acts in this situation is not established. An enzyme in the rat pineal, presumably the tryptophan hydroxylase, is capable of converting phenylalanine to tyrosine; this conversion is inhibited in vivo by the administration of pCPA or tryptophan (213).

MELATONIN   The rate at which cultured rat pineals synthesize ^{14}C-melatonin from ^{14}C-tryptophan is increased by a number of compounds structurally related to L-norepinephrine—i.e., D-norepinephrine, L-epinephrine, dopamine, tyramine, octopamine, tryptamine (111)—as well as by amphetamine (214), and the monoamine oxidase inhibitors Catron® (111) and harmine (215). It is unaffected by morphine (216) and decreased by cyclohexamide (111). The increase in melatonin synthesis caused by adding norepinephrine to the culture medium can be blocked by propranolol, but not by phenoxybenzamine (178); the increase caused by dibutyryl cyclic AMP is unaffected by either receptor blocking agent (178), but is blocked by cyclohexamide or actinomycin D (189).

ENZYMES   A number of compounds have been shown to inhibit HIOMT activity in vitro, but apparently none of them blocks melatonin synthesis in vivo. Such inhibitors include substituted N-benzoyltryptamines and N-phenylacetyltryptamines (217), haloperidol (218, 219), fluphenazine, GABA (218), and oxypertine (219). L-Norepinephrine in concentrations of 10^{-5} M increases the HIOMT activity of rat pineals maintained in organ culture (175), possibly by accelerating formation of the enzyme. The addition of dimethyltryptamine (DMT) to pineal homogenates accelerates the O-methylation of N-acetylserotonin as well (220).

Pineal tryptophan hydroxylase is inhibited by pCPA in vivo, in vitro, or when added to organ cultures (203, 221, 222).

The administration of L-DOPA to rats causes a rapid and major increase in pineal melatonin content in vivo (223); it also increases the activities of the melatonin-forming enzymes, SNAT (179) and HIOMT (223). Presumably, the mechanism by which L-DOPA acts involves either the release of norepinephrine from pineal sympathetic nerve terminals, or the intravascular conversion of the catechol amino acid to dopamine, which acts directly on pineal parenchymal cells to stimulate melatonin synthesis (111). The latter is more consistent with the finding that pineal sympathetic denervation potentiates the DOPA-induced increase in pineal melatonin (223). Now that an assay is available for measuring the melatonin excreted in human urine, the increase in pineal melatonin synthesis after L-DOPA administration might provide the basis for an in vivo "pineal function test" in humans.

The SNAT activity of cultured rat pineals is increased by the addition of norepinephrine (179, 186, 188, 190, 198, 224–226); this effect may or may not be potentiated by prior pineal denervation (224, 225) and blocked by adding cyclohexamide or propranolol to the media (227). One group of investigators observed a similar change in SNAT after adding dibutyryl cyclic AMP to cultures (190); another did not (179). SNAT activity in cultured pineal organs is also increased by epinephrine, L-DOPA, octopamine (198), isoproterenol, theophylline, and the monoamine oxidase inhibitors pargyline and Catron (179), but not by serotonin or 5-hydroxytryptophan (179, 198). The magnitude of the increase in SNAT activity caused by isoproterenol depends upon the time of day that the pineal organ was taken from the donor animal (228). Cocaine and procaine also increase SNAT activity in cultured rat pineals (229). That this effect is mediated by the release of norepinephrine from surviving sympathetic nerve terminals is indicated by its failure to occur in pineals taken from animals previously subjected to bilateral superior cervical ganglionectomy, and its blockade by propranolol and phentolamine.

The nocturnal rise in pineal SNAT activity is suppressed in rats treated with reserpine, propranolol, or cyclohexamide, but not by phenoxybenzamine, pCPA, or, paradoxically, actinomycin D (227). Isoproterenol administration elevates SNAT activity in vivo; this effect is blocked by propranolol, but not by phenoxybenzamine (179) or phentolamine (230). The increase in SNAT activity is associated with a fall in pineal serotonin content, which can be blocked by giving rats pargyline, a monoamine oxidase inhibitor (230), or by adding cyclohexamide or propranolol to the media (227). Isoproterenol raises N-acetylserotonin levels in vivo; this effect is reversed by propranolol but not by phentolamine (231). Pargyline also first decreases, then increases, SNAT activity in vivo, if given during the light period of a diurnal cycle (232).

Pineal SNAT activity increases rapidly in rats under stress from immobilization, or made hypoglycemic with insulin (199). These increases are mediated by the release of catecholamines from three loci: sympathetic nerve terminals in the pineal, sympathetic nerve terminals in other organs that are not susceptible to damage by 6-hydroxydopamine, and the adrenal medulla. They are blocked by propranolol.

Effects of Drugs on Pineal Cyclic AMP and Adenylate Cyclase

L-Norepinephrine activates the adenylate cyclase in pineal homogenates (180) and accelerates the synthesis of cyclic AMP in both homogenates (181) and cultures (182) of rat pineals. Cyclic AMP levels in the pineal are also elevated by D-norepinephrine, L-epinephrine, and isoproterenol (181). The effect of L-norepinephrine is blocked by propranolol and dichloroisoproterenol and partially inhibited by trifluoperazine and chlorpromazine, but it is not influenced by phenoxybenzamine or phentolamine (181, 184). It is potentiated by exposing donor animals to continuous light for three days prior to taking the pineal—probably because this treatment decreases the occupancy of pineal receptors by endogenous norepinephrine (183)—or by adding theophylline, a phosphodiesterase inhibitor, to the medium (185). Deguchi (233) found that isoproterenol administration produced an elevation in pineal cyclic AMP content and, 1 hr later, in SNAT activity. Pretreatment with propranolol blocked both increases; administration of the β-blocker subsequent to isoproterenol after cyclic AMP had returned to baseline blocked the increase in SNAT activity. Pretreatment with cyclohexamide blocked only the rise in SNAT activity.

Effects of Drugs on Pineal Phospholipids

In concentrations of $1–300 \times 10^{-6}$ M, L-norepinephrine increases the rate at which cultured pineal organs incorporate inorganic ^{32}P into phosphatidyl inositol (PI) (234), monophosphoinositide (235), and phosphatidyl glycerol (PG) (236), and decreases the synthesis of phosphatidylethanolamine (235). The synthesis of pineal PI and PG are also accelerated by D-norepinephrine, L-epinephrine, dopamine, tyramine, and octopamine (236), as well as phenylephrine and propranolol (237), while monophosphoinositide synthesis is accelerated by acetylcholine plus eserine or by serotonin. An α-receptor blocker, phenoxybenzamine, has also been reported to block the phospholipid stimulatory effects of norepinephrine and phenylephrine, but not of propranolol (237), suggesting two distinct components to phospholipid stimulation in the pineal. Local anesthetics such as dibucaine accelerate the degradation of phospholipids in the pineal (238).

Effects of Drugs on Pineal Morphology

Using electron microscopy and autoradiography to localize the ^{3}H-norepinephrine taken up and retained within rat pineal organs, Wolfe and his colleagues showed in 1962 (239) that the pineal norepinephrine is stored in granulated vesicles of postganglionic sympathetic neurons. This granularity is decreased by reserpine and increased by iproniazid administration (240). The cellular localization of pineal serotonin was examined using histochemical fluorescence technology; about half of this amine was found within pineal parenchymal cells, and half within sympathetic nerve endings (241). Recently, pCPA has been shown to decrease the number of yellow-fluorescing pineal cells thought to contain this amine (242). Parenchymal serotonin is depleted by α-methyltyrosine; neural serotonin is depleted when tryptophan hydroxylase is inhibited by α-propyldopacetamide (243). In general, drugs that modify the storage of norepinephrine within sympathetic nerve terminals elsewhere in the body act similarly in the pineal, for example, metaraminol (241), desmethylimipramine (244), 6-hydroxydopamine (245), tyramine (246), and anti-nerve-growth factor (247), and both norepinephrine and dibutyryl cyclic AMP cause morphologic changes in pineals compatible with increased biosynthetic activity (248).

Effects of Hormones on the Pineal

Estradiol administration may (249) or may not (250) affect HIOMT activity. Paradoxically, estradiol increases pineal protein content and protein synthesis (251). Progesterone also reportedly decreases HIOMT activity, but without affecting pineal weight (249). In castrated rats, estradiol decreases pineal HIOMT, while norepinephrine partially reverses this decrease (252). Testosterone also decreases HIOMT activity, and norepinephrine has also been demonstrated to partially reverse this effect (253, 254). Testosterone also increases pineal protein synthesis in castrated male rats. Superior cervical ganglionectomy blocks this effect (255) and decreases pineal uptake of both testosterone and estradiol (256), suggesting a possible role of sympathetic transmission in the effects of these hormones on the pineal. Thyroxine and cortisol allegedly stimulate the Krebs and Embden-Meyerhof enzymes in vivo, as well as pineal aryl sulfatase (257). Epinephrine and melatonin increase the uptake of thyroxine by the pineal in culture, while TSH and aldosterone are without effect (113). Estradiol administration (500 mg/kg for three days) decreases pineal adenylate cyclase activity assayed in vitro; testosterone and progesterone are without effect in this system (258).

SUMMARY

Considerable evidence is now available that melatonin, a methoxyindole synthesized in, and secreted from, the mammalian pineal organ, is responsible for many, if not all, of the biological activities attributed to this gland. The best-studied effects of melatonin are those involving actions on the brain (and possibly elsewhere) to suppress the maturation and functional activity of the gonads. Melatonin synthesis exhibits a 24-hr rhythmicity, and melatonin levels in human urine are correspondingly greatest during the hours of darkness. The synthesis of melatonin in vivo and in vitro is stimulated by drugs that enhance the interactions of norepinephrine with pineal β-receptors, and suppressed by β-receptor blocking agents. Pineal extracts may contain additional biologically active compounds besides melatonin; these include peptides and other methoxyindoles. It seems likely that a number of experimental and, perhaps, clinical uses will be found for pineal constituents.

ACKNOWLEDGMENTS

This work was supported in part by a grant from the US Public Health Service (AM-11709).

Literature Cited

1. Kitay, J., Altschule, M. 1954. *The Pineal Gland.* Cambridge, Mass: Harvard Univ. Press
2. Lerner, A., Case, J., Takahashi, Y., Lee, T., Mori, W. 1958. *J. Am. Chem. Soc.* 80:2587
3. Wurtman, R., Axelrod, J., Chu, E. 1963. *Science* 141:277–78
4. Lynch, H., Wurtman, R., Moskowitz, M., Archer, M., Ho, M. 1975. *Science* 187:169–71
5. Wurtman, R., Axelrod, J., Phillips, L. 1963. *Science* 142:1071–73
6. Wurtman, R., Axelrod, J., Kelly, D. 1968. *The Pineal Gland.* New York: Academic
7. Wade, J. 1937. *Endocrinology* 21: 681–83
8. Fischer, O. 1938. *Arch. Int. Pharmacodyn. Ther.* 59:340
9. Engel, P. 1939. *Endocrinology* 25: 144–45
10. Fischer, E. 1943. *Endocrinology* 33: 116–17
11. Kitay, J., Altschule, M. 1954. *Endocrinology* 55:782–84
12. Wurtman, R., Altschule, M., Holmgren, U. 1959. *Am. J. Physiol.* 197: 108–10
13. Moszkowska, A. 1963. *Ann. Endocrinol.* 24:215–26
14. Smith, M. 1971. *Anat. Rec.* 169:432–33
15. Benson, B., Matthews, M., Orts, R. 1972. *Life Sci.* 11(I):669–77
16. Fiske, V., Bryant, K., Putnam, J. 1960. *Endocrinology* 66:489–91
17. Browman, L. 1937. *J. Exp. Zool.* 75:375–88
18. Hemmingsen, A., Krarup, N. 1937. *K. Dan. Vidensk. Selsk. Biol. Medd.* 13:7
19. Fiske, V. 1941. *Endocrinology* 29: 187–96
20. Wurtman, R., Roth, W., Altschule, M., Wurtman, J. 1961. *Acta Endocrinol.* 36:617–24
21. Ifft, J. 1962. *Endocrinology* 71:181–82
22. Reiss, M., Davis, R., Sideman, M., Mauer, I., Plichta, E. 1963. *J. Endocrinol.* 27:107–18
23. Meyer, C., Wurtman, R., Altschule, M., Lazo-Wasem, E. 1961. *Endocrinology* 68:795–800
24. Soffer, L., Fogel, M., Rudavsky, A. 1965. *Acta Endocrinol.* 48:561–64
25. Hipkin, L. 1970. *Nature London* 228: 1201
26. Schnitman, M., Debeljuk, L. 1971. *J. Reprod. Fertil.* 26:397–99
27. Davis, R. 1971. *J. Reprod. Fertil.* 26:383–85
28. Matthews, M., Benson, B., Rodin, A. 1971. *Life Sci.* 10(I):1375–79
29. Benson, B., Matthews, M., Rodin, A. 1971. *Life Sci.* 10(I):607–12
30. Benson, B., Matthews, M., Rodin, A. 1972. *Acta Endocrinol.* 69:257–66
31. Orts, R., Benson, B. 1973. *Life Sci.* 12(II):513–19
32. Vaughan, M., Reiter, R. 1972. *Gen. Comp. Endocrinol.* 18:372–77
33. Bensinger, R., Vaughan, M., Klein, D. 1973. *Fed. Proc.* 32:252
34. Debeljuk, L. 1970. *J. Reprod. Fertil.* 23:161–63
35. Moszkowska, A., Scemama, A., Lombard, M., Hery, M. 1973. *J. Neural Transm.* 34:11–22
36. Moszkowska, A., Citharel, A., L'Heritier, A., Ebels, I., Laplante, E. 1974. *Experientia* 30:964–65
37. Citharel, A., Ebels, I., L'Heritier, H., Moszkowska, A. 1973. *Experientia* 29: 718–19
38. Hayes, M. M., Knight, B. K., Warton, C. R. 1973. *Cent. Afr. J. Med.* 9:193–94
39. Cassano, C., Torsoli, C. 1961. *Folia Endocrinol.* 14:755–59
40. Roldan, R., Anton-Tay, F. 1968. *Brain Res.* 11:238–45
41. Dickson, K., Hasty, D. 1972. *Acta Endocrinol.* 70:438–44
42. Wurtman, R., Axelrod, J., Fischer, J. 1964. *Science* 143:1328–30
43. Wurtman, R., Axelrod, J. 1966. *Life Sci.* 5:655–59
44. Wurtman, R., Anton-Tay, F. 1969. *Recent Prog. Horm. Res.* 25:493–522
45. Moszkowska, A. 1965. *Rev. Suisse Zool.* 72:145–60
46. Chu, E., Wurtman, R., Axelrod, J. 1964. *Endocrinology* 75:238–42
47. McIsaac, W., Taborsky, R., Farrell, G. 1964. *Science* 145:63–64
48. Collu, R., Fraschini, F., Martini, L. 1971. *Separatum Exper.* 27:844–45
49. Ying, S., Greep, R. 1973. *Endocrinology* 92:333–35
50. Thorpe, P. A., Herbert, J. 1974. *J. Endocrinol.* 63:56P–57P
51. Vaughan, M. K., Vaughan, G. M. 1974. *Endokrinol. Exp.* 8:261–66
52. Vaughan, M., Benson, B., Norris, J. 1970. *J. Endocrinol.* 47:397–98
53. Vaughan, M., Reiter, R., Vaughan, G. 1971. *J. Endocrinol.* 51:787–88
54. Konig, A., Wulff, K. 1973. *Acta Endocrinol.* 173:15

55. Hipkin, L. 1970. *J. Endocrinol.* 48: 287–88
56. Reiter, R., Sorrentino, S. 1971. *Contraception* 4:385–92
57. Longenecker, D., Gallo, D. 1971. *Proc. Soc. Exp. Biol. Med.* 137:623–25
58. Ota, M., Hsieh, K. 1968. *J. Endocrinol.* 41:601–2
59. Fiske, V., Macdonald, G. 1972. *Proc. 4th Int. Congr. Endocrinol.* 880–85
60. Rust, C., Meyer, R. 1969. *Science* 165:921–22
61. Konig, A., Hofmann, R., Wirths, A., Von Wnuck, E. 1971. *J. Neuro Vis. Relat.* 10:177–86
62. Hoffmann, K. 1972. *Naturwissenschaften* 5:218–19
63. Kappers, J. 1962. *Gen. Comp. Endocrinol.* 2:610–11
64. Motta, M., Fraschini, F., Martini, L. 1967. *Proc. Soc. Exp. Biol. Med.* 126:431–35
65. Kinson, G., Peat, F. 1971. *Life Sci.* 10:259–69
66. Sorrentino, S., Reiter, R., Schalch, D. 1971. *J. Endocrinol.* 51:213–14
67. Ewig, J. 1971. *Diss. Abstr.* 32:2–3
68. Kinson, G., Liu, C. 1973. *Life Sci.* 12:173–84
69. Ellis, L. 1972 *Endocrinology* 90: 17–28
70. Debeljuk, L., Vilchez, J., Schnitman, M., Pauluccio, O., Feder, V. 1971. *Endocrinology* 89:1117–19
71. Kinson, G., MacDonald, N., Liu, C. 1973. *Can. J. Physiol. Pharmacol.* 51: 313–18
72. Frehn, J., Urry, R., Ellis, L. 1974. *J. Endocrinol.* 60:507–15
73. Reiter, R., Vaughan, M. K., Blask, D. E., Johnson, L. Y. 1975. *Endocrinology* 96:206–13
74. Reiter, R., Vaughan, M. K. Blask, D. E., Johnson, L. Y. 1974. *Science* 185:1169–71
75. Ebels, I., Prop, N. 1965. *Acta Endocrinol.* 49:567–77
76. DeProspo, N., Hurley, J. 1971. *J. Endocrinol.* 49:545–46
77. Prop, N., Ebels, I. 1968. *Acta Endocrinol.* 57:585–94
78. Thieblot, L., Berthelay, J., Blaise, S. 1966. *Ann. Endocrinol.* 27:65–68
79. Macphee, A., Cole, F., Rice, B. 1974. *Endocrinol. Soc. 56th Meet.* A169
80. Adams, W., Wan, L., Sohler, A. 1965. *J. Endocrinol.* 31:295–96
81. Clementi, F., De Virgiliis, G., Fraschini, F., Mess, B. 1966. *Proc. 6th Int. Congr. Electron Micros.* Tokyo: Maruzen
82. Clementi, F., De Virgiliis, G., Mess, B. 1969. *J. Endocrinol.* 44:241–46
83. Fraschini, F., Mess, B., Piva, F., Martini, L. 1968. *Science* 159:1104–5
84. Fraschini, F., Mess, B., Martini, L. 1968. *Endocrinology* 82:919–24
85. Debeljuk, L., Feder, V., Pauluccio, O. 1970. *Endocrinology* 87:1358–60
86. Roche, J., Foster, D., Karsch, F., Dziuk, R. 1970. *Endocrinology* 87: 1205–10
87. Fraschini, F., Collu, R., Martini, L. 1971. *The Pineal Gland.* Ciba Found. Symp. 259–73
88. Talbot, J., Reiter, R. 1973–1974. *Neuroendocrinology* 13:164–72
89. Narang, G., Singh, D., Turner, C. 1967. *Proc. Soc. Exp. Biol. Med.* 125:184–88
90. Vaughan, M., Vaughan, G., O'Steen, W. 1971. *J. Endocrinol.* 51:211–12
91. Debeljuk, L. 1969. *Endocrinology* 84: 937–39
92. Sorrentino, S. 1968. *Anat. Rec.* 160:432
93. Kamberi, I., Mical, R., Porter, J. 1971. *Endocrinology* 88:1288–93
94. Lu, K., Meites, J. 1973. *Endocrinology* 93:152–55
95. Baschieri, C. et al 1963. *Experientia* 19:15–18
96. Panda, J., Turner, C. 1968. *Acta Endocrinol.* 57:363–73
97. Singh, D., Turner, C. 1971. *Acta Endocrinol.* 68:597–604
98. Reiter, R., Hofman, R., Hester, R. 1965. *Am. Zool.* 5:727–28
99. DeProspo, N., DeMartino, L., McGuinness, E. 1968. *Life Sci.* 7: 183–88
100. DeProspo, N., Safinski, R., DeMartino, L., McGuinness, E. 1969. *Life Sci.* 8:837–42
101. DeProspo, N., Hurley, J. 1971. *Agents Actions* 2:14–17
102. Ishibashi, T., Hahn, D., Srivastava, L., Kumaresan, P., Turner, C. 1966. *Proc. Soc. Exp. Biol. Med.* 122:644–47
103. Singh, D., Narang, G. D., Turner, C. 1969. *J. Endocrinol.* 43:489–90
104. Singh, D., Turner, C. 1972. *Acta Endocrinol.* 69:35–40
105. Gromova, E., Kraus, M., Krecek, J. 1967. *J. Physiol.* 39:345–50
106. Barchas, J., Conner, R., Levine, S., Vernikos-Danellis, J. 1969. *Experientia* 15:413–14
107. Giordano, G., Balestreri, R., Jacopino, G., Foppiani, E., Bertolini, S. 1970. *Ann. Endocrinol.* 31:1071–80
108. Vaughan, M., Vaughan, G., Reiter, R., Benson, B. 1972. *Neuroendocrinology* 10:139–54

109. Bailey, C., Matty, A. 1973. *J. Endocrinol.* 58:17–18
110. Bailey, C., Atkins, T., Matty, A. 1974. *Hormone Res.* 5:21–28
111. Axelrod, J., Shein, H., Wurtman, R. 1969. *Proc. Natl. Acad. Sci. USA* 62:544–49
112. Fiske, V., Huppert, L. 1968. *Science* 162:279–80
113. Cady, P., Dillman, R. 1971. *Neuroendocrinology* 8:228–34
114. Pavel, S. 1973. *Nature London New Biol.* 246:183–84
115. Smythe, G., Lazarus, L. 1973. *Nature London* 244:230–31
116. Smythe, G., Lazarus, L. 1973. *Horm. Metab. Res.* 5:227–31
117. Anton-Tay, F., Choi, C., Anton, S., Wurtman, R. 1968. *Science* 162:277–278
118. Smythe, G. A., Stuart, M. C., Lazarus, L. 1974. *Experientia* 30:1356–1357
119. Smythe, G., Lazarus, L. 1974. *J. Clin. Invest.* 54:116–121
120. Chazov, E. et al 1972. *Vopr. Med. Khim.* 18:3–7
121. Wurtman, R., Axelrod, J., Potter, L. 1964. *J. Pharmacol. Exp. Ther.* 143:314–18
122. Piezzi, R., Wurtman, R. 1970. *Science* 169:285–86
123. Anton-Tay, F., Sepulveda, J., Gonzalez, S. 1970. *Life Sci.* 9:1283–88
124. Fernstrom, J., Wurtman, R. 1974. Serotonin—new vista. *Advances in Psychopharmacology* 11:133–42 New York: Raven
125. Collu, R., Fraschini, F., Visconti, P., Martini, L. 1972. *Endocrinology* 90:1231
126. Kordon, C., Balke, C., Terkel, J., Sawyer, C. 1973/1974. *Neuroendocrinology* 13:213–23
127. Wendel, O., Waterbury, L., Pearce, L. 1974. *Experientia* 30:1167–68
128. Cardinali, D., Nagle, C., Rosner, J. 1973. *Life Sci.* 13:823–33
129. Orsi, L., Denari, J., Nagle, C., Cardinali, D., Rosner, J. 1973. *J. Endocrinol.* 58:131–32
130. Anton-Tay, F., Wurtman, R. 1969. *Nature London* 221:474–75
131. Kopin, I., Pare, C., Axelrod, J., Weissbach, H. 1961. *J. Biol. Chem.* 236:3072–75
132. Reiss, M., Davis, R., Sideman, M., Plichta, E. 1963. *J. Endocrinol.* 28:127–28
133. Wong, R., Whiteside, C. 1968. *J. Endocrinol.* 40:383–84

134. Cotzias, G., Tang, L., Miller, S., Ginos, J. 1971. *Science* 173:450–53
135. Kastin, A., Miller, M., Ferrell, L., Schally, A. 1973. *Physiol. Behav.* 10:399–401
136. Marczynski, T., Yamaguchi, N., Ling, G., Gradzinska, L. 1964. *Experientia* 20:435–37
137. Lerner, A., Case, J. 1960. *Fed. Proc.* 19:590–92
138. Anton-Tay, F., Diaz, J., Fernandez-Guardiola, A. 1971. *Life Sci.* 10:841–50
139. Papavasilou, P. et al 1972. *J. Am. Med. Assoc.* 221:88–89
140. Barchas, J. 1968. *Proc. West. Pharmacol. Soc.* 11:22
141. Arutyunyan, G., Mashkovskii, M., Roshchina, L. 1964. *Fed. Proc.* 23:T1330–32
142. Izumi, K., Donaldson, J., Minnich, J., Barbeau, A. 1973. *Gen. Comp. Endocrinol.* 51:572–78
143. Quastel, M., Rahamimoff, R. 1965. *Br. J. Pharmacol.* 24:455–61
144. Hertz-Eschel, M., Rahamimoff, R. 1965. *Life Sci.* 4:1367–72
145. Davis, R., McGowan, L., Uroskie, T. 1971. *Proc. Soc. Exp. Biol. Med.* 138:1002–4
146. Bruderman, J., Rahamimoff, R. 1967. *J. Appl. Physiol.* 23:938–43
147. Burns, J. 1973. *J. Physiol.* 229:38P–39P
148. Hamilton, T. 1969. *Br. J. Surg.* 56:764–66
149. Buswell, R. S. 1975. *Lancet* i:34–35
150. Shani, J., Knaggs, G., Tindal, J. 1971. *J. Endocrinol.* 50:543–44
151. Burns, J. 1972. *J. Endocrinol.* 226:106P–7P
152. Burns, J. 1973. *J. Endocrinol.* 232:84P–85P
153. Heldmaier, G., Hoffmann, K. 1974. *Nature London* 247:224–25
154. Sandler, J. A., Clyman, R. I., Manganiello, V. C., Vaughan, M. 1975. *J. Clin. Invest.* 55:431–55
155. McIsaac, W. M., Farrell, G., Taborsky, R. G., Taylor, A. N. 1965. *Science* 148:102–3
156. Collu, R., Fraschini, F., Martini, L. 1971. *J. Endocrinol.* 50:679–83
157. Feldstein, A., Chang, F., Kucharski, J. 1970. *Life Sci.* 9:323–29
158. Milcu, S., Pavel, S., Neascu, C. 1962. *Endocrinology* 72:563–66
159. Pavel, S. 1965. *Endocrinology* 77:812–17
160. Pavel, S., Petrescu, S. 1966. *Nature London* 212:1054
161. Cheesman, D., Fariss, B. 1970. *Proc. Soc. Exp. Biol. Med.* 133:1254–56

162. Pavel, S., Petrescu, M., Vicoleanu, N. 1973. *Neuroendocrinology* 11:370–374
163. Pavel, S., Dimitru, I., Klepsh, I., Dorcescu, M. 1973/1974. *Neuroendocrinology* 13:41–46
164. Pavel, S., Matrescu, L., Petrescu, M. 1973. *Neuroendocrinology* 12:371–75
165. Moszkowska, A., Ebels, I. 1968. *Experientia* 24:610–11
166. Vaughan, M. K., Vaughan, G. M., Klein, D. C. 1974. *Science* 186:938–39
167. Vaughan, M. K., Reiter, R. J., McKinney, T., Vaughan, G. M. 1974. *Intern. J. Fertil.* 19:103–6
168. White, W. et al 1974. *Endocrinology* 94:1422–26
169. Rudman, D. et al 1970. *Endocrinology* 87:27
170. Kappers, J. 1960. *Z. Zellforsch. Mikrosk. Anat.* 52:163–215
171. Milofsky, A. 1957. *Anat. Rec.* 127:435–36
172. Giarman, N., Day, M. 1959. *Biochem. Pharmacol.* 1:235
173. Owman, C. 1965. *Prog. Brain Res.* 10:423–52
174. Schon, F., Beart, P., Chapman, D., Kelly, J. 1975. *Brain Res.* 85:479–90
175. Klein, D. 1969. *Fed. Proc.* 28:734
176. Shein, H., Wurtman, R. 1969. *Science* 166:519–20
177. Wurtman, R., Shein, H., Axelrod, J., Larin, F. 1969. *Proc. Natl. Acad. Sci. USA* 62:749–55
178. Wurtman, R., Shein, H., Larin, F. 1971. *J. Neurochem.* 18:1683–87
179. Deguchi, T., Axelrod, J. 1972. *Proc. Natl. Acad. Sci. USA* 69:2208–11
180. Weiss, B., Costa, E. 1967. *Science* 156:1750–52
181. Weiss, B., Costa, E. 1968. *J. Pharmacol. Exp. Ther.* 161:310–19
182. Weiss, B. 1969. *J. Pharmacol. Exp. Ther.* 166:330–38
183. Weiss, B. 1969. *J. Pharmacol. Exp. Ther.* 168:146–52
184. Uzunov, P., Weiss, B. 1971. *Neuropharmacology* 10:697–708
185. Strada, S., Klein, D., Weller, J., Weiss, B. 1972. *Endocrinology* 90:1470–75
186. Strada, S., Weiss, B. 1974. *Arch. Biochem. Biophys.* 160:197–204
187. Klein, D., Berg, G., Weller, J., Glinsmann, W. 1970. *Science* 167:1738–40
188. Klein, D., Berg, G. 1970. *Adv. Biochem. Psychopharmacol.* 3:241–63
189. Berg, G., Klein, D. 1971. *Endocrinology* 89:453–64
190. Klein, D., Berg, G., Weller, J. 1970. *Science* 168:979–80
191. Nakamura, S., Ichiyama, A., Hayaishi, O. 1965. *Fed. Proc.* 24:604
192. Shein, H., Wurtman, R., Axelrod, J. 1967. *Nature London* 217:953–54
193. Snyder, S., Fischer, J., Axelrod, J. 1965. *Biochem. Pharmacol.* 14:363–64
194. Quay, W., Halvey, A. 1962. *Physiol. Zool.* 35:1–7
195. Quay, W. 1963. *Gen. Comp. Endocrinol.* 3:473–79
196. Quay, W. 1964. *Proc. Soc. Exp. Biol. Med.* 121:946–48
197. Taylor, A., Wilson, R. 1970. *Experientia* 26:267–69
198. Klein, D., Weller, J. 1970. *Science* 169:1093–95
199. Lynch, H., Eng, J., Wurtman, R. 1973. *Proc. Natl. Acad. Sci. USA* 70:1704–7
200. Lynch, H. 1971. *Life Sci.* 10:791
201. Vollrath, L., Kantarijan, A., Howe, C. 1975. *Experientia* 31:458–60
202. Wurtman, R., Larin, F., Axelrod, J., Shein, H., Rosaco, K. 1967. *Nature London* 217:953–54
203. Bensinger, R., Klein, D., Weller, J., Lovenberg, W. 1974. *J. Neurochem.* 23:111–17
204. Klein, D., Berg, G., Weller, J. 1973. *J. Neurochem.* 21:1261–71
205. Shein, H., Wilson, S., Larin, F., Wurtman, R. 1971. *Life Sci.* 10:273–82
206. Snyder, S., Axelrod, J. 1965. *Science* 149:542–44
207. Zweig, M., Axelrod, J. 1969. *J. Neurobiol.* 1:87–97
208. Deguchi, T., Barchas, J. 1972. *Nature London New Biol.* 235:92–93
209. Wurtman, R., Larin, F., Mostafapour, S., Fernstrom, J. 1974. *Science* 185:183–84
210. Hyyppa, M., Lehtinen, P., Rinne, U. 1971. *Brain Res.* 30:265–72
211. Snyder, S., Axelrod, J., Zweig, M. 1967. *J. Pharmacol. Exp. Ther.* 158:206–13
212. Merritt, J., Sulkowski, T. 1969. *J. Pharmacol. Exp. Ther.* 166:119–24
213. Bagchi, S., Zarycki, E. 1971. *Res. Commun. Chem. Pathol. Pharmacol.* 2:370–81
214. Backstrom, M., Wetterberg, L. 1973. *Acta Physiol. Scand.* 87:113–20
215. Klein, D., Rowe, J. 1970. *Mol. Pharmacol.* 6:164–71
216. Shein, H., Larin, F., Wurtman, R. 1970. *Life Sci.* 9(I):29–33
217. Ho, B., Fritchie, G., Noel, M., McIsaac, W. 1971. *J. Pharm. Sci.* 60:634–37
218. Hartley, R., Padwick, D., Smith, J. 1972. *J. Pharm. Pharmacol.* 24:100P–102P

219. Ho, B., Gardner, P., McIsaac, W. 1973. *J. Pharm. Sci.* 62:508–9
220. Hartley, R., Smith, J. 1973. *J. Pharm. Pharmacol.* 25:751–52
221. Lovenberg, W., Jequier, E., Sjoerdsma, A. 1967. *Science* 155:217–19
222. Deguchi, T., Barchas, J. 1972. *Mol. Pharmacol.* 8:770–79
223. Lynch, H., Wang, P., Wurtman, R. 1973. *Life Sci.* 12:141–51
224. Klein, D., Weller, J., Moore, R. 1971. *Proc. Natl. Acad. Sci. USA* 68:3107–10
225. Deguchi, T., Axelrod, J. 1973. *Mol. Pharmacol.* 9:612–18
226. Klein, D., Weller, J. 1973. *J. Pharmacol. Exp. Ther.* 186:516–27
227. Deguchi, T., Axelrod, J. 1972. *Proc. Natl. Acad. Sci. USA* 69:2547–2550
228. Romero, J., Axelrod, J. 1974. *Science* 184:1091–92
229. Holz, R., Deguchi, T., Axelrod, J. 1974. *J. Neurochem.* 22:205–9
230. Brownstein, M., Holz, R., Axelrod, J. 1973. *J. Pharmacol. Exp. Ther.* 186:109–13
231. Brownstein, M., Saavedra, J., Axelrod, J. 1973. *Mol. Pharmacol.* 9:605–11
232. Illnerova, H. 1974. *Neuroendocrinology* 16:202–11
233. Deguchi, T. 1973. *Mol. Pharmacol.* 9:184–90
234. Muraki, R. 1972. *Biochem. Pharmacol.* 21:2536–39
235. Basinska, J., Sastry, P., Stancer, H. 1973. *Endocrinology* 92:1588–95
236. Eichberg, J., Shein, H., Schwartz, M., Hauser, G. 1973. *J. Biol. Chem.* 248:3625–32
237. Hauser, G., Shein, H. M., Eichberg, J. 1974. *Nature London* 252:482–83
238. Eichberg, J., Hauser, G. 1974. *Biochem. Biophys. Res. Commun.* 60:1460–67
239. Wolfe, D., Potter, L., Richardson, K., Axelrod, J. 1962. *Science* 138:440–42
240. Pellegrino de Iraldi, A., De Robertis, E. 1963. *Int. J. Neuropharmacol.* 2:251–59
241. Bertler, A., Falck, B., Owman, C. 1964. *Acta Physiol. Scand.* 63:Suppl. 23, 1–18
242. Smith, A. R., Kappers, J. A. 1975. *Brain Res.* 86:353–71
243. Falck, B., Owman, C., Rosengren, E. 1966. *Acta Physiol. Scand.* 67:300–305
244. Jaim-Etcheverry, G., Zieher, L. 1971. *J. Pharmacol. Exp. Ther.* 178:42–48
245. Eranko, A. 1971. *Histochem. J.* 3:357–63
246. Pellegrino de Iraldi, A., Suburo, A. 1972. *Eur. J. Pharmacol.* 19:251–59
247. Schott, H., Masuoka, D., Vivonia, C. 1970. *Life Sci.* 9:713–20
248. Karasek, M. 1974. *Endokrinologie* 64:106–14
249. Houssay, A., Barcelo, A. 1972. *Experientia* 28:478–79
250. Wurtman, R., Axelrod, J., Snyder, S., Chu, E. 1965. *Endocrinology* 76:778–80
251. Nir, I., Kaiser, N., Hirschmann, N., Sulman, F. 1970. *Life Sci.* 9:851–58
252. Nagle, C., Neuspillar, N., Cardinali, D., Rosner, J. 1972. *Life Sci.* 11:1109–16
253. Houssay, A., Barcelo, A. 1972. *Acta Physiol. Lat. Am.* 22:274–75
254. Nagle, C., Cardinali, D., Rosner, J. 1974. *Neuroendocrinology* 14:14–23
255. Nagle, C., Cardinali, D., Rosner, J. 1975. *Life Sci.* 16:81–92
256. Cardinali, D., Nagle, C., Rosner, J. 1975. *Life Sci.* 16:93–106
257. Milcu, S., Petrescu, R., Tasca, C. 1968. *Histochemie* 15:312–17
258. Weiss, B., Crayton, J. 1970. *Endocrinology* 87:527–33

THERAPEUTIC IMPLICATIONS ❖6635
OF BIOAVAILABILITY[1]

Daniel L. Azarnoff
Departments of Medicine and Pharmacology, The University of Kansas Medical Center,
Kansas City, Kansas 66103

David H. Huffman
Veterans Administration Hospital, Kansas City, Missouri 64128

There is no longer any doubt that the bioavailability of drug products may vary.
Rather, the question now is whether the variation in the absorption of marketed
products has any therapeutic consequences, be they production of toxic effects or
reduction in therapeutic effects. These alterations in effect may be due either to
changes in the rate and/or extent of absorption from the dosage form, that is,
bioavailability.

Previous reviews (1–3) have concentrated on the biopharmaceutical and methodological aspects of bioavailability testing. Instead, we plan to document any therapeutic consequences that have occurred as a result of alterations in bioavailability.
The expert panel on drug bioequivalence of the Office of Technology Assessment
(4) recently stated there were few documented reports of clinical problems associated with bioavailability. They cautioned, however, that since the vast majority of
products had not been studied, it could not a priori be stated no problems exist. The
latter point should be emphasized in any review on the therapeutic implications of
bioavailability.

How much change is needed in the bioavailability of a product before clinical
consequences will ensue? The answer to this question will vary with the drug. Small
differences in bioavailability are more likely to alter the therapeutic response of
drugs that have either a steep dose-response curve or a small therapeutic-toxicity
ratio. Most clinically useful drugs have relatively flat dose-response curves making
it likely that only marked differences in bioavailability will alter the therapeutic

[1]Studies by authors were supported, in part, by grant GM 15956 from the United States
Public Health Service.

53

response. Variation in bioavailability will produce a greater alteration in the therapeutic response at the lower than at the upper end of the curve (5). Bioavailability differences also become more important with drugs that have significant first-pass effects or capacity-limited absorption or metabolism.

Except for an occasional example, we do not intend to discuss variations due to chemical differences, such as salt or ester formation, since it is assumed that when a physician prescribes by generic name the pharmacist will fill the prescription with the same chemical form prescribed. Likewise, although controlled-release preparations pose significant bioavailability problems, they will not be discussed to any extent. An example of both types of problems can be seen in the studies of Svedmyr, Harthon & Lundholm (6) who demonstrated a direct relationship between the plasma concentration and pharmacological effects of nicotinic acid. Nicotinic acid given orally as regular tablets was absorbed and eliminated rapidly, resulting in large fluctuations in plasma nicotinic acid concentrations. In contrast, irregular and transitory elevations of nicotinic acid levels in the plasma occurred 5 hr after administration of an enteric coated tablet. A third preparation, pentaerythritol tetranicotinate produced moderate but consistent and prolonged levels. With equivalent doses of nicotinic acid, the acid form produced a greater free fatty acid (FFA) decrease of shorter duration as well as a more pronounced flush than the ester (7). The decrease of FFA produced by the acid form was followed by a secondary prolonged FFA elevation which was not seen with the ester. There is also evidence that the sodium salt of most barbiturates is more rapidly absorbed than the acid form (8).

ANTIBIOTICS AND CHEMOTHERAPEUTIC AGENTS

A number of investigations have been reported demonstrating varying degrees of bioavailability inequivalence of antibiotics determined by the area under the plasma concentration x time curve (AUC), peak plasma levels, or excretion in urine. However, documentation of therapeutic inequivalence is not readily available and must be inferred. Even infectious disease specialists have not decided whether the peak height or AUC is the important determinant of therapeutic efficacy. The clinical trial is not sensitive enough to determine significant differences in relative efficacy of antibiotics (9), since it is not possible in many studies to determine if the antibiotic had an effect on the course of the disease in as many as one fourth of the patients.

The purpose of chemotherapy is to hinder bacteria from multiplying for an initial period during which the animals' natural defenses are inadequate (10). After this initial period of low resistance, antibiotic therapy becomes less important as animals acquire a greater endogenous resistance to infection. With bacteriostatic agents the results of studies in mice are consistent with the hypothesis proposed by Krüger-Thiemer & Burger (11) that an adequate concentration of drug must be maintained uninterruptedly. The optimal effect with bactericidal antibiotics, however, is to be expected even if the level intermittently falls below the minimum inhibitory concentration (MIC).

The MIC range for common pathogens is 0.10–12.5 μg/ml (12–14). For a given organism, the in vitro MIC is thought to be a rough index of in vivo serum levels required for satisfactory therapeutic response (12). Comparing in vitro sensitivity of bacteria to antibiotics and the concentration of these drugs in serum with clinical results, Pullen (15) stated therapeutic blood levels should be maintained 2–5 times in vitro MIC. When the peak titer of bacteriostatic activity in serum was equal to or greater than 1:8, the infection was cured in at least 80% of the cases. The cure in patients with urinary tract infections was 90% if the titer of bacteriostatic activity in urine was equal to or greater than 1:4 (16). However, efficacy also depends on the ability of a drug to reach the site of inflammation. The peak blood level gives little indication of tissue levels, the latter often being as much as 50% less (17). If the antibiotic is rapidly excreted, the concentration in tissue fluid is particularly unpredictable. With drugs of this type, constant serum levels should be maintained to assure that tissue concentration is satisfactory (17).

The therapeutic response to isoniazid (INH) is better with a moderate dose (400 mg) than a small dose (200 mg); a single 400 mg dose is better than the same dose given as 200 mg twice a day (18). The higher peak level and better therapeutic response with the single dose are compatible with animal studies in which the best bacteriostatic and bactericidal effect is obtained when actively growing organisms are exposed to high concentrations of the drug (19). In treatment with INH alone, increasing the dosage enough to raise the peak concentrations 600% only produced a 50% improvement in therapeutic response (18). A complicating factor in the therapeutic use of INH is that some patients are slow and some fast acetylators of this drug. In one study (20), by six months, mycobacteria were still found in the sputum of only a few patients receiving INH, PAS, and intermittent streptomycin. The only significant difference among the patients occurred at 2–3 months when more than 50% of the patients with an INH blood level greater than 0.4 μg/ml at 6 hr following a dose had converted to a bacteriologically negative sputum, whereas only approximately 35% of those with levels less than 0.4 μg/ml had converted. The higher levels were found in the slow acetylators and the lower levels in the rapid acetylators.

Slow and fast acetylators may respond differently depending upon the dosage form. Controlled-release tablets given at 30 mg/kg in fast acetylators produced the same blood level as 10 mg/kg of the regular formulation in slow acetylators. The matrix preparation had a lower peak level, however, than regular INH in the slow acetylators (21). Levy & Gelber (22) in an excellent review declared 50% greater dosage is needed for fast acetylators and that the greatest efficacy with the least toxicity will be obtained when the absorption characteristics of the formulation maximizes the peak while minimizing the AUC. No difference in AUC or peak levels was observed in an evaluation of six commercial INH formulations (23). Efficacy of any INH regimen in the treatment of tuberculosis is increased by additional drugs, making it unlikely that any but the most marked bioavailability differences in INH formulation will be therapeutically significant.

In a study by Barr et al (24) brand A of tetracycline produced blood levels of 3–5 μg/ml compared to 2–3 μg/ml for brand B. The authors stated that if the MIC were greater than 3.0 μg/ml, patients would respond better to A than B. They also found marked variation in absorption between subjects and felt the poor absorbers would do better with A than B. They also suggested that more drug remained within the gastrointestinal tract with product B, increasing the possibility of nausea, local irritation, and alteration in normal flora with overgrowth of nonsusceptible organisms. Poor and good absorbers of tetracycline have been noted by others (25) and with drugs other than antibiotics (26, 27) and may be particularly important with drugs of marginal bioavailability.

Peak plasma levels below the usually accepted 0.6 μg/ml MIC were observed with 7 of 16 lots of 250 mg oxytetracycline dosage forms given to fasting subjects. In 6 of the 7 the levels were lower than the Terramycin® standard at all four time points studied (28). Seven comparison products were also markedly lower and more variable than Terramycin at 2, 3, and 6 hr after ingestion in another study (29). Although the mean level attained with all six products being compared to Terramycin in another study (30) was above the MIC, mean levels can be misleading as demonstrated in the evaluation of 7 oxytetracycline and 2 tetracycline products marketed in Norway (31). Even though the mean value appeared satisfactory, insignificant or nondetectable levels were found in 2–3 of the 10 volunteers with some products.

Mean peak chloramphenicol plasma levels were 2.7, 6.3, 5.2, and 10.9 μg/ml and AUC 34, 61, 53, and 100% (Chloromycetin®) in a study of four formulations of this antibiotic (32). The peak levels attained by Chloromycetin ranged from 8.9–12.9 μg/ml, whereas the product with the poorest absorption was 0.7–5.1 μg/ml. This study was in healthy volunteers, but one can assume that poor therapeutic results have occurred in an occasional patient using the latter product since levels greater than 10 μg/ml are required for in vitro bacteriostasis of the majority of sensitive organisms (33, 34). However, single-dose studies may also be misleading. When Chloromycetin was compared with Amphicol, the mean concentration of chloramphenicol was greater following Chloromycetin than following Amphicol® for the initial 1–2 hr of the initial two dosing periods. With continued dosing, however, Amphicol produced higher levels than Chloromycetin (35).

Suspensions of micronized and "regular" sulfadiazine produced considerable differences in single-dose blood levels in humans (36), but again therapeutic differences can only be inferred. In another study, Van Petten et al (37) found differences in the bioavailability among four different brands of sulfadiazine and a suspension they did not consider therapeutically important. These investigators, however, stressed that at least during the loading phase of treatment in patients with a life-threatening infection, a completely and rapidly bioavailable product should be used.

Studies with griseofulvin have included correlations of bioavailability with clinical effects. One hundred and twenty-five mg tablets of griseofulvin particles with a specific surface area of 1.0 m^2/g given twice daily for 4 weeks produced a 95% cure rate in patients treated for favus. A similar dose of griseofulvin with a specific surface activity of 0.4 produced cures in only 65% ($P < 0.02$) (38). Similar results were reported by others (39) utilizing a historical comparison to the product containing the coarser material rather than a comparative trial.

Pascorbic® (PAS crystallized from a solution of ascorbic acid) supposedly has fewer gastrointestinal side effects and greater AUC than other forms of PAS permitting lower doses in the treatment of tuberculosis. However, Pentikäinen et al demonstrated that the AUC was less for Pascorbic (40) than for rapid dissolution sodium *p*-aminosalicylic acid tablets. The faster rate of absorption allows more PAS to escape acetylation by the capacity-limited enzyme activity during the first pass.

Other substances in the tablet besides active ingredients may result in therapeutic problems. Renal tubular acidosis may result from chemical changes that occur with prolonged storage of tetracycline. Degradation may be accelerated by citric acid and decreased by lactose (41), substances frequently found in dosage forms. Contaminants, such as allergenic residues in penicillin preparations, may also vary among products (42).

The concentration of nitrofurantoin in urine, not blood, is paramount in importance in the effective use of this drug. In contrast, nausea and vomiting are adverse effects which appear to be related to dose and blood level (43). Since nitrofurantoin has limited water solubility, dissolution and the rate of absorption are directly related to crystal size. Therefore, the administration of the macro crystal should decrease the peak concentration in plasma as well as the incidence of nausea and vomiting without significantly altering the concentration of the drug in the urinary tract. Less gastrointestinal intolerance was reported with the large crystal preparation in 112 patients with a previous history of this side effect. A direct comparison was not done and these complaints are quite subjective; therefore, one must wonder about the validity of the interpretation because in 287 patients without previous intolerance, no difference was observed in the incidence with regular and macronitrofurantoin (14 vs 8%). The cure rate was better than 80% with both (44). Significantly greater amounts of nitrofurantoin were found in the urine after ingestion of tablet than after a capsule formulation; however, both achieved a concentration of at least 30 μg/ml, a level that will eradicate at least 90% of most strains of *Escherichia coli* (45). This concentration was achieved within 4 hr regardless of whether the formulation consisted of regular or macro crystals (46). Two of 14 nitrofurantoin products, however, did not produce minimally acceptable concentrations of the drug in urine (47).

MacLeod et al (48) evaluated three brands of ampicillin in a crossover study in healthy volunteers. Brands B and C had 78% and 72% of the mean AUC of Brand A. The peak levels were 4.21 μg/ml for A and 3.13 and 2.87 for B and C respectively. These authors point out that the Canadian Health Protection Branch considers 80% or more of a reference standard as satisfactory (49). We cannot determine the therapeutic basis for such a standard. This statement is interesting in view of the observation that a minor modification in the fraction of dispersing agent improved the performance of Novoampicillin® (B) so that it became 17% better than Penbritin® (A) (50). Obviously, the product with the best absorption should be the reference standard since products that are incompletely absorbed have the greatest potential for erratic absorption, even within the same individual. It has been suggested that pro drug forms of ampicillin (hetacillin) could be utilized to improve ampicillin absorption since the former is hydrolyzed to ampicillin in the plasma (51).

Variable results have been reported for the bioavailability of erythromycin formulations studied in a variety of ways (single vs chronic dosing, food vs fasting, etc) (52–57). In general, the estolate is better absorbed than the stearate in single- and multiple-dosing schedules (53) and food does not appreciably alter estolate absorption whereas the absorption of the stearate is significantly reduced. In some instances, differences may be seen after a single dose such as in a study of various formulations of erythromycin stearate, 250 mg every 6 hr before meals. However, after 5 doses no differences were seen in steady state (57). Even though higher serum levels of erythromycin were obtained with the proprionate than the stearate, the authors' clinical impression was that both drugs were equally satisfactory (58). In view of the high natural cure rates of infections for which erythromycin is appropriate therapy, it is unlikely a single comparative therapeutic trial for efficacy would reveal a difference between formulations. We must keep in mind, however, that only the estolate appears to be associated with significant hepatotoxicity (59).

If a physician does not observe a satisfactory clinical response when treating patients for infections with an antibiotic he is more likely to change the antibiotic than adjust the dose upward. This approach to treatment somewhat reduces the importance of differences in bioavailability of antibiotics except in the critically ill patient.

L-DOPA

Lander (60) reported three parkinsonian patients who were well controlled with minimal nausea on capsules on L-DOPA (Synodopa®). When deterioration in the patients' condition occurred over a 3- to 5-week period, it was found that they had been changed to a tablet dosage form (Larodopa®). In one patient a return to the original satisfactory effect was obtained by increasing the dose of Larodopa from 3 to 4 g per day.

STEROIDS

Campagna et al (61) reported a patient with familial Mediterranean fever who had repeated attacks of peritonitis in which the clinical symptoms were routinely aborted by the prompt use of 20 mg prednisone taken orally daily for 2–3 days. On one occasion after taking 20 mg daily for 3 days there was no improvement. It was noted that the patient had received a generic brand of prednisone, so he was again given the brand used previously with "almost complete resolution of the clinical syndrome" within 24 hr. In another report (62), a patient adequately controlled with prednisolone tablets for arthritic pain failed to respond when a generic form was dispensed even though the patient increased the dose fourfold. His arthritis again responded when tablets of the original brand were administered.

THYROID

Lack of a clinical effect of USP thyroid tablets was noted by Catz et al (63) in a number of patients over a 9-month period. Several patients became euthyroid when tablets of another brand were administered; the effect was substantiated by changes in the protein bound iodine (PBI). In another report, two myxedematous patients had relapses traced to substitution of enteric coated thyroid tablets for the uncoated tablets that had been prescribed (64).

DIURETICS

Tannenbaum and his associates (65) studied a fixed ratio combination of hydrochlorothiazide and triamterene formulated in tablets and capsules with quite different pharmaceutical ingredients. Absorption of both diuretics was twofold greater from the tablet than from the capsule. The tablets consistently produced an effect on sodium excretion that was greater than the capsule ($P < 0.01$). Although the 12 hr sodium excretion was greater following the tablets, the rapid onset and marked effect of this dosage form invoked compensatory mechanisms for conservation of the sodium. A similar situation was not observed with capsules. As a result, the 24 hr naturetic effect of the two dosage forms was essentially the same.

In 1963, Shaldon et al (66) demonstrated in eight patients with stable ascites secondary to cirrhosis of the liver controlled by administration of chlorothiazide and spironolactone (Aldactone®) that a preparation of smaller particles (Aldactone A®) was effective at one fourth the dose. Plasma levels and excretion in the urine of the major metabolite, canrenone, were also equivalent at the reduced dose. The importance of particle size was further defined in a study in dogs by utilizing the appearance of canrenone in blood as well as the ratio of sodium/potassium excreted in urine (67). These studies make it obvious that dose-related therapeutic and adverse effects may be affected by significant differences in bioavailability of products of spironolactone.

Potassium supplementation is frequently required with chronic diuretic use. Tablets of KCl have been associated with more than 300 cases of severe ulceration, hemorrhage, and stenosis of the small bowel thought to be due to the local effect of a high concentration of KCl in the bowel following release from the tablet (68). Solutions of KCl are available but patient compliance is poor because of the unpleasant taste and minor gastrointestinal complaints. Solutions of potassium gluconate, bicarbonate, citrate, and acetate taste better, but chloride is essential for effective supplementation of potassium (69). Ben-Ishay & Engleman (70) compared a single 40 meq dose of a 10% KCl solution and a slow-release tablet (Slow-K) in ten normal subjects. The amount of K^+ in the urine increased sooner and to a greater peak with the solution. However, after four days of administration no difference in net potassium excretion in urine was noted following equivalent doses. Although much better tolerated, under unusual circumstances, an occasional case of stenosis still occurs with the slow-release preparations (71).

ANTICONVULSANTS

Unusual central nervous system symptoms in patients receiving one brand of phenytoin sodium (Dilantin®) were described in letters to the *Medical Journal of Australia* in 1968. The symptoms occurred primarily in patients stabilized on a high dose of this drug product (72–75). In 87% of the patients, plasma phenytoin levels were above the therapeutic range and reduction of the dose ameliorated the symptoms (76). Subsequently, it was determined that the excipient in the capsules had been changed from $CaSO_4$ dihydrate to lactose and the amount of magnesium silicate and magnesium stearate increased slightly. Direct evidence for the increased absorption of phenytoin from the new formulation was obtained by measuring blood levels in a crossover study of 13 subjects (77). This study further demonstrated an increased fecal loss of phenytoin, apparently secondary to decreased solubility of phenytoin in the presence of calcium sulfate.

ANTI-INFLAMMATORY DRUGS

Katz and co-workers (78) carried out an extensive therapeutic trial with indomethacin in 97 patients with rheumatoid arthritis and other rheumatoid disorders. They noted a 37% incidence of adverse reactions including six patients who developed peptic ulcers. Doses of 100–400 mg of hard-pressed tablets later shown to have variable and erratic absorption were used in this study. Subsequent studies were done with a 25 mg capsule containing ultrafine milled powder. This formulation was associated with a more uniform rate of absorption and more predictable blood levels (79). Doses of 75–150 mg of this preparation produced 61% improvement compared to 42% in the previous high-dose studies. The adverse reactions decreased from 37 to 12% and no serious complications occurred.

The bioavailability of nine brands of phenylbutazone was studied in 10 healthy volunteers given a light, standard breakfast 1–1.5 hr before dosing (80). The percent absorption relative to an oral solution varied from 56.8 (Brand E) to 100.6 (Brand A). Based on theoretical considerations, the authors concluded that with chronic dosing all brands would achieve peak levels between 94 and 155 μg/ml by 36 hr. Brand E was the only brand significantly lower than A. Because of induction of its own metabolism, Burns et al (81) found that the limit of the plasma concentration with chronic dosing is 60–150 μg/ml. Five brands did not achieve peak levels until 4–8 hr so that the first dose of these preparations might not relieve the patients' discomfort satisfactorily. Otherwise, all tablets tested produced blood levels considered within the therapeutic range. Two of 23 brands of phenylbutazone tablets resulted in what the authors considered inadequate blood levels; this interpretation is questionable and based on only two healthy volunteers. Therefore, it is impossible to extrapolate the results to therapeutic response (82).

In 1963, a series of letters to the editor appeared in the *Canadian Medical Association Journal* reporting experiences with diabetic patients whose blood sugars were controlled by brand name tolbutamide preparations. A change to generic tolbutamide preparations was associated with hyperglycemia (83, 84). As a result, doubt was cast on the efficacy of three brands of tolbutamide sold in Canada by nonproprietary name. To evaluate this problem, two brand and three generic products were studied in a crossover design in 22 diabetic patients given 1–2 g tolbutamide per day (85). Fasting, midmorning and midafternnon blood sugar and tolbutamide levels were measured in addition to excretion of carboxytolbutamide in a 24 hr urine. The only difference observed was better control of the fasting blood sugar by one brand. No clinical differences were observed by the investigators. It must be remembered that secondary failures (8% per year) as well as temporary resistance to tolbutamide occur not uncommonly in response to a variety of emotional and physical stresses (86).

Variation in tolbutamide bioavailability caused by minor pharmaceutic variation has been demonstrated by Varley (87). Ten healthy and 9 diabetic volunteers were studied in a double-blind, crossover study comparing a tablet of Orinase® with a similar tolbutamide tablet containing half as much Vee Gum®. The 8 hr AUC for Orinase was 3.57 times greater than the other tolbutamide tablet ($P < 0.001$). The pharmacological effect determined as the AUC of blood sugar lowering was 2.09 times greater with Orinase, the difference in effect occurring, however, only in the first 3 of the 8 hr. It must be remembered the tablets with inadequate bioavailability were not a marketed product.

ANALGESIA

Two dosage forms of naproxen suppositories were found essentially the same except for the rate of absorption, which may be important if rapid analgesia is required (88). Phenacetin produces central nervous system side effects in volunteers, which were well correlated with phenacetin blood levels and bioavailability of the preparation. The adverse effects came on rapidly, primarily after administration of a fine suspension (less than 75 μ) of the drug and seldom after the preparations containing particles greater than 150 μ (89).

No difference was found in buffered and unbuffered aspirin in either efficacy or gastrointestinal tolerance in 160 patients receiving the products acutely and chronically (90). Similar results were obtained in a study of 1434 patients (91). A soluble form of aspirin (Alka Seltzer®) did cause less gastrointestinal bleeding than plain aspirin (92). Physiological differences secondary to variation in aspirin formulations were found by Pfeiffer et al (93) utilizing monopolar-integrated electroencephalographic changes to quantitate effect.

It is difficult to evaluate the efficacy of drugs that influence the central nervous system since even the color of the product may influence the effect (94). The evaluation process is further complicated by the presence of slow and fast absorbers of acetaminophen (26) and aspirin (27). Bioavailability differences between acetaminophen products were only detected in the slow absorbers (95).

TOPICAL PREPARATIONS

Bioavailability problems are also likely with topical preparations. Aware that there is a good correlation between blanching and alleviation of inflammation (96), Woodford & Barry (97) tested 30 proprietary hydrophylic topical corticosteroid preparations for their ability to produce blanching in 10 volunteers. All the preparations were within 90% of each other except for one with 78% and one with 54% effectiveness. In 50 patients with chronic bilateral inflammatory dermatoses (eczema and psoriasis) a solution of fluocinolone acetonide in propylene glycol dispersed in soft paraffin (A) was compared to a microcrystalline powder (B) suspended in soft paraffin (98). In 32% of the patients with eczema there was no difference between the two preparations, whereas 82% of the remaining patients had better results with A compared to 12% with B ($P < 0.02$). Fifty-two percent of patients with psoriasis did equally well with A or B. However, 36% of the remaining patients did better with A compared to 12% with B ($P < 0.15$). Overall there was no difference in 42% of the patients. In the remaining patients 79% did better with A than B ($P < 0.005$).

CARDIAC GLYCOSIDES

Following the report by Lindenbaum et al (99) of variation in the bioavailability of digoxin tablets from different manufacturers and even different lots of the same manufacturer, there have been other studies demonstrating that digoxin tablets are incompletely (20–75%) and variably absorbed (100–108). A good correlation exists between the serum digoxin concentration and the patient's clinical response to the drug (109). Since a narrow margin exists between the therapeutic and toxic digoxin levels (110–112), differences in bioavailability may have significant therapeutic consequences.

A prime example of the therapeutic consequences of variation in bioavailability of digoxin tablets occurred in the United Kingdom where in 1969 a "minor change" in the manufacturing process of Lanoxin® was installed. During the latter half of 1971 a number of patients with atrial fibrillation developed either congestive heart failure or a rapid ventricular response despite continuing the same dose of Lanoxin (113–116), which previously controlled their cardiac disorders satisfactorily (117). Considerable variation in absorption from the "new" and "old" tablets was manifested by an unpredictable increase in digoxin levels when the patients were changed from one to the other (114). The experience in Great Britain leaves little doubt that changes in bioavailability of digoxin tablets result in important alterations in the therapeutic response to digoxin (116).

The bioavailability of digoxin is also altered by certain types of malabsorption (118) and the coadministration of other drugs (119), particularly those that affect gastrointestinal motility (120). The administration of either metaclopramide and propantheline significantly alter the absorption of digoxin tablets; the altered absorption of digoxin secondary to the latter drugs is not significantly affected when the digoxin is given as a solution or a rapidly dissolving tablet (121). Similarly, Jusko et al (122) reported a low serum digoxin concentration in a patient maintained on digoxin tablets following radiation therapy to the small bowel. The concentration was increased to the therapeutic range when the same dose of digoxin was administered orally as an elixir.

ANTICOAGULANTS

Bleeding during treatment with oral coumarin anticoagulants is directly related to an excessive decrease in prothrombin activity (123) or to inhibition of platelet aggregation in an anticoagulated patient. Because of the poor solubility of dicumarol in water, formulation changes may markedly affect the therapeutic effect as measured by the prothrombin time. Both hemorrhage and ineffectiveness of previously satisfactory doses have occurred in some patients. Simply adding filler to change the tablet size to make it easier to break in half led to bioavailability problems due to differences in the dispersion and thus the rate of dissolution of the drug (124). Even when comparing one manufacturer's product it was found that five 5 mg warfarin sodium tablets were absorbed twice as fast as one 25 mg tablet; the latter tablet was only 80% absorbed compared to the five smaller tablets (125). However, bioavailability problems are less likely with warfarin sodium than with dicumarol because of the significant water solubility and long plasma elimination $T_{1/2}$ of the former.

VITAMINS

There are several reports of marked differences in the bioavailability of water- and fat-soluble vitamins (126–128). The therapeutic importance of such differences is difficult to assess since vitamins are usually taken in great excess of actual requirements and by individuals who are not actually deficient.

We have limited this review primarily to single-entity products, to similar chemical entities, and to similar-dosage forms. Controlled-release dosage forms are a special problem. We conclude that documentation of therapeutic consequences of differences in bioavailability have been few. However, a significant number of studies in healthy volunteers clearly demonstrate that the potential for alteration of therapeutic effect due to variation in bioavailability is quite significant. The lack of documentation of therapeutic alterations may be due to (*a*) the flat dose-response curve of many therapeutic agents, (*b*) physicians' lack of awareness of the potential effects of alterations in bioavailability, (*c*) the small number of patients any physician sees using one drug product, (*d*) the similarity of toxic effects of some drugs and the disease being treated (e.g. cardiac arrhythmias due to myocardial disease and digitalis), (*e*) concomitant use of more than one drug or mode of treatment (e.g. digitalis and diuretics for congestive heart failure), and (*f*) use of specially prepared, nonmarketed products in healthy volunteers in many of the studies designed to show differences.

The potential for therapeutic inequivalence of dosage forms due to variation in bioavailability emphasizes the need for compendial standards to minimize the problem.

Literature Cited

1. Barr, W. H. 1969. *Drug Inf. Bull.* Jan./June:27–45
2. Chasseaud, L. F., Taylor, T. 1974. *Ann. Rev. Pharmacol.* 14:35–46
3. Schumacher, G. E. 1973. *Am. J. Hosp. Pharm.* 30:150–54
4. Drug Bioequivalence Study Panel—Office Technol. Assessment. 1974. Drug Bioequivalence. Washington DC: GPO
5. Levy, G. 1972. *Pharmacology* 8:33–43
6. Svedmyr, N., Harthon, L., Lundholm, L. 1969. *Clin. Pharmacol. Ther.* 10:559–70
7. Svedmyr, N., Harthon, L. 1970. *Acta Pharmacol. Toxicol.* 28:66–74
8. Sjögren, J., Sjövell, L., Karlsson, I. 1965. *Acta Med. Scand.* 178:553–59
9. Waisbren, B. A. 1965. *Am. J. Med. Sci.* 250:406–23
10. Sackmann, W. 1971. *Chemotherapy* 16:203–10
11. Krüger-Thiemer, E., Burger, P. 1965. *Chemotherapia* 10:61–73
12. Kunin, C. M., Finland, M. 1961. *Clin. Pharmacol. Ther.* 2:51–69
13. Steigbigel, N. H., Reed, C. W., Finland, M. 1968. *Am. J. Med. Sci.* 225:296–312
14. Hirsch, H. A., Finland, M. 1960. *Am. J. Med. Sci.* 239:288–94
15. Pullen, F. W. 1960. *Arch. Surg. Chicago* 81:942–52
16. Klastersky, J., Daneau, D., Swings, G., Weerts, D. 1974. *J. Infect. Dis.* 129:187–93
17. Chisholm, G. D., Waterworth, P. M., Calnan, J. S., Garrod, L. P. 1973. *Br. Med. J.* 1:569–73
18. Fox, W. 1962. *Lancet* 2:413–17
19. Gangadharam, P., Cohn, M. L., Middlebrook, G. 1963. *Am. Rev. Resp. Dis.* 88:558–62
20. Harris, W. 1961. *Trans. VA-AF Chemother. Conf.* 20:39–45
21. Eidus, L., Hodgkin, M. M., Hsu, A. H. E. 1973. *Int. J. Clin. Pharmacol.* 8:154–59
22. Levy, L., Gelber, R. 1969. *Drug Inf. Bull.* Jan./June:82–92
23. Gelber, R., Jacobsen, P., Levy, L. 1969. *Clin. Pharmacol. Ther.* 10:841–48
24. Barr, W. H., Gerbracht, L. M., Letcher, K., Plaut, M., Strahl, N. 1972. *Clin. Pharmacol. Ther.* 13:97–108
25. Davis, C. M., Vandersarl, J. V., Kraus, E. W. 1973. *Am. J. Med. Sci.* 265:69–74
26. Gwilt, J. R., Robertson, A., Goldman, L., Blanchard, A. W. 1963. *J. Pharm. Pharmacol.* 15:445–53
27. Levy, G., Hollister, L. E. 1964. *NY State J. Med.* 64:3002–5
28. Brice, G. W., Hammer, H. F. 1969. *J. Am. Med. Assoc.* 208:1189–90
29. Blair, D. C., Barnes, R. W., Wildner, E. L., Murray, W. J. 1971. *J. Am. Med. Assoc.* 215:251–54
30. Butler, K. 1973. *Rev. Can. Biol.* 32: Suppl., 53–67
31. Bergan, T., Oydvin, B., Lunde, I. 1973. *Acta Pharmacol. Toxicol.* 33:138–56
32. Glazko, A. J., Kinkel, A. W., Alegnani, W. C., Holmes, E. L. 1968. *Clin. Pharmacol. Ther.* 9:472–83
33. Hewitt, W. L., Williams, B. Jr. 1950. *N. Engl. J. Med.* 242:119–27
34. Roy, T. E. et al 1952. *Antibiot. J. Chemother.* 2:505–16
35. Bartelloni, P. J., Calia, F. M., Minchew, B. H., Beisel, W. R., Ley, H. L. 1969. *Am. J. Med. Sci.* 258:203–8
36. Reinhold, J. G., Phillips, F. J., Flippin, H. F. 1945. *Am. J. Med. Sci.* 210:141–47
37. Van Petten, G. R., Becking, G. C., Withey, R. J., Lettau, H. F. 1971. *J. Clin. Pharmacol.* 11:27–34
38. Pettit, J. H. S. 1962. *Br. J. Dermatol.* 74:62–65
39. Harvey, G., Alexander, J. O'D. 1967. *Lancet* 1:327–28
40. Pentikäinen, P., Wan, S. H., Azarnoff, D. L. 1973. *Am. Rev. Respir. Dis.* 108:1340–70
41. Fulop, M., Drapkin, A. 1965. *N. Engl. J. Med.* 272:986–89
42. Stewart G. T. 1967. *Lancet* 1:1177–83
43. Halliday, A., Jawetz, E. 1961. *Antimicrob. Agents Chemother.*, pp. 317–23
44. Hailey, F. J., Glascock, H. W. 1967. *Curr. Ther. Res.* 9:600–605
45. Barry, A. L., Thrupp, L. D. 1968. *Antimicrob. Agents Chemother.*, pp. 415–22
46. Twick, M., Ronald, A. R., Petersdorf, R. G. 1966. *Antimicrob. Agents Chemother.* 446–52
47. Meyer, M. C. et al 1974. *J. Pharm. Sci.* 63:1693–98
48. MacLeod, C. et al 1972. *Can. Med. Assoc. J.* 107:203–9
49. Davies, R. O., Zarowny, D. P., Robin, H. R. 1972. *Can. Med. Assoc. J.* 107:183–84
50. Mayersohn, M., Endrenyi, L. 1973. *Can. Med. Assoc. J.* 109:989–93
51. Jusko, W. J., Lewis, G. P., Schmitt, G. W. 1973. *Clin. Pharmacol. Ther.* 14:90–99, 1973

52. Clapper, W. E., Mostyn, M., Meade, G. H. 1960. *Antibiot. Med. Clin. Ther.* 7:91–96
53. Blough, H. A., Hall, W. H., Hong, I. 1960. *Am. J. Med. Sci.* 239:539–47
54. Griffith, R. S., Black, H. R. 1964. *Am. J. Med. Sci.* 247:69–74
55. Perry, D. M., Hall, G. A., Kirby, W. M. 1958–1959. *Antibiot. Ann.*, pp. 375–81
56. Hirsch, H. A., Finland, M. 1959. *Am. J. Med. Sci.* 237:55–71
57. Bell, S. M. 1971. *Med. J. Aust.* 2:1280–83
58. Triggs, E., Neaverson, M. A. 1973. *Med. J. Aust.* 2:334
59. Aust. Drug Eval. Comm. 1971. *Med. J. Aust.* 1:1203–8
60. Lander, H. 1971. *Med. J. Aust.* 2:984
61. Campagna, F. A., Cureton, G., Mirigian, R. A., Nelson, E. 1963. *J. Pharm. Sci.* 52:605–6
62. Levy, G., Hall, N. A., Nelson, E. 1964. *Am. J. Hosp. Pharm.* 21:402
63. Catz, B., Ginsburg, E., Salenger, S. 1962. *N. Engl. J. Med.* 266:136–37
64. Corbus, H. F. 1964. *Calif. Med.* 100:364–65
65. Tannenbaum, P. J., Rosen, E., Flanagan, T., Crosley, A. P. Jr. 1968. *Clin. Pharmacol. Ther.* 9:598–604
66. Shaldon, S., Ryder, J. A., Garsenstein, M. 1963. *Gut* 4:16–19
67. Kagawa, C. M., Bouska, D. J., Anderson, M. L. 1964. *J. Pharm. Sci.* 53:450–51
68. Allen, A. C., Boley, S. J., Schultz, L., Schwartz, S. 1965. *J. Am. Med. Assoc.* 193:1001–6
69. Nordin, B. E., Wilkinson, R. 1970. *Br. Med. J.* 1:433
70. Ben-Ishay, D., Engelman, K. 1973. *Clin. Pharmacol. Ther.* 14:250–58
71. Pemberton, J. 1970. *Br. Heart J.* 32:267–68
72. Rail, L. 1968. *Med. J. Aust.* 2:339
73. Balla, J. 1968. *Med. J. Aust.* 2:480–81
74. Eadie, M. J., Sutherland, J. M., Tyrer, J. H. 1968. *Med. J. Aust.* 2:515
75. Landy, P. J. 1968. *Med. J. Aust.* 2:639
76. Tyrer, J. H., Eadie, M. J., Sutherland, J. M., Hooper, W. D. 1970. *Br. Med. J.* 4:271–73
77. Bochner, F. R., Hooper, W. D., Tyrer, J. H., Eadie, M. J. *J. Neurol. Sci.* 16:481–87
78. Katz, A. M., Pearson, C. M., Kennedy, J. M. 1965. *Clin. Pharmacol. Ther.* 6:25–30
79. Pearson, C. M. 1966. *Clin. Pharmacol. Ther.* 7:416
80. Van Petten, G. R., Feng, H., Withey, R. J., Lettau, H. F. 1971. *J. Clin. Pharm.* 11:177–86
81. Burns, J. J. et al 1953. *J. Pharmacol. Exp. Ther.* 109:346–57
82. Searl, R. O., Pernarowski, M. 1967. *Can. Med. Assoc. J.* 96:1513–20
83. Caminetsky, S. 1963. *Can. Med. Assoc. J.* 88:950
84. Carter, A. K. 1963. *Can. Med. Assoc. J.* 88:98
85. McKendry, J. B. R., Lu, F. C., Bickerton, D., Hancharyk, G. 1965. *Can. Med. Assoc. J.* 92:1106–9
86. McKendry, J. B. R., Kuwayti, K., Sagle, L. A. 1957. *Can. Med. Assoc. J.* 77:429–38
87. Varley, A. B. 1968. *J. Am. Med. Assoc.* 206:1745–48
88. Sevelius, H. et al 1973. *Eur. J. Clin. Pharmacol.* 6:22–25
89. Prescott, L. F., Steel, R. F., Ferrier, W. R. 1970. *Clin. Pharmacol. Ther.* 11:496–504
90. Batterman, R. C. 1958. *N. Engl. J. Med.* 258:213–19
91. Cronk, G. A. 1958. *N. Engl. J. Med.* 258:219–21
92. Leonards, J. R. 1963. *Gastroenterology* 44:617–19
93. Pfeiffer, C. C., Goldstein, L., Murphree, H. B., Hopkins, M. 1967. *J. Pharm. Sci.* 56:1338–40
94. Schapira, K., McClelland, H. A., Griffiths, N. R., Newell, J. 1970. *Br. Med. J.* 2:446–49
95. Prescott, L. F., Nimmo, J. 1971. *Acta Pharmacol. Toxicol.* 29:288–303
96. Place, V. A., Velazquez, J. G., Burdick, K. H. 1970. *Arch. Dermatol.* 101:531–37
97. Woodford, R., Barry, B. W. 1973. *J. Pharm. Pharmacol.* 25:Suppl, 123P
98. Portnoy, B. 1965. *Br. J. Dermatol. Syph.* 77:579–81
99. Lindenbaum, J., Mellow, M. H., Blackstone, M. O., Butler, V. P. 1971. *N. Engl. J. Med.* 285:1344–47
100. Manninen, V., Melin, J., Härtel, G. 1971. *Lancet* 2:934–35
101. Huffman, D. H., Azarnoff, D. L. 1972. *J. Am. Med. Assoc.* 222:957–60
102. Wagner, J. G. et al 1973. *J. Am. Med. Assoc.* 224:199–205
103. Johnson, B. F., Greer, H., McCrerie, J., Bye, C., Fowle, A. 1973. *Lancet* 1:1473–75
104. Shaw, T. R. D., Howard, M. R., Haner, J. 1972. *Lancet* 2:303–7
105. Steiner, B., Christensen, V., Johansen,

H. 1973. *Clin. Pharmacol. Ther.* 14: 949–54
106. Shaw, T. R. D., Raymond, K., Howard, M. R., Haner, J. 1973. *Br. Med. J.* 4:763–66
107. Manninen, V., Korhonen, A. 1973. *Lancet* 2:1268
108. Butler, V. P. Jr., Lindenbaum, J. 1975. *Am. J. Med.* 58:460–69
109. Huffman, D. H., Crow, J. W., Pentikäinen, P., Azarnoff, D. L. 1976. *Am. Heart J.* In press
110. Smith, T. W., Butler, V. P. Jr., Haber, E. 1969. *N. Engl. J. Med.* 281:1212–16
111. Beller, G. A., Smith, T. W., Abelwann, W. H., Haber, E., Hood, W. E. 1971. *N. Engl. J. Med.* 284:979–89
112. Grahame-Smith, D. G., Everett, M. D. 1969. *Br. Med. J.* 1:286–89
113. Falch, D., Teien, A., Bjerkelund, C. J. 1973. *Br. Med. J.* 1:695–98
114. Shaw, T. R. D., Howard, M. R., Haner, J. 1974. *Br. Heart J.* 36:85–89
115. Shaw, T. R. D. 1974. *Postgrad. Med. J.* 50:Suppl 6,24–29
116. Shaw, T. R. D. 1974. *Am. Heart J.* 87:399–401
117. Chamberlain, D. A., White, R. J., Howard, M. R., Smith, T. W. 1970. *Br. Med. J.* 3:429–36
118. Heizer, W. D., Smith, T. W., Goldfinger, S. E. 1971. *N. Engl. J. Med.* 285:257–59
119. Lindenbaum, J., Manlitz, R. M., Saha, J. R., Shea, N., Butler, V. P. Jr. 1972. *Clin. Res.* 20:410
120. Manninen, V., Apajalahti, A., Melin, J., Karesoja, M. 1973. *Lancet* 1:398–99
121. Manninen, V., Apajalahti, A., Simonen, H., Reissel, P. 1973. *Lancet* 1:1118–19
122. Jusko, W. J., Conti, D. R., Molson, A., Kreitzky, P., Giller, J., Schultz, R. 1974. *J. Am. Med. Assoc.* 230:1554–55
123. Rabiner, S. F. 1965. *Am. J. Med. Sci.* 249:404–11
124. Lozinski, R. 1960. *Can. Med. Assoc. J.* 83:117–18
125. Wagner, J. G., Welling, P. G., Lee, K. P., Walker, J. E. 1971. *J. Pharm. Sci.* 60:666–77
126. Chapman, D. G., Crisafio, R., Campbell, J. A. 1954. *J. Am. Pharm. Assoc. Sci. Ed.* 43:297–304
127. Middleton, E. J., Davies, J. M., Morrison, A. B. 1964. *J. Pharm. Sci.* 53: 1378–80
128. Sobel, A. E., Rosenberg, A. A. 1952. *Am. J. Dis. Child.* 84:609–15

TOXICOLOGY OF INHALATION ANESTHETICS AND METABOLITES

♦6636

Ethard W. Van Stee

National Institute of Environmental Health Sciences,
Research Triangle Park, North Carolina 27709

Several reviews that bear on the subject of the toxicology of inhalation anesthetics have appeared in recent years. A partial list includes biotransformation (1–4), the biochemical basis of chemical injury (5–9), and anesthetic toxicity (10–13). The proceedings of two symposia (14, 15) and another monograph in the series of the *Handbook of Experimental Pharmacology* (16) have been published.

Patterns of exposure to inhalation anesthetics may be divided into two broad groups: (*a*) acute, single or multiple exposures to relatively high levels, typical of the clinical application of general anesthetics, and (*b*) chronic, low-level exposure to which operating room personnel are subjected.

This review is divided into three sections: (*a*) biotransformation of anesthetics, (*b*) mechanism of toxic injury, and (*c*) toxicology of chronic exposure to anesthetic gases.

BIOTRANSFORMATION

Halothane

Species differences in the biotransformation of halothane ($CF_3CHBrCl$) have been demonstrated to be largely quantitative. No firm evidence of significant qualitative differences has been published at this writing.

Halothane at anesthetic concentrations has been demonstrated to inhibit its own dehalogenation (17). The rate of halothane metabolism in miniature swine has been equated with the rate of hepatic extraction and suggested to be related inversely to the rate of delivery of halothane to the liver (18). The implication was that the anesthetic impaired its own metabolism. Topham & Longshaw (19) conducted related studies but measured the biliary excretion of halothane in rats and dogs as well as the accumulation of nonvolatile metabolites in the whole bodies and organs of rats and mice. They concluded that a significant fraction of hepatic halothane extraction may be accounted for by the biliary excretion of unchanged halothane, thus calling for cautious interpretation of data equating hepatic extraction with

67

metabolism. They further offered support for a postulated enterohepatic circulation of halothane and/or metabolites that would contribute to a prolongation of the half-time of hepatic excretion. Halothane in trace amounts was identified in venous blood 44 hr after the induction of anesthesia in humans (17). Such persistence could be attributable to a combination of enterohepatic circulation and redistribution of the anesthetic. An enterohepatic cycle would not seem likely to be of great significance for the highly lipid-soluble halothane and the putative polar conjugates of its metabolites. Even if the conjugates were hydrolyzed in the gut, the principal non-volatile metabolite of halothane, trifluoroacetate (20, 21), would not be likely to be reabsorbed by the gut, since it remains mostly ionized at body pH (pK = 0.25) unless a carrier-mediated mechanism were involved in its reabsorption.

No evidence has been presented to date that any species tested is able to defluorinate halothane. Fiserova-Bergerova (22) detected no increase in bone fluoride levels following the intraperitoneal (i.p.) injection of halothane in olive oil to mice and rats. One would hope that similar studies would be pursued using the inhalational route of exposure. The lung represents the usual route of clinical exposure, and recognition of the potential significance of this organ as a site of xenobiotic biotransformation suggests the possibility of a role for it in the formation and disposition of metabolites of anesthetics as well as the fate of the parent compounds themselves (23, 24).

Creasser & Stoelting (25) detected no increase in serum fluoride levels in five patients anesthetized with halothane-N_2O.

Current concepts in the biotransformation of halothane are summarized in Figure 1.

Dechlorination (26) and debromination (27) require NADPH, are mediated by enzymes of the hepatic endoplasmic reticulum, and may be stimulated by the prior administration of phenobarbital. In the presence of O_2, dehalogenation is assumed to be oxidative (1).

Trifluoroacetate has been recovered from the urine of men (20, 21, 28) and squirrel monkeys (29) following exposure to halothane. Trifluoroacetaldehyde has been proposed as an intermediate in the formation of trifluoroacetate during the oxidative dehalogenation of halothane (12). Implicit in this scheme is the participation of liver dehydrogenase systems following the model of the biotransformation of trichloroethylene (30). Once the concept of the participation of these enzymes has been invoked, the formation of trifluoroethanol from trifluoroacetaldehyde or trifluoroacetate reduction by liver dehydrogenases (31) becomes reasonable (1).

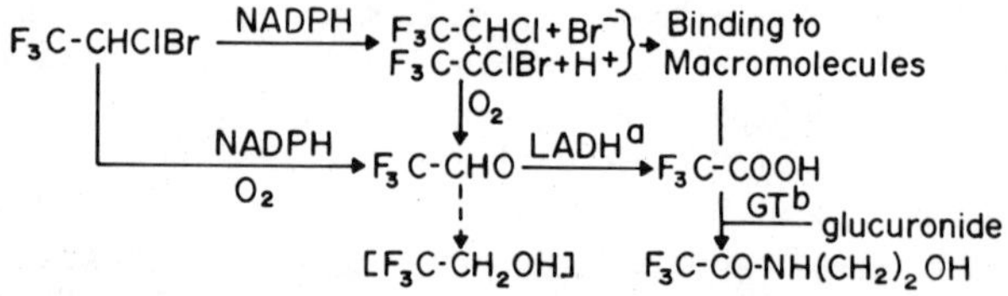

Figure 1 Current concepts in the biotransformation of halothane: (*a*) liver alcohol dehydrogenase, and (*b*) glucuronyl transferase.

The fact that neither trifluoroethanol nor its glucuronide has ever been identified in any species as a metabolite of halothane weakens the force of this argument. Were the alcohol formed in significant quantity it probably would have been detected by now as it has been following the administration of fluroxene (32). It is unlikely that trifluoroethanol is an endproduct of halothane metabolism in man (33), but that trifluoroethanol is not formed cannot be excluded absolutely. Nonvolatile metabolites of halothane are formed that remain to be identified.

The possibility that halothane undergoes reductive dehalogenation is being investigated by Van Dyke (34). He is following the lead of Stier (35) who suggested a pathway involving formation of a radical that is converted directly to trifluoroacetate. The possibility that enzymes of the hepatic endoplasmic reticulum mediate reductive dehalogenation in the absence of O_2 is being investigated (34).

Cohen & Trudell (29) have presumptive evidence in the squirrel monkey exposed to halothane of the urinary excretion of trifluoroacetate and glucuronic acid, although not necessarily as a single molecule. Blake et al (28) have provided evidence that in man trifluoroacetate is excreted in the free form rather than conjugated with glucuronic acid. Other glucuronides, possibly that of trifluoroethanol, could be involved. The significance of the inhibition of UDP glucuronyl transferase that has been shown to occur in the presence of not only halothane, but also of methoxyflurane, chloroform, and diethyl ether (36) is uncertain.

Trifluoroacetyl ethanolamide has been reported in the urine of men exposed to halothane (3). The implications of this observation as well as the binding of halothane metabolites to macromolecules are discussed later.

Methoxyflurane

A scheme for the biotransformation of methoxyflurane ($H_3C\text{-}O\text{-}CF_2CHCl_2$) that includes the known metabolites identified by both in vitro and in vivo studies of mammalian systems is presented in Figure 2.

Holaday et al (37) identified products of the biotransformation of methoxyflurane in man as CO_2, inorganic fluoride, dichloroacetic acid, and methoxyfluoroacetic acid. Formaldehyde that is rapidly oxidized to CO_2 has been shown to be formed by human and rat hepatic microsomes in the presence of methoxyflurane (38).

The bones of rats and mice accumulated fluoride following the intraperitoneal injection of methoxyflurane in olive oil (22). The apparent defluorination of methoxyflurane in this series of experiments was enhanced by the prior administration of phenobarbital. Blood serum levels of inorganic fluoride have been demonstrated to

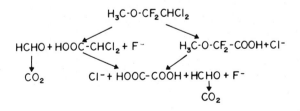

Figure 2   Proposed pathways for the metabolism of methoxyflurane.

become elevated during and after surgical anesthesia in man (25, 39, 40). Mice, rats, guinea pigs, rabbits, dogs, and monkeys also defluorinate methoxyflurane (41).

Blood oxalate levels increased (42), calcium oxalate crystals were detected in renal biopsy specimens (43), and urinary oxalate excretion was increased significantly (43, 44) after methoxyflurane anesthesia in man.

Fluroxene

The principal metabolites of fluroxene (F_3CCH_2–O–CH=CH_2) in mice, dogs, and man are CO_2 (derived exclusively from the vinyl moiety), trifluoroethanol (largely as the glucuronide), and trifluoroacetic acid (32, 45). No inorganic fluoride is liberated from the trifluoromethyl group (25, 32, 45). The principal urinary metabolite in the mouse and dog is trifluoroacetate (32).

The probable scheme for the biotransformation of fluroxene is illustrated in Figure 3.

Enflurane and Isoflurane

Enflurane (F_2HC–O–CF_2CHClF) and isoflurane (F_2HC–O–CHClCF$_3$) are structural isomers and will be considered together.

Of the nonflammable halogenated agents isoflurane represents the clinically useful general anesthetic that has most nearly approached the "ideal" with respect to biotransformation in man. Isoflurane has been reported to be only minimally defluorinated (46, 47) or not defluorinated (48; D. A. Holaday et al, personal communication) in man, minimally defluorinated in the Fischer 344 rat (47, 49, 50), and not defluorinated in the miniature pig (51), C-57 and white Swiss mice, and Wistar rat (22).

Enflurane, on the other hand, is apparently defluorinated to a somewhat greater extent than isoflurane. Elevated serum fluoride levels have been reported in man (48, 52), the Fischer 344 rat (53), and in an unidentified species (4). Halsey et al (51) inferred from hepatic extraction studies in the miniature pig that enflurane was not metabolized.

Nonionic fluoride has been detected in the urine of man (46, 47) and the Fischer 344 rat (47) following exposure to isoflurane, and in the Fischer 344 rat (53) following exposure to enflurane.

Animal pretreatment with phenobarbital has been shown to stimulate the defluorination in vitro of both isoflurane and methoxyflurane by Fischer 344 rat liver microsomes, but only of methoxyflurane when tested in vivo (50). This apparent

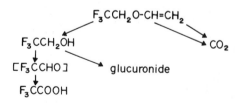

Figure 3 Proposed pathway for the biotransformation of fluroxene.

inconsistency was suggested to be a consequence of the difference in lipid solubilities of the respective compounds. Ostwald solubility coefficients for methoxyflurane in blood at 37°C have been reported to be 8–14, depending on the species, and 1.0–1.4 for isoflurane in human blood (54). The implication was that the relatively lower lipid solubility of isoflurane limited its delivery to the site(s) of biotransformation.

In this connection it is appropriate to point out an often overlooked physiological adaptation to the metabolic demands placed on the liver by the stimulation of drug-metabolizing enzyme systems. Liver blood flow was shown to increase within 24 hr in rats treated with phenobarbital, antipyrine, but not benzpyrene, and to remain elevated for 2–8 days after treatment (55). Increases amounted to 33–175% of control rates. Increases in liver perfusion would have the effect of increasing the rates of delivery of all blood-borne substances to the liver and should therefore be expected to influence the processes of xenobiotic biotransformation as well as their measurement in vivo. The potential effects of hepatic hypoperfusion, on the other hand, have been considered by Van Dyke & Wood (34).

Unidentified fluoro-organic metabolites of enflurane and isoflurane are known to be produced in man and the rat (46, 47). In an interesting theoretical study Loew et al (56) have proposed pathways of biodegradation for the respective compounds (Figures 4 and 5) within the context of their structural relationship to methoxyflurane (Figure 2).

Loew et al (56) concluded that the susceptibility of the three anesthetics to O-dealkylation or dechlorination was methoxyflurane > enflurane > isoflurane. This agreed with observed behavior. The rank order correlation was based on the insertion of active oxygen into C–H bonds, which is more likely to occur the more electron-rich each atom is.

THE MECHANISM OF TOXIC INJURY

The results of the national halothane study (57) did not rule out the possibility that massive, postoperative hepatic necrosis might, in rare instances, be attributable to halothane anesthesia. The study did reveal, however, that the highest incidence of

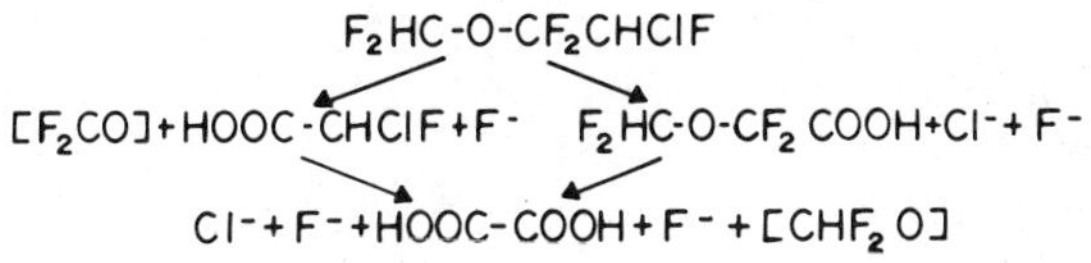

$$F_2HC\text{-}O\text{-}CF_2CHClF$$

$$[F_2CO]+HOOC\text{-}\overset{}{C}HClF+F^- \qquad F_2\overset{}{H}C\text{-}O\text{-}CF_2\,COOH+Cl^-+F^-$$

$$Cl^-+F^-+HOOC\text{-}\overset{}{C}OOH+F^-+[CHF_2O]$$

Figure 4   Proposed pathway for the biotransformation of enflurane (56).

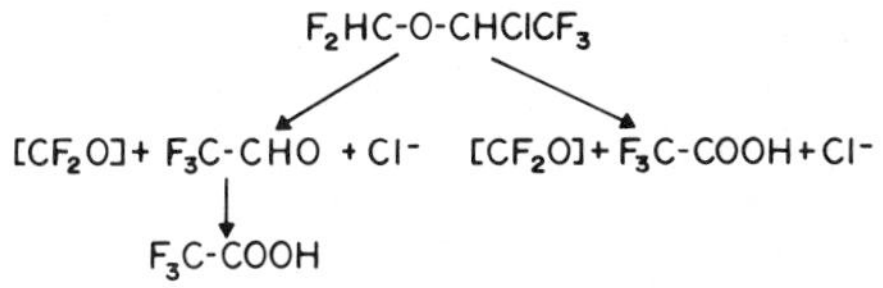

$$F_2HC\text{-}O\text{-}CHClCF_3$$

$$[CF_2O]+F_3C\text{-}CHO+Cl^- \qquad [CF_2O]+F_3C\text{-}COOH+Cl^-$$

$$F_3C\text{-}COOH$$

Figure 5   Proposed pathway for the biotransformation of isoflurane (56).

postoperative liver complications not otherwise explicable, occurred following the use of cyclopropane.

"Halothane hepatitis" remains an enigma. Various etiologic factors contributing to, and theories explaining the occurrence of hepatic failure attributable to halothane have been proposed (10, 58). Among these are liver hypoxia, liver disease, impaired liver nutrition, sepsis, viral hepatitis, multiple exposures, obesity, factors affecting biotransformation, direct hepatotoxicity, immunosuppression, toxic metabolites, and hypersensitivity. In spite of massive efforts to solve this problem, the diagnosis of halothane hepatitis still cannot be made with certainty and remains "a diagnosis of exclusion" (58).

Dykes et al (11) found little support for the hypothesis that an immunologic mechanism is important in the development of halothane hepatitis. Some animal studies fail to support the notion that a toxic mechanism is involved (59, 60); indeed, the failure to detect any dose-response relationship in man further undermines the argument for a toxic mechanism.

Whether or not halothane hepatitis is a genuine clinical entity remains to be determined. That halothane is metabolized, though, is beyond doubt. Nonvolatile metabolites, presumably bound to macromolecules, are known to remain in animal bodies for weeks following exposure (29).

The tissue binding of drugs and their products of biotransformation is presumed to be a necessary prerequisite for not only drug-receptor interactions, but also for the metabolism and potential manifestations of toxicity (8, 9). The multiplicity of physicochemical properties of the wide variety of macromolecules that occur in the body confers a highly variable specificity on the potential drug-metabolite-receptor interactions. This leads to the requirement of considering interactive schemes such as the one represented in Figure 6.

Radioautographic and fractionation studies in mice (29) have shown that several halothane metabolites are accumulated in the liver and that these seem to be preferentially distributed to the mitochondria. Possible halothane metabolites have been demonstrated to decrease hepatic ATP/ADP ratios in mice (61). Reduced ATP/ADP, AMP ratios could interfere with protein synthesis (62), which would be accompanied by the disaggregation of polyribosomes. This has been observed in rat liver cells following exposure to halothane (63).

The inhibition of protein synthesis could lead to a failure of the synthesis of lipoproteins (64) and result in the inability of the liver to transport triglycerides. Such a mechanism has been proposed for the development of fatty livers following ethionine and CCl_4 (65), and has not been ruled out for halogenated anesthetics. The connection, if any, between fatty livers and necrosis is uncertain. Fatty infiltration is often a prelude to necrosis but the degree of insult sufficient to cause cellular death remains unknown (5).

If a nonvolatile metabolite of an anesthetic is able to accumulate in the mitochondria to concentrations sufficient to interfere with respiration and/or phosphorylation (66–68), this process might, under certain circumstances, result in the disruption of the mitochondrial membranes with the release of serologically active phospholipids (69, 70) or lipoproteins (71). Furthermore, anesthetic metabolites could be bound to liberated fragments of subcellular membranes, whether of mito-

Binding of metabolites to macromolecules

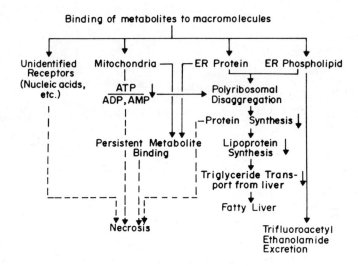

Figure 6   Possible mechanisms of the toxic action of the metabolites of inhalation anesthetics.

chondrial or endoplasmic reticular origin (34) and acting as haptens give rise to other immunologically active species (72–74). Thus, the trifluoroacetyl ethanolamide excreted by man following halothane anesthesia (3) would be expected to be of a subcellular membrane origin.

Recent work suggests that the condition of the liver determines its response to the presence of anesthetics (59). Centrolobular necrosis has been observed in rats pretreated with phenobarbital followed by exposure to halothane (75). Another model of liver injury has been investigated in which rats were pretreated with polychlorinated biphenyls prior to exposure to halothane (E. S. Reynolds, personal communication).

Possible interactions among halothane metabolite free radical formation, glutathione, and lipoperoxidation are illustrated in Figure 7.

Hepatic NADPH and reduced glutathione (GSH) levels decreased following i.p. injection of very large doses of halothane (2000 mg/kg) and proposed halothane metabolites (76, 77). The decrease in tissue levels of NADPH and GSH could have been attributable to the formation of glutathione-metabolite conjugates with GSH in the role of a free-radical scavenger (77). A proposed inhibition of glutathione reductase (77) would not account for the NADPH depletion, but the profound respiratory insufficiency that undoubtedly accompanied the injection of 2000 mg/kg of liquid halothane could.

Excess free radical formation from halothane, accelerated by pretreatment with phenobarbital (75), could result in the covalent binding of metabolites to macromolecules (Figure 6) and the triggering of peroxidation of phospholipids of subcellular membranes (78). This would explain the detection of diene conjugates in the urine of animals exposed to halothane (59, 75, 78).

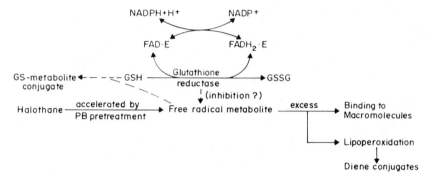

Figure 7   Possible interactions of halothane metabolites with glutathione and their relationships to lipoperoxidation.

Not only has a methoxyflurane-induced nephropathy been identified as a clinical entity, but the etiology also has been defined with a reasonable degree of certainty (79). Of the principal metabolites, inorganic fluoride has been incriminated as the probable cause of the usually reversible, vasopressin-resistant polyuria associated with methoxyflurane anesthesia (79–81). Oxalate probably is not formed in sufficient quantity to be of clinical significance in the pathogenesis of clinical methoxyflurane nephropathy (79, 82, 83). A persistent renal insufficiency has been reported following methoxyflurane, but the pathogenesis is not well understood (84).

The impairment of the ability of the kidney to concentrate urine is thought to be the consequence of a reduction of the corticomedullary concentration gradient (80).

TOXICOLOGY OF CHRONIC EXPOSURE TO ANESTHETIC GASES

Overview

The report by Vaisman (85) in 1967 of an increased incidence of reproductive failure in women working in the operating room (OR) has sparked a growing interest in the potential consequences of occupational exposure to anesthetic gases. Linde & Bruce (86) measured an average of 1.8 ppm of halothane in the end-expired air of 24 anesthetists within 1 hr of leaving the OR following exposures of 1–2 hr. In another series involving eight subjects they detected end-expired mean levels of halothane of 3.7 ppm after an average exposure to 5.3 ppm for 2 hr. A significant correlation ($r = 0.79$) existed between the end-expired levels of the anesthetic and the room air concentration times the duration of exposure. Corbett & Ball (87) made similar observations on personnel exposed to methoxyflurane and further detected significant elevations in urinary fluoride excretion within 5 hr after exposure. They also were able to reduce OR air levels of 1.3–9.8 ppm of methoxyflurane to 0.015–0.095 ppm through the use of a waste anesthetic gas scavenging system. Halothane was detected in the expired air of anesthesiologists for 7–64 hr after exposure to 1–10 ppm for 20–390 min (88).

Table 1 Methoxyflurane-induced nephrotoxicity; dose-response relationships

Serum inorganic F⁻ μmol/liter	MAC-Hr[a]	Toxic response	Reference
< 40	—	0/11, none	83
< 40	< 2.0	0/7, none	81
50–80	2.5–3.0	3/4, subclinical	81
		1/4, mild clinical	
80–175	> 5.0	3/7, mild clinical	81
		3/7, clinical	

[a]Minimum (alveolar) anesthetic concentration (end-expiratory) times duration of anesthesia.

Bruce et al (89) in a retrospective study of mortality among anesthesiologists over a period of 20 yr found significantly higher death rates from malignancies of lymphoid-reticuloendothelial origin, but no difference in death rates from leukemia when compared to rates among US males in general. Corbett et al (90) reported a higher than expected incidence of malignancies among Michigan nurse-anesthetists during 1971.

Reproductive histories of operating-room personnel have been surveyed (91, 92), and the results of two such studies are summarized in Table 2. In addition to higher incidences of spontaneous miscarriage among the OR personnel, both studies revealed that the miscarriages occurred earlier in pregnancy in the exposed versus the control groups. The conclusion by one group (92) that the increased rate of abortion among the exposed women was probably attributable to stress rather than to some other variable such as exposure to traces of anesthetic gases was not well supported by their evidence, particularly in view of the fact that they took reasonable care to match their controls on the basis of occupational stress.

Corbett et al (93) have suggested the possibility of a teratogenic hazard associated with occupational exposure to anesthetic gases. A significantly higher than expected incidence of cavernous skin hemangiomas and musculoskeletal anomalies appeared in the offspring of 641 female nurse-anesthetists surveyed.

Pregnant hamsters (94) and pregnant rats (95) have been exposed repeatedly late in the first third of gestation to anesthetic concentrations of N_2O-halothane. Results from both studies suggested that exposure to halothane early in pregnancy may have

Table 2 Incidence of spontaneous abortion among operating-room personnel

Occupationally exposed	Controls	Reference
29.7%[a] (67)[b]	8.8% (92)	91
37.8%[a] (50)[b]	10.3% (81)	92
19.5%[a] (182)[b]	11.4% (118)	92

[a]Incidence among total number of pregnancies occurring during periods of employment in OR.
[b]Number of individuals surveyed.

increased the incidence of reproductive failure. These results cannot be extrapolated directly to man, but along with the foregoing discussion they should serve to alert the medical community to the possible harmful effects of inhalation anesthetics on human reproductive biology.

Report of the American Society of Anesthesiologists Ad Hoc Committee on Effects of Trace Anesthetic Agents on Health of Operating Room Personnel

This retrospective study (96) was based on the responses to 73,496 mailed questionnaires. Of these, 49,585 represented exposed operating room personnel and 23,911 represented the control group. The survey provided statistically significant evidence that the risk of spontaneous abortion was increased by exposure to the operating-room environment during the first trimester of pregnancy. The liveborn offspring of both the women directly exposed and the wives of men exposed to the OR environment had an increased incidence of congenital abnormalities. Higher rates of cancer and hepatic and renal diseases were found in exposed females but not in exposed males. The committee concluded that the hypothesis that exposure to the OR atmosphere posed a significant health hazard to operating room personnel be weighed carefully.

Central Nervous System Correlates of Chronic Exposure to Inhalation Anesthetics

An interesting and thus far totally inexplicable finding in the study by Bruce et al (89) was that anesthesiologists had a higher than expected death rate from suicide during the period of 1947–1966. Whether or not any connection exists between this observation and their occupational exposure to waste anesthetic gases is a matter of conjecture. Exposure of volunteers to trace levels of N_2O-halothane for 4 hr caused six of twenty to fall asleep during psychological testing and significantly increased psychomotor reaction time (97).

Chronic exposure of young rats to 90 ppm of halothane resulted in deficits in responses to negatively and positively reinforced operant training (98). Exposure as adults was without a similar effect. Acute exposure of volunteers to higher, but subanesthetic, levels of methoxyflurane, enflurane, or isoflurane suggested that the anesthetics as a group caused impairment of memory functions (99). The evidence supports the idea that the possibility of behavioral modification in the presence of very low levels of anesthetic gases is a matter deserving critical examination.

Furthermore, it is possible that a connection between structure and function ultimately will be found. Ultrastructural changes in the rat central nervous system were detected after exposure for 8 wk to 10 ppm halothane (100), and differentiation in cultured mouse neuroblastoma cells exposed for 72 hr to 0.3–2.1% halothane was impaired (101).

On Cleaning Up the Environment

Evidence has been presented suggesting that chronic exposure to traces of anesthetic gases may constitute a significant occupational hazard to operating-room personnel. It would, therefore, seem prudent to take steps to reduce such pollution in the operating room pending further investigation. Escape of significant quantities of anesthetic gases from both closed and open systems is inevitable. This may be controlled by active scavenging systems (102, 103) that capture waste gases to be disposed of through venting systems or by the incorporation of activated charcoal adsorbent cannisters to the expiratory circuit (104). Such measures are easily instituted, and the hardware is relatively cheap to install. The potential benefit would certainly seem to be worth the investment while we are waiting for the results of further studies of the problem.

CONCLUSION

A large fraction of the halothane absorbed by the liver is strongly bound to subcellular fractions. The halothane is presumably in the form of metabolites and probably covalently bound. Furthermore, liver injury sustained in the presence of halothane may be dependent on the prior condition of the liver, that is, macromolecular constitution as an expression of genotype and the effects of chemical agents other than halothane. The identification of metabolites and their interaction with subcellular constituents may provide the basis for the future resolution of the problem of "halothane hepatitis."

The search continues for a better general anesthetic. All tested so far are biotransformed to a measurable extent. Isoflurane is apparently metabolized to a lesser extent than the others and in this respect may represent a step forward in the search for the "ideal" inhalation anesthetic.

Presumptive evidence has been presented that exposure to trace levels of anesthetic gases may adversely affect human reproductive and behavioral processes. The further investigation of these potential problems is of paramount importance. Meantime the prudent course of action would seem to be to institute measures to reduce the contamination of the operating-room atmosphere by waste anesthetic gases.

ACKNOWLEDGMENTS

The author wishes to thank Drs. J. R. Fouts and M. B. Chenoweth for wise counsel and thoughtful criticism during the preparation of this review.

Literature Cited

1. Van Dyke, R. A., Chenoweth, M. B. 1965. *Anesthesiology* 26:348–57
2. Brown, B. R., Vandam, L. D. 1971. *Ann. NY Acad. Sci.* 179:235–43
3. Cohen, E. N. 1971. *Anesthesiology* 35:193–202
4. Van Dyke, R. A. 1973. *Can. Anaesth. Soc. J.* 20:21–33
5. Farber, E. 1971. *Ann. Rev. Pharmacol.* 11:71–96
6. Orlandi, F., Jezequel, A. M., eds. 1972. *Liver and Drugs.* New York: Academic. 267 pp.
7. Slater, T. F. 1972. *Free Radical Mecha-*
nisms in Tissue Injury. London: Pion. 283 pp.
8. Gillette, J. R. 1974. *Biochem. Pharmacol.* 23:2785–94
9. Gillette, J. R. 1974. *Biochem. Pharmacol.* 23:2927–38
10. Carney, F. M. T., Van Dyke, R. A. 1972. *Anesth. Analg. Cleveland* 48: 135–60
11. Dykes, M. H. M., Gilbert, J. P., Schur, P. H., Cohen, E. N. 1972. *Can. J. Surg.* 15:1–22
12. Rosenberg, P. H., Airaksinen, M. M. 1973. *Fluoride* 6:41–48

13. Gottlieb, L. S., Trey, C. 1974. *Ann. Rev. Med.* 25:411–29
14. Lofstrom, J. B., ed. 1971. *Acta Anaesthesiol. Scand. Suppl.* 49:1–43
15. Fink, B. R., ed. 1972. *Cellular Biology and Toxicity of Anesthetics.* Baltimore: Williams & Wilkins. 328 pp.
16. Chenoweth, M. B., ed. 1972. *Modern Inhalation Anesthetics. Handbook of Experimental Pharmacology,* Vol. 30. New York: Springer. 591 pp.
17. Atallah, M. M., Geddes, I. C. 1973. *Br. J. Anaesth.* 45:464–70
18. Sawyer, D. C., Eger, E. I., Bahlman, S. H., Cullen, B. F., Impelman, D. 1971. *Anesthesiology* 34:230–35
19. Topham, J. C., Longshaw, S. 1972. *Anesthesiology* 37:311–23
20. Stier, A. 1964. *Biochem. Pharmacol.* 13:1544
21. Rehder, K., Forbes, J., Alter, H., Hessler, O., Stier, A. 1967. *Anesthesiology* 28:711–15
22. Fiserova-Bergerova, V. 1973. *Anesthesiology* 38:345–51
23. Brown, E. A. B. 1974. *Drug Metab. Rev.* 3:33–87
24. Orton, T. C., Anderson, M. W., Pickett, R. D., Eling, T. E., Fouts, J. R. 1973. *J. Pharmacol. Exp. Ther.* 186:482–97
25. Creasser, C., Stoelting, R. K. 1973. *Anesthesiology* 39:537–40
26. Van Dyke, R. A. 1966. *J. Pharmacol. Exp. Ther.* 154:364–69
27. Clauberg, G. 1970. *Anaesthesist* 19:387–92
28. Blake, D. A., Barry, J. Q., Cascorbi, H. F. 1972. *Anesthesiology* 36:152–54
29. Cohen, E. N., Trudell, J. R. 1972. See Ref. 15, pp. 205–14
30. Smith, G. F. 1966. *Bri. J. Ind. Med.* 23:249–62
31. Goldstein, A., Aronow, L., Kalman, S. M. 1974. *Principles of Drug Action.* New York: Wiley. 854 pp. 2nd ed.
32. Blake, D. A., Rozman, R. S., Cascorbi, H. F., Krantz, J. C. Jr. 1967. *Biochem. Pharmacol.* 16:1237–48
33. Cascorbi, H. F., Blake, D. A. 1971. *Anesthesiology* 35:493–95
34. Van Dyke, R. A., Wood, C. L. 1975. *Drug Metab. Dispos.* 3:51–57
35. Stier, A. 1968. *Anesthesiology* 29:388–89
36. Brown, B. R. Jr. 1972. *Anesthesiology* 37:483–88
37. Holaday, D. A., Rudofsky, S., Treuhaft, P. S. 1970. *Anesthesiology* 33:579–93
38. Van Dyke, R. A., Wood, C. L. 1973. *Anesthesiology* 39:613–18
39. Dobkin, A. B., Levy, A. A. 1973. *Can. Anaesth. Soc. J.* 20:81–93
40. Fry, B. W., Taves, D. R., Merin, R. G. 1973. *Anesthesiology* 38:38–44
41. Murray, W. J., Fleming, P. J. 1972. *Anesthesiology* 37:620–25
42. McIntyre, J. W. R., Russell, J. C., Chambers, M. 1973. *Anesth. Analg. Cleveland* 52:946–50
43. Franscino, J. A., Vanamee, P., Rosen, P. P. 1970. *New Engl. J. Med.* 283:676–79
44. Silverberg, D. S. et al 1971. *Can. Anaesth. Soc. J.* 18:496–504
45. Gion, H., Yoshimura, N., Holaday, D. A., Fiserova-Bergerova, V., Chase, R. E. 1974. *Anesthesiology* 40:553–62
46. Mazze, R. I., Cousins, M. J., Barr, G. A. 1974. *Anesthesiology* 40:536–42
47. Hitt, B. A. et al 1974. *Anesthesiology* 40:62–67
48. Dobkin, A. B., Kim, D., Choi, J. K., Levy, A. A. 1973. *Can. Anaesth. Soc. J.* 20:494–98
49. Cousins, M. J., Mazze, R. I., Barr, G. A., Kosek, J. C. 1973. *Anesthesiology* 38:557–63
50. Mazze, R. I., Hitt, B. A., Cousins, M. J. 1974. *J. Pharmacol. Exp. Ther.* 190:523–29
51. Halsey, M. J., Sawyer, D. C., Eger, E. I. II, Bahlman, S. H., Impelman, D. 1971. *Anesthesiology* 35:43–47
52. Maduska, A. L. 1974. *Anesth. Analg. Cleveland* 53:351–53
53. Barr, G. A., Cousins, M. J., Mazze, R. I., Hitt, B. A., Kosek, J. C. 1974. *J. Pharmacol. Exp. Ther.* 188:257–64
54. Steward, A., Allott, P. R., Cowles, A. L., Mapleson, W. W. 1973. *Br. J. Anaesth.* 45:282–93
55. Ohnhaus, E. E., Thorgeirsson, S. S., Davies, D. S., Breckenridge, A. 1971. *Biochem. Pharmacol.* 20:2561–70
56. Loew, G., Motulsky, H., Trudell, J., Cohen, E. N., Hjelmeland, L. 1974. *Mol. Pharmacol.* 10:406–18
57. Bunker, J. P., Forrest, W. H. Jr., Mosteller, F., Vandam, L. D., ed. 1969. *The National Halothane Study.* Bethesda, Md.: NIH
58. Reves, J. G. 1974. *Postgrad. Med.* 56:65–70
59. Brown, B. R., Sipes, I. G., Sagalyn, A. M. 1974. *Anesthesiology* 41:554–61
60. Rosenberg, P., Wahlstrom, T. 1971. *Acta Pharmacol. Toxicol.* 29:9–19
61. Rosenberg, P. H., Airaksinen, M. M., Tammisto, T. 1970. *Acta Pharmacol. Toxicol.* 28:327–33

62. Freudenberg, H., Mager, J. 1971. *Biochim. Biophys. Acta* 232:537–54
63. Ross, W. T. Jr., Cardell, R. R. Jr. 1972. *Am. J. Anat.* 135:5–22
64. Glaser, G., Mager, J. 1972. *Biochim. Biophys. Acta* 261:487–99
65. Glaser, G., Mager, J. 1972. *Biochim. Biophys. Acta* 261:500–7
66. Miller, R. N., Smith, E. E., Hunter, F. E. Jr. 1972. See Ref. 15, pp. 93–108
67. Cohen, P. J., McIntyre, R. 1972. See Ref. 15, pp. 109–16
68. Taylor, C. A. et al 1972. See Ref. 15, pp. 117–27
69. Schiefer, H. G. 1973. *Z. Physiol. Chem.* 354:722–24
70. Schiefer, H. G. 1973. *Z. Physiol. Chem.* 354:725–28
71. Doniach, D., Walker, G. 1974. *Gut* 15:664–68
72. Rodriguez, M., Paronetto, F., Schaffner, F., Popper, H. 1969. *J. Am. Med. Assoc.* 208:148–50
73. Cohen, A. B., Rosenthal, W. S., Stenger, R. J. 1973. *Proc. Soc. Exp. Biol. Med.* 142:817–19
74. Mathieu, A., DiPadua, D., Mills, J., Kahan, B. 1974. *Anesthesiology* 40:385–90
75. Reynolds, E. S., Moslen, M. T. 1974. *Biochem. Pharmacol.* 23:189–95
76. Airaksinen, M. M., Rosenberg, P. H., Tammisto, T. 1970. *Acta Pharmacol. Toxicol.* 28:299–304
77. Rosenberg, P. H. 1971. *Ann. Med. Exp. Biol. Fenn.* 49:84–88
78. Brown, B. R. Jr. 1972. *Anesthesiology* 36:458–65
79. Cousins, M. J., Mazze, R. I., Kosek, J. C., Hitt, B. A., Love, F. V. 1974. *J. Pharmacol. Exp. Ther.* 190:530–41
80. Whitford, G. M., Taves, D. R. 1973. *Anesthesiology* 39:416–27
81. Cousins, M. J., Mazze, R. I. 1973. *J. Am. Med. Assoc.* 225:1611–16
82. Dryden, G. E. 1974. *Anesth Analg. Cleveland* 53:383–85
83. Tobey, R. E., Clubb, R. J. 1973. *J. Am. Med. Assoc.* 223:649–52
84. Churchill, D. et al 1974. *Am. J. Med.* 56:575–82
85. Vaisman, A. I. 1967. *Eksp. Khir. Anesteziol.* 3:44–49
86. Linde, H. W., Bruce, D. L. 1969. *Anesthesiology* 30:363–68
87. Corbett, T. H., Ball, G. L. 1971. *Anesthesiology* 34:532–37
88. Corbett, T. H. 1973. *Anesth. Analg. Cleveland* 52:614–18
89. Bruce, D. L., Eide, K. A., Linde, H. W., Eckenhoff, J. E. 1968. *Anesthesiology* 29:565–69
90. Corbett, T. H., Cornell, R. G., Lieding, K., Endres, J. L. 1973. *Anesthesiology* 38:260–63
91. Cohen, E. N., Bellville, J. W., Brown, B. W. Jr. 1971. *Anesthesiology* 35:343–47
92. Rosenberg, P., Kirves, A. 1973. *Acta Anaesthesiol. Scand. Suppl.* 53:37–42
93. Corbett, T. H., Cornell, R. G., Endres, J. L., Lieding, K. 1974. *Anesthesiology* 41:341–44
94. Bussard, D. A., Stoelting, R. K., Peterson, C., Ishaq, M. 1974. *Anesthesiology* 41:275–78
95. Wittman, R., Doenicke, A., Heinrich, H., Pausch, H. 1974. *Anaesthesist* 23:30–35
96. Am. Soc. Anesthesiol. 1974. *Anesthesiology* 410:321–40
97. Bruce, D. L., Bach, M. J., Arbit, J. 1974. *Anesthesiology* 40:453–58
98. Quimby, K. L., Aschkenase, L. J., Bowman, R. E., Katz, J., Chang, L. W. 1974. *Science* 185:625–27
99. Adam, N. 1973. *J. Comp. Physiol. Psychol.* 83:294–305
100. Chang, L. W., Dudley, A. W. Jr. Lee, Y. K., Katz, J. W. 1974. *Exp. Neurol.* 45:209–19
101. Hinkley, R. E., Telser, A. G. 1974. *J. Cell Biol.* 63:531–40
102. Whitcher, C. E., Cohen, E. N., Trudell, J. R. 1971. *Anesthesiology* 35:348–53
103. Lane, J. R. 1974. *Proc. R. Soc. Med.* 67:34–36
104. Vaughan, R. S., Mapleson, W. W., Mushin, W. W. 1973. *Br. Med. J.* 220:727–29

ORGANIC NITRATE METABOLISM[1],[2]

❖6637

Philip Needleman
Department of Pharmacology, Washington University Medical School,
St. Louis, Missouri 63110

OVERVIEW

The biotransformation of organic nitrates is initiated by a redox reaction and is manifest by the conversion of potent lipid-soluble vasodilator compounds into water-soluble metabolites which have much lower biological potency and are readily excreted in the urine. Studies by numerous workers have indicated that destruction of organic nitrates is rapidly and specifically catalyzed by hepatic glutathione-organic nitrate reductase. Blood clearance data explicitly demonstrate that the parent nitrate ester (following intravenous administration) has a very transient lifetime, whereas the nitrate metabolites circulate for hours. The duration of the vasodilator effectiveness of organic nitrates is in direct temporal correlation with blood levels of the intact ester and is completely out of phase with circulating metabolites. Thus, the parent compound appears to be the active species. On the other hand, experiments in rats, dogs, and humans indicate that after oral administration of various organic nitrates, essentially none of the parent compound is present in the circulation. A growing number of clinical studies indicate that many orally administered organic nitrates are ineffective in the treatment of angina pectoris, which is consistent with the metabolic data.

ISOLATION AND CHARACTERIZATION OF ORGANIC NITRATE REDUCTASE

The investigation of organic nitrate biotransformation began with the observation that inorganic nitrite appeared after incubation of GTN and other organic nitrates

[1]The following abbreviations are used in this review: BTTN, butanetrioltrinitrate; EGDN, ethylene glycol dinitrate; EGMN, ethylene glycol mononitrate; ETN, erythrityl tetranitrate; GDN, glyceryl dinitrate; GLUC, glucuronide; GMN, glyceryl mononitrate; GTN, glyceryl trinitrate; IS, isosorbide; ISD, isosorbide dinitrate; 2-ISMN, isosorbide-2-exomononitrate; 5-ISMN, isosorbide-5-endomononitrate; MHN, mannitol hexanitrate; ONR, organic nitrate reductase; PE, pentaerythritol; PEDN, pentaerythrityl dinitrate; PEMN, pentaerythrityl mononitrate; PETN, pentaerythrityl tetranitrate; PE-tri-N, pentaerythrityl trinitrate.

[2]Additional reviews on some aspects of this topic have previously appeared (1–3).

81

with blood (4–7). Inorganic nitrite formation was also observed when nitrate esters were incubated with rabbit liver homogenates (8). Furthermore, GTN administered intravenously was demonstrated to disappear rapidly from the circulation with the concurrent appearance of inorganic nitrite (5).

GTN and ETN reacted nonenzymatically with GSH to form inorganic nitrite and oxidized glutathione (9). The reduction of GTN (and ETN) by GSH was catalyzed by a hog liver enzyme in which 2 μmol of GSH were oxidized for every micromole of nitrite ion formed (9). The stoichiometry of the reaction was demonstrated by coupling the GTN transformation reaction to glutathione reductase, which catalyzed the reduction of oxidized glutathione by $NADPH_2$ (10). The coupled reaction proceeded as follows:

$$GTN + 2\ GSH \longrightarrow GSSG + NO_2^- + \text{other products}$$

$$NADPH_2 + GSSG \xrightarrow{\text{glutathione reductase}} 2\ GSH + NADP$$

with the $NADPH_2$ consumed equivalent to the nitrite formed (10).

Continuous perfusion of isolated rat livers with GTN resulted in a concentration-dependent depletion of hepatic GSH and ATP (10–12). The dependence of the denitration reaction on GSH was demonstrated in an experiment in which pretreatment of rats with bromobenzene caused a 70% reduction in hepatic glutathione and resulted in a marked inhibition (90% decrease) of GTN degradation by the perfused liver (11).

The contribution of hepatic inactivation of organic nitrates was further evaluated in eviscerated rats (13, 14). GTN administered intravenously underwent rapid disappearance from the blood ($T_{1/2} <$ 1 min) of normal rats with the concurrent rapid appearance of GTN metabolites in the blood (peaked at 2–5 min). GTN disappeared from the blood of eviscerated animals much more slowly than in controls, with an apparent $T_{1/2}$ of 7–8 min. Furthermore, there was no increase in GTN metabolites in the blood with time (13). Similarly, rabbits that were functionally hepatectomized had prolonged elevated blood level of nitrates after GTN administration (14). These results were consistent with the notion that the liver was the primary site for the degradation of GTN.

The primary subcellular site of the hepatic GTN-metabolizing enzyme was in the 100,000 $\times$ g soluble fraction (15, 16). The enzyme preparation purified 100-fold from hog liver acetone powder was inhibited by cupric sulfate, stimulated by cyanide, and unaffected by dialysis or anoxia, and its optimal substrate concentrations were 5×10^{-3} M GSH and 3×10^{-3} M GTN (9). Fresh liver extracts were partially purified and yielded two distinct peaks of enzymatic activity (14,000 and 43,700 mol wt) with different relative activities toward organic nitrates (17, 18). The K_m for GSH was 1.5×10^{-5} M with GTN, 5×10^{-5} M with ETN, and 3.7×10^{-5} M with MHN (17).

Linear-chain polynitrate esters (e.g. MHN, ETN, and GTN) were rapidly transformed by rat liver 100,000 $\times$ g supernatant in the presence of GSH whereas branched-chain alcohol nitrates (e.g. PETN, PE-tri-N, and trimethylol ethane trinitrate) and anhydrides (e.g. ISD) were only slowly transformed (10). Replacement of the nitrate by hydrogen (ETN vs 1,2,4-butanetriol trinitrate; or BTTN vs 1,4-butanediol dinitrate) or a hydroxyl (GTN > GDN >> GMN) markedly decreased the velocity of enzymatic degradation (10).

The in vitro destruction of GTN by rat liver homogenates (15, 19) or perfused rat livers (11) was markedly increased in tissue removed from animals chronically treated with phenobarbital. Similarly, the rate of disappearance of intact GTN and the appearance and excretion of metabolites of GTN were accelerated in phenobarbital-treated rats (20, 21), rabbits (22), and humans (23). The enhanced rate of nitrate degradation was apparently the result of induction of organic nitrate reductase, for inhibition of protein synthesis by DL-ethionine or inhibition of RNA synthesis by actinomycin D completely inhibited the enhancement of organic nitrate metabolism by phenobarbital pretreatment (24). On the other hand, SKF-525A pretreatment has been reported to inhibit organic nitrate metabolism in dogs and rabbits without affecting the vascular changes (25) while others could not demonstrate inhibition of nitrate metabolism whether the SKF-525A was administered in vivo or added directly to rat liver homogenates (19, 20).

The denitration of GTN by rat blood serum was independent of GSH and proceeded at a slow rate with a half-time of about 20 min (14, 18, 21, 26–28). The pH optimum was 7.8 with maximum activity at 50–57° (26, 28). The slow rate of organic nitrate degradation in vitro coupled with the apparent lack of denitration in eviscerated rats (13, 20) indicates that blood plays only a minor role in the disappearance of GTN and other organic nitrates from the circulation. The exception was MHN, which was rapidly metabolized in blood (27).

ISOLATION AND CHARACTERIZATION OF ORGANIC NITRATE METABOLITES

Metabolic Pathway in the Degradation of Glyceryl Trinitrate

Incubation of GTN with liver homogenates from several species led to inorganic nitrite formation (8, 9, 15, 16, 29). The transformation of GTN in the presence of GSH produced two organic nitrate products which were less lipid soluble than the parent molecule (15). Chromatographically, there were no differences in the GTN metabolites produced by (a) the nonenzymatic reaction between GTN and GSH, (b) the liver enzyme–catalyzed reaction of GTN and GSH, (c) the urinary excretion products following GTN administration to adult rats, and (d) synthetic 1,3- and 1,2-glyceryl dinitrate (10, 15). The time course for degradation of GTN in the rat liver homogenate was similar to the rate of the formation of 1,3- and 1,2-GDN (10). Traces of glyceryl mononitrate but no glycerol were found. The total of the nitrate groups found in GDN and inorganic nitrite accounted for 90% of the nitrate groups in the GTN that had undergone enzymatic reaction (10). Recirculation of GTN through an isolated perfused rat liver resulted in an extremely rapid disappearance ($T_{1/2}$, 1 min) of the parent compound consistent with its V_{max} for GSH-organic nitrate reductase. The total of the GDN, GMN, and inorganic nitrite that rapidly appeared during the liver perfusion accounted for all the GTN metabolized (11). In summary, the major route for GTN transformation appeared to be denitration in the presence of GSH. One molecule of GTN reacted with two GSH to release one inorganic nitrite ion from either the 2- or 3-position to form 1,3- or 1,2-GDN. The denitration of GDN proceeded at only 2–5% of the rate for GTN (10). GMN was practically unaltered by the liver enzyme; this was in agreement with the finding that no glycerol was found after GTN degradation (9, 10, 20, 29).

Administration of ^{14}C-GTN to intact rats resulted in the appearance of ^{14}C carbon dioxide in the exhaled air, which reflected the total in vivo degradation of the parent molecule (20, 30). Pretreatment of rats with phenobarbital of SKF-525A had no effect on GTN oxidation, nor was there an enhancement of CO_2 released in GTN-tolerant animals (11). Eviscerated rats with or without nephrectomy were unable to oxidize GTN to CO_2. Because eviscerated rats readily oxidized glycerol to CO_2, the interruption in the GTN degradative pathway must lie somewhere in the denitration sequence (20). No CO_2 production was detected following incubation of GTN with homogenates of brain, heart, intestine, kidney, liver, lung, skeletal muscle, spleen, stomach, and blood (20). On the other hand, kidney, brain, liver, and muscle were capable of oxidizing glycerol to CO_2 (20). Thus, if GTN would have been degraded to glycerol it would have been converted to readily detectable CO_2. Furthermore, when GTN was incubated with GSH in the presence of liver homogenates, no glycerol could be detected (9, 20). Thus, there did not appear to be active enzyme system in liver (or the other tissues tested) capable of catalyzing the complete denitration of GTN metabolites of glycerol.

The GTN degradation and elimination sequence is illustrated in Figure 1. Intravenous administration of GTN to rats was associated with an extremely transient blood level of the unchanged parent compound [$T_{1/2}$ of 1 min (27)]. The GTN was apparently rapidly degraded by GSH-ONR to 1,3- and 1,2-GDN (10, 15). The disappearance of GTN from the blood proceeded at the same rate as rose bengal (^{131}I-labeled), which is a marker of hepatic function and is normally cleared from the plasma in one transit across the liver (27). GDN in turn was degraded to GMN by the same liver enzyme but at a much slower rate than the intact nitrate ester (10). The blood metabolite level consisted of 1,3-GDN and GMN. The half-time to reach the peak blood level of the nitrate metabolites was about 30 sec for GTN. The rate of disappearance of organic nitrate metabolites from the blood, after intravenous administration to rats, was slower than the appearance rate by several orders of magnitude (27). Metabolites of GTN disappeared at a first-order rate, with a clearance $T_{1/2}$ of 4 hr. The blood disappearance of the organic nitrate was regulated by the rate at which the metabolites were excreted by the kidney into the urine (31). The urinary metabolites detected after treatment of rats with GTN were identified as GMN, 1,3-GDN, and 1,2-GDN (15, 20, 21, 30). The major urinary metabolite was GMN, and the total GMN and water-soluble metabolites (presumably including glycerol) made up 80% of the excreted label (20). After intravenous administration to rabbits of 1,3-GDN, 1,3-GDN and GMN were found in the urine, whereas after intravenous administration of 1,2-GDN only GMN was detected (21). Thus, the enzymatic denitration of glyceryl trinitrate and other organic nitrates led to the generation of water-soluble metabolites that were readily elminated in the urine. A portion of the labeled compound was converted to CO_2, which was then exhaled;

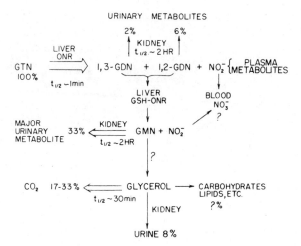

Figure 1   Schematic representation of the in vivo metabolism, clearance, and excretion of glyceryl nitrates following the administration of ^{14}C-GTN to rats. The percentage indicates the fraction of the original ^{14}C-radioactivity administered as GTN. The urinary metabolites were from pooled 24-hr samples (20). The exhaled CO_2 data represent the total for 24 hr (20, 30). The blood disappearance and urine appearance data were taken from references (27, 31). All the half-times ($T_{1/2}$) were from in vivo experiments.

thus less than 100% of the original label appeared in the urine (20, 30). Finally, the fate of the formed inorganic nitrite has not been extensively studied. Rat liver and kidney homogenates have been demonstrated to catalyze the oxidation of inorganic nitrite to inorganic nitrate (32).

GTN administered sublingually to humans produced peak plasma levels of the parent compound in the first blood sample at 4 min, and the rate at which at least half of the intact GTN was cleared from the blood was 1–3 min (33). A transient tachycardia was associated with the transient duration of circulating GTN.

Metabolic Pathway in the Degradation of Isosorbide Dinitrate

The plasma levels following intravenous administration of unchanged ISD to dogs, rats, and rabbits peaked at 2 min and then disappeared rapidly with a half-time of about 5 min (27, 34, 35) (Figure 2). The initial biotransformation occurred by denitration in the presence of hepatic GSH-organic nitrate reductase (10, 27). The blood clearance rate of the ISD metabolites was very slow ($T_{1/2}$ of 2.5 hr) (17, 34). The major plasma metabolite was 5-isosorbide mononitrate (5-ISMN-isosorbide-5-endomononitrate) (Figure 2). The plasma clearance of 2-isosorbide mononitrate (isosorbide-2-exomononitrate) paralleled that of the 5-isomer but at only approximately one seventh the concentration, thereby indicating a stereospecificity in the biotransformation (34). Low levels of isosorbide also appeared in the plasma. The primary metabolite in the plasma was 5-ISMN (65% of the administered ISD) which had only one thirtieth the coronary-dilating activity of the parent compound

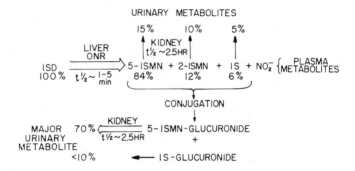

URINARY METABOLITES

Figure 2   Metabolic pathway in the degradation of ISD. After intravenous administration, ISD is rapidly cleared from the blood (27, 34, 35) following denitration by organic nitrate reductase (10,27) with the appearance of 5-ISMN, 2-ISMN, and free IS. The relative ratio of ISD metabolites in the blood is 14:2:1 for 5-ISMN:2-ISMN:IS (34); thus about 65% of the administered drug in the plasma is 5-ISMN, which has only one thirtieth to one hundredth the coronary-dilating activity of the parent compound (63, 64) but circulates 20–50 times longer than the ISD. The slow clearance from plasma (27, 34) is the result of renal filtration and conjugate formation. In 24 hr, 80–100% of the administered dose appears in the urine (33). Essentially no parent ISD was detected in the plasma after oral administration (34). The percentages indicated the portion of the total radioactivity originally administered (34, 38, 39). GSH-ONR is the abbreviation for GSH-organic nitrate reductase.

but circulated 20-50 times longer than the ISD (34). Unlike GTN, the disappearance of the metabolites of ISD from the blood was not only determined by renal filtration but also required conjugation leading to the formation of glucuronides of 5-ISMN and of IS (36). A quantitatively different blood clearance pattern was observed following oral administration of ISD to dogs (34). Only trace amounts of the unchanged material appeared in the circulation. The major metabolite 5-ISMN reached its peak concentration at a later time (30 min); 2-ISMN was again found to parallel 5-ISMN but at a much lower concentration. Five human volunteers treated sublingually with ISD had peak blood levels of intact ISD by 6 min, and the blood clearance rate of the parent compound was rapid, with 60% disappearance occurring by 15 min or less (37). An oral dose of ^{14}C-ISD was rapidly absorbed and 99% eliminated principally as the isosorbide glucuronide in the urine by human subjects (38).

The rate of appearance of urinary metabolites of ISD reflected the rate of blood clearance of the metabolites (Figure 2). The accumulated sum of the ISD urinary metabolites approached 100% of the administered radioactive ISD at 24 hr (31). A similar pattern was observed in dogs treated orally or intravenously with ISD (34). No unchanged ISD was found in the urine. Twenty to thirty percent of the carbon skeleton of ISD was excreted as neutral metabolites, principally IS, 5-ISMN, 2-ISMN, and isoidide (34, 36, 39). The remainder primarily consisted of the ether glucuronide of 5-ISMN and ether monoglucuronides of IS.

Rats orally treated with the dinitrates of isosorbide and its stereoisomers isomannide and isoidide had only trace amounts of the parent compounds in the urine (40). The mononitrates, the denitrated alcohols, and large amounts of conjugated mononitrates were qualitatively identified. Evidence for inversion from the endo- to the exo-position was provided by the finding that following ISD administration, isoiodide mononitrate and isoidide were also in the urine. Similarly, following isomannide dinitrate treatment, 5-isosorbide mononitrate and isosorbide were found.

Metabolic Pathway in the Degradation of Pentaerythrityl Nitrates

Incubation of PETN with rat liver homogenate and GSH resulted in a slow rate of formation of three metabolites (10) that were identified as the tri-, di-, and mononitrates of PE (28, 41, 42) (Figure 3). PE and its mono- (42%) and di- (33%) nitrate accounted for the major radioactivity in the blood but PETN and PE-tri-N were not detected in blood at any time interval studied following oral administration of PETN to mice and rats (42–45). The first urine collection (at 2 hr) following oral administration of PETN to rats contained PEMN (52% of administered dose), PEDN (33%), and PE (16%) (44). By 18 hr only PEMN (27%) and PE (73%) were present. There was no detectable PETN or PE-tri-N in the urine. Fifteen human volunteers were treated with ^{14}C-PETN and the pattern of metabolites in blood or urine of humans was the same as in experimental animals (46). PETN and PE-tri-N were not detected in blood. The major circulating metabolite was PE with lower levels of PEMN and trace amounts of PEDN (46–49). PE and PEMN were the major urinary metabolites. There was no qualitative or quantitative difference in the

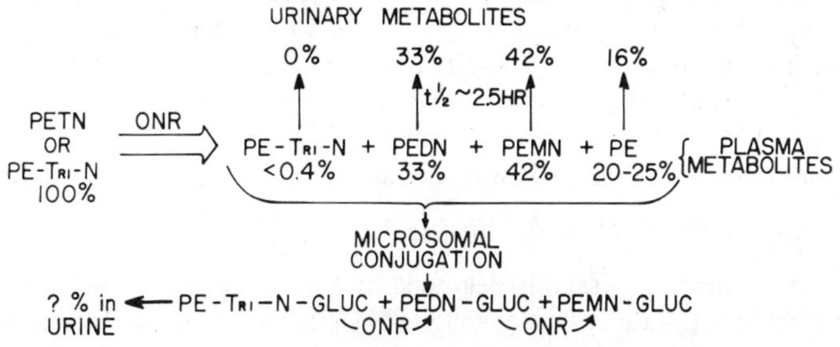

Figure 3 Metabolic pathway in the degradation of PETN or PE-trinitrate. The following abbreviations are used: PE-trinitrate (PE-tri-N), PE-dinitrate (PEDN), PE-mononitrate (PEMN), glucuronide (GLUC), and GSH-organic nitrate reductase (ONR). Two hours after oral PETN administration to rats there was no parent compound or PE-tri-N in the blood, and the major plasma metabolites were PEDN, PEMN, and PE. The percentages indicate the portion of the originally administered dose (42, 45, 49, 51, 55). The clearance of PE-tri-N metabolites from blood was 2–3 hr (43). The PE-nitrates are converted to glucuronides by liver microsomes (45, 52–54); then these PE-nitrate-glucuronides undergo further denitration by ONR (49, 53). The urinary metabolites are those found 2 hr after oral administration, and the percentage represents the fraction of the totally excreted radioactivity in the urine at 2 hr (44).

excretion patterns and blood levels exhibited by coronary artery disease patients and controls (Figure 3). PEDN, PEMN, and PE have little or no peripheral or coronary vasodilator activity and cannot account for the biological activity of the parent compound (50).

In a very recent paper intact PETN and PE-trinitrate were claimed to be present in plasma and to disappear slowly ($T_{1/2}$, 2 and 3 hr respectively) following oral administration of ^{14}C-PETN to rats (45). Their own data indicate that only 0.0006% and 0.008% of the circulating drug exist as PETN and PE-trinitrate. Furthermore, in numerous previous papers by these authors (using the same conditions as in the above report) they have concluded that "PETN and PE-trinitrate were not detected in blood at any time interval studied" in rats (44, 51), dogs (55), and humans (47, 49).

The lack of aqueous solubility of PETN has generated interest in studying the properties of the more soluble PE-tri-N. PE-tri-N administered orally was found to be absorbed faster than PETN (48, 51). PE-tri-N was partially metabolized by hepatic glutathione organic nitrate reductase (10) and by perfused rat livers (11). PE tri-, di-, and mononitrates are converted to glucuronides by liver microsomes (45, 52), and these nitrates and their glucuronides undergo further denitration by organic nitrate reductase (52–54). Following oral administration of PE-trinitrate to various species, there was little or no unchanged parent compound present in the circulation (51, 55). Even at the earliest sampling time (1 hr), there was only a trace amount of the PE-dinitrate (4%), some PE-mononitrate (28%), and predominantly PE (67%). The primary urinary metabolites following the oral administration of PE trinitrate were: PE > PE-mononitrate > PE-dinitrate (51). Biliary excretion of PE-trinitrate metabolites has been demonstrated (52). The contribution of the enterohepatic circulation was indicated by the observation that bile collection caused a 60% reduction in the radioactivity that appeared in the urine of PE-trinitrate-treated rats (52). ^{14}C PE-trinitrate was administered to humans by either the oral or sublingual route (48). No intact PE-trinitrate appeared in the blood, PE-dinitrate was present only briefly, and PE was the major circulating form of the drug.

Degradation of Other Organic Nitrate Esters

Mannitol hexanitrate was rapidly degraded by hepatic glutathione-organic nitrate reductase about seven times faster than GTN (10). The in vivo clearance of MHN from the blood of rats was extremely rapid ($T_{1/2}$, 10 sec) (27). In addition, a significant rate of blood metabolism of MHN ($T_{1/2}$, 1–2 min) further accelerated the blood clearance rate. Metabolites of MHN disappeared very slowly from rat blood after intravenous administration; the $T_{1/2}$ for clearance from the blood into the urine was 2 hr (27).

Erythrityl tetranitrate was metabolized three times faster than GTN by liver homogenates or by isolated perfused rat livers (10, 27), and the total amount of organic nitrate metabolized in the perfusion correlated closely to the previously measured V_{max} with GSH-organic nitrate reductase (10).

Ethylene glycol dinitrate subcutaneously injected in rats produced peak blood levels of the parent compound in 30 min and fell to zero by 8 hr; the metabolites ethylene glycol mononitrate, inorganic nitrite, and inorganic nitrate were rapidly produced reaching a peak at about 1–3 hr and falling to zero in 12 hr (56). Mostly inorganic nitrate was present in the urine; there was no EGDN, a trace of EGMN, no inorganic nitrite.

Propylene glycol 1,2-dinitrate was degraded in vitro (rat blood) or in vivo (rats, s.c.) into 1- and 2-isomers of propylene glycol mononitrate, inorganic nitrite, and inorganic nitrate (57). The mononitrates are further metabolized in vivo with the result that only small amounts were excreted and the major urinary metabolite was inorganic nitrate.

1,-Chloro-2,3-propanediol dinitrate was metabolized in dogs (orally administered) to 1-chloropropyl-3-glucuronide-2-nitrate and 1-chloropropyl-2-glucuronide-3-nitrate (58). Presumably the initial degradation was hepatic denitration and subsequent formation of the glucuronide prior to urinary excretion.

RELATIONSHIP BETWEEN ORGANIC NITRATE METABOLISM AND BIOLOGICAL ACTIVITY

Temporal Relationship Between Plasma Levels and Biological Activity

Administration of organic nitrates into jugular veins of anesthetized rats resulted in a transient vasodepression, usually of a 1- to 4-min duration, depending on the dose (31). There was essentially no difference in the duration of the fall in blood pressure produced by intravenous injection of GTN or by the so-called longer-acting nitrates, MHN, PETN, ISD, or ETN. On the other hand, injection of the above nitrates into the portal vein produced no blood pressure fall, suggesting that the liver has the capacity in a single passage to prevent organic nitrate-induced vasodepression by destroying the intact vasoactive ester. The only exception found was 1,2,4-butanetriol trinitrate, which in high doses exceeded the liver capacity and produced a vasodepression (31). This compound was previously found to be more slowly degraded by glutathione-organic nitrate reductase than the other drugs tested (10). In different investigations in rats, GTN and PE-trinitrate were 50 to 100 times more potent as a vasodepressor when intravenously administered than when administered through the portal vein (59). Extremely high doses of GTN or PE-trinitrate given by intraduodenal or oral administration were reported to cause a vasodepression, but there was only a very transient (1–2 min) decrease in coronary vessel resistance with the PE-trinitrate. However, there was no evidence of blood levels of intact parent compound (i.e. either PETN or PE-trinitrate) nor substantial amounts of the initial metabolite (PE-dinitrate) following oral administration of either PE-tetranitrate or PE-trinitrate (47, 48). The oral administration of very high doses of organic nitrates to overcome hepatic inactivation would probably exaggerate side effects and induce tolerance to the administered agent and cross-tolerance to GTN (60).

The clearance of intact GTN, ISD, and MHN from the blood proceeded very rapidly ($T_{1/2} < 1$ min) following intravenous injection in rats (31). The blood was cleared of more than 80% of the parent nitrate in 1 min. The rates of disappearance of the metabolites were slower than their appearance by several orders of magnitude.

The approximate half-times for metabolite clearance from the blood were 2 hr for MHN, 2.5 hr for ISD, and almost 4 hr for GTN (31). Following injection of radioactive organic nitrates directly into the portal vein, little of the intact parent compound passed through the liver as an intact molecule, but there was an immediate appearance of metabolites in the circulation; however, there was no systemic vasodepression (31). The blood clearance data following intravenous administration of organic nitrates indicate that the transient duration (1–4 min) of the biological response (vasodepression) correlated directly with the transient circulation time (80% removed in 1 min) for the parent compound. The vasodepression (1–4 min) was completely out of phase with the circulation time for the nitrate metabolites ($T_{1/2}$, about 2 hr) (31).

Biological Activity of Metabolites

The comparisons of the vasodilator potency of intact organic nitrates on blood pressure or vascular resistance indicated that the denitrated metabolites were less potent than the parent compounds (49, 61–64).

GLYCERYL TRINITRATE   Organic nitrates were compared as blood pressure depressants in dogs and guinea pigs (61, 62). GTN was at least 10 times more potent than glyceryl dinitrate and 40 times more potent than inorganic nitrite, and GMN and inorganic nitrate were inactive (61). Compared with GTN, GDN was only 2% as active in lowering guinea pig blood pressure, 0.2% as active in relaxing rabbit aorta strips, and 5% as active in decreasing dog hindleg resistance (62). PETN and butanetriol trinitrate were also more potent than their denitrated metabolites (62). In general, the more active vasodepressor compounds were the nitrates with high oil/water partition coefficients. The less lipid-soluble compounds (i.e. denitration replaces lipid-soluble nitrate ester group with a water-soluble hydroxyl group) required progressively higher doses to elicit an equivalent fall in blood pressure (61).

ISOSORBIDE DINITRATE   The order of the coronary vasodilator potency (i.e. the dose required to produce a 10 ml/min change in blood flow in the circumflex coronary artery in dogs) was as follows: GTN, 1 μg; ISD, 100 μg; 2-ISMN, 300 μg; and 5-ISMN, 3000 μg (63). The order of potency required to reduce pressure by 10 mm Hg in the perfused dog hindlimb was GTN, 0.1 μg; ISD, 2 μg; 2-ISMN, 10 μg; and 5-ISMN, 200 μg (63, 64). 5-ISMN was demonstrated to be the predominant circulating metabolite in blood after either oral or intravenous administration of ISD (34). Much lower concentrations of the 2-ISMN metabolite were present. 5-ISMN was only one thirtieth to one hundredth as potent as ISD (63, 64). These observations strongly supported the evidence that the intact parent nitrate ester was the biologically active species and that denitration inactivated the compound.

PENTAERYTHRITOL TRINITRATE   An explanation to justify the use of PETN or PE-trinitrate as long-acting compounds was the demonstrated presence of persisting levels of PE-dinitrate or mononitrate metabolites in blood (42, 43, 45, 49, 51, 55). However, these metabolites proved to be without significant vasodilator activity in comparison to the parent compound; "therefore their persistent plasma levels cannot be responsible for the sustained action of PE-trinitrate in man" (65). PE-trinitrate was one fifth as potent as GTN as a coronary vasodilator and as a systemic vasodepressor. PE-dinitrate was only one fiftieth as potent as the PE-trinitrate, PE-mononitrate was one hundredth the potency of PE-trinitrate, and PE was completely inactive (50, 65). Furthermore, cross tolerance occurred between the active nitrate, PE-trinitrate, and its nearly inactive metabolites (65). Thus, accumulation of inactive metabolites in the plasma following chronic drug treatment might be expected to diminish response to an active agent needed acutely (e.g. GTN during angina).

CONCLUSIONS

The qualitative and quantitative pattern of biotransformation of organic nitrates in humans was the same as in experimental animals. The primary route of degradation of organic nitrates was enzymatic denitration by hepatic GSH-organic nitrate reductase. Fresh human liver biopsy samples had the same maximum enzyme velocity for GSH-dependent denitration as did rat liver, which was the model species for many of the nitrate biotransformation studies (31). Since these comparisons were on a liver weight basis, humans actually had at least 200 times more enzyme available than rats.

The principal finding of nitrate metabolism experiments in rats, dogs, and humans was that following oral administration of various organic nitrates, little if any of the parent compound was present in the circulation to relax vascular smooth muscle. Thus, following oral administration, the nitrates were absorbed into the portal circulation and were rapidly and completely degraded by the liver (GSH-organic nitrate reductase) before reaching the systemic circulation; therefore, they could have little chance of producing vasodilation.

Consistent with these observations are a large number of clinical studies that indicate that orally administered organic nitrates are ineffective. According to Modell (66), "The history of failure with so-called long-acting nitrates is an unbroken one." One would anticipate that long-term effects of a "long-lasting" vasodilator would be associated with sustained blood levels of the active compound. This has not proven to be the case. After oral administration or shortly after intravenous administration of intact nitrates, the predominant circulating species have been metabolites. The primary circulating metabolites of GTN, PETN, PE-trinitrate, or ISD are much too low in potency to account for the biological effect. The only other metabolite thus far tested was mannitol pentanitrate (67), which has very weak vasodilator activity in dogs. The circulating metabolites although unassociated with the time course of the nitrate-induced vasodilation would still be involved in provoking side effects. Severe headaches, which were out of time phase with biological effects and not accompanied by any change in blood pressure or heart rate, were noted following GTN treatment of human volunteers (23).

The sublingual administration of organic nitrates still represents a rational approach to the acute relief of an angina pectoris attack. ETN, MHN, and triethanola-

92   NEEDLEMAN

mine trinitrate were effective when administered sublingually instead of orally (68). Buccal adsorption of drug initially avoids hepatic destruction, and since only about 15% of the cardiac output is delivered to the liver, a transient but effective circulating level of intact organic nitrate would occur prior to inactivation. Little difference in the duration of action of various organic nitrates taken by the sublingual route should be anticipated because the hepatic organic nitrate reductase is highly active in humans (31). Such a comparison was carried out by adjusting the sublingual dosage of ISD and GTN to be equipotent regarding circulatory changes in triple product and in exercise tolerance in patients (69). Under these conditions there was no significant difference in the duration of action of these nitrates in the patients tested. Hepatic destruction of organic nitrates following sublingual administration should be dependent only on the rate at which they are delivered to the liver. It is conceivable that different patients could vary in their time course of response to sublingual nitrates. The amount of drug delivered to the liver could be influenced by such conditions as differential volumes of distribution for the various organic nitrates or radically altered (by stress, exercise, or angina) hepatic blood flow.

ACKNOWLEDGMENT

The research performed by the author was supported by USPHS grant from the NIH, HE-11771, and NIH Research Career Development Award HL-19586.

Literature Cited

1. Litchfield, M. H. 1971. *J. Pharm. Sci.* 60:1599–1607
2. Litchfield, M. H. 1973. *Drug Metab. Rev.* 2:239–64
3. Needleman, P. 1975. *Organic Nitrates, Handbook of Experimental Pharmacology,* 40:57–96. Berlin: Springer
4. Hay, M. 1883. *Practitioner* 30:422–33
5. Crandall, L. A. Jr., Leake, C. D., Loevenhart, A. S., Muehlberger, C. W. 1929. *J. Pharmacol. Exp. Ther.* 37:283–96
6. Crandall, L. A. Jr. 1933. *J. Pharmacol. Exp. Ther.* 48:127–40
7. Yagoda, H., von Oettingen, W. F. 1944. *Toxicology and Potential Dangers of Pentaerythritol Tetranitrate, Pub. Health Bull. No. 282,* p. 8
8. Oberst, F. W., Snyder, F. H. 1948. *J. Pharmacol. Exp. Ther.* 93:444–50
9. Heppel, L. A., Hilmoe, R. J. 1950. *J. Biol. Chem.* 183:129–38
10. Needleman, P., Hunter, F. E. Jr. 1965. *Mol. Pharmacol.* 1:77–86
11. Needleman, P., Harkey, A. B. 1971. *Biochem. Pharmacol.* 20:1867–76
12. Hunter, F. E. Jr., Kahana, S., Ford, S. 1953. *Fed. Proc.* 12:221
13. Lang, S., Johnson, E. M. Jr., Needle-
man, P. 1972. *Biochem. Pharmacol.* 21:422–24
14. Bogaert, M. G., Rosseel, M. T., De Schaepdryver, A. F. 1969. *Arch. Int. Pharmacodyn. Ther.* 179:480–89
15. Needleman, P., Krantz, J. C. Jr. 1965. *Biochem. Pharmacol.* 14:1225–30
16. Hunter, F. E. Jr., Ford, L. 1955. *J. Pharmacol. Exp. Ther.* 113:186–91
17. Posadas del Rio, F. 1970. *Fed. Proc.* 29:412
18. Posadas del Rio, F., Hunter, F. E. Jr. 1973. *Fed. Proc.* 32:733
19. Lee, N. H., Belpaire, F. M. 1972. *Arch. Int. Pharmacodyn. Ther.* 196:165–67
20. Needleman, P., Blehm, D. J., Harkey, A. B., Johnson, E. M. Jr., Lang, S. 1971. *J. Pharmacol. Exp. Ther.* 179:347–53
21. Di Carlo, F. J., Melgar, M. D. 1970. *Biochem. Pharmacol.* 19:1371–79
22. Bogaert, M. G., Rosseel, M. T., De Schaepdryver, A. F. 1969. *Arch. Int. Pharmacodyn Ther.* 177:487–91
23. Bogaert, M. G., Rosseel, M. T., Belpaire, F. M. 1971. *Arch. Int. Pharmacodyn. Ther.* 192:198–99
24. Lee, N. H., Belpaire, F. M. 1972. *Biochem. Pharmacol.* 21:3171–77
25. Bogaert, M. G., Rosseel, M. T., De

Schaepdryver, A. F. 1970. *Eur. J. Pharmacol.* 12:224–30
26. Di Carlo, F. J., Melgar, M. D. 1969. *Proc. Soc. Exp. Biol. Med.* 131:406–8
27. Johnson, E. M. Jr., Harkey, A. B., Blehm, D. J., Needleman, P. 1972. *J. Pharmacol. Exp. Ther.* 182:56–62
28. Di Carlo, F. J., Hartigan, J. M. Jr., Phillips, G. E. 1965. *Proc. Soc. Exp. Biol. Med.* 118:514–16
29. Lee, N. H. 1973. *Biochem. Pharmacol.* 22:3122–24
30. Di Carlo, F. J., Crew, M. C., Haynes, L. J., Melgar, M. D., Gala, R. L. 1968. *Biochem. Pharmacol.* 17:2179–83
31. Needleman, P., Lang, S., Johnson, E. M. Jr. 1972. *J. Pharmacol. Exp. Ther.* 181:489–97
32. Heppel, L. A., Porterfield, V. T. 1949. *J. Biol. Chem.* 178:549–56
33. Bogaert, M. G., Rosseel, M. T. 1972. *J. Pharm. Pharmacol.* 24:737–38
34. Sisenwine, S. F., Ruelius, H. W. 1971. *J. Pharmacol. Exp. Ther.* 176:296–301
35. Sherber, D. A., Marcus, M., Kleinberg, S. 1970. *Biochem. Pharmacol.* 19:607–12
36. Reed, D. E., May, J. F., Hart, L. G., McCurdy, D. H. 1971. *Arch. Int. Pharmacodyn* 191:318–36
37. Rosseel, M. T., Bogaert, M. G. 1973. *J. Pharm. Sci.* 62:754–58
38. Down, W. H., Chasseaud, L. F., Grundy, R. K. 1974. *J. Pharm. Sci.* 63:1147–49
39. Dietz, A. J. Jr. 1967. *Biochem. Pharmacol.* 16:2447–48
40. Rosseel, M. T., Bogaert, M. G. 1973. *Biochem. Pharmacol.* 22:67–72
41. Di Carlo, F. J., Coutinho, C. B., Sklow, N. J., Haynes, L. J., Crew, M. C. 1965. *Proc. Soc. Exp. Biol. Med.* 120:705–9
42. Di Carlo, F. J., Hartigan, J. M., Coutinho, C. B., Phillips, G. E. 1965. *Proc. Soc. Exp. Biol. Med.* 118:311–15
43. Di Carlo, F. J., Coutinho, C. B., Crew, M. C. 1967. *Arch. Int. Pharmacodyn.* 167:163–70
44. Di Carlo, F. J., Crew, M. C., Coutinho, C. B., Haynes, L. J., Sklow, N. J. 1967. *Biochem. Pharmacol.* 16:309–16
45. Crew, M. C., Melgar, M. D., Di Carlo, F. J. 1975. *J. Pharmacol. Exp. Ther.* 192:218–23
46. Davidson, I. W. F., Miller, H. S., Jr. Di Carlo, F. J. 1971. *J. Pharm. Sci.* 60:274–77
47. Davidson, I. W. F., Miller, H. S. Jr., Di Carlo, F. J. 1970. *J. Pharmacol. Exp. Ther.* 175:42–50
48. Davidson, I. W. F., Rollins, F. O., Di Carlo, F. J., Miller, H. S. Jr. 1971. *Clin. Pharmacol. Ther.* 12:972–81
49. Di Carlo, F. J., Crew, M. C., Sklow, N. J., Coutinho, C. B., Nonkin, P., Simon, F., Bernstein, A. 1966. *J. Pharmacol. Exp. Ther.* 153:254–58
50. Parker, J. C., Chang, Y., Davidson, I. W. F. 1973. *Fed. Proc.* 32:794
51. Di Carlo, F. J., Crew, M. C., Haynes, L. J., Wilson, M. 1969. *Biochem. Pharmacol.* 18:1985–90
52. Crew, M. C., Gala, R. L., Haynes, L. J., Di Carlo, F. J. 1971. *Biochem. Pharmacol.* 20:3077–89
53. Melgar, M. D., Leinweber, F. J., Crew, M. C., Di Carlo, F. J. 1974. *Drug Metab. Dispos.* 2:46–52
54. Leinweber, F. J., Melgar, M. D., Crew, M. C., Di Carlo, F. J. 1974. *Drug Metab. Dispos.* 2:40–45
55. Di Carlo, F. J., Melgar, M. D., Haynes, L. J., Gala, R. L., Crew, M. C. 1969. *J. Pharmacol. Exp. Ther.* 168:235–39
56. Clark, D. G., Litchfield, M. H. 1967. *Bri. J. Ind. Med.* 24:320–25
57. Clark, D. G., Litchfield, M. H. 1969. *Toxicol. Appl. Pharmacol.* 15:175–84
58. Dietz, A. J. Jr. 1967. *J. Pharm. Sci.* 56:1664–65
59. Commarato, M. A., Winbury, M. M., Kaplan, H. R. 1973. *J. Pharmacol. Exp. Ther.* 187:300–307
60. Schelling, J., Lasagna, L. 1967. *Clin. Pharmacol. Ther.* 8:256–60
61. Needleman, P., Blehm, D. J., Rotskoff, K. S. 1969. *J. Pharmacol. Exp. Ther.* 165:286–88
62. Bogaert, M. G., Rosseel, M. T., De Schaepdryver, A. F. 1968. *Arch. Int. Pharmacodyn.* 176:458–60
63. Wendt, R. L. 1972. *J. Pharmacol. Exp. Ther.* 180:732–42
64. Bogaert, M. G., Rosseel, M. T. 1972. *Arch. Pharmacol.* 275:339–42
65. Parker, J. C., Di Carlo, F. J., Davidson, I. W. F. 1975. *Eur. J. Pharmacol.* 31:29–37
66. Modell, W., Ed. 1970. *Drugs of Choice, 1970–1971*, p. 376. St. Louis, Mo: Mosby
67. Blum, S. W., Quinn, J. B., Howe, B. B., Hefner, M. A., Winbury, M. M. 1971. *J. Pharmacol. Exp. Ther.* 176:684–91
68. Riseman, J. E. F., Altman, G. E., Koretsky, S. 1958. *Circulation* 17:22–39
69. Goldstein, R. E., Douglas, M. D., Rosing, M. D., Redwood, D. R., Beiser, G. D., Epstein, S. E. 1971. *Circulation* 43:629–40

ARSENIC TOXICOLOGY AND INDUSTRIAL EXPOSURE

❖6638

Sherman S. Pinto and Kenneth W. Nelson
ASARCO, Incorporated, P. O. Box 1677, Tacoma, Washington 98401

The Occupational Safety and Health Act of 1970 tremendously enlarged the field of health care in industry in the United States. It directs the Secretary of Labor "to set the standard which most adequately assures . . . that no employee will suffer material impairment of health or functional capacity even if such employee has regular exposure to the hazard dealt with by such standard for the period of his working life" (1).

The secretary's task in setting standards involves great problems, because it assumes knowledge of pharmacology and toxicology of substances not yet developed in spite of the cumulative experience of centuries in some cases and of scientific research for decades. Arsenic is an example of a substance for which it has been difficult to set standards. In this paper we review the challenging and divergent views met with when an attempt is made to set a standard for airborne inorganic arsenic.

Inorganic arsenic is widely used in industry. The National Institute of Safety and Health (NIOSH) has estimated that about 1.5 million people in industry are potentially exposed to arsenic at least part of the time during the course of their work. (2) NIOSH is authorized to "conduct such research and experimental programs . . . as are necessary for the development of criteria for . . . improved health standards" and to "make recommendations concerning new . . . health standards." NIOSH has been most concerned with the possibility of inorganic airborne arsenic acting as a respiratory carcinogen. This, or course, is just part of a larger question, that is, does arsenic cause cancer?

Buchanan (3) and Vallee (4) have reviewed the problem and state that the idea was first proposed in the publications of Paris in 1820. However, Paris's work has not been confirmed. In 1887 Hutchinson showed a relationship between prolonged oral administration of arsenical preparations and skin cancer. Neubauer (5) in 1947 brilliantly reviewed all prior literature on the question of arsenical cancer and stated that only a very few persons of the thousands receiving oral arsenical preparations ever developed epitheliomas. He suggests that "in arsenical cancer, arsenic is not the only aetiological factor." Neubauer collected 143 published cases of medicinal

95

arsenical epithelioma in man. Many of these cases had an "affection of the skin, and especially psoriasis [which] gives a predisposition for arsenical cancer although there is no real definite proof." The great majority of the cases developed after the drug had been given for about 15 years, and the average patient received 28 grams of arsenic during the entire course of treatment. Roth (6) studied cancer in German vintners who were exposed to arsenic from inhalation of insecticide sprays and dusts as well as from drinking a wine that contained a high level of arsenic (0.2–8.9 mg/100 ml). He estimated that the workers had a 12–17 year exposure and an intake of about 53 grams of arsenic over a 12 year period. The latent period for tumor development was estimated to be 13–22 years after first exposure.

Regelson (7) described an instance of hemangioendothelial sarcoma of the liver seven years after the discontinuation of treatment with Fowler's solutions. In this report, a case of psoriasis is described which had been treated with Fowler's solution for 17 years.

Hill & Fanning (8) studied mortality data on employees working in a factory that produced sodium arsenate. Mortality data for workers in the factory between 1910 and 1943 were compared with mortality data for other workers in the community. Among 75 deceased factory workers there were 22 deaths from cancer (29.3%), while workers in other occupations in the community showed 157 deaths from cancer in 1216 deceased workers (12.9%). Workers engaged in handling sodium arsenate had an increased percentage of their deaths from cancer of the respiratory system. Thus 31.3% of their deaths from cancer were in the respiratory system while 15.9% of the control group had respiratory cancer. The factory workers also had an increase in skin cancer compared to the control group.

Perry et al (9) investigated the clinical and environmental aspects of the factory and its employees in 1946. Appreciable arsenic absorption was evidenced by skin changes (pigmentation and warts), which were observed clinically in all chemical workers. Atmospheric concentrations of arsenic in different parts of the factory were found to range from a high of 1034 μg per cubic meter, to a low of 384 μg of arsenic per cubic meter.

Hill & Fanning describe their conclusions as "guarded but suggestive." A twofold excess of deaths from all cancer was observed in the factory workers; the organ systems especially affected were the respiratory and skin.

Snegireff & Lombard in 1951 (10) published a study of deaths from cancer in two plants, one in which arsenic trioxide was produced, the other in which no arsenic was handled. No apparent difference between the two plants in cancer death experiences was found, but NIOSH has suggested that the lack of inter-plant differences could be due to an unsuspected arsenic exposure in the control plant. (11) In the arsenic-exposed plant 39% of all cancer deaths were due to lung cancer while 50% of all cancer deaths in the non-arsenic exposure plant were due to lung cancer. The sample size limitations in this study make it of questionable significance in evaluating the problem of arsenic and cancer.

Pinto & Bennett (12) in 1963 studied the mortality data in the deaths of 229 individuals who worked at a copper smelter where arsenic trioxide was produced as a by-product. The deaths covered the period 1946–1960. The total number of deaths from lung cancer in this group was compared with a list of such deaths prepared by the Washington State Division of Vital Statistics. The cases that were classed as lung cancer cases by the state were the same cases of lung cancer used in the Pinto-Bennett study, and there was no under-reporting of cases as has been suggested (11).

The study showed that workers in the plant had the same total incidence of cancer as in the state of Washington for the population of the same sex and age. However, within the cancer group there was a twofold increase in respiratory cancer for both the group exposed to high arsenic levels and the group exposed to low arsenic levels. In a previous study Pinto & McGill (13) had studied two groups of employees in the plant. One group worked in an area of high potential arsenic exposure, and the other in an area with presumably minimal arsenic exposure. The high exposure group had an average urinary arsenic value of 820 μg/liter, while the minimal exposure group had an average urinary excretory value of 130 μg/liter.

In a more recent study Pinto & Enterline (14) analyzed the causes of death among 530 male retirees from the same smelter who retired between January 1, 1949 and December 31, 1973. Pensioners were specifically studied because each member of the group had been exposed to arsenic trioxide for a definite period of time that ended with retirement. Thus, exposure and follow-up period did not overlap. Total arsenic exposure for each individual was calculated from personnel records, and was obtained by multiplying the average arsenic exposure in each department by the time spent in that department. An excess of respiratory cancer deaths was found and there appeared to be a linear relationship between the increase in deaths from respiratory cancer and degree of exposure to arsenic or some closely related material. No excess in deaths from lymphatic cancer was found.

Further analysis of the data indicated that there was a measure of arsenic exposure below which no excess respiratory cancer was found if the period of exposure was shorter than 25 years. The safe level of exposure to arsenic was indicated to be of the order of 100 μg per m^3 of air. It was noted there were other air contaminants in the industrial atmosphere and that their possible synergistic action cannot be overlooked. The proposed exposure level cannot be considered as based solely on arsenic trioxide. Rather, arsenic trioxide is used as an indicator of a complex industrial airborne exposure. After 25 or more years of exposure, there were statistically significant respiratory cancer excesses that were related to the intensity of exposure.

This study also developed histories of the smoking patterns of 377 men in the total pensioner group who were alive on January 1, 1961. Their mortality experience was followed through 1973. Analyses showed some interaction between smoking and arsenic exposure but not the multiplying effect observed for some other substances. The figures indicate that the excess mortality ratio due to respiratory cancer in the group was not due entirely to smoking.

Weir (14) has pointed out a number of factors that must be considered in evaluating lung cancer presumably due to occupational factors. These include smoking pattern, urban-rural residence, foreign born/native born population proportions, and socioeconomic variations. He further pointed out that the age-adjusted lung cancer rate for white males for 1950–1969 in the state of Washington is 34.61 per 100, 000 yet the county rates for this same period range from 10.4–46.0. It is evident that a variety of factors influencing rates of death from lung cancer fluctuate by county of residence and account for this variation in death rate.

Lee & Fraumeni (15) in 1969 compared the mortality data of 8047 white male smelter workers who were exposed to both arsenic trioxide and sulfur dioxide from 1933 to 1963. They found 1877 deaths compared to 1634 expected deaths. Classifying the deaths into three groups according to intensity of arsenic exposure, Lee & Fraumeni found that deaths from lung cancer increased with higher degrees of arsenic trioxide exposure. When workers were grouped according to duration and degree of exposure to sulfur dioxide, excess lung cancer mortality was found with increasing exposure to sulfur dioxide. Lee & Fraumeni's studies also indicated that there was more respiratory cancer among the foreign-born sample than in the native-born sample. However, figures on the incidence of lung cancer for the two groups are not presented in the paper and cannot be generated from the published tables.

The authors conclude that their findings are "consistent with the hypothesis that exposure to high levels of arsenic trioxide, perhaps in interaction with sulfur dioxide or unidentified chemicals in the work environment, is responsible for the threefold excess of respiratory cancer deaths among smelter workers." In an attempt to find the levels of arsenic that might have been present in this smelter, air analyses were made in various departments of a smelter in 1965. The validity of applying an air-contamination figure of 1965 to a similar operation in 1940 is open to question. It has been our experience that air contamination in the non-ferrous smelting industry was less in 1965 than it was in the period before 1948. After 1948, structural building material was available, and the processes learned for reducing harmful air contaminants in industry during World War II were applied more widely throughout the United States smelting industry.

Nelson et al (16) studied the long-term effect of lead arsenate spray on the users rather than on the producers. This was a follow-up mortality study for a cohort of 1231 individuals who had participated in a 1938 mortality survey of the effects of exposures to lead arsenate insecticide spray. Over 97% of the original 1938 group were located. The authors concluded that excess mortality did not occur. In fact, the orchardists, the most highly exposed group, had the lowest standard mortality ratio of the three groups analyzed. It should be noted that the authors report having used as cause-of-death the primary cause listed on death certificates. This action usually results in underestimating the true frequency of death due to lung cancer.

Ott et al (17) in 1974 presented a study of exposure to lead arsenate and calcium arsenate occurring between 1919 and 1956. Arsenic trioxide was the basic material from which the arsenates were made. The relationship between cumulative arsenic exposure and the ratio of observed to expected respiratory malignancy deaths was estimated by the method of least squares. The predicted ratio was 7:1 for individuals exposed for more than eight years to compounds that contained an equivalent level of 1 mg/m^3 arsenic. In the more heavily exposed individuals, an excess of respiratory cancer was observed 35+ years after the initial exposure. An increase in malignant neoplasms of the lymphatic and hematopoietic tissues, except leukemia, was also found in the exposed group. No clear dose-response relationship was found.

Baetjer, Levin & Lillienfield (11) studied the mortality experience of retirees from an Allied Chemical plant that had been engaged in manufacturing dry arsenicals for pesticides. Arsenic trioxide was the starting compound for the subsequent syntheses of lead arsenate and calcium arsenate. Analysis of the death rates among male retirees of this plant showed an increase of observed over expected deaths from all cancer, as well as respiratory and leukemia-lymphatic cancers. It should be noted that a survey of materials used in the manufacturing processes of this plant was made. Several of these materials are well recognized as being carcinogenic, but no significance seems to have been attached to their presence.

Kuratsune et al (18) in 1974 reported on lung cancers in some employees of a Japanese copper smelter. The most significant information presented was that all the workers who died of lung cancer were "engaged in the dirtiest pre-war operations," when the amount of arsenic contained in the ores processed was estimated to be four to eight times higher than in recent years.

Newman et al (19) studied the histologic characteristics of lung cancers found in a copper-mining city and in a group of copper smelter workers in another city. Both areas had a higher than normal lung cancer rate. Poorly differentiated epidermoid bronchogenic carcinomas were found among the smelter workers. The authors believe that such a cell type may be related to exposure to arsenic. In the area presumably not exposed to arsenic, the predominant cell type of the cancer was "well differentiated" in the majority of the cases studied. The authors believe this type of cancer may have been caused by exposure to finely ground dust containing biotite, sericite, chlorite, and hornblende. These results should be of significant help in charting a course for further studies of lung cancer and its possible relationship to environmental factors.

Toxicologists who are concerned with the occupational cancer problem are anxious to find experimental confirmation of their theory by producing cancers in one animal or another. At the OSHA fact-finding hearing (September 1974), Dr. Herman Kraybill (11) said "arsenic stands out as the one substance for which human carcinogenicity has been demonstrated but for which an animal model has yet to be found to reproduce this effect."

The work of Milner (20) on arsenic and experimentally induced skin tumors in mice shows the problems encountered in this field. Cutaneous tumors were initiated by topical methylcholanthrene and promoted by transplantation. In one strain of mice the number of papillomas produced appeared to increase after feeding arsenic although the effect was not statistically significant. In another strain of mice the arsenic treatment resulted in a decrease in the number of papillomas produced, and the result was statistically significant.

DISCUSSION

These papers almost uniformly point to some low-grade carcinogenic activity by arsenic although not confirmed by any animal model (11) yet suggest that various cocarcinogenic factors must be studied much more thoroughly (2).

Regelson (7) points out that the antimitotic effect of arsenic is clinically useful since it is used in treating psoriasis and chronic myelocytic leukemia. Arsenic also is an antiparasitic agent and is an inhibitor of insect fecundity. Arsenic possesses both carcinogenic- and tumor-inhibitory properties, a characteristic seen in other clinically useful antimitotics.

We feel it is highly unlikely that a single scientifically sound level for all inorganic compounds of arsenic in air can be established from the data at hand. Arsenical compounds differ in toxicity, so why not in carcinogenicity? Fields of investigation that should be pursued in developing an understanding of the arsenic-respiratory cancer problem include (a) smoking history of subject as well as amount of arsenic exposure; (b) level and chemical nature of respirable arsenic compounds in the air; (c) investigation of other airborne contaminants that may be present, including such materials as sulfur dioxide, chromium, asbestos, and recognized organic carcinogens; (d) more histological studies of types of lung cancer and their relationship to known occupational carcinogens; (e) socioeconomic variations of lung cancer incidence. Although the academician trained in toxicology has become very important in helping to develop the rules and regulations for modern industry, his awareness of the pressing nature of the problem should be further increased.

Literature Cited

1. Congr. Rec. 1970. *USA Proc. Debates 91st Congr. 2nd Sess.* Vol. 116, S20270-20279
2. US Dep. Health Educ. Welfare, Nat. Inst. Occup. Safety Health. 1973. *Criteria for a Recommended Standard: Occupational Exposure to Inorganic Arsenic,* pp. 1–105. Washington DC: GPO.
3. Buchanan, W. D. 1962. *Toxicity of Arsenic Compounds,* pp. 101–26. London: Elsevier
4. Vallee, B. L., Ulmer, D. D., Wacker, W. E. C. 1960. *Arch. Ind. Health* 21:132–51
5. Neubauer, O. 1947. *Br. J. Cancer* I:192–251
6. Roth, F. 1959. *Zentralbl. Allg. Pathol.* 100-529-30
7. Regelson, W., Kim, U., Ospina, J., Holland, F. J. 1968. *Cancer* 21:514–22
8. Hill, A. B., Fanning, E. L. 1948. *Br. J. Ind. Med.* 5:1–6
9. Perry, K., Bowler, R. G., Buckell, H. M., Druett, H. A., Schilling, R. S. F. 1948. *Br. J. Ind. Med.* 5:6–15
10. Snegireff, L. S., Lombard, O. M. 1951. *Arch. Ind. Hyg. Occup. Med.* 4:199–205
11. Dep. Labor, Occup. Safety Health Admin. 1975. *Fed. Regist.* 40:3392–3403
12. Pinto, S. S., Bennett, B. M. 1963 *Arch. Environ. Health* 7:583–91
13. Pinto, S. S., McGill, C. M. 1953. *Ind. Med. Surg.* 22:281–87
14. Pinto, S. S., Enterline, P. E. 1975. *Occup. Safety Health Admin. Conf. Inorg. Arsenic Stand.* Washington DC: US Dep. Labor
15. Lee, A. M., Fraumeni, J. P. 1969. *J. Nat. Cancer Inst.* 42:1045–53
16. Nelson, W. C. et al 1973. *J. Chron. Dis.* 26:105–13
17. Ott, M., Holder, B., Gordon, H. 1974. *Arch. Environ. Health* 29:250–55
18. Kuratsune, M. et al 1974. *Cancer* 13:552–58
19. Newman, J. A. et al 1975. *Conf. Occup. Carcinogenesis,* New York: NY Acad. Sci.
20. Milner, J. E. 1969. *Arch Environ. Health* 18:7–11

NEUROTOXIC INDOLEAMINES ♦6639
AND MONOAMINE NEURONS[1]

H. G. Baumgarten
Department of Neuroanatomy, University of Hamburg, Hamburg,
German Federal Republic

A. Björklund
Department of Histology, University of Lund, Lund, Sweden

INTRODUCTION

In 1968 Thoenen & Tranzer (1) discovered that the long-lasting depletion of NA
in sympathetically innervated organs by 6-OH-DA is due to degeneration of NA
terminals. This provided the basis for the development of a new concept in neurobiological research: the method of selective chemical neurodegeneration. The successful
application of this method to produce degeneration of DA and NA neurons in brain
(2, 3) stimulated a search for compounds with comparable effects on central 5-HT
neurons. In studies with a restricted number of 5-HT analogs, we were able to show
that certain dihydroxylated tryptamines caused toxic damage to serotonin terminals. The recent findings by Björklund, Baumgarten & Rensch (4) and Gerson &
Baldessarini (5) that DMI treatment prior to intraventricular 5,7-DHT injection
prevents the damaging effect of the latter drug on NA but not on 5-HT neurons
indicate that powerful and probably rather selective destruction of central indoleamine–containing axons and terminals can be achieved.

BIOCHEMICAL EFFECTS

Effects on Monoamine Levels

Table 1 depicts those tryptamines that have been found to cause substantial long-
term depletion of 5-HT in the brain and spinal cord (6, 7). A standard dose of 50
μg free-base 5,6-DHT, 5,7-DHT, N-m-5,6-DHT, N-m-5,7-DHT, or 5,6-DAcOT

---

[1]Abbreviations used: CA, catecholamine(s); DA, dopamine; 5,6-DAcOT, 5,6-diacetoxytryp-
tamine; DHT, dihydroxytryptamine(s); DMI, desmethylimipramine; 5-HIAA, 5-hydroxyin-
dole acetic acid; HT, hydroxytryptamine(s); IC, inhibitory concentration; 6-OH-DA,
6-hydroxydopamine; MAO, monoamine oxidase; NA, noradrenaline; N-m-, N-methyl-.

Table 1 Effects of five potent neurotoxic indoleamines on whole brain and spinal cord serotonin and catecholamine content[a,b]

| | 5-HT content (% control) | | NA content (% control) | | DA content (% control) |
	Brain	Spinal cord	Brain	Spinal cord	Brain
5,6-DHT (50 μg)	56	12	84	121	70
5,6-DAcOT (50 μg)	59	21	117	158	93
N-m-5,6-DHT (50 μg)	76	24	104	115	98
5,7-DHT (50 μg)	48	12	52	42	91
5,7-DHT (150 μg)	17	10	48	16	*[c]
5,7-DHT (150 μg) + + DMI (25 mg/kg)	21	10	124	95	*[c]
N-m-5,7-DHT (50 μg)	63	16	65	68	90

[a] Each drug (calculated as the free-base) was given in a single intraventricular injection (student's t-test).

[b] Data from references 4, 6, and 8.

[c] *, not assayed.

results in a 25 to 50% reduction of brain 5-HT and a loss of 80–90% of 5-HT from the spinal cord 8–12 days after injection. Other mono- or dihydroxylated indoleamines, including the α-methylated derivatives of 5,6- and 5,7-DHT, were found to be less efficient long-term depletors of brain 5-HT. All nonsubstituted DHTs tested (5,6-, 5,7-, 4,5-, and 6,7-DHT) also decrease brain CA levels, indicating a relative nonselectivity in the action of these compounds (6,7). While 6,7- and 4,5-DHT deplete NA even more efficiently than 5-HT (6,7), 5,7-DHT (in doses up to 75 μg) has similar depleting effects on NA and 5-HT in the brain (8,9). Besides its strong depleting action on brain and spinal cord 5-HT, 5,6-DHT produces marginal, though significant, long-term reductions of both NA and DA in brain (16 and 30% reduction, respectively, at 8–12 days after 50 μg 5,6-DHT; references 6, 7). The acetic acid ester derivative of 5,6-DHT, 5,6-DAcOT, is more specific than 5,6-DHT when given in doses up to 50 μg (6). Increasing the dose of 5,6-DAcOT fails to enhance its long-term action on brain 5-HT but tends to impair its selectivity for 5-HT neurons.

The long-term effect of 5,6-DHT on brain 5-HT is maximal after a dose of 50–75 μg (free base). Increasing the dose above 75 μg fails to cause any further reduction in 5-HT, but results in enhancement of its nonspecific toxic effects as well as in increased depletion of brain CA (10, 11). 5,7-DHT depletes brain 5-HT in a dose-related manner up to a dose of about 200 μg (8), and this is true also for spinal cord NA. By contrast, the depletion of NA in the brain is maximal already after 50 μg. From fluorescence histochemical observations it seems likely that this latter phenomenon is due to a failure of 5,7-DHT to penetrate to NA fiber systems remote from the ventricles in sufficiently high concentrations to produce toxic damage. Thus, after 50 μg, there is, in the brain, a zone of efficient damage to NA axons of about 1 to 2 mm from the ventricular surface, and this zone does not increase appreciably at higher doses of 5,7-DHT (12).

Time-course analysis of the 5-HT depletion pattern following 5,6- or 5,7-DHT reveals that minimum amine levels are not reached until 4 to 12 days after drug injection in some brain regions and in the spinal cord (9, 11). This points to the importance of anterograde degeneration of nerve terminals following primary lesions to the nonterminal axons as an important mechanism of damage in the central 5-HT neurons (8, 9, 11, 13). Generally, the reduction in 5-HT levels is smallest in cell body–rich CNS regions, which reflects the resistance of the neuronal pericarya to the acute toxic effects of 5,6- or 5,7-DHT (see below).

It has been shown that the extent and specificity of 5-HT depletion in the adult rat brain by 5,6-DHT depends on the route of administration, the speed of injection, and the type of anesthesia used (10). Generally, intracisternal injections yield less 5-HT depletion than intraventricular ones (14–17). This difference is greater the more autoxidizable the drug. Thus, larger differences are noted with 5,6-DHT, which is more rapidly autoxidized, than with 5,7-DHT. Low doses of 5,7-DHT, when administered intracisternally in newborn rats, have been found to cause long-lasting, profound reductions in CNS 5-HT and 5-HIAA with little effect on brain NA (19). These findings indicate that the intracisternal route of administration is very useful in developing animals, probably because of the relatively large size of the ventricular system, facilitating rapid distribution of the drug in the cerebrospinal fluid and efficient penetration into the small brain.

As shown by Björklund et al (18) the neurotoxic indoleamines are highly suitable for direct intracerebral administration by local stereotaxic injection of small amounts of the drugs. This offers a very useful tool for localized selective lesioning of 5-HT-containing axon bundles or terminal systems. The intracerebral route of administration may also help to circumvent problems of nonselectivity and general toxicity encountered after intraventricular or intracisternal injections (for discussion, see references 9 and 18).

Uptake Site Affinity

Table 2 compares, for the five most potent neurotoxic tryptamines, the IC-50 values for the inhibition of the uptake of ^{3}H-5-HT into brain homogenates, with the relative percentage inhibition of ^{3}H-5-HT, ^{3}H-NA, and ^{3}H-DA uptake, measured at fixed concentrations of the tryptamines (20, 21). Two compounds, N-methyl-5,6-DHT and 5,6-DHT, have affinities to the 5-HT uptake system close to 5-HT itself. (IC-50 for 5-HT, 10^{-7}M; for 5,6-DHT, 6.0×10^{-7}M; for N-methyl-5,6-DHT, 3.7×10^{-7}M). 5,7-DHT is approximately 7 times weaker as an inhibitor of 5-HT transport than 5,6-DHT (20, 21). The IC-50 of 5,7-DHT indicates, however, that this compound competes more successfully for the 5-HT uptake sites than does 6-OH-DA for the NA or DA uptake sites (22). As revealed by the studies referred to earlier, the uptake of 5,7-DHT into noradrenergic neurons can be counteracted by pretreatment with the potent inhibitor of NA uptake, DMI, thereby improving its selectivity of action on 5-HT neurons (4, 5). Similarly, it has been reported that side effects of 5,6-DHT can be counteracted, and its selectivity increased by DMI (23). It is evident from these findings that the uptake of neurotoxic indoleamines is mediated by the same transport mechanism that mediates reuptake of the natural transmitter.

Table 2 Uptake site affinity and neurotoxic potency of five neurotoxic indoleamines, as evaluated in vitro[a]

	Affinity for 5-HT uptake sites[b]	Percentage inhibition of uptake[c]			In vitro toxicity at 10^{-6} M[d]	
		5-HT	NA	DA	^{3}H-5-HT uptake (% reduction)	^{3}H-NA uptake (% reduction)
5,6-DHT	6.0×10^{-7} M	59.0 (1 μM)	43.3 (1 μM)	44.7 (1 μM)	-57	+9
5,6-DAcOT	7.4×10^{-5} M	53.9 (10 μM)	23.0 (10 μM)	31.6 (10 μM)	-48	-11
N-methyl-5,6-DHT	3.7×10^{-7} M	72.3 (1 μM)	39.1 (1 μM)	37.4 (1 μM)	-64	-26
5,7-DHT	4.0×10^{-6} M	27.5 (1 μM)	32.5 (1 μM)	15.4 (1 μM)	-65	-24
N-methyl-5,7-DHT					-63	-18

[a] Data from reference 21.

[b] Measured as the concentration of the compound causing 50% inhibition of the ^{3}H-5-HT uptake by synaptosomes prepared from rat hypothalamus.

[c] Measured in synaptosomes from rat hypothalamus (^{3}H-5-HT and ^{3}H-NA) or striatum (^{3}H-DA). The inhibition was measured at a fixed concentration of the added compound (10^{-6} or 10^{-7} M).

[d] Measured in thin cortical slices as the effect of a 30 min incubation at +37°C (in the presence of 10^{-6} M of the various compounds) on the uptake of ^{3}H-5-HT (0.5×10^{-7} M) or ^{3}H-NA (10^{-7} M) during a subsequent incubation for 10 min.

Impairment of Amine Uptake In Vitro

Reduction in the capacity of the tissue to accumulate tritiated amines is an early and sensitive sign of axonal damage in monoaminergic neurons. We have taken advantage of this fact in a series of in vitro studies in which the tissue was preincubated with the neurotoxic indoleamines at concentrations of 10^{-7} to 10^{-5} M for up to 60 min. After thorough rinsing of the tissue, the ^{3}H-5-HT or ^{3}H-NA uptake capacity was then measured in a subsequent 10 min incubation (21). The extent of reduction in ^{3}H-amine uptake measured in this way is considered to reflect the "neurotoxic potency" of the indoleamine analyzed. Monohydroxylated tryptamines, such as 4-HT, 5-HT, 6-HT, and 7-HT do not cause uptake impairment under these conditions, whereas all dihydroxylated analogs (4,5-DHT, 5,6-DHT, 5,7-DHT, and 6,7-DHT, as well as the N-methylated derivatives of 5,6- and 5,7-DHT) are active (Table 2). 5,6-, 5,7-DHT, and their N-methylated analogs are the most potent compounds. Maximum impairment in ^{3}H-5-HT uptake (60-65% reduction after a 30 min exposure to the drugs) is obtained at 10^{-6}M, and the effect is almost negligible with 10^{-7}M. This suggests that their toxicity depends on reaching a critical concentration. At the same time, these experiments demonstrate that the neurotoxicity develops rapidly: a 5 min exposure to 10^{-5}M 5,6-DHT, followed by a 20 min rinsing in buffer, is sufficient to produce maximum impairment of the subsequent ^{3}H-5-HT uptake. From a comparison with the data of Sachs (24) on the in vitro effects of 6-OH-DA it is evident that the concentrations of the 5,6- or 5,7-DHTs required to produce damage to serotonin terminals in vitro are much lower than the concentrations of 6-OH-DA required to produce damage to CA terminals. This points to a high intrinsic neurotoxic potency of the hydroxylated indoleamines.

Reduction in ^{3}H-Amine Uptake In Vivo

It is generally believed that the uptake of ^{3}H-amines into brain slices or homogenates is related to the amount of intact monoaminergic nerve terminals in the tissue. Therefore, the extent of terminal degeneration induced by treatment with neurotoxic amines can be evaluated by measuring ^{3}H-amine uptake at various intervals after drug administration. Such measurements have been performed at 8–14 days after intraventricular 5,6-, 5,7-DHT, or 5,6-DAcOT (6, 8, 9, 25). The reduction of ^{3}H-5-HT and ^{3}H-NA uptake induced by these compounds parallels fairly well the percentage depletion of endogenous 5-HT and NA, strongly supporting the idea that these compounds cause axonal degeneration of monoamine neurons in brain and spinal cord.

Effects on Enzymes of Monoamine Biosynthesis

In the CNS, tryptophan hydroxylase is supposed to be selectively confined to 5-HT neurons (26). Activities of this enzyme following administration of 5,6- or 5,7-DHT may, therefore, reflect the functional state of the neurons in response to a chemical injury. A complicated, mostly biphasic, depletion and recovery pattern is disclosed in many CNS regions after 5,6-DHT treatment (27). These changes can be interpreted as an initial, direct enzyme inactivation, a subsequent loss of activity due to direct terminal degeneration, an intermediate rise of enzyme activity due to increased pericaryal synthesis, and finally, a retarded loss of activity due to anterograde loss of terminals. A further long-term recovery of enzyme in some regions is consistent with the idea of functional recovery and/or axonal regeneration in the central 5-HT systems (28–30). A dramatic reduction of tryptophan hydroxylase is seen after 5,7-DHT in the adult rat (31) concomitant with a slight reduction in regional dopamine-β-hydroxylase, but not tyrosine hydroxylase activity (32), in accordance with the unselective effect of 5,7-DHT on NA neurons. The unchanged activity of tyrosine hydroxylase in all forebrain regions analyzed is thought to reflect the integrity of the dopaminergic neurons. Similar findings have been obtained in developing rats (33).

MORPHOLOGICAL EFFECTS

Central Nervous System

Shortly after the intraventricular injection of 5,6-DHT, an indoleamine fluorophore (induced by 5,6-DHT itself) can be visualized that is preferentially confined to monoaminergic axons, terminals, and cell bodies, provided they have a ventricle-near location. The 5,6-DHT fluorophore is no longer detectable in these monoaminergic fibers after 24 hr. By this time, the indoleamine axons have developed signs of damage, that is, numerous grotesque enlargements resembling axonal dilatations after mechanical injury (9, 13, 18, 25, 34, 35). Concomitantly, there is a loss of many ventricle-near indoleamine terminals. Additional indoleamine terminals, not acutely affected by 5,6-DHT, disappear from brain after a latency of four days or more, reflecting anterograde degeneration processes. Although no acute toxic effects of 5,6-DHT on cell bodies have been demonstrated, some pericarya disintegrate by retrograde injury (13, 36). A few days after 5,6-DHT injection, sprouting of indoleamine axons is noted in the vicinity of the drug-damaged axonal stumps. These sprouting fibers regrow during the subsequent months (see section on regeneration of the drug-lesioned central neurons).

In principle, 5,7-DHT produces similar pathological changes in central 5-HT neurons as 5,6-DHT does but, in addition, 5,7-DHT damages NA axons and terminals (8, 18, 35–37). Even after moderate intraventricular doses, 5,6-DHT causes bilaterally a reduction in the number of ventricle-near DA terminals of the caudate whereas the NA systems seem morphologically intact (25).

Terminal degeneration and axonal injury induced by 5,6-DHT have been observed in the electron microscope. In addition, it has been shown that 5,6-DHT is capable of unselectively damaging myelinated axons (38). 5,7-DHT seems to be largely devoid of such unspecific toxic side effects (35).

Peripheral Nervous System

A partial chemical axotomy of sympathetic adrenergic neurons can be achieved by high doses of 5,6-DHT in combination with MAO inhibition (39). To prevent the animals from getting severe cardiovascular side effects (a 5-HT-like intense vasoconstriction), α-adreno receptor and 5-HT receptor blockers have to be administered before intravenous or intraperitoneal 5,6-DHT injections. 5,7-DHT is, on the other hand, well tolerated in doses up to 60 mg/kg and causes degeneration of NA terminals in many target organs (40). Its potency on peripheral sympathetic neurons, at the 60 mg/kg dose level, resembles that of 6-OH-DA.

REGENERATION OF THE DRUG-LESIONED CENTRAL NEURONS

Following the initial lesion of the serotonin systems by an intraventricular dose of 75 μg 5,6-DHT, and to a lesser extent after 150 μg 5,7-DHT, there is a regrowth of the damaged axons during the subsequent months. After 5,6-DHT this is reflected in a significant recovery of 5-HT in all regions analyzed, except the spinal cord, between 1 and 6 months (28–30). Separate analysis of lower and higher segments of the spinal cord has shown that a significant recovery of the 5-HT levels occurs also in most cranial spinal cord segments. This is paralleled by an extensive development of new, sprouting indoleamine fibers, as visualized in the fluorescence microscope (28, 29, 36), and by a recovery of the ^{3}H-5-HT uptake capacity in several brain regions (28). The fluorescence histochemical analysis of the 5,6-DHT-treated animals has revealed that the regenerating axons are able to partly regrow to their original terminal areas. In addition, apparently abnormal fiber patterns are formed in many regions where no or only few indoleamine-containing fibers can be detected normally; in still other areas, normally supplied with indoleaminergic fibers, there is an overgrowth of 5-HT axons leading to a hyperinnervation (28, 29, 36).

Regeneration in the serotonin systems occurs also after a high dose of 5,7-DHT but is more restricted than after 5,6-DHT and primarily confined to the lower brain stem (36). This difference has been explained by the fact that the high dose of 5,7-DHT produces lesions in the indoleamine axons that lie closer to the cell bodies, resulting in a higher incidence of retrograde cell loss and in an impaired regeneration. The most active and extensive regeneration after 5,7-DHT takes place in the NA systems (12, 37, 41). Thus, many diencephalic and telencephalic centers initially denervated by the drug treatment are efficiently reinnervated by the regrowing, sprouting NA fibers. This is accompanied by a recovery of brain NA levels and ^{3}H-NA uptake (12, 37).

The regrowth phenomena in the 5,6- and 5,7-DHT-lesioned neurons have to be taken into consideration when interpreting behavioral or functional data in treated animals. It is highly probable that the regenerated fibers reestablish synaptic contacts, either in the initially denervated areas or in abnormal sites, and these may well be of critical importance for recovery of function in the lesioned animals. A detailed knowledge of the degeneration-regeneration processes is obviously necessary for an understanding of the functional consequences of a neurotoxic lesion.

THE USE OF DRUGS FOR MODIFYING THE ACTIONS OF NEUROTOXIC INDOLEAMINES

Because of the small difference in their affinity to the 5-HT and CA uptake sites (see section on uptake site affinity), almost all neurotoxic indoleamines tested cause unselective damage to CA neurons in addition to their effects on 5-HT neurons. Among the several possibilities for improving their specificity of action against CNS indoleamine neurons two methods have been found satisfactory: (a) interference with the unspecific uptake of 5,6- or 5,7-DHT into CA neurons by inhibitors of catecholamine transport, such as DMI (4, 5, 23, 41), and (b) counteraction of the toxic effects of 5,7-DHT on central NA neurons by prior monoamine oxidase inhibition (41, 42). Such combined treatments thus render 5,7-DHT a tool for powerful, long-lasting, and remarkably selective degeneration of 5-HT neurons in the rat CNS.

BEHAVIORAL AND NEUROENDOCRINE EFFECTS

Intraventricular 5,6- or 5,7-DHT injections, when given alone or in combination with DMI, produce characteristic behavioral alterations in adult male rats, consisting of transitory deficits in themoregulation; persistent increases in irritability; hyperresponsiveness and failure to adapt to tactile, optic, acoustic, and pain stimuli; hypersexuality; enhanced aggressiveness and bizarre social interaction; and changes in sleep pattern and cortical EEG (10, 15, 17, 41, 43). Similar though much less dramatic behavioral disturbances have been documented after p-chlorophenylalanine, a well-established, long-lasting inhibitor of tryptophan hydroxylase (44), and may thus reflect interference with serotonergic transmission in brain.

The effects induced by selective degeneration of 5-HT axons and terminals in brain have gained particular interest for the elucidation of the role of serotonergic neurons in the control of secretion of anterior pituitary hormones. The results obtained with 5,7-DHT suggest a serotonergic inhibitory control of serum growth hormone levels in the developing male and female rat, but no clear role in the adult rat (45, 46). The findings in developing animals are, however, complicated by the strong, though transitory, anorexigenic effects of neonatally administered 5,7-DHT. Other recent data obtained with 5,7-DHT suggest that contrary to published concepts serotonergic neurons may furnish stimulatory inputs to LH secretion, as judged from the depression of serum LH in adult male rats following treatment with DMI plus 5,7-DHT (47). Serotonin appears also to be involved in the inhibition of the pituitary release of prolactin in the adult male rat (47). The specificity of this latter effect is, however, difficult to assess, since serotonin-deficient rats are extremely stress-sensitive.

It should be emphasized that the analysis of functional changes in animals lesioned with neurotoxic indoleamines is extremely complicated. Such analysis should ideally include a correlation between the behavioral or neuroendocrine data with a number of biochemical and structural parameters, such as the extent and selectivity of the drug-induced lesion, the drug-induced changes in the activity of the serotonergic neurons, the changes in receptor sensitivity, the extent and location of degeneration, and the time course of the drug-induced effects. It seems particularly important to remember that a reduction in serotonin in the CNS induced by a neurotoxic indoleamine is very different from a reduction induced, say, by synthesis inhibitors or amine-depleting drugs. Thus, for example, a partial reduction in brain 5-HT induced by 5,6- or 5,7-DHT reflects the removal of part of the 5-HT fibers, whereas remaining fibers are intact, In fact, such a denervation is probably complete in certain nuclei and partial or absent in others. Moreover, in a brain with a partial destruction of the terminal networks, the functioning of the remaining, intact fibers are likely to change in response to the damage, for example, by an increased or decreased activity.

MODE OF ACTION OF NEUROTOXIC INDOLEAMINES

In order to produce selective neurotoxic effects on central 5-HT neurons, the toxic tryptamines must be provided with a reasonable affinity to the 5-HT uptake sites in brain. The lack of affinity to the 5-HT transport mechanism coincides with a lack of toxicity on serotonin neurons, but, at the same time, with potential toxicity for all nonserotonergic structures in brain. All compounds that have been found to be toxic to monoamine neurons are capable of forming quinone-like metabolites. These metabolites are most likely involved in the molecular mechanism of action of all neurotoxic indoleamines. Based on our present-day understanding of the physico-chemical properties of quinones and quinoneimines, the following hypotheses concerning the molecular mechanism of action of the indoleneurotoxins may be formulated: the cytotoxicity may depend on (a) formation of hydrogen peroxide, (b) covalent irreversible binding of indolequinones to nucleophilic groups of proteins, particularly their SH-groups, and subsequent denaturation of the proteins (48, 49), (c) uncoupling of oxidation and phosphorylation and/or arrest of electron transport in respiratory chain enzymes due to replacement of ubiquinones by cytotoxic indolequinones with subsequent block of ATP formation. Irreversible binding of radioactive metabolites of 6-OH-DA, 5,6-, and 5,7-DHT to proteins has been verified in vitro and in vivo, suggesting that protein denaturation may be important for the toxicity of certain indole- and catecholneurotoxins (48–50). The binding of 5,6-DHT, and particularly 5,7-DHT, to monoamine oxidase seems to be an important step in the events leading to toxicity, since monoamine oxidase-resistant α-methylated analogs have reduced in vivo and in vitro effects on NA and 5-HT neurons (6, 21), and since monoamine oxidase inhibitors counteract the toxic effects of 5,7-DHT on NA neurons.

SUMMARY

Taken together, the available data indicate that 5,7-DHT, in combination with ip DMI or monoamine oxidase inhibitors, can be considered a tool for selective lesioning of central 5-HT axons and terminals, useful for the analysis of function of serotonin neurons in various forms of behavior, in neuroendocrine regulation, and in drug interaction. The neurotoxic indoleamines are also important new tools for studies on neuronal ontogeny, regeneration, and plasticity in the CNS.

ACKNOWLEDGMENTS

This review is based mainly on work supported by grants from the Deutsche Forschungsgemeinschaft and the Swedish Medical Research Council (04X-3874, 04X-56).

110 BAUMGARTEN & BJÖRKLUND

Literature Cited

1. Thoenen, H., Tranzer, J. P. 1968. *Arch. Pharmacol. Exp. Pathol.* 261:271–88
2. Uretsky, N. J., Iversen, L. L. 1970. *J. Neurochem.* 17:269–78
3. Ungerstedt, U. 1968. *Eur. J. Pharmacol.* 5:107–10
4. Björklund, A., Baumgarten, H. G., Rensch, A. 1975. *J. Neurochem.* 24: 833–35
5. Gerson, S., Baldessarini, R. J. 1975. *Brain Res.* 85:140–45
6. Baumgarten, H. G., Björklund, A., Nobin, A., Rosengren, E., Schlossberger, H. G. 1975. *Acta Physiol. Scand. Suppl.* 429:1–27
7. Baumgarten, H. G., Björklund, A., Horn, A. S. Schlossberger, H. G. 1974. *Dynamics of Degeneration and Growth in Neurons,* ed. K. Fuxe, L. Olson, and Y. Zotterman, 153–67. Oxford & New York: Pergamon
8. Baumgarten, H. G., Björklund, A., Lachenmayer, L., Nobin, A. 1973. *Acta Physiol. Scand. Suppl.* 391:1–9
9. Björklund, A., Baumgarten, H. G., Nobin, A. 1974. *Adv. Biochem. Psycho. Pharmacol.* 10:13–33
10. Baumgarten, H. G., Evetts, K. D., Holman, R. B., Iversen, L. L., Vogt, M., Wilson, G. 1972. *J. Neurochem.* 19: 1587–97
11. Baumgarten, H. G., Björklund, A., Lachenmayer, L., Nobin, A., Stenevi, U. 1971. *Acta Physiol. Scand. Suppl.* 373:1–15
12. Björklund, A., Lindvall, O. 1975. Unpublished observations
13. Nobin, A., Baumgarten, H. G., Björklund, A., Lachenmayer, L., Stenevi, U. 1973. *Brain Res.* 56:1–24
14. Baumgarten, H. G., Björklund, A., Nobin, A., Rosengren, E. 1975. Unpublished observations
15. Vogt, M. 1974. *J. Physiol. London* 236:483–98
16. Costa, E., Lefevre, H., Meek, J., Revuelta, A., Spano, F., Strada, S., Daly, J. 1972. *Brain Res.* 44:304–8
17. Breese, G. R., Cooper, B. R., Grant, L. D., Smith, R. D. 1974. *Neuropharmacology* 13:177–87
18. Björklund, A., Nobin, A., Stenevi, U. 1973. *Z. Zellforsch.* 145:479–501
19. Lytle, L. D., Jacoby, J. H., Nelson, M. F., Baumgarten, H. G. 1975. *Life Sci.* 15:1203–17
20. Horn, A. S., Baumgarten, H. G., Schlossberger, H. G. 1973. *J. Neurochem.* 21:231–36

21. Björklund, A., Horn, A. S., Baumgarten, H. G., Nobin, A., Schlossberger, H. G. 1975. *Acta Physiol. Scand.* 429: 30–60
22. Iversen, L. L., Uretsky, N. J. 1971. *6-Hydroxydopamine and Catecholamine Nurons,* ed. T. Malmfors and H. Thoenen, 171–86. Amsterdam: North-Holland
23. Gerson, S., Baldessarini, R. J., Wheeler, S. C. 1974. *J. Neuropharmacol.* 13:987–1004
24. Sachs, C. 1971. See Ref. 22, pp. 59–74
25. Björklund, A., Nobin, A., Stenevi, U. 1973. *Brain Res.* 53:117–27
26. Clineschmidt, B. V., Pierce, J. E., Lovenberg, W. 1971. *J. Neurochem.* 18:1593–96
27. Victor, S. J., Baumgarten, H. G., Lovenberg, W. 1974. *J. Neurochem.* 22:541–46
28. Björklund, A., Nobin, A., Stenevi, U. 1973. *Brain Res.* 50:214–20
29. Nobin, A., Baumgarten, H. G., Björklund, A., Lachenmayer, L., Stenevi, U. 1973. *Brain Res.* 56:1–24
30. Baumgarten, H. G., Lachenmayer, L., Björklund, A., Nobin, A., Rosengren, E. *Life Sci.* 12:357–64
31. Baumgarten, H. G., Victor, S. J., Lovenberg, W. 1973. *J. Neurochem.* 21:251–53
32. Baumgarten, H. G., Victor, S. J., Bruckwick, E., Lovenberg, W. 1975. Unpublished observations
33. Baumgarten, H. G., Victor, S. J., Lovenberg, W. 1975. *Psychopharmacol. Commun.* 1:75–88
34. Baumgarten, H. G., Lachenmayer, L., Schlossberger, H. G. 1972. *Z. Zellforsch.* 125:535–69
35. Baumgarten, H. G., Lachenmayer, L. 1972. *Z. Zellforsch.* 135:395–414
36. Baumgarten, H. G., Björklund, A., Lachenmayer, L., Rensch, A., Rosengren, E. 1974. *Cell. Tiss. Res.* 152:271–81
37. Björklund, A., Baumgarten, H. G., Lachenmayer, L., Rosengren, E. 1975. *Cell Tissue Res.* 161:145–55
38. Baumgarten, H. G., Björklund, A., Holstein, A. F., Nobin, A. 1972. *Z. Zellforsch.* 129:256–71
39. Baumgarten, H. G., Göthert, M., Holstein, A. F., Schlossberger, H. G. 1972. *Z. Zellforsch.* 128:115–34
40. Baumgarten, H. G., Groth, H. P., Göthert, M., Manian, A. 1974. *Arch. Pharmacol.* 282:245–54

41. Breese, G. R., Cooper, B. R. 1975. *Brain Res.* 98:517-28
42. Baumgarten, H. G., Björklund, A. 1975. Unpublished observations
43. Longo, V. G., Scotti de Carolis, A., Liuzzi, A., Massotti, M. 1974. *Adv. Biochem. Psychopharmacol.* 10:109-20
44. Koe, B. K., Weissman, A. 1968. *Adv. Pharmacol.* 6B:29-47
45. Müller, E. E., Baumgarten, H. G., Gil-Ad, I., Udeschini, G., Cocchi, D. 1975. Unpublished observations
46. Skyler, J., Baumgarten, H. G., Lovenberg, W. 1975. Unpublished observations

47. Wuttke, W., Baumgarten, H. G., Björklund, A. 1975. Unpublished observations
48. Victor, S. J., Baumgarten, H. G., Bogdanski, D. F., Lovenberg, W. Schlossberger, H. G., 1975. Unpublished observations
49. Baumgarten, H. G., Björklund, A., Bogdanski, D. F. 1975. *Chemical Tools in Catecholamine Research,* ed. G. Jonsson, T. Malmfors, Ch. Sachs, 59-66. Amsterdam: North-Holland
50. Saner, A., Thoenen, H. 1971. *Mol. Pharmacol.* 7:147-54

CENTRAL NORADRENERGIC CONTROL OF BLOOD PRESSURE

◆6640

A. Scriabine, B. V. Clineschmidt, and C. S. Sweet

Merck Institute for Therapeutic Research, West Point, Pennsylvania 19486

The importance of central catecholaminergic neurons in the control of systemic arterial pressure has been revealed to a great extent through pharmacological studies, for example, investigations on the mechanisms of action of antihypertensive drugs such as methyldopa and clonidine. The use of pharmacological tools like 6-hydroxydopamine has also yielded important information that probably was unattainable by any other means. Our intention is to review pertinent studies that were basically pharmacological in nature, after first briefly considering the distribution of catecholaminergic neurons in the brain and spinal cord.

DISTRIBUTION

The distribution of norepinephrine-containing nerve terminals and cell bodies in the central nervous system (CNS) provides in itself sufficient reason for seriously considering that this monoamine participates in the central integration and regulation of systemic arterial blood pressure. With the Falck-Hillarp histochemical fluorescence method, groups of cell bodies containing norepinephrine were visualized principally in the medulla and pons, the A1, A2, and A4-7 cell groups of Dahlström & Fuxe's classification (1). Axons emanating from these cell bodies, as visualized also by the Falck-Hillarp technique, organize into ascending dorsal and ventral bundles (2) and a descending bulbospinal system. Practically all noradrenergic cell groups in the medulla and pons contribute fibers to the ventral bundle (3), whereas the bulbospinal system receives input only from the two most caudal cell groups, A1 and A2 (4). The organization of the ascending noradrenergic fibers as revealed by the more recent and more sensitive glyoxylic acid fluorescence method (5) indicates a greater degree of complexity than previously described, but the details are beyond the scope of the present review. Of particular importance with regard to the control of arterial pressure is the demonstrated (6) high density of norepinephrine-containing terminals in the nucleus tractus solitarii (NTS), nucleus dorsalis motorius nervi vagi, and sympathetic intermediolateral columns, as well as a varying density of noradrener-

113

gic terminals throughout the hypothalamus. The terminals close to preganglionic sympathetic neurons in the spinal cord originate from cell bodies situated in the ventrolateral part of the reticular formation (A1 group) and from cell bodies lying in the area of the solitary-vagal complex, including the nucleus commissuralis (A2 group). Thus, the NTS contains noradrenergic cell bodies and receives a noradrenergic input. The origin of the noradrenergic neurons terminating in the NTS remains somewhat vague but their possible significance is clear since one of the primary relay points for baroreceptor afferents is in the NTS (7). The hypothalamus, which exerts well-known and important influences on baroreceptor reflexes and sympathetic nervous outflow, receives its highly complex noradrenergic input from the ascending noradrenergic fiber systems (2, 5).

Recently the possibility has arisen that epinephrine, in addition to norepinephrine, could also be involved in the central control of arterial pressure. Epinephrine in mammalian brain accounts for approximately only 10% of the total amount of norepinephrine and epinephrine. However, results from recent studies support the proposal of an independent neuronal network containing epinephrine in the rat brain. The distribution of these putative adrenergic neurons has been explored indirectly by the immunocytochemical localization in neurons of phenylethanolamine-N-methyltransferase (PNMT) (8–10), the enzyme that catalyzes conversion of norepinephrine to epinephrine, and with a sensitive radio-enzymatic assay for PNMT (11). The distribution of epinephrine has also been examined more directly in some nuclei and other areas of rat brain using mass fragmentography (12). Based on the immunohistochemical studies of Hökfelt and co-workers (9, 10), epinephrine-containing cell bodies have so far been located in two cell clusters, termed C1 and C2, and their locations correspond to the A1 and A2 cell groups of Dahlström & Fuxe. Furthermore, the density of adrenergic terminals (specifically PNMT positive terminals) is high in NTS, nucleus dorsalis motorius nervi vagi, and the lateral sympathetic columns, whereas the density of terminals varies in different regions of the hypothalamus. Thus, the putative adrenergic neurons are well placed for exerting control over the cardiovascular system.

NORADRENERGIC NEURONS IN EXPERIMENTAL HYPERTENSION

Two recent extensive reviews covered this topic in detail (13, 14); therefore, only the most pertinent reports are dealt with here. Hypertension in the rat can be produced by bilateral lesions of NTS (15). Noradrenergic neurons are apparently involved, because 6-hydroxydopamine administered intracisternally prevented this form of hypertension (16). 6-Hydroxydopamine administered centrally has also been reported to prevent other forms of hypertension including neurogenic hypertension produced by sinoaortic denervation (17), hypertension in spontaneously hypertensive (SH) rats, DOCA-salt, and renal hypertension (18). Lewis and co-workers (19) reported that depletion of brain catecholamines by intracisternal 6-hydroxydopamine in rabbits significantly attenuated the rise in arterial pressure following wrapping the kidney in cellophane. Because the early phase in arterial renal hypertension is under the control of the renin-angiotensin system, Lewis's study suggested an interrelationship between the kidney and the central nervous system. Of interest was their observation that the pressor response to intraventricular angiotensin was significantly reduced by 6-hydroxydopamine. Severs & Daniels-Severs (20) have recently reviewed the effects of angiotensin II on the CNS. Currently it is understood that the site of the central hypertensive effects of angiotensin II is the nucleus mesencephalicus in the midbrain and/or the area postrema in the caudal half of the medulla. These sites are heavily innervated by noradrenergic nerves.

CENTRAL CARDIOVASCULAR EFFECTS OF α-ADRENERGIC AGONISTS

Norepinephrine and Related Substances

Norepinephrine elicits a fall in systemic pressure and bradycardia following intracerebroventricular (i.c.v.) administration in the anesthetized dog (21–23), cat (24–26), rat (27), and rabbit (28). Prior i.c.v. injection of phentolamine (22) or phenoxybenzamine (23) markedly diminishes these actions of norepinephrine, suggesting that central receptors similar to the peripheral α-adrenergic receptor are involved. Moreover, other α-adrenergic receptor agonists such as α-methyl-norepinephrine (29), dopamine (27), epinephrine (24), and phenylephrine (23) have also been reported to produce hypotension and bradycardia after i.c.v. administration. Using unanesthetized cats, Day & Roach (30) reported hypotensive and cardiac-slowing effects following i.c.v. administration of norepinephrine or α-methylnorepinephrine; both effects were abolished after i.c.v. administration of phentolamine. Similar results were obtained when epinephrine was given i.c.v., but only if the β-adrenergic receptor blocking agent, propranolol, was first injected centrally. Of importance was Baum & Shropshire's (27) finding of reduced electrical activity in lumbar sympathetic chains after i.c.v. injection of norepinephrine or dopamine. These observations suggest that activation of α-adrenergic receptors in the CNS leads to hypotension and bradycardia. The location of these receptors is an important point that has received attention only recently. Struyker Boudier et al (31) surveyed several sites in the rat hypothalamus, extending in a caudal-rostral direction from the mammillary area to the preoptic region, to determine whether arterial pressure and heart rate were reduced upon injection of norepinephrine. Hypotension and bradycardia were consistently elicited from the anterior hypothalamic/preoptic region (AH/PO) and phentolamine applied locally was an effective antagonist. Phenylephrine was more effective than oxymetazoline in reducing blood pressure and heart rate when microinjected into the AH/PO area (32) even though both agents were approximately equal as stimulants of peripheral α-adrenergic receptors. This observation may reflect a subtle difference between typical peripheral α-adrenergic receptors and the central α-adrenergic receptors mediating hypotension and bradycardia. Such an explanation could perhaps account for the finding (33) that epinephrine was about ten times more potent than norepinephrine upon application to the AH/PO region. De Jong (34) microinjected norepinephrine into the NTS in rats and found a decrease in systemic arterial pressure and heart rate, an effect susceptible to blockade by locally administered phentolamine.

According to Neumayr et al (35), electrical stimulation in cats near the areas of the solitary-vagal complex (i.e. near the A2 cell group) or in the ventrolateral reticular region (i.e. close to the A1 group) produces pressor responses and sympathetic discharge. These investigators proposed that the bulbospinal noradrenergic pathway excites preganglionic sympathetic neurons. This proposal is consistent with an accelerated turnover of norepinephrine in the thoracolumbar cord in rabbits with neurogenic hypertension (36). However, Coote & Macleod (37) reached the opposite conclusion. They suggest that the descending noradrenergic pathway arising from A1 cell cluster is inhibitory to sympathetic outflow. Furthermore, in the rat, electrical stimulation near the NTS region was recently reported to lower arterial pressure and heart rate (38).

Methyldopa

The possible relationship between central α-adrenergic receptors and the mode of action of methyldopa was reviewed recently by Van Zwieten (39) and Day & Roach (40). Upon entering the central nervous system, methyldopa undergoes decarboxylation via L-aromatic amino acid decarboxylase and hydroxylation via dopamine-β-hydroxylase to form α-methyldopamine and α-methylnorepinephrine (41). The dependence of the antihypertensive effect of methyldopa on the formation of these metabolites in the CNS was first clearly demonstrated by Henning & Van Zweiten (42, 43). Inhibition of decarboxylase in peripheral tissues with carbidopa did not substantially alter the hypotensive effect of methyldopa in renal hypertensive rats, whereas inhibition of both peripheral and central decarboxylase with benserazide (RO 4–4602) abolished the response. Evidence has also been obtained indicating that conversion of α-methyldopamine to α-methylnorepinephrine is important for the full expression of the hypotensive effect of methyldopa (44–47). It is well established that the central nervous system is the principal site of action of methyldopa. Furthermore, it is clear that α-methylnorepinephrine is the active metabolite. It has been hypothesized that α-methylnorepinephrine released from monoaminergic neurons interacts with central α-adrenergic receptors more strongly than norepinephrine itself, thus effecting a reduction in blood pressure—a variation of the original "false transmitter" hypothesis (40). α-Methylnorepinephrine and norepinephrine appear to be equiactive with respect to decreasing arterial pressure following i.c.v. administration (30, 47), although the α-methylated compound may have a longer duration of action (30). Injection of α-methylnorepinephrine into the AH/PO region in the rat induced depressor effects at doses lower than those needed to obtain depressor effects with norepinephrine (48). α-Methylnorepinephrine also appears to be more effective than norepinephrine in decreasing blood pressure and heart rate following injection into the NTS of the medulla oblongata (49). The greater efficacy of α-methylnorepinephrine may be the result of less effective inactivation mechanisms for the α-methylated compound or of some difference in the ability of α-methylnorepinephrine and norepinephrine to activate central α-adrenergic receptors. Whether α-methylnorepinephrine acts on postjunctional receptors to facilitate synaptic transmission or on prejunctional α-adrenergic receptors (see below) to inhibit noradrenergic or adrenergic transmission remains to be ascertained.

Clonidine

The first clinical observation suggesting a utility for α-adrenergic stimulants in the treatment of hypertension was made in 1957 by Finnerty et al (50). They observed that a nasal decongestant, tetrahydrozoline, an imidazoline with α-adrenergic stimulant properties, given orally lowered arterial pressure in hypertensive patients. The mechanism of antihypertensive action of tetrahydrozoline was not established. Subsequent pharmacological studies characterized this drug as a peripheral α-adrenergic stimulant that lowered cardiac output and heart rate possibly by a central action (51, 52). Numerous related imidazolines had similar activity (53). The importance of α-adrenergic receptors in the control of arterial pressure has been revealed largely by studies on the mode of action of clonidine (54). Van Zwieten reviewed the earlier pharmacological and clinical studies with clonidine emphasizing its central site of action (55).

According to Schmitt et al (56), clonidine decreased the sympathetic activity in the splanchnic and cardiac nerves in normal animals as well as in animals with denervated carotid sinuses. Clonidine had pronounced hypotensive activity when injected or infused into the vertebral artery of cats or dogs (57, 58); it also reduced arterial pressure by intracisternal administration of doses that were ineffective when injected intravenously (59). In cross-circulation experiments, clonidine administered into the arterial inflow of neurally intact but vascularly isolated heads of recipient dogs led to a decrease in arterial pressure in both the recipient and donor dogs (60).

Several studies suggest that the hypotensive and cardiac-slowing effects of clonidine involve α-adrenergic receptors. For example, it has been shown that the hypotensive effect of clonidine in rabbits was reduced by α-adrenergic blocking agents, tolazoline, and phenoxybenzamine (61). Also, an α-adrenergic blocking agent, piperoxane, by either intravenous or intracisternal administration antagonized the hypotensive and cardiac-slowing effects of clonidine in cats (62). These and other studies (63, 64) on the interaction of clonidine with α-adrenergic blocking drugs led to the conclusion that clonidine interacts with α-adrenergic receptors to decrease blood pressure and heart rate.

In addition to reducing sympathetic outflow to the heart, clonidine was also shown to enhance pressure-sensitive compensatory reflexes (65–68). This effect was found to be vagally mediated. Further studies of this phenomenon (69–71) indicated that clonidine acted on the central nervous system to enhance vagal activity and that this action also involved central α-adrenergic receptors.

The site of central hypotensive action of clonidine has been the subject of numerous investigations. Destruction of a medullary depressor area in cats and dogs antagonized the hypotensive effect of clonidine (72). Because the effects of clonidine were, however, never completely abolished, other sites of action of clonidine must be considered (72). Further studies on localization of the site of central hypotensive action of clonidine in cats led to the conclusion that clonidine exerts its action on "chemosensitive zones" located on the ventral surface of the brain stem (73). There is also evidence that an additional site of action of clonidine may be the spinal cord. In spinal cats, stimulation of the dorsal lateral column below the transection caused sympathetic discharge that was reduced by clonidine (74). Klevans et al (75) have also presented some evidence that supramedullary structures are involved in central cardiovascular effects of clonidine. On the basis of studies discussed above, it can be concluded that clonidine acts at multiple sites within the central nervous system.

Several investigators have considered the possibility that dopaminergic or serotonergic systems might be involved in the mechanism of the hypotensive action of clonidine. The hypotensive effect of clonidine in cats was not blocked by dopaminergic blocking agents, pimozide and spiroperidol (76).

According to other investigators, however, dopamine and clonidine, but not norepinephrine, lowered arterial pressure when applied to the ventral surface of the brain stem in cats. These effects of clonidine and dopamine were blocked by pimozide (77). In DOCA-saline hypertensive rats, the antihypertensive effect of clonidine was not modified by 5, 6-dihydroxytryptamine or p-chloro-N-methylamphetamine, drugs that destroy central serotonin-containing neurons, but was antagonized by desipramine, piperoxane, or phentolamine (78).

In addition to previously described effects of clonidine on the central nervous system, the drug also inhibits sympathetic transmission at a peripheral site or sites. Scriabine et al (79, 80) reported that clonidine reduced heart rate in dogs with spinal cord sectioned at the level of the second cervical vertebra, antagonized the pressor and positive chronotropic effects of a muscarinic ganglionic stimulant, McN A-343 (4-(m-chlorophenylcarbamoyloxy)-2-butynyltrimethylammonium chloride), blocked cardiac acceleration caused by low frequency electrical stimulation of right postganglionic cardiac sympathetic nerve in dogs (with or without vagotomy), and slowed the heart rate by direct administration into the artery supplying the sinus node. In isolated rabbit hearts, clonidine also antagonized release of norepinephrine caused by electrical stimulation of intact sympathetic nerves (81). This inhibitory effect of clonidine on norepinephrine release was not due to its local anesthetic activity and was inversely related to overflow of norepinephrine caused by control electrical stimulation prior to administration of clonidine (82, 83). This negative correlation was thought to reflect competition between clonidine and liberated norepinephrine for a receptor site. On the basis of these findings, Starke hypothesized the existence of a presynaptic α-adrenergic receptor mediating feedback control of norepinephrine release (84). According to this concept, the release of norepinephrine by nerve impulses is inhibited by a feedback system; the feedback loop consists of released norepinephrine and α-adrenergic receptors on the nerve endings. α-Adrenergic antagonists block the access of norepinephrine and other α-stimulants to the receptors at the nerve membrane, thereby interrupting the feedback loop and facilitating the release of norepinephrine.

This concept of α-adrenergic receptor–mediated feedback control of norepinephrine release has been extended to central noradrenergic neurons. Clonidine was found to diminish the stimulation-evoked tritium overflow from slices of rat cerebral cortex preincubated with ^{3}H-norepinephrine. The extent of this inhibition was greater at a low than at a high frequency of stimulation. α-Adrenergic blocking agents, phentolamine and phenoxybenzamine, increased the stimulation-induced release of norepinephrine from the cerebral cortical slices (85).

These observations raise the question as to the possible importance of prejunctional α-adrenergic receptors to the central hypotensive action of clonidine. The destruction of noradrenergic neurons by 6-hydroxydopamine reduced the hypotensive effect of clonidine in rabbits (86). In rats, however, Haeusler & Finch (87) found that 6-hydroxydopamine given i.c.v. did not alter the hypotensive effect of clonidine. In cats pretreated with reserpine and α-methyl-p-tyrosine at doses sufficient to produce marked depletion of norepinephrine in the central and peripheral nervous systems, clonidine produced its usual inhibitory effect on sympathetic nerve activity but higher doses were required (88).

Drugs Related to Clonidine

Among other α-adrenergic stimulants with central hypotensive activity, xylazine, 2-(2,6-dimethylphenylamino)-4H-5,6-dihydro-1,3-thiazine (Bayer 1470), is probably the most thoroughly investigated compound. In the initial pharmacological studies (89) xylazine inhibited the response to adrenergic as well as cholinergic nerve stimulation and had peripheral adrenergic stimulant and central hypotensive effects. It was also highly potent as an analgesic and sedative; as such it found application in veterinary medicine (90).

Central hypotensive activity was also observed in a series of oxazoline derivatives. The most active were Bay a6781, 2-[2-(e)-methyl-6(e)-methylcyclohexyl]-1-(e)-amino-2-oxazoline (91), and LD 2855, 2-(2,6-dimethylphenylamino)-1,3-oxazol-2-ine (92). The mechanism of their antihypertensive action appeared to be similar to clonidine.

Extensive pharmacological studies with guanabenz (WY 8678; BR 750; 2,6-dichlorobenzylideneamino guanidine acetate) indicated that this compound is also, in some respects, similar to clonidine. It was shown to lower arterial pressure by at least two mechanisms, i.e. centrally mediated reduction in sympathetic nerve activity and peripheral adrenergic neuron blockade (93–95).

Another α-adrenergic stimulant with antihypertensive activity is N-amidino-2-(2,6-dichlorophenyl) acetamide hydrochloride or BS 100/141 (96). BS 100/141 was shown to have peripheral α-adrenergic stimulant action in cats, dogs, and rats. By infusion into the vertebral artery or by injection into the lateral cerebral ventricle of anesthetized cats, BS 100/141 produced a marked reduction in arterial pressure and heart rate at doses that were ineffective intravenously. BS 100/141 also reduced norepinephrine turnover rate in the brain stem of rats apparently by virtue of its α-adrenergic stimulant activity. The site of central antihypertensive action of BS 100/141 has been claimed to be different from clonidine. Clonidine reduced arterial pressure by topical application to the ventral surface of medulla oblongata of cats; under similar experimental conditions, BS 100/141 was ineffective.

Desipramine-Clonidine Interaction

Of considerable interest in relation to the site and the mechanism of hypotensive action of clonidine and of other α-adrenergic stimulants is the interaction between clonidine and desipramine, a tricyclic antidepressant and a neuronal uptake inhibitor of norepinephrine. According to Reid et al (97) the hypotensive activity of clonidine given intracisternally to rabbits was antagonized by desipramine. This interaction was confirmed in cats (98) and in man (99) but not in rabbits (100). Other tricyclic antidepressants also antagonized the hypotensive effects of clonidine in cats (98). The interaction of clonidine with desipramine is of clinical and also of theoretical significance. If inhibition of the uptake mechanism at the presynaptic sites of noradrenergic neurons is responsible for the interaction between clonidine and desipramine, a presynaptic site must be involved in the mode of antihypertensive action of clonidine.

CENTRAL β-ADRENERGIC RECEPTORS

Not only α- but also β-adrenergic receptors may be involved in the central regulation of arterial pressure. The presence of β-adrenergic receptors within the central nervous system was first suggested by Share & Melville (101) who found that intraventricular injection of the β-adrenergic blocking drug, dichloroisoproterenol (DCI) attenuated the cardiac acceleration resulting from an intraventricular injection of picrotoxin. Subsequently, a number of investigators demonstrated that isoproterenol, administered intraventricularly, will either raise or lower arterial pressure depending on the species and experimental conditions. Thus, in anesthetized cats (102), dogs (23, 103, 104), rabbits (28, 105, 106), and rats (107), an i.c.v. injection of isoproterenol has been reported to cause hypotension and tachycardia. Day & Roach (108), however, found that isoproterenol caused a pressor response and tachycardia in conscious cats. In a more extensive subsequent study (30), this effect was observed in only about one half of the cats examined; in the remaining animals, isoproterenol produced hypotension and tachycardia. A number of investigators have been able to block the effects of i.c.v. injections of isoproterenol by i.c.v. administration of β-adrenergic blocking agents (23, 30, 102, 105, 106, 108). The effects of isoproterenol are of central origin because section of the spinal cord (23, 102) and ganglion blockade (108) abolished the cardiovascular effects of i.c.v. injection of isoproterenol. Taken collectively, the available data indicate that centrally mediated cardiovascular effects of isoproterenol can be demonstrated in animals but the variability observed has not been satisfactorily explained.

Clinical studies have clearly demonstrated that β-adrenergic blocking drugs have antihypertensive activity. Early studies in man suggested that propranolol may have central nervous system side effects. A number of investigators tried to determine whether the central nervous system is involved in mediating the hypotensive effects of β-adrenergic blocking drugs. Kelliher & Buckley (109) were the first to provide evidence for a central site of action. Other workers, using various techniques and animal species, have observed a fall in arterial pressure after central administration of β-adrenergic blocking drugs (30, 106, 108, 110, 111). The usual response to an i.c.v. injection of a β-adrenergic blocking agent is a transient rise in arterial pressure followed by a sustained fall. This early rise in arterial pressure has been attributed to the local anesthetic action of β-adrenergic blocking drugs (105, 106) but hypertensive response to timolol i.c.v. (110), a β-adrenergic blocking agent devoid of local anesthetic properties, has also been observed. Reports on the cardiovascular effects of vertebral artery injections of propranolol are conflicting (111, 112). Stern et al (111) observed a difference between intravenous versus intravertebral injections of propranolol, but Offerhaus & Van Zwieten (112) found similar hypotensive effects regardless of which route of administration was used. It has not been clearly shown that the cardiovascular effects of centrally administered propranolol are mediated through central noradrenergic neurons. However, according to one report (105), propranolol administered i.c.v. does not produce a fall in arterial pressure in rabbits pretreated with intracisternal 6-hydroxydopamine, an observation suggesting that noradrenergic neurons must be intact for the drug to exert its central hypotensive effect.

CONCLUSIONS

In recent years, it has become apparent that central noradrenergic neurons are involved in the regulation of arterial pressure. Areas in the central nervous system known to be involved in the control of arterial pressure and heart rate are densely innervated by noradrenergic neurons. Destruction of these neurons with 6-hydroxydopamine prevents the development of certain forms of hypertension in animals. Noradrenergic control of arterial pressure is mediated at least partially through central α-adrenergic receptors. β-Adrenergic receptors in the central nervous system have been identified, but their importance in the regulation of arterial pressure remains to be defined. The main site of antihypertensive action of methyldopa and clonidine is the central nervous system. The evidence suggests that their effects are mediated through α-adrenergic receptors at a pre- or postsynaptic site.

Further understanding of central noradrenergic control of arterial pressure will provide a basis for development of novel and more selective antihypertensive drugs.

Literature Cited

1. Dahlström, A., Fuxe, K. 1964. *Acta Physiol. Scand.* 62:Suppl. 232, 1–55
2. Ungerstedt, U. 1971. *Acta Physiol. Scand.* 82:Suppl. 367, 1–48
3. Bolme, P., Fuxe, K., Lidbrink, P. 1972. *Res. Commun. Chem. Pathol. Pharmacol.* 4:657–97
4. Dahlström, A., Fuxe, K. 1965. *Acta Physiol. Scand.* 64:Suppl. 247, 1–36
5. Lindvall, O., Björklund, A. 1974. *Acta Physiol. Scand.* 92:Suppl. 412, 1–48
6. Fuxe, K. 1965. *Acta Physiol Scand.* 64:Suppl. 247, 37–85
7. Crill, W. E., Reis, D. J. 1968. *Am. J. Physiol.* 214:269–76

8. Hökfelt, T., Fuxe, K., Goldstein, M. 1973. *Brain Res.* 62:461–69
9. Hökfelt, T., Fuxe, K., Goldstein, M., Johansson, O. 1973. *Acta Physiol. Scand.* 89:286–88
10. Hökfelt, T., Fuxe, K., Goldstein, M., Johansson, O. 1974. *Brain Res.* 66:235–51
11. Saavedra, J. M., Palkovits, M., Brownstein, M. J., Axelrod, J. 1974. *Nature London* 248:695–96
12. Koslow, S. H., Schlumpf, M. 1974. *Nature London* 251:530–31
13. Reis, D. J., Doba, N. 1974. *Prog. Cardiovasc. Dis.* 17:51–71

14. Chalmers, J. P. 1975. *Circ. Res.* 36:469–80
15. Doba, N., Reis, D. J. 1973. *Circ. Res.* 32:584–93
16. Doba, N., Reis, D. J. 1974. *Circ. Res.* 34:293–301
17. Chalmers, J. P., Reid, J. L. 1972. *Circ. Res.* 31:789–804
18. Haeusler, G., Finch, L., Thoenen, H. 1972. *Experientia* 28:1200–1203
19. Lewis, P. J., Reid, J. L., Chalmers, J. P., Dollery, C. T. 1973. *Clin. Sci. Mol. Med.* 45:115S–18S
20. Severs, W. B., Daniels—Severs, A. E. 1973. *Pharmacol. Rev.* 25:415–49
21. McCubbin, J. W., Kaneko, Y., Page, I. H. 1960. *Circ. Res.* 8:849–58
22. Kaneko, Y., McCubbin, J. W., Page, I. H. 1960. *Circ. Res.* 8:1228–34
23. Bhargava, K. P., Mishra, N., Tangri, K. K. 1972. *Br. J. Pharmacol.* 45:596–602
24. Nashold, B. S., Mannarino, E., Wunderlich, M. 1962. *Nature London* 193:1297–98
25. Share, N. N., Melville, K. I. 1963. *J. Pharmacol. Exp. Ther.* 141:15–21
26. Smookler, H. H., Severs, W. B., Kinnard, W. J., Buckley, J. P. 1966. *J. Pharmacol. Exp. Ther.* 153:485–94
27. Baum, T., Shropshire, A. T. 1973. *Neuropharmacology* 12:49–56
28. Toda, N., Matsuda, Y., Shimamoto, K. 1969. *Int. J. Neuropharmacol.* 8:451–61
29. Heise, A., Kroneberg, G. 1972. *Eur. J. Pharmacol.* 17:315–17
30. Day, M. D., Roach, A. G. 1974. *Br. J. Pharmacol.* 51:325–33
31. Struyker Boudier, H. A. J., Smeets, G. W. M., Brouwer, G. M., van Rossum, J. M. 1974. *Neuropharmacology* 13:837–46
32. Struyker Boudier, H., Smeets, G., Brouwer, G., van Rossum, J. 1974. *Life Sci.* 15:887–99
33. Struyker Boudier, H. A. J., Bekers, A. 1975. *Eur. J. Pharmacol.* 31:153–55
34. De Jong, W. 1974. *Eur. J. Pharmacol.* 29:179–81
35. Neumayr, R. J., Hare, B. D., Franz, D. N. 1974. *Life Sci.* 14:793–806
36. Chalmers, J. P., Wurtman, R. J. 1971. *Circ. Res.* 28:480–91
37. Coote, J. H., Macleod, V. H. 1974. *J. Physiol.* 241:453–75
38. De Jong, W., Zandberg, P., Bohus, B. 1975. *Prog. Brain Res.* 42:In press
39. Van Zwieten, P. A. 1973. *J. Pharm. Pharmacol.* 25:89–95
40. Day, M. D., Roach, A. G. 1974. *Clin. Exp. Pharmacol. Physiol.* 1:347–60
41. Carlsson, A., Lindqvist, M. 1962. *Acta Physiol. Scand.* 54:87–94
42. Henning, M., Van Zwieten, P. A. 1968. *J. Pharm. Pharmacol.* 20:409–17
43. Henning, M. 1969. *Acta Pharmacol. Scand.* 27:135–48
44. Henning, M., Rubenson, A. 1971. *J. Pharm. Pharmacol.* 23:407–11
45. Day, M. D., Roach, A. G., Whiting, R. L. 1973. *Eur. J. Pharmacol.* 21:271–80
46. Torchiana, M. L., Lotti, V. J., Clark, C. M., Stone, C. A. 1973. *Arch. Int. Pharmacodyn. Ther.* 205:103–13
47. Heise, A., Kroneberg, G. 1973. *Arch. Pharmacol.* 279:285–300
48. Struyker Boudier, H., Smeets, G., Brouwer, G., van Rossum, J. M. 1975. *Arch. Int. Pharmacodyn. Ther.* 213:285–93
49. De Jong, W., Nijkamp, F. P., Bohus, B. 1975. *Arch. Int. Pharmacodyn. Ther.* 213:272–84
50. Finnerty, F. A., Buchholz, J. H., Guillaudeu, R. L. 1957. *Proc. Soc. Exp. Biol. Med.* 94:376–79
51. Hutcheon, D. E., P'an, S. Y., Gardocki, J. F., Jaeger, D. A. 1955. *J. Pharmacol. Exp. Ther.* 113:341–52
52. Hutcheon, D. E., Scriabine, A., Niesler, V. N. 1958. *J. Pharmacol. Exp. Ther.* 122:101–9
53. Hutcheon, D. E., Scriabine, A., Ling, J. S., P'an, S. Y., Bloom, B. M. 1964. *Arch. Int. Pharmacodyn. Ther.* 147:146–55
54. Hoefke, W., Kobinger, W. 1966. *Arzneim. Forsch.* 16:1038–50
55. Van Zwieten, P. A. 1968. *Klin. Wochenschr.* 46:77–80
56. Schmitt, H., Schmitt, H., Boissier, J. R., Giudicelli, J. F. 1967. *Eur. J. Pharmacol.* 2:147–48
57. Sattler, R. W., Van Zwieten, P. A. 1967. *Eur. J. Pharmacol.* 2:9–13
58. Constantine, J. W., McShane, W. K. 1968. *Eur. J. Pharmacol.* 4:109–23
59. Schmitt, H., Schmitt, H., Boissier, J. R., Giudicelli, J. F., Fichelle, J. 1968. *Eur. J. Pharmacol.* 2:340–46
60. Sherman, G. P., Grega, G. J., Woods, R. J., Buckley, J. P. 1968. *Eur. J. Pharmacol.* 2:326–28
61. Toda, N., Fukuda, N., Shimamoto, K. 1969. *Jpn. J. Pharmacol.* 19:199–210
62. Schmitt, H., Schmitt, H., Fénard, S. 1971. *Eur. J. Pharmacol.* 14:98–100
63. Schmitt, H., Schmitt, H. 1970. *Eur. J. Pharmacol.* 9:7–13
64. Anden, N. E., Corrodi, H., Fuxe, K.,

Hökfelt, B., Hökfelt, T., Rydin, C., Svensson, T. 1970. *Life Sci.* 9:513–24
65. Robson, R. D., Kaplan, H. R., Laforce, S. 1969. *J. Pharmacol. Exp. Ther.* 169:120–31
66. Robson, R. D., Kaplan, H. R. 1969. *Eur. J. Pharmacol.* 5:328–37
67. Nayler, W. G., Stone, J. 1970. *Eur. J. Pharmacol.* 10:161–67
68. Korner, P. I., Oliver, J. R., Sleight, P., Chalmers, J. P., Robinson, J. S. 1974. *Eur. J. Pharmacol.* 28:189–98
69. Haeusler, G. 1973. *Arch. Pharmacol.* 278:231–46
70. Kobinger, W., Walland, A. 1972. *Eur. J. Pharmacol.* 19:203–9
71. Kobinger, W., Walland, A. 1972. *Eur. J. Pharmacol.* 19:210–17
72. Schmitt, H., Schmitt, H., Fénard, S. 1973. *Experientia* 29:1247–49
73. Bousquet, P., Guertzenstein, P. G. 1973. *Br. J. Pharmacol.* 49:573–79
74. Sinha, J. N., Atkinson, J. M., Schmitt, H. 1973. *Eur. J. Pharmacol.* 24:113–19
75. Klevans, L. R., Kepner, K., Kovacs, J. L. 1973. *Eur. J. Pharmacol.* 24:262–65
76. Bolme, P., Fuxe, K. 1971. *Eur. J. Pharmacol.* 13:168–74
77. Bloch, R., Bousquet, P., Feldman, J., Velly, J., Schwartz, J. 1974. *Thérapie* 29:251–59
78. Finch, L., Buckingham, R. E., Moore, R. A., Bucher, T. J. 1975. *J. Pharm. Pharmacol.* 27:181–86
79. Scriabine, A., Stavorski, J., Wenger, H. C., Torchiana, M. L., Stone, C. A. 1970. *J. Pharmacol. Exp. Ther.* 171:256–64
80. Scriabine, A., Stavorski, J. M. 1973. *Eur. J. Pharmacol.* 24:101–4
81. Starke, K., Schümann, H. J. 1971. *Experientia* 27:70–71
82. Starke, K., Wagner, J., Schümann, H. J. 1972. *Arch. Int. Pharmacodyn. Ther.* 195:291–308
83. Starke, K., Altmann, K. P. 1973. *Neuropharmacology* 12:339–47
84. Starke, K. 1973. *Frontiers in Catecholamine Research*, ed. E. Usdin, S. Snyder, 561–65. New York: Pergamon
85. Starke, K., Montel, H. 1973. *Neuropharmacology* 12:1073–80
86. Dollery, C. T., Reid, J. L. 1973. *Br. J. Pharmacol.* 47:206–16
87. Haeusler, G., Finch, L. 1972. *J. Pharmacol.* 3:544–45
88. Haeusler, G. 1974. *Arch. Pharmacol.* 286:97–111

89. Kroneberg, G., Oberdorf, A., Hoffmeister, F., Wirth, W. 1967. *Arch. Pharmacol.* 256:257–80
90. Simon, P., Chermat, R., Puech, A. J., Goujet, M. A., Boissier, J. R. 1973. *Thérápie* 28:735–51
91. Jacobs, F., Werner, U., Schümann, H. J. 1972. *Arzneim Forsch.* 22:1124–26
92. Giudicelli, R., Schmitt, H. 1970. *J. Pharmacol.* 1:339–58
93. Baum, T. et al 1969. *Experientia* 25:1066–67
94. Baum, T. et al 1970. *J. Pharmacol. Exp. Ther.* 171:276–87
95. Baum, T., Shropshire, A. T. 1970. *Neuropharmacology* 9:503–6
96. Scholtysik, G., Jerie, P. 1976. *New Antihypertensive Drugs,* ed. A. Scriabine, C. S. Sweet. Holliswood, NY: Spectrum. In press
97. Reid, J. L., Briant, R. H., Dollery, C. T. 1973. *Life Sci.* 12:459–67
98. Van Spanning, H. W., Van Zwieten, P. A. 1973. *Eur. J. Pharmacol.* 24:402–4
99. Briant, R. H., Reid, J. L., Dollery, C. T. 1973. *Br. Med. J.* 1:522–23
100. Hoefke, W., Warnke-Sachs, E. 1974. *Arzneim. Forsch.* 24:1046–47
101. Share, N. N., Melville, K. I. 1965. *Int. J. Neuropharmacol.* 4:149–56
102. Gagnon, D. J., Melville, K. I. 1967. *Int. J. Neuropharmacol.* 6:245–51
103. Schmitt, H., Fénard, S. 1971. *Arch. Int. Pharmacodyn. Ther.* 190:229–40
104. Conway, E. L., Lang, W. J. 1974. *Clin. Exp. Pharmacol. Physiol.* 1:59–64
105. Myers, M. G., Lewis, P. J., Reid, J. L., Dollery, C. T. 1975. *Neuropharmacology* 14:221–26
106. Reid, J. L., Lewis, P. J., Myers, M. G., Dollery, C. T. 1974. *J. Pharmacol. Exp. Ther.* 188:394–99
107. Ito, A., Schanberg, S. M. 1974. *J. Pharmacol. Exp. Ther.* 189:392–404
108. Day, M. D., Roach, A. G. 1973. *Nature London New Biol.* 242:30–31
109. Kelliher, G. J., Buckley, J. P. 1970. *J. Pharm. Sci.* 59:1276–80
110. Sweet, C. S., Scriabine, A., Wenger, H. C., Ludden, C. T., Stone, C. A. 1976. *Regulation of Blood Pressure by the Central Nervous System,* ed. G. Onesti, M. Fernandes, K. Kim. New York: Grune & Stratton. In press
111. Stern, S., Hoffman, M., Braun, K. 1971. *Cardiovasc. Res.* 5:425–30
112. Offerhaus, L., Van Zwieten, P. A. 1974. *Cardiovasc. Res.* 8:488–95

CHEMICALS, DRUGS, AND LIPID PEROXIDATION

❖6641

Gabriel L. Plaa and Hanspeter Witschi

Département de Pharmacologie, Université de Montréal, Montréal, Québec, Canada

INTRODUCTION

Lipid peroxidation is the oxidative deterioration of polyunsaturated lipids. Peroxidative reactions for nonbiological olefinic substances are known. The peroxidative process leads to the formation of free radical intermediates, which can lead to autocatalysis. The effects of free radical formation in radiation-induced reactions are reasonably well recognized. However, the eventual results of free radicals generated during chemically induced lipid peroxidation in vivo are less well understood. Lipid peroxidation in vivo has been said to be of basic importance in aging, in damage to cells by air pollution, in some phases of atherosclerosis, in some forms of liver injury, and in oxygen toxicity (1). However, much of the evidence is indirect and based largely on in vitro findings or the use of antioxidants in vivo. The interpretations made with experiments involving the use of antioxidants have been questioned (2). Nevertheless, lipid peroxidation is a subject of current interest to pharmacologists and toxicologists. The purpose of this review is not to provide an exhaustive treatment of the subject, but to treat sectors of research that are currently receiving considerable attention.

MEASUREMENT OF LIPID PEROXIDATION

The detection and especially the quantitative determination of lipid peroxidation in biological material is not an easy task. Over the last few years, essentially three procedures have gained practical use in measuring lipid peroxidation: the thiobarbituric acid (TBA) reaction, the detection of conjugated dienes, and the measurement of fluorescent products formed by the interaction of peroxidized lipids and other tissue constituents. Among the three methods, the TBA reaction is the most widely used. Since malonaldehyde is a degradation product of peroxidized lipids, the development of a color with the same absorption characteristics (absorption maximum at 532 nm) as a TBA-malonaldehyde chromophore has been taken as an index of lipid peroxidation in a given biological sample. There seems to be general

125

agreement that the TBA reaction gives a reliable index of lipid peroxidation in tissue extracts. The method has been extensively reviewed and discussed by Barber & Bernheim (3) and Slater (4). Several investigators have attempted to improve the reliability or reproducibility of the test while analyzing biological material (5–10). Failure to detect TBA-reacting material in tissue extracts is not an indication of the absence of lipid peroxidation. Malonaldehyde, if injected, disappears within a few hours from the serum (11) and is metabolized by liver homogenates and fractions thereof (12, 13).

A second method for the detection of lipid peroxidation is to examine tissue extracts for the presence of conjugated dienes by ultraviolet spectrophotometry. The spectra of peroxidized lipids show an absorption at 233 nm, with a shoulder due to ketone dienes between 260 and 280 nm. It is possible, by observing suitable precautions, such as analysis of tissue extracts under strictly anaerobic conditions, to detect the presence of conjugated dienes after treatment in vivo with lipid peroxidizing agents. The methods have been described in detail (14–16).

A comparatively new approach to the measurement of products of lipid peroxidation in tissue is to measure the occurrence of fluorescent products. A variety of molecules that occur commonly in tissue may react with malonaldehyde and yield characteristic fluorescent chromophores (17, 18). Malonaldehyde undergoes decomposition and the decomposition products may also cause production of fluorescent products when they react with proteins (19). Formation of a fluorescent product was observed when DNA was reacted with malonaldehyde (20), or peroxidizing arachidonic acid (21), during peroxidation of phosphatidylethanolamine and phosphatidylcholine and from the reaction of polyunsaturated fatty acids with synthetic phosphatidylethanolamine and phenylalanine (22, 23). Both aqueous and lipid soluble fluorescent products were found in systems that contained peroxidizing polyunsaturated fatty acids and amines; there was good correlation between the formation of fluorescence and oxygen consumption and the formation of TBA reactants. Measurement of these fluorescent products seems to offer a workable way for detecting lipid peroxidation in biological systems and tissues (24–26). Data on the properties and the molecular structures required to produce fluorescence are available (27).

Other methods available for measurement of lipid peroxidation are the iodimetric procedure as described by Bunyan et al (28). An interesting suggestion for measuring lipid peroxidation was made in 1966 by Lieberman & Hochstein (29). In an in vitro system, it was found that the formation of malonaldehyde was paralleled by formation of ethylene, but only when ascorbate and cupric ions were present. Later, it was observed that ethane production was a characteristic of spontaneously peroxidizing mouse tissue, and was found in mice injected with CCl_4 (30). Ethane evolution might therefore be a useful new index of lipid peroxidation in vivo.

LIPID PEROXIDATION AND MICROSOMES

In 1963, Hochstein & Ernster (31) reported that isolated rat liver microsomes formed TBA-reacting material in vitro when they were incubated in the presence of NADPH and ADP. Antioxidants inhibited its formation. These observations strongly implicated that microsomes would catalyze an ADP-activated peroxidation of lipids, coupled to the NADPH oxidase system (32). The presence of iron in the form of Fe^{2+} seemed essential to activate microsomal lipid peroxidation by ADP and other pyrophosphates (33). The dependence of microsomal lipid peroxidation on the partial oxygen pressure was examined (34). Minimal lipid peroxidation in the presence of NADPH and ADP has a K_m for oxygen of $3 \times 10^{-5}M$, i.e. close to the critical oxygen partial pressure of the living cell. CO had no effect on microsomal lipid peroxidation; therefore, it appeared unlikely that cytochrome P450 was involved in the process. The extent of in vitro stimulation of lipid peroxidation depends upon the age and sex of the animal supplying the liver microsomes (35).

The mechanism of in vitro lipid peroxide formation in several tissues was extensively studied (36). Total homogenates from liver, kidney, spleen, heart, or subcellular fractions (nuclear, mitochondrial, microsomal, and soluble) all formed lipid peroxides upon incubation in vitro; they were also active in peroxidizing unsaturated fatty acids. Lipid peroxide formation in microsomes was studied in greater detail (37) and compared to ascorbate-induced lipid peroxidation. Microsomes were fractionated into a supernate, a fluffy layer fraction composed of membranes with a high lipid content, and a sediment. Both NADPH- and ascorbate-induced lipid peroxidation were most pronounced in the fluffy layer fraction. This suggested that the unsaturated fatty acids of the membranes were the substrate for peroxidation in both systems. The role of nonheme iron in lipid peroxidation was more closely analyzed (38). Evidence was found that at least some of the active iron had to be present, as a phosphate complex, and that adenine or adenosine helped to stabilize or orient it in an active configuration. This raised the interesting possibility that iron might be bound to the nucleic acids of the microsomal fraction.

More recent studies have drawn attention to some other features of microsomal lipid peroxidation. Incubation of liver microsomes in the presence of NADPH has led to a loss of cytochrome P450 (39–41). The presence of an antioxidant, butylated hydroxytoluene (BHT), prevented lipid peroxidation and preserved cytochrome P450 (40). Decrease of cytochrome P450 in microsomes under in vitro incubation can be enhanced by CCl_4 and also can be brought about by irradiation of microsomes with ultraviolet light (41). All these changes were parallel to a loss of microsomal polyunsaturated fatty acids and a formation of malonaldehyde. Inhibition of lipid peroxidation by chelating agents, heavy metals, and free-radical trapping agents prevented breakdown of cytochrome P450, and so did some drug substrates; however, other drugs were ineffective in preventing lipid peroxidation (42). Evidence therefore suggests that breakdown of cytochrome P450 is the result of lipid peroxidation and not a prerequisite, although other investigators have reached somewhat different conclusions (43, 44). Electron micrographs of liver and kidney microsomes after in vitro lipid peroxidation are available (45, 46).

Enzymes located within microsomal membranes are affected by lipid peroxidation (46, 47). However, there is no uniform pattern: cytochrome P450 concentration decreases parallel lipid peroxidation. Whereas UDP glucuronyl transferase is activated if lipid peroxidation is moderate, it returns to normal if lipid peroxidation is extensive. Glucose-6-phosphatase may be affected late during peroxidation, but activity may be preserved in the presence of the substrate, glucose-6-phosphatase.

NADPH–cytochrome c reductase, plays an essential role in the peroxidation of microsomal lipids (48). Antibodies prepared against the isolated and partially purified enzyme, which requires EDTA in an optimal concentration for maximum activity, can completely inhibit the NADPH-dependent peroxidation of lipids. Another enzyme involved in the initiation of the reaction is cytochrome b_5 reductase (49). Microsomal lipid peroxidation can be catalyzed not only by NADPH, but as readily by NADH, provided EDTA-Fe is present in the reaction mixture together with ADP-Fe (50). The data suggest that the NADPH-dependent peroxidation of microsomal lipids involved not only NADPH–cytochrome c reductase but possibly an additional, not yet identified microsomal electron transport component, which may be replaced by EDTA. On the other hand, in vitro microsomal lipid peroxidation can be inhibited by superoxide dismutase (49, 51). This suggests that superoxide anion and possibly singlet oxygen is instrumental in microsomal lipid peroxidation. Some recent experimental evidence supports this conclusion (52).

It was recognized early that drugs that undergo oxidative demethylation may interfere with and inhibit the NADPH-mediated peroxidation of microsomal lipids. Orrenius et al (53) found that codeine and aminopyrine would strongly prevent the formation of malonaldehyde in rat liver microsomes incubated in the presence of NADPH. Gram & Fouts (54) also observed that aminopyrine, zoxazolamine, aniline, and benzpyrene markedly reduced NADPH-stimulated lipid peroxidation in microsomal membranes. The same authors found that there was a species difference; in rat liver microsomes, considerably more TBA-reacting material was found than in rabbit liver microsomes. Wills (55) suggested that the system involved in lipid peroxidation was at least partially identical with the drug-hydroxylating system. He found a close parallelism between formation of malonaldehyde and loss of activity of certain microsomal enzymes. The following enzymes were sensitive to lipid peroxidation: glucose-6-phosphatase, oxidative demethylation of aminopyrine, and p-chloromethylaniline, hydroxylation of aniline, NADPH-oxidation, and menadione-dependent NADPH-oxidation; on the other hand, NAD-NADP glycohydrolase, ATPase, esterase, and NADPH-cytochrome c reductase were insensitive or only slightly inhibited (47). Therefore, certain substrates may actually protect microsomes against lipid peroxidation. A recent, interesting example is the potent carcinogen aflatoxin B_1; oxidative metabolism of aflatoxin B_1 retards lipid peroxidation (56).

Induction of lipid peroxidation with Fe^{2+} in isolated microsomes leads to an immediate sharp decline of ethylmorphine demethylase activity (57), and preincubation of microsomes with ascorbic acid or a NADPH-generating system reduces aminopyrine, ethylmorphine, and codeine demethylase (58). Contrary to other observations (39–41) the content of the microsomes in cytochrome P450 and the activities of NADPH–cytochrome c reductase and NADPH–neotetrazolium diaphorase apparently were only slightly affected by the stimulation of lipid peroxidation in these experiments. Treatment of the microsomes with CO inhibited aminopyrine N-demethylation, but increased lipid peroxidation; this observation seems to contradict the earlier findings by Hrycay & O'Brien (43, 44) that cytochrome P450 would be instrumental in inducing lipid peroxidation.

More recently, Jacobson et al (59) examined the kinetics of acetanilide hydroxylation and pentobarbital oxidation by rat liver microsomes and found that the deviation from linearity for product formation was attributable at least in part, to lipid peroxidation and the associated breakdown of cytochrome P450, an idea originally put forth by Gram & Fouts (54). They also confirmed that rat liver microsomes underwent rapid lipid peroxidation in vitro, whereas in microsomes from rabbit liver, practically no malonaldehyde formation occurred and the loss of cytochrome P450 was less than 10%. Similar species differences were also observed by Kamataki & Kitagawa (60); in rat liver microsomes, lipid peroxidation was most extensive; then came guinea pigs, mice, and rabbits. There was no good correlation between the extent of lipid peroxidation and the loss of microsomal activity.

LIPID PEROXIDATION AND LUNG INJURY

During the last few years, considerable attention has been focused on the pathological and biochemical changes brought about in lung tissue by oxygen and oxidant gases nitrogen dioxide and ozone. Nitrogen dioxide and ozone are essential ingredients in the so-called photochemical smog. Pulmonary oxygen toxicity may be a serious complication in the prolonged treatment of certain cardiorespiratory diseases and may also be a problem in aerospace technology. There are several recent reviews on the mechanism and the anatomo-pathological and functional consequences of oxygen toxicity in the lung (61–63), and it is generally thought that lipid peroxidation may be an important consequence of exposure to normobaric or hyperbaric oxygen. Lipid peroxides are readily formed during incubation of homogenates from many tissues under oxygen (36). In lung homogenates obtained from α-tocopherol-deficient animals, significantly greater lipid peroxidation occurred during a 2-hr incubation period than did in lung homogenates obtained from normal animals (64). However, prior to the incubation, identical amounts of TBA-reacting material were found in the lungs from the deficient animals compared to nondeficient animals. Exposure of both normal and α-tocopherol-deficient animals to hyperbaric oxygen failed to raise the concentrations of lipid peroxides in the lung in vivo, although formation was enhanced in deficient lungs upon in vitro incubation. However, if homogenates of normal animals exposed to hyperbaric oxygen were incubated in vitro, lipid peroxidation was inhibited. No inhibition was observed if Fe^{2+} and ascorbic acid were added to the homogenates prior to the incubation; lipid peroxidation proceeded at a normal rate. The possibility was raised that in vivo hyperbaric oxygen would oxidize ascorbic acid and Fe^{2+}, leaving the lungs too depleted of these elements, thus permitting the occurrence of in vitro lipid peroxidation.

Direct evidence for the in vivo production of lipid peroxides in lung has been obtained from experiments with nitrogen dioxide and ozone. In vitro experiments established that both gases are capable of oxidizing fatty acid methyl esters (65). The lungs of rats exposed to NO_2 (1 ppm for 4 hr) were analyzed for peroxidized polyenoic fatty acids (66). Difference spectra were obtained which were characteristic of diene conjugation. The changes reached a maximum between 24 and 48 hr after exposure. Pretreatment of the animals with large doses of α-tocopherol partially prevented the development of lipid peroxidation. Ultraviolet absorption spectra characteristic of diene conjugation were also found in the lipids extracted from the lungs of mice exposed to ozone (0.4–0.7 ppm for 4 hr) (67). It was pointed out that the levels of both the ozone (67) and the nitrogen dioxide (66) to which the animals were exposed were not above concentrations to which populations in major urban centers may frequently be exposed. However, in vitro exposure of erythrocytes to ozone is also a procedure that enhances formation of lipid peroxides, as measured by the TBA reaction (68). It is conceivable that other oxidant gases will have similar effects. Since exposure to ozone may cause considerable blood stasis within the pulmonary vasculature, it has to be recognized that at least part of the observed lipid peroxidation might not actually occur in the lung cells themselves, but could be due to an increased presence of red blood cells.

In another series of experiments, it was observed that animals exposed to various concentrations of ozone had substantially more TBA-reacting material in their lung homogenates than had animals not exposed to ozone. Supplementing the diet with α-tocopherol decreased, but did not completely abolish the observed increase in lipid peroxidation (69, 70). In the same experiments, it was found that although the TBA reaction detected the formation of lipid peroxides, analysis of lung tissue with the fluorescent techniques developed by Tappel and his associates (17–26) gave negative results. Mustafa et al (71) examined the respiration of lung homogenates and isolated mitochondria from the lungs of ozone-exposed rats, and also exposed mitochondria in vitro to ozone. Acute in vivo exposure or in vitro exposure decreased the respiratory rate of mitochondria; increased production of TBA-reacting material and evidence for diene conjugation was observed if mitochondria were exposed to ozone in vitro. However, in homogenates of lungs from animals exposed to ozone in vivo, no increased amount of lipid peroxidation could be detected. This made it questionable whether the decreased rate of mitochondrial respiration was indeed due to lipid peroxidation in the mitochondrial membranes. Later work (72) confirmed that in vitro exposure of lung mitochondrial suspension to ozone results in a 5- to 6-fold greater production of TBA-reacting material, whereas no such evidence was found in the homogenates subsequent to in vivo ozone exposure. Presence of vitamin E did not protect against in vitro lipid peroxidation by ozone, but the presence of ascorbate and glutathione greatly enhanced it. Indication for in vivo peroxidation of lung lipids, as measured by increased ultraviolet absorption at 235 nm, was also observed in the lungs of rabbits exposed to 1 ppm of ozone for 4 hr (73). Indexes of erythrocyte lysis and membrane damage were not observed under these circumstances, and the ozone lesion seemed to be confined to lung tissue only. Exposure of rabbits to 1 ppm of ozone for 90 min produced an appreciable decrease in lung microsomal cytochrome P450 content, which was evident immediately following ozone exposure and persisting for about 5 days. In vitro studies confirmed the in vivo results inasmuch as ozone produced a loss of cytochrome P450, together with the production of TBA-reacting material (74).

Studies on the effects of oxidant gases upon lung biochemistry now begin to show that the lung has an effective mechanism with which it may protect itself against oxidant-induced lipid peroxidation (75–78). The most prominent features are increases in the activities of the enzymes 6-phosphogluconate dehydrogenase (6PGDH), glucose-6-phosphate dehydrogenase (G6PDH), glutathione reductase, and glutathione peroxidase. Nitrogen dioxide has essentially similar effects, as did ozone, although it changed glutathione peroxidase activity only insignificantly. Increased activities of the same enzymes were also observed during exposure to oxygen (77). It is possible that the observed changes in enzyme activity represent a protective mechanism. Increased activity of G6PDH and of 6PGDH most probably reflects an increased activity of the pentose pathway. One consequence of this might be to maintain adequate concentrations of cellular NADPH and glutathione. Thus the cells would be protected against lipid peroxidation. The view that increased production of NADPH seems to be vital to protect lung cells of ozone-exposed animals also comes from the observation that the addition of α-tocopherol to the diet practically prevents an increase in the NADPH-generating enzyme system, but had practically no effect on the activity of other enzymes involved in glucose metabolism. However, increases in the enzymes involved in the pentose pathway and the maintenance of adequate glutathione supply are probably not the only protective mechanisms the lung disposes of for protecting itself against oxidant-inflicted lipid peroxidation. Crapo & Tierney (79) found recently that tolerance to oxygen is accompanied by an increase in pulmonary superoxide dismutase. This enzyme transforms the free radical superoxide anion to a less toxic form and, by doing so, might prevent the formation of lipid peroxides.

Lipid peroxidation in lung need not necessarily be produced by oxidant gases only. The herbicide paraquat, if ingested or injected parenterally, will produce extensive lung damage (80). The lesion is characterized by acute edema, death of alveolar epithelial cells and, in later stages, by a progressive interstitial fibrosis of the lung. In rats, paraquat toxicity is greatly enhanced by oxygen (81). This prompted Bus et al (82) to examine whether the toxicity of paraquat might be due to lipid peroxidation. Incubation of paraquat with liver microsomes or a system containing NADPH-cytochrome c reductase, NADPH, and microsomal lipid greatly increased the formation of malonaldehyde; the amount of malonaldehyde formed was dependent upon the concentration of paraquat in the incubation mixture. Jlett et al (83), on the other hand, found that paraquat inhibited in vitro lipid peroxidation. However, in more recent experiments, Bus et al (84) were able to provide additional evidence that paraquat might, in vivo, peroxidize pulmonary lipids. Paraquat toxicity was significantly enhanced in selenium- or vitamin E–deficient mice or mice pretreated with diethyl maleate. Other evidence that paraquat may exert its toxic action through formation of singlet oxygen and subsequent lipid peroxidation has been provided (85); rats can be partially protected against paraquat toxicity by petreatment with the enzyme superoxide dismutase. Lipid peroxidation in lung may therefore occur also by drugs that reach the lung via the bloodstream.

LIPID PEROXIDATION AND LIVER INJURY

Injury Resulting in Necrosis

Since 1965 there has been considerable work by several investigators that indicates that lipid peroxidation could be one of the principal causes for the hepatotoxicity produced by CCl_4. Earlier investigators had demonstrated that the liver injury produced by CCl_4 could be prevented or greatly modified by pretreating animals with various antioxidants. This work was reviewed in detail by Recknagel (86). In vitro CCl_4 could accelerate the lipid peroxidation of rat liver homogenate (87, 88) and exhibited a prooxidant effect on rat liver microsomes (87, 89); this increase in lipid peroxidation was associated with a loss in glucose-6-phosphatase activity. Subsequently it was shown that in vivo lipid peroxidation also occurred shortly after the administration of CCl_4 to rats. These data have been reviewed in detail by Slater (4) and by Recknagel & Glende (90). It is now reasonably established that CCl_4 is activated to a free radical in vivo, that lipid peroxidation occurs very quickly in microsomes prepared from damaged livers, that this lipid peroxidation occurs within minutes after the administration of CCl_4 in vivo, that the lipid peroxidation is associated with loss of enzyme activity of microsomes prepared from livers, and that various antioxidants or free radical-trapping agents can protect animals against the hepatotoxic effects of CCl_4. Slater & Sawyer (91) compared the prooxidant effect of CCl_4 to those obtained with $CBrCl_3$, $CFCl_3$, and $CHCl_3$. They found that $CBrCl_3$ was much more potent as a prooxidant than CCl_4. $CFCl_3$ although much weaker than CCl_4 was more potent than $CHCl_3$. The relative order of activity in this in vitro system was what would be expected if homolytic bond fission of the halomethane had stimulated lipid peroxidation. CHI_3 has been found to produce liver injury which is quite similar to that produced by CCl_4; with this substance it has also been possible to demonstrate the lipid peroxidation in vivo by the formation of conjugated dienes (92).

Although it seems reasonably established that lipid peroxidation does occur with CCl_4-induced liver injury, there is still some controversy regarding the relative importance of this effect in the subsequent pathologic changes. Some of the various points of controversy are contained in the reviews by Slater (4) and by Recknagel & Glende (90). Recknagel and his co-workers, who have been the chief proponents of the lipid peroxidation hypothesis, do recognize that there are a number of unknown factors that can contribute to cell death after lipid peroxidation has occurred. They state that there is not a one-to-one correspondence between the initial lipid peroxidation and the eventual development of necrosis. Unfortunately in a number of experiments that have been used to unravel the relative importance of lipid peroxidation, death of the animal has been used as the biological end point. As Slater (4) points out, the cause of death in acute CCl_4 intoxication is not known; CCl_4 can affect the central nervous system, the cardiovascular system, and kidney function. Therefore, conclusions drawn on survival of animals can be precarious unless the actual cause of death is established.

Comporti et al (93) have reported that N,N'-diphenyl-*p*-phenylenediamine (DPPD), an antioxidant that protects against CCl_4-induced necrosis, did not prevent the production of conjugated dienes in microsomal lipids in vivo. Cystamine, cysteine, and pyrazole, which decrease the binding of CCl_4 to cellular components, do not change the extent of lipid peroxidation, although necrosis is partially prevented (94–97). Recently Díaz Gómez et al (98) have studied species differences in CCl_4-induced hepatotoxicity. They found that the degree of necrosis decreased in the following order: mouse, guinea pig, hamster, rat. The chicken was resistant to CCl_4. The degree of irreversible binding of CCl_4 to cellular components decreased in the same order. However, the intensity of CCl_4-induced lipid peroxidation decreased in a different order: rat, hamster, guinea pig, chicken, mouse. There was a better correlation between the intensity of the process of irreversible binding of CCl_4 to cellular components and necrosis than there was between lipid peroxidation and necrosis. In the mouse, the necrotic process was seen in the absence of lipid peroxidation during the 3- to 24-hour period of observation. These authors could find no evidence of lipid peroxidation in mice.

Recently, the effects of vitamin E on CCl_4-induced lipid peroxidation and the increase in liver triglycerides have been studied (99). With a large dose of CCl_4, there was a good correlation between the amount of lipid peroxidation in the liver and the degree of triglyceride accumulation; vitamin E treatment could partially reduce lipid peroxidation and also reduced steatosis in rats. However with low doses of CCl_4 there was no correlation between these events; administration of vitamin E did not affect the incorporation of CCl_4 into microsomal lipids nor did it affect the reduction in glucose-6-phosphatase activity induced by CCl_4. de Ferreyra et al (100) studied the protective effects of a number of antioxidants (DPPD, α-tocopherol, promethazine). At doses that protected against CCl_4, these antioxidants had no effect on the production of conjugated dienes in microsomal lipids after the administration of CCl_4. Therefore, caution is urged in the use of antioxidant protection as supporting evidence for lipid peroxidation.

Torrielli et al (101), on the other hand, were able to show that the antioxidant DPPD could reduce the amount of lipid peroxidation which occurs in liver microsomes after intoxicating doses of CCl_4. The amount of conjugated dienes were markedly reduced 30 min after the administration of the hepatotoxin; they also showed that recovery from the peroxidative alterations seemed to occur more quickly in DPPD-protected rats. The metabolic activation of CCl_4, however, was unaffected by pretreatment with DPPD. They found that DPPD could also act as an inhibitor of enzymes bound to the endoplasmic reticulum and that this substance has properties other than antioxidant ones.

Selenium can reduce significantly the amount of malonaldehyde present in the livers of animals treated with CCl_4 (102). This is consistent with the known antioxidant properties of selenium. However, selenium treatment apparently has no effect on the formation of conjugated dienes 2 hr after administration of CCl_4. The protective effects of selenium have been attributed to enhanced activity of glutathione peroxidase, which brings about the destruction of excess lipid peroxides by reducing them to hydroxy acids, thus diminishing the formation of malonaldehyde; the lack of effect of selenium on conjugated dienes was attributed to the enhanced formation of hydroxy acids. Benedetti et al (102) found that CCl_4 did not affect glutathione peroxidase activity.

When the lipid peroxidation hypothesis was introduced it appeared that a universal mechanism for the production of liver injury might have been uncovered. It was expected that the halogenated hydrocarbons related to CCl_4, which also produce liver necrosis, would also exhibit prooxidant activity. With $CHCl_3$ this has not been found to occur. In vitro $CHCl_3$ does not exert a prooxidant effect on the liver microsomal lipids (90, 103, 104). Klaassen & Plaa (104) attempted to find evidence for the formation of conjugated dienes in microsomes from animals treated with $CHCl_3$; in parallel studies they were able to demonstrate conjugated dienes following CCl_4. However they could never find increased conjugated dienes after $CHCl_3$ administration, regardless of the time period studied. These authors and others (104–106) also failed to detect a decrease in hepatic glucose-6-phosphatase activity after the administration of $CHCl_3$ in vivo.

Recently it has been reported that rats pretreated with phenobarbital will produce conjugated dienes in hepatic microsomal lipids after 2 hr of $CHCl_3$ anesthesia (103, 107); however, rats not treated with phenobarbital did not show this response to $CHCl_3$ anesthesia. Lavigne & Marchand (108) reported that hepatic glucose-6-phosphatase activity was depressed in phenobarbital-pretreated rats given $CHCl_3$ but that this response was absent in rats not treated with phenobarbital.

These data have been difficult to reconcile with the lipid peroxidation theory because $CHCl_3$ produces the same extensive liver injury seen after CCl_4. Slater (4) has argued that the amount of conjugated dienes formed following $CHCl_3$ administration might occur at a rate considerably slower than that produced by CCl_4 and well within the limits of the biotransformation capacity of the hepatocyte. He proposed that the lack of evidence for conjugated dienes in vivo may merely indicate that the products of lipid peroxidation are metabolized too rapidly to permit accumulation and detection by the present analytical tests. Klaassen & Plaa (104) have also pointed out the possibility that the techniques devised for the determination of conjugated dienes in vivo might be too insensitive to detect that degree of lipid peroxidation necessary to produce liver injury. In effect, the possibility occurs that the conjugated dienes that are measured after CCl_4 administration represent an amount of lipid peroxidation that is much greater than that necessary to produce the degenerative changes. Therefore, the question whether $CHCl_3$ produces lipid peroxidation or not depends upon the devising of more sensitive analytical techniques for the detection of lipid peroxidation in vivo. In this regard it should also be noted that even with CCl_4 the cells responsible for the production of conjugated dienes in vivo have not been identified histochemically. The cell type and their location in the hepatic lobule are yet to be determined.

Recently the effects of 1,1-dichloroethylene have been studied in rats (109). This chlorinated hydrocarbon causes liver injury that is quite comparable to that produced by CCl_4. It was found that 1,1-dichloroethylene causes reduction of hepatic glucose-6-phosphatase activity, causes an increase in hepatic triglycerides, and appears to inhibit microsomal mixed function oxidases; these effects are all similar to those of CCl_4. 1,1-Dichloroethylene does not produce lipid peroxidation in vitro or in vivo; conjugated dienes were not increased over a 20-hr span after the administration of the substance.

Ethylene dibromide can produce liver injury in rats; however, the accumulation of triglycerides is considerably less than that obtained with CCl_4 (110); this substance also produces the appearance of conjugated dienes in rat liver microsomal lipids 2 hr after its administration in vivo. However, this compound does not produce a prooxidant effect on microsomal lipids in vitro (111); it was concluded that the lipid peroxidation after ethylene dibromide did not seem to be directly related to its toxicity. Dimethylnitrosamine, which also produces liver injury, has been shown to be a prooxidant of rat liver microsomes in vitro (112) but does not cause production of conjugated dienes in vivo. Thioacetamide has also been found not to produce enhanced lipid peroxidation in hepatic microsomes in doses that produced liver injury (113). Brown et al (103, 107) have studied the effects of halothane on conjugated diene contents of rat liver following anesthesia by inhalation. Two hours after anesthesia no increase in conjugated dienes was observed in the microsomal lipids in any of the animals. However, when the rats were subjected to phenobarbital treatment for 5 days prior to the anesthesia, halothane was found to cause noticeable increases in conjugated dienes. The maximum increase in conjugated dienes occurred 1 hr after anesthesia, and the concentration was back to normal by 16 hr. Halothane, when added to incubations of hepatic microsomes, did not cause an increase in TBA reactants in vitro.

Injury Resulting in Lipid Accumulation

In 1964, DiLuzio (114) reported that ethanol-induced fatty liver could be modified by treating animals with antioxidants. This led to the formulation of the hypothesis that lipid peroxidation was an important factor in the production of fatty liver caused by ethanol. The subject is still rather controversial. Hashimoto & Recknagel (115) carried out studies to show whether there was any direct evidence for the formation of lipid peroxides; they concluded that there was no chemical evidence for hepatic lipid peroxidation in acute ethanol toxicity. However, DiLuzio (116, 117) has summarized evidence that is consistent with the idea that enhanced lipid peroxidation occurs with acute ethanol intoxication. Rats pretreated with ethanol exhibited an increased amount of peroxides in lipids (118); the peroxides were measured by an iodimetric method using purified lipid extracts. The applicability of this technique for measuring lipid peroxides in tissues has been questioned (4, 115). The intravenous administration of coenzyme Q_4 was shown (118) to abolish the elevation in liver triglycerides and also diminish the peroxide content of the liver lipid. It was later demonstrated (119) that various other antioxidants could protect animals against the ethanol-induced fatty liver. Subsequently, lipid peroxidation, as estimated by the TBA reaction in liver homogenates obtained from animals treated with ethanol, was shown to be significantly increased (120). Enhanced TBA reactants could be detected for 6 and 12 hr after the oral administration of ethanol; the greatest concentration was observed in the 12-hr ethanol-treated group. In vitro the addition of ethanol to rat liver homogenates resulted in enhanced lipid peroxidation. The suitability of the TBA reaction for measuring in vivo lipid peroxidation has also been questioned (115). While Recknagel's group has been unable to find increased formation of conjugated dienes in microsomal and mitochondrial liver lipids following ethanol administration, DiLuzio has reported (116, 117) that ethanol administration results in an increase in conjugated dienes in liver mitochondria but not in liver microsomal lipids; these increases were observed 1 hr after the administration of ethanol in vivo. In the same experiments DiLuzio was able to show that CCl_4 caused increases in conjugated dienes only in microsomal lipids but not in mitochondrial lipids, thus confirming Recknagel's observations. Scheig & Klatskin (121) were also unable to show increased formation of malonaldehyde in homogenates of rat liver containing cell sap and microsomes but no mitochondria, following treatment with ethanol.

More recently Comporti et al (122) were able to show that liver homogenates from animals treated with ethanol exhibited increased malonaldehyde formation. The increase in activity seemed to be due to a component present in the soluble supernatant fraction of the homogenates rather than one that was from the mitochondria or from the microsomes. MacDonald (123) measured conjugated dienes in mitochondrial and microsomal lipids from livers of rats 3 hr after treatment with ethanol. This author confirmed the finding that mitochondrial lipids showed enhanced conjugated diene formation whereas microsomal lipids did not; however, lipid peroxidation was found to occur in only one half of the animals treated with ethanol. The other animals showed no evidence of conjugated dienes; the reason for this variation is unknown.

Evidence for enhanced formation of lipid peroxides has been obtained in rats fed alcohol for 1 month (124). In these experiments microsomes obtained from livers were found to form more malonaldehyde in vitro than control livers. A decrease in polyenoic fatty acids in the microsomes of the ethanol-treated animals was observed, which would be consistent with a peroxidative destruction of membrane lipids.

DiLuzio & Hartman (125) have postulated that ethanol causes lipid peroxidation by reducing the endogenous antioxidant activity of the tissue. They envisaged a balance between autoxidation and antioxidant activity occurring in normal tissue. They postulated that ethanol administration would result in a decrease in endogenous antioxidant activity and that this would be found particularly in the mitochondria of ethanol-treated livers. Experimentally this seems to have been confirmed; ethanol administration produced a significant reduction in endogenous lipid-soluble antioxidant content of hepatic mitochondria, but not in microsomes. In the same experiments, CCl_4 resulted in a significant reduction in lipid-soluble antioxidant activity in microsomes but not in the mitochondrial fraction. They suggested that the losses observed in the antioxidant content of the subcellular particles were directly attributable to a free radical attack on the lipoprotein membranes of the respective subcellular components.

Orotic acid when added to the diet of rats will cause fatty livers. The addition of 1.5% orotic acid to the diet will produce a three-fold increase in liver lipids within 4 days. This increase in liver lipids is prevented by pretreating animals with DPPD (126). Liver lipids obtained from animals fed orotic acids will undergo lipid peroxidation, as measured by the TBA reaction, much more rapidly in vitro than liver lipids from control animals (127, 128). The composition of the lipids obtained from these animals was unchanged; in particular no reduction in polyunsaturated fats was observed (128). Torrielli et al (129) demonstrated that the pretreatment of animals with DPPD prevented the enhanced formation of lipid peroxides. However, these investigators also searched for the presence of conjugated dienes in microsomal lipids from animals treated with orotic acid; 2–8 days after the dietary administration of orotic acid, it was not possible to detect the enhanced formation of conjugated dienes. They, therefore, concluded that orotic acid does not function like CCl_4 in that conjugated dienes are not formed more rapidly in animals fed orotic acid. They proposed that perhaps orotic acid interferes with endogenous antioxidants present in the liver and thereby alters the rate of the TBA reaction in vitro. They also proposed that the protective effect of DPPD on hepatic triglyceride accumulation did not necessarily indicate that peroxidation was the initiating event in this response. They proposed that DPPD could be protecting by some other mechanisms, because they had demonstrated that this antioxidant is also capable of decreasing enzyme activity in the endoplasmic reticulum. While it now appears that animals fed orotic acid do seem to have some enhanced formation of lipid peroxide, this process does not seem to be the major reason for the initiation of fatty livers.

Peroxidative decomposition of microsomal lipids has also been demonstrated to occur in rats given yellow phosphorus (130). In these experiments, conjugated dienes were found to be elevated in microsomal lipids obtained from animals 4 hr after the administration of phosphorus. At this time liver lipids had not increased significantly. It was also found that the vesiculation of the endoplasmic reticulum and ribosomal dispersion was prominent 12 hr after the administration of phosphorus. Mitochondria were still normal at this time. In this situation, therefore, it appears that lipid peroxidation could be a factor in the fatty liver induced by phosphorus because the appearance of conjugated dienes occurred rapidly, preceded the changes in hepatic ultrastructure, and preceded the increase in liver lipids. In this regard the sequence of events with phosphorus is qualitatively similar to that observed after CCl_4. DiLuzio (131) has shown that an antioxidant can protect animals against the effect of phosphorus.

There has been some interest in determining whether the fatty liver caused by choline-deficient diets can also be explained by enhanced lipid peroxidation. Ghoshal et al (132) measured the presence of diene conjugation in microsomal liver lipids and in mitochondria of rats 3 to 12 hr after the administration of a choline-deficient diet. They also measured conjugated dienes in the fraction of weanling rats 5 days after the commencement of the choline-deficient diet. The concentration of hepatic triglycerides progressively increased in these animals and by the twelfth hour was significantly higher than those obtained in controls. However, there was no evidence in microsomes or in mitochondria that enhanced formation of conjugated dienes had occurred. There was an absence of enhanced lipid peroxidation in the livers of weanling rats fed a choline-deficient diet for 5 days; these authors therefore concluded that lipid peroxidation is not a factor in the development of hepatic changes associated with early choline deficiency.

CONCLUSION

In this article, we review some experiments, all of which were designed to shed some light on the question whether peroxidation of structural and functional lipids by drugs and chemicals can cause cell and tissue damage. A sound and critical appraisal of the significance and implications of this concept seems more than overdue. However, the data reviewed, as well as many others omitted for lack of space, do not yet seem to allow this.

Peroxidation of unsaturated lipids by molecular oxygen is a straightforward chemical process, well understood and well analyzed. In artificial or natural membrane systems, chemicals may readily produce changes associated with lipid peroxidation. Under appropriate in vitro conditions, microsomal membranes in particular, but also mitochondrial and lysosomal membranes, do show loss of functional integrity when lipid peroxidation appears to occur. However, the seemingly most crucial piece of evidence, the presence of peroxidized lipids in vivo, is more often lacking than not. This, of course, does not mean that lipid peroxidation does not occur in vivo. Absence of evidence is not necessarily evidence of absence. But, it has to be realized that much of the most convincing evidence for the role of lipid peroxidation in vivo, in the final analysis, is mostly indirect evidence and that many of our conclusions have been drawn by inference.

Nevertheless, the concept of lipid peroxidation is one of the truly important concepts of current experimental pathology and toxicology. It has created discussion, stimulated the planning of careful and ingenious experiments, and given us many sound data. To us, it appears to be a hypothesis that remains, and deserves, to be tested extensively.

Literature Cited

1. Tappel, A. L. 1973. *Fed. Proc.* 32: 1870–74
2. Green, J. 1972. *Ann. NY Acad. Sci.* 203:29–44
3. Barber, A. A., Bernheim, F. 1967. *Adv. Gerontol. Res.* 2:355–403
4. Slater, T. F. 1972. *Free Radical Mechanisms in Tissue Injury.* London: Pion. 283 pp.
5. Singh, H., Pritchard, E. T. 1962. *Can J. Biochem. Physiol.* 40:317–18
6. Wills, E. D. 1964. *Biochim. Biophys. Acta* 84:475–77
7. Schoenmakers, A. W., Tarladgis, B. G. 1966. *Nature London* 210:1153
8. McKnight, R. C., Hunter, F. E. Jr. 1965. *Biochim. Biophys. Acta* 98:643–46
9. Placer, Z. A., Cushman, L. L., Johnson, B. C. 1966. *Anal. Biochem.* 16:359–64
10. Sawicki, E., Stanley, T. W., Johnson, H. 1963. *Anal. Chem.* 35:199–205
11. Placer, Z., Veselková, A., Rath, R. 1965. *Experientia* 21:19–20
12. Recknagel, R. O., Ghoshal, A. K. 1966. *Exp. Mol. Pathol.* 5:108–17
13. Horton, A. A., Packer, L. 1970. *Biochem. J.* 116:19P–20P
14. Haase, G., Dunkley, W. L. 1969. *J. Lipid Res.* 10:555–60
15. Recknagel, R. O., Ghoshal, A. K. 1966. *Lab. Invest.* 15:132–48
16. Sell, D. A., Reynolds, E. S. 1969. *J. Cell Biol.* 41:736–52
17. Chio, K. S., Tappel, A. L. 1969. *Biochemistry* 8:2821–27
18. Chio, K. S., Tappel, A. L. 1969. *Biochemistry* 8:2827–32
19. Shin, B. C., Huggins, J. W., Carraway, K. L. 1972. *Lipids* 7:229–33
20. Reiss, U., Tappel, A. L., Chio, K. S. 1972. *Biochem. Biophys. Res. Commun.* 48:921–26
21. Reiss, U., Tappel, A. L. 1973. *Lipids* 8:199–202
22. Bidlack, W. R., Tappel, A. L. 1973. *Lipids* 8:203–7

23. Dillard, C. J., Tappel, A. L. 1973. *Lipids* 8:183–89
24. Chio, K. S., Reiss, U., Fletcher, B., Tappel, A. L. 1969. *Science* 166:1535–36
25. Dillard, C. J., Tappel, A. L. 1971. *Lipids* 6:715–21
26. Fletcher, B. L., Dillard, C. J., Tappel, A. L. 1973. *Anal. Biochem.* 52:1–9
27. Malshet, M. G., Tappel, A. L. 1973. *Lipids* 8:194–98
28. Bunyan, J., Murrell, E. A., Green, J., Diplock, A. T. 1967. *Br. J. Nutr.* 21:475–95
29. Lieberman, M., Hochstein, P. 1966. *Science* 152:213–14
30. Riely, C. A., Cohen, G., Lieberman, M. 1974. *Science* 183:208–10
31. Hochstein, P., Ernster, L. 1963. *Biochem. Biophys. Res. Commun.* 12:388–94
32. Hochstein, P., Nordenbrand, K., Ernster, L. 1964. *Biochem. Biophys. Res. Commun.* 14:323–28
33. Marks, F., Hecker, E. 1967. *Z. Physiol. Chem.* 348:727–29
34. Lumper, L., Plock, H. J., Staudinger, N. 1968. *Z. Physiol. Chem.* 349:4485–90
35. Utley, H. G., Bernheim, F., Hochstein, P. 1967. *Arch. Biochem. Biophys.* 118:29–32
36. Wills, E. D. 1966. *Biochem. J.* 99:667–76
37. Wills, E. D. 1969. *Biochem. J.* 113:315–24
38. Wills, E. D. 1969. *Biochem. J.* 113:325–32
39. Schacter, B. A., Marver, H. S., Meyer, U. A. 1972. *Biochim. Biophys. Acta* 279:221–27
40. Welton, A. F., Aust, S. D. 1972. *Biochem. Biophys. Res. Commun.* 49:661–66
41. Reiner, O., Athanassopoulos, S., Hellmer, K. H., Murray, R. E., Uehleke, H. 1972. *Arch. Toxicol.* 29:219–33
42. Levin, W., Lu, A.Y.H., Jacobson, M., Kuntzman, R., Poyer, J. L., McCay, P. B. 1973. *Arch. Biochem. Biophys.* 158:842–52
43. Hrycay, E. G., O'Brien, P. J. 1971. *Arch. Biochem. Biophys.* 147:28–35
44. Hrycay, E. G., O'Brien, P. J. 1971. *Arch. Biochem. Biophys.* 147:14–27
45. Arstila, A. U., Smith, M. A., Trump, B. F. 1972. *Science* 175:530–33
46. Högberg, J., Bergstrand, A., Jakobsson, S. V. 1973. *Eur. J. Biochem.* 37:51–59
47. Wills, E. D. 1971. *Biochem. J.* 123:983–91
48. Pederson, T. C., Aust, S. D. 1972. *Biochem. Biophys. Res. Commun.* 48:789–95
49. Pederson, T. C., Buege, J. A., Aust, S. D. 1973. *J. Biol. Chem.* 248:7134–41
50. Bidlack, W. R., Okite, R. T., Hochstein, P. 1973. *Biochem. Biophys. Res. Commun.* 53:459–65
51. Zimmermann, R., Flohé, L., Weser, U., Hartmann, H. J. 1973. *FEBS Lett.* 29:117–20
52. Pederson, T. C., Aust, S. D. 1973. *Biochem. Biophys. Res. Commun.* 52:1071–78
53. Orrenius, S., Dallner, G., Ernster, L. 1964. *Biochem. Biophys. Res. Commun.* 14:329–34
54. Gram, T. E., Fouts, J. R. 1966. *Arch. Biochem. Biophys.* 114:331–35
55. Wills, E. D. 1969. *Biochem. J.* 113:333–41
56. Raj, H. G., Santhanam, K., Gupta, R. P., Venkitasubramanian, T. A. 1974. *Res. Commun. Chem. Pathol. Pharmacol.* 8:703–6
57. Kamataki, T., Kitagawa, H. 1973. *Biochem. Pharmacol.* 22:3199–3207
58. Kitada, M., Kamataki, T., Kitagawa, H. 1974. *Chem. Pharm. Bull.* 22:752–56
59. Jacobson, M., Levin, W., Lu, A. Y. H., Conney, A. H., Kuntzman, R. 1973. *Drug Metab. Dispos.* 1:766–74
60. Kamataki, T., Kitagawa, H. 1974. *Biochem. Pharmacol.* 23:1915–18
61. Haugaard, N. 1968. *Physiol. Rev.* 48:311–73
62. Clark, J. M., Lambertsen, C. J. 1971. *Pharmacol. Rev.* 23:37–133
63. Pfister, A., Nogues, C. 1974. *Pathol. Biol.* 22:89–98
64. Raskin, P., Lipman, R. L., Oloff, C. M. 1971. *Aerosp. Med.* 42:28–30
65. Roehm, J. N., Hadley, J. G., Menzel, D. B. 1971. *Arch. Intern. Med.* 128:88–93
66. Thomas, H. V., Mueller, P. V., Lyman, R. L. 1967. *Science* 159:532–34
67. Goldstein, B. D., Lodi, C., Collinson, C., Balchum, O. J. 1969. *Arch. Environ. Health* 18:631–35
68. Goldstein, B. D., Balchum, O. J. 1967. *Proc. Soc. Exp. Biol. Med.* 126:350–58
69. Fletcher, B. L., Tappel, A. L. 1973. *Environ. Res.* 6:165–75
70. Chow, C. K., Tappel, A. L. 1972. *Lipids* 7:518–24
71. Mustafa, M. G., de Lucia, A. J., York, G. K., Arth, C., Cross, C. E. 1973. *J. Lab. Clin. Med.* 82:357–65

72. Mustafa, M. G., Cross, C. E. 1974. *Arch. Biochem. Biophys.* 162:585–94
73. Kyei-Aboagye, K., Hazucha, M., Wyszogrodski, I., Rubinstein, D., Avery, M. E. 1973. *Biochem. Biophys. Res. Commun.* 54:907–13
74. Goldstein, B. D., Solomon, S., Pasternack, B. S., Bicker, D. R. 1975. *Res. Commun. Chem. Pathol. Pharmacol.* 10:754–62
75. Chow, C. K., Tappel, A. L. 1973. *Arch. Environ. Health* 26:205–8
76. Chow, C. K., Dillard, C. J., Tappel, A. L. 1974. *Environ. Res.* 7:311–19
77. Tierney, D., Ayers, L., Herzog, S., Yang, J. 1973. *Am. Rev. Respir. Dis.* 108:1348–51
78. Mustafa, M. G., de Lucia, A. J., Hussain, M. Z., Chow, C. K., Cross, C. E. 1974. *Am. Rev. Respir. Dis.* 109:721
79. Crapo, J. D., Tierney, D. F. 1974. *Am. J. Physiol.* 226:1401–7
80. Conning, D. M., Fletcher, K., Swan, A. A. B. 1969. *Br. Med. Bull.* 25: 245–49
81. Fisher, H. K., Clements, J. A., Wright, R. R. 1973. *Am. Rev. Respir. Dis.* 107:246–52
82. Bus, J. S., Aust, S. D., Gibson, J. E. 1974. *Biochem. Biophys. Res. Commun.* 58:749–55
83. Jlett, K. F., Stripp, B., Menard, R. H., Reid, W. D., Gillette, J. R. 1974. *Toxicol. Appl. Pharmacol.* 28:216–26
84. Bus, J. S., Aust, S. D., Gibson, J. E. 1975. *Res. Commun. Chem. Pathol. Pharmacol.* 11:31–38
85. Autor, A. P. 1974. *Life Sci.* 14:1309–19
86. Recknagel, R. O. 1967. *Pharmacol. Rev.* 19:145–208
87. Ghoshal, A. K., Recknagel, R. O. 1965. *Life Sci.* 4:1521–30
88. Comporti, M., Saccocci, C., Dianzani, M. U. 1965. *Enzymologia* 29:185–204
89. Ghoshal, A. K., Recknagel, R. O. 1965. *Life Sci.* 4:2195–2209
90. Recknagel, R. O., Glende, E. A. Jr. 1973. *CRC Crit. Rev. Toxicol.* 2:263–97
91. Slater, T. F., Sawyer, B. C. 1971. *Biochem. J.* 123:805–14
92. Sell, D. A., Reynolds, E. S. 1969. *J. Cell Biol.* 41:736–52
93. Comporti, M., Benedetti, A., Casini, A. 1974. *Biochem. Pharmacol.* 23:421–32
94. D'Acosta, N., Castro, J. A., de Ferreyra, E. C., Díaz Gómez, M. I., de Castro, C. R. 1972. *Res. Commun. Chem. Pathol. Pharmacol.* 4:641–50
95. Castro, J. A., Cignoli, E. V., de Castro, C. R., de Fenos, O. M. 1972. *Biochem. Pharmacol.* 21:49–57
96. Castro, J. A., de Ferreyra, E. C., de Castro, C. R., Díaz, Gómez, M. I., D'Acosta, N., de Fenos, O. M. 1973. *Toxicol. Appl. Pharmacol.* 24:1–9
97. de Ferreyra, E. C., Castro, J. A., Díaz Gómez, M. I., D'Acosta, N., de Castro, C. R., de Fenos, O. M. 1974. *Toxicol. Appl. Pharmacol.* 27:558–68
98. Díaz Gómez, M. I., de Castro, C. R., D'Acosta, N., de Fenos, N., de Ferreyra, E. C., Castro, J. A. 1975. *Toxicol. Appl. Pharmacol.* 34:102–14
99. Benedetti, A., Ferrali, M., Chieli, E., Comporti, M. 1974. *Chem. Biol. Interact.* 9:117–34
100. de Ferreyra, E. C., Castro, J. A., Díaz Gómez, M. I., D'Acosta, N., de Castro, C. R., de Fenos, O. M. 1975. *Toxicol. Appl. Pharmacol.* 32:504–12
101. Torrielli, M. V., Ugazio, G., Gabriel, L., Burdino, E. 1974. *Agents Actions* 4/5:383–90
102. Benedetti, A., Ferrali, M., Casini, A., Comporti, M. 1974. *Res. Commun. Chem. Pathol. Pharmacol.* 9:711–22
103. Brown, B. R. 1972. *Anesthesiology* 36:458–65
104. Klaassen, C. D., Plaa, G. L. 1969. *Biochem. Pharmacol.* 18:2019–27
105. Reynolds, E. S., Yee, A. G. 1968. *Lab. Invest.* 19:273–81
106. Cawthorne, M. A., Palmer, E. D., Bunyan, J., Green, J. 1971. *Biochem. Pharmacol.* 20:494–96
107. Brown, B. R., Sipes, I. G., Sagalyn, A. M. 1974. *Anesthesiology* 41:554–61
108. Lavigne, J. G., Marchand, C. 1974. *Toxicol. Appl. Pharmacol.* 29:312–26
109. Jaeger, R. J., Trabulus, M. J., Murphy, S. D. 1973. *Toxicol. Appl. Pharmacol.* 24:457–67
110. Nachtomi, E., Alumot, E. 1972. *Exp. Mol. Pathol.* 16:71–78
111. Nachtomi, E. 1972. *Exp. Mol. Pathol.* 17:171–75
112. Jose, P. J., Slater, T. F. 1970. *Biochem. J.* 117:66P–67P
113. Castro, J. A., D'Acosta, N., de Ferreyra, E. C., de Castro, C. R., Díaz Gómez, M. I., de Fenos, O. M. 1974. *Toxicol. Appl. Pharmacol.* 30:79–86
114. DiLuzio, N. R. 1964. *Life Sci.* 3:113–18
115. Hashimoto, S., Recknagel, R. O. 1968. *Exp. Mol. Pathol.* 8:225–42
116. DiLuzio, N. R. 1968. *Exp. Mol. Pathol.* 8:394–402
117. DiLuzio, N. R. 1973. *Fed. Proc.* 32: 1875–81
118. Kalish, G. H., DiLuzio, N. R. 1966. *Science* 152:1390–92

119. DiLuzio, N. R., Costales, F. 1965. *Exp. Mol. Pathol.* 4:141–54
120. DiLuzio, N. R., Hartman, A. D. 1967. *Fed. Proc.* 26:1436–42
121. Scheig, R., Klatskin, G. 1969. *Life Sci.* 8:855–65
122. Comporti, M., Benedetti, A., Chieli, E. 1973. *Lipids* 8:498–502
123. MacDonald, C. M. 1973. *FEBS Lett.* 35:227–30
124. Reitz, R. C. 1975. *Biochim. Biophys. Acta* 380:145–54
125. DiLuzio, N. R., Hartman, A. D. 1969. *Exp. Mol. Pathol.* 11:38–52
126. Torrielli, M. V., Ugazio, G. 1970. *Life Sci.* 9: Part II, 1–7
127. Kinsella, J. E. 1967. *Biochim. Biophys. Acta* 137:205–7
128. Kinsella, J. E. 1967. *Can. J. Biochem.* 45:1206–11
129. Torrielli, M. V., Dianzani, M. U., Ugazio, G. 1971. *Life Sci.* 10: Part II, 99–111
130. Ghoshal, A. K., Porta, E. A., Hartroft, W. S. 1969. *Am. J. Pathol.* 54:275–91
131. DiLuzio, N. R. 1966. *Life Sci.* 5: 1467–78
132. Ghoshal, A. K., Monserrat, A. J., Porta, E. A., Hartroft, W. S. 1970. *Exp. Mol. Pathol.* 12:31–35

PHARMACOLOGY OF DRUGS THAT AFFECT INTRACELLULAR MOVEMENT

❖6642

Frederick E. Samson

Ralph L. Smith Mental Retardation Research Center, University of Kansas
Medical Center, Kansas City, Kansas 66106

1 INTRODUCTION

Although the movements of cellular constituents on first glance often appear to be random in character, they are more often highly controlled, and the concept that emerges is that the cell is organized even at the molecular level. Indeed, a function of intracellular membranes, granules, vesicles, and organelles is to segregate functionally related molecules. Further, if these assemblies are scrambled, the cell has a considerable capability for sorting them out again. What this amounts to is a segregation of "unit processes" into increasing levels of organization and performances. To coordinate these levels, the traffic within the cell must move under a high degree of control.

In a recent review, Allen (1) classifies cytoplasmic movements into three basic types: (*a*) bulk cytoplasmic transport that accompanies pseudopodia formation and ameboid locomotion; (*b*) bulk cytoplasmic transport that is unrelated to cell locomotion and serves to circulate cytoplasm; (*c*) selective transport of cytoplasmic constituents (such as nuclear movements) unrelated to any bulk transport. Allen points out that the endoplasm of cells is variably resistant to the displacement of particulates within it, behaving as a gel of cross-linked polymers undergoing sol ⇌ gel transformations.

This review focuses on the selective transport of cytoplasmic constituents in neuronal processes, for the neuron has proven to be suitable for the study of the action of pharmacological agents on these movements. Pharmacological research has contributed substantially to the understanding of these intracellular events, and in turn such studies have shed light on the mechanism of some drug actions.

2 THE NEURON AS A MODEL

Neurons as a class of cells have a great range in size, from 20 μm to greater than several meters long (in the whale for example) and a corresponding heterogeneity of shapes. They are characterized by a high degree of functional segregation (2) with the spatial separation for example of impulse reception, action potential conduction, and synaptic transmitter release. Such functional segregation is not unique to neurons of course, but the segregation of particular importance here is the almost complete restriction of protein synthesis and many types of organelles to the perikaryon. The axon itself is entirely lacking in ribosomes and with increasing distance from the cell body the ribosomes selectively disappear in dendrites (2). Therefore, those neurons with long axonal processes, which depend upon components manufactured in the perikaryon, make accessible for study the traffic that moves within them. These movements of cytoplasmic components within the neuron are referred to as axoplasmic transport (AXT) or less correctly, axoplasmic flow, and more correctly as neuroplasmic transport. Although the neuron is specialized in its own way, it seems reasonable to assume that the general principles of intracellular movement (ICM) in neurons are essentially the same for all eukaryotic cells.

3 NEUROPLASMIC TRANSPORT (AXOPLASMIC TRANSPORT)

3.1 Anterograde Neuroplasmic Transport (Away From the Cell Body)

There are a number of excellent reviews of axoplasmic transport (3–9) and an overview of the effect of drugs upon axoplasmic transport (10). The movement of axoplasmic components from the cell bodies to the terminals is an old concept but the classical studies of Weiss & Hiscoe (11) gave the first direct demonstration. A major breakthrough was provided by Droz & Leblond's demonstration that the movements of proteins could be traced by labeling them with radioactive precursors (12). Recently a number of nonradioactive markers have been developed. The subject may be summarized as follows: a wide variety of transported materials have been identified (enzymes, proteins, phospholipids, catecholamine-containing granules, glycoproteins, 5-hydroxytryptamine, dopamine-β-hydroxylase, etc). The most extensively studied are labeled proteins, some of which move at rates in the order of 1 mm/day (slow transport) and another group that move about 400 mm/day (fast transport). However, there is a wide spectrum of rates reported for various types of cytoplasmic components (see reference 5 for summary). Among the most rapidly moving are the neurosecretory granules of the preoptic nucleus, calculated to move 2000 mm/day (13).

The transport processes bring not only materials for maintenance and renewal of the axon, but also some of the molecules released at the terminals. Recently the important trophic action that nerves have on striated muscles was shown to be related to axoplasmic transport (14, 15).

The movements of intracellular particles have been studied in a wide variety of cells with specialized light microscope techniques, and there is a large literature on the subject (16–18). There is an increased interest recently in the use of dark-field microscopy and the optical sectioning quality of Nomarski optics in observing the movements within axons (19, 20), and computer analyses of the movements have been carried out (21). The particles visualized by these techniques appear to move in channels in a saltatory fashion. They move in directions both toward and away from the cell body (see section 3.2 below). The particles have a range of velocities with the fastest ones moving at speeds comparable with fast axonal transport (FAXT). This method is limited in that only the particles visible can be studied, but it provides another very important window to the events of intraaxonal movements.

3.2 Retrograde Neuroplasmic Transport (Toward the Cell Body)

In Section 3.1, the movements of neuronal constituents synthesized in the cell body out to the terminals are briefly summarized. Probably as important and extensive as the anterograde movements is the traffic of axoplasmic constituents toward the cell bodies. Indeed, the particulates visible with Nomarski microscopy that move retrograde outrumber those that move anterograde (20). It has been recently recognized that the retrograde intraaxonal transport provides a major route for substances from the periphery to the central nervous system. A wide variety of macromolecules, including proteins exogenous to the neuron, as well as some viruses, move to the cell body from the terminals (22–24). The rate of these movements is in the order of 75–90 mm/day. Research has been carried out with markers such as horseradish peroxidase, which are taken up by pinocytosis into axon terminals and move intraaxonally, and have great potential for studies of this interesting transport (25, 26). The exciting concept that this retrograde transport may serve as a communication mechanism between the terminals and their microenvironment and the genetic apparatus in the cell body has been supported by the recent demonstration that nerve growth factor is specifically transported toward the cell body in adrenergic neurons (27).

4 MECHANISMS OF INTRACELLULAR MOVEMENTS

The mechanism(s) underlying ICM are no doubt the work of complicated machinery. Most of the ICM are not driven by diffusion and thus require metabolically generated energy. Therefore, drugs that interfere with the flow of free energy in the cell generally will arrest the movements. For example, FAXT depends on a local supply of energy: anoxia, dinitrophenol, and other energy flow inhibitors have been shown to inhibit FAXT (19, 28–30).

There are two major considerations with regard to the ICM mechanisms: one, what are the chemomechanical energy–coupling components that harness metabolically generated energy to drive them and, two, what are the components that give specificity such that certain cytoplasmic constituents are moved to particular intracellular locations? The implicated structures are extended surfaces such as the plasma membrane; tubular organelles such as the endoplasmic reticulum and microtubular channels; and linear fibrillar elements such as actomyosin, microfilaments, neurofilaments, and microtubules (external surface of MT). It is likely that each plays a part in some of the various types of ICM.

4.1 Plasma Membrane

The movements of the plasma membrane and in particular the peristaltic waves, which were shown by Weiss to sweep down the axonal membranes (9), have been proposed to have a role in ICM. There are reasons, however, that might rule out this proposition. The movements observed in "skinned" amoeba (plasma membrane removed) by Allen and his colleagues show that at least the class of ICM studied required neither a plasma membrane nor hydrostatic pressure generated by an ectoplasmic tube (1, 31). In myelinated nerves, the analysis of axoplasmic movement and myelin movement revealed no evidence to support the idea that axoplasmic flow results from peristalsis in the myelin covering the axon (32). Further, it is difficult to see how peristalsis could provide the specificity or sufficient intracellular hydrostatic pressure for the movements within the axoplasm of, say, large invertebrate axons.

4.2 Endoplasmic Reticulum

In some cell localities, proteins, lipids, and probably other materials are known to be distributed through the endoplasmic reticulum (ER). These substances may accumulate within the ER and, in addition, may be modified while within the ER. The path of secretory material from the polysome to the lumen in exocrine cells and the packaging of material for transport involve the ER. The movement of protein and other constituents within the ER is a major subject in its own right and from the viewpoint of future research, pharmacology could give insight into these important transport events. The smooth ER frequently seen in axons may be involved in axoplasmic transport but no clear-cut hypothesis has emerged that is backed by any compelling experimental evidence.

4.3 Microtubule Channels

The internal diameter of microtubules (MTs) is about 15 nm and could accommodate sizable molecules. When appropriately stained, dense particles, which some authors have interpreted as macromolecules, are revealed in the central core of the MT (33). Whether this is a stationary structure or material in transit is unknown. (See section 7.)

4.4 Actomyosin

Actin has been shown to exist in a wide variety of nonmuscle cells (34) and is probably a universal constituent of eukaryotic cells. The properties of the actin in nonmuscle cells are remarkably similar to those of muscle actin, and this actin is probably involved in the cellular movements, ICM, and other mechanical events. Where contractile systems are known in detail an interaction of actin with myosin is involved. Myosins, in contrast with actins, are more diverse in their properties. It is now clear that myosin also is present in a number of nonmuscle vertebrate cells (34). Actomyosin complexes have been identified in brain (35). Further, the related protein tropomyosin has been identified in nervous tissue (36). An attractive, unifying concept is the idea that actomyosin is universal in eukaryotic cells and, with some individual modification or specialization, underlies most if not all of the movements, both cellular and intracellular. The evidence is compelling although the details of the activation of the force generation and exertion are less well known in nonmuscle cells than in striated muscle (1, 34). The extensive studies in protozoa emerge as almost conclusive that many of the intracellular movements are driven by an actomyosin system (16). In particular, the class of ICM described as bulk cytoplasmic transport by Allen (1) is probably motivated by actomyosin.

4.5 Microfilaments

Microfilaments are identified as a class primarily on the basis of their size (about 4–5 nm). They are a heterogeneous class; for example some are clearly actin-like (bind heavy meromyosin) and some are not, and some are cytochalasin B sensitive (see Section 6). Those that are actinoid probably are part of an actomyosin system.

4.6 Neurofilaments and Other 10 nm Filaments

The 10 nm filaments may be a distinct class of filaments that occur in a number of types of cells. The neurofilaments are typically abundant in myelinated axons and less abundant in unmyelinated axons, and the component protein has been characterized by Davison (37). From time to time the suggestion is made that the neurofilaments are involved in axoplasmic transport; however, there is no evidence as to the function of any of the 10 nm filaments. If a reasonably specific pharmacological agent that interacts with those filaments were found, it would give a major impetus to understanding their function as colchicine has done for microtubules.

4.7 Microtubules

Microtubules are proteinaceous, intracellular tubular structures that are found in varying numbers in almost every type of animal and plant cell. They have a characteristic tube structure with an outside diameter of 25 nm and an inside diameter or channel of 15 nm. They are abundant in neurons, where they may run unbranched in dendritic and axonic processes for several micrometers. They are the principal fibrous protein of the mitotic spindle and dominant components of cilia and flagella. They often occur in highly ordered arrays. Indeed, as methods for ultrastructural studies improve it seems likely they will be revealed as components of larger systems in which a number of MTs are linked and function in a coordinated way. Since the widespread use of glutaraldehyde as a fixative for electron microscopy (which preserves MT structure better than previous fixation methods do) and the discovery that colchicine binds specifically to tubulin, a component protein of MTs, interest in the MT as an entity for research has greatly increased. This research has enlarged the understanding of many cellular functions, and there are a number of excellent reviews that cover the various aspects of the biochemistry (38, 39) and biology (40, 41) of microtubule protein.

Among the functions proposed for MTs, which now constitute a sizable list, the most convincing has been their role in the development and maintenance of an isometric cell form (42) and in intracellular movements. The effects of the pharmacologic agents colchicine and the vinca alkaloids have played a leading role in these findings. The evidence implicating MTs as a necessary component of the biological machinery that moves chromosomes and other cytoplasmic constituents in Allen's class 3 type of movements may be outlined as follows: the MTs are often oriented in the right way for transport, especially in extended processes such as axons; their location with respect to large cellular inclusions (such as pigment granules and mitochondria) reveals that they at least act as guides, if not directly, in the propulsion; their characteristic, universal presence in motile processes such as flagella and sperm tails suggests that chemomechanical energy coupling is part of their physiological function. But among the best arguments are the findings that pharmacological agents that have a strong affinity for the MT protein subunits, and in many cases that disrupt MTs, arrest cytoplasmic translocations (see section 5).

Although a few papers have questioned the essential role that MTs have in ICM, they are not persuasive enough to outweigh the contrary evidence. One paper (43) is weakened by the small number of observations (of two animals) and by the sampling problems of electron microscopy. In another study the shuttling movements of the kinetocysts in heliozoan axopods, and the movements of nonmotile bacteria adhering externally to the axopods were analyzed, and it was concluded that the plasma membrane of the axopods rather than the MTs mediates these movements (44). The different average velocities and variances of the inward movements contrasted with the outward, suggested two fundamentally different mechanisms for "in versus out" (as in the case of the melanophores where inward and outward movements of the granules are differentially sensitive to drugs pointed out in section 6). When the MTs were destroyed by colchicine, similar movements persisted but were not in straight lines. This implies that the MTs do not provide the impelling force but rather the directionality. It is relevant that actin filaments (at least in cultured neuroblastoma cells) tend to be a network immediately beneath the plasma membrane (45) and may provide the driving force rather than the plasma membrane itself, which would not seem to have sufficient mass to accomplish such a large mechanical energy requirement.

Given that MTs are involved in transport, the question is "how." The actinoid character of tubulin has not been overlooked and it has been proposed that the mechanism is similar to the sliding filaments of actin and myosin of muscle contraction, with tubulin behaving akin to actin, interacting with a myosinoid protein associated with the particulates (46). Bridges directly connecting vesicles and MTs have been illustrated in several preparations (47).

Another mechanism that has been proposed takes into account the layer of anionic polyelectrolyte, which ensheaths axonal MTs and also extends to form a network through the axoplasm (48). This material is associated with MTs in axons and stains with alcian blue (49), ruthenium red, alkaline bismuth (50), and lanthanum (51). These methods under the conditions used have some specificity for mucopolysaccharides, or at least for polyanionic molecules with high charge density. In this minimal model, the MTs are the anchor points of a network composed of macroanionic molecules (macroions). The branching molecular units would specifically attach to the transported molecules or organelles. It is well known that linear flexible macroions characteristically extend and contract with small ionic changes in their immediate environment (52). Indeed, polyelectrolyte gels can be made to act as transformers of chemical energy to mechanical work (52). The expansion-contraction movements of the anionic polyelectrolyte network might be expected to be discontinuous and generate the saltatory character of cytoplasmic movements. A dynein-like protein with ATPase activity has been reported to be associated with neuronal MTs (55).

5 ANTIMITOTIC DRUGS

Certain antimitotic drugs are now known to block mitosis by interfering with the movements of the chromosomes. Further, the molecular mechanism of the blockade is the disruption of the microtubules of the mitotic spindle by the binding of the drug to the microtubule protein (53). The drugs for which this mechanism is best established are colchicine and some of its derivatives, the vinca alkaloids (vinblastine and vincristine), and podophyllotoxin. The importance of these findings should not be underestimated for they have led to substantial advances in a wide spectrum of research from biochemistry to medicine. The escalation of knowledge about the microtubules is an example. The interaction of these drugs with microtubule protein has been comprehensively reviewed in reference 54.

5.1 Colchicine

Because colchicine binds specifically to tubulin, the protein subunit of the spindle microtubules, it can be considered a prototype of a class of antimitotic drugs known as spindle poisons (56, 57). The details of the interaction of colchicine with tubulin are covered in reference 54.

Colchicine blocks ICM in addition to those of chromosomes in a wide variety of cells. It has been shown to block the axoplasmic transport of axoplasmic constituents such as acetylcholinesterase in sciatic nerve (58), amine storage granules (59, 60), proteins (61–63), and sulfated mucopolysaccharide protein (64). Further, colchicine blocks the movements of pigment granules in chromophore cells (65), nuclear migrations in fused cells (66), in other words, a wide variety of cytoplasmic movements. Although some work suggests that colchicine blocks only the rapidly transported axonal constituents, a greater number of studies show that the slow transport (1 mm/day) is also blocked (7, 61, 63, 67).

Colchicine also blocks the retrograde transport of horseradish peroxidase (26), nerve growth factor (27), and optically observed particulate movements (19). In many preparations the blockade of transport is associated with a disappearance of the microtubules. The specific binding of colchicine to the microtubule protein and the microtubule disruption has been the major contributing evidence to the conclusion that microtubules are an essential component of the biological machinery for ICM.

An increasing variety of cellular responses affected by colchicine (and also by the vinca alkaloids) are appearing in the literature. Included in these are the glucose-stimulated release of insulin (68); nerve-stimulated release of norepinephrine and dopamine-β-hydroxylase from sympathetic nerves (69); TSH-stimulated release of thyroxin (70); acetylcholine-stimulated release of catecholamines from the adrenal medulla (71); release of histamine from mast cells (72) and leukocytes (73); release of growth hormone and prolactin induced by prostaglandin E (74). The inference drawn from these experiments generally is that the MTs are involved in the mechanical movements leading to release of the secretory products contained in granules. Still other intracellular events such as the conversion of proparathyroid hormone to parathyroid hormone (75) have been shown to be influenced by colchicine (and the vinca alkaloids). The *stimulation* of steroid secretion by colchicine and other antimicrotubular agents has been interpreted by Temple & Wolff (76) to mean that access of cholesterol to the mitochondria is ordinarily restricted by the MTs and that stimulation occurs when this restriction is removed by the antimicrotubular agents.

The antimicrotubular agents (but not cytochalasin B, which does not bind to MT) have been shown to affect plasma membrane topographical responses (77). These agents reverse the inhibition by concanavalin A of patch formation and immunoglobulin receptor mobility in lymphocytes (78). Also, lymphocyte mitogenesis induced by the binding of antigen to the cell surface receptors is inhibited by colchicine at a step prior to spindle formation. It is not known whether the colchicine-binding protein in this case is tubulin, but the similarity of effects of a variety of antimicrotubular drugs suggests that it is. The hypothesis proposed by Edelman postulates a subsurface protein (tubulin?) in association-dissociation equilibrium with certain cell receptors that anchors the receptors and modulates their mobility. Further, he proposes that this protein assembly may be involved in a signaling process for mitogenesis (78).

The question of the specificity of colchicine for microtubule protein in some responses continues to be raised (79). In an attempt to resolve this, Zweig & Chignell (80) have suggested that a stronger case for the participation of MTs in these processes could be made if the effect were directly related to the ability of a given analog to bind to tubulin. To illustrate their approach, they have compared the ranking of the binding of seventeen colchicine analogs, podophyllotoxin, and vinblastine to tubulin with the ranking in the mouse sarcoma test and in anti-inflammatory activity (80). They found a good correlation between the binding of these drugs and their efficacy as both antimitotic and antigout agents. This supports the theory of Malawista (81) that the binding of colchicine to tubulin is responsible for its antigout as well as its antimitotic activities. The lumicolchicines are also useful tools for such studies since these derivatives do not bind to tubulin (54) and are not antimitotic. Lumicolchicine does not affect FAXT under conditions where colchicine does (82).

The blockade of transport by the tubulin-binding drugs is sometimes reported as occurring without detectable changes in the ultrastructure of MTs. However, the sample of tissue in electron microscopy is small and flaws in the MTs could escape attention. Furthermore, the ultrastructural appearance of the MTs may not always be a reliable index of their functional integrity. This would be particularly true if the dynamic polymerization-depolymerization of pool subunits and MTs is necessary for functioning. Colchicine binds to the tubulin subunits and not to the polymerized MT itself, so it causes the disappearance of the MT only when there is an ongoing polymerization-depolymerization by drawing the equilibrium away from the polymerized state.

5.2 Vinca Alkaloids

The interaction of the vinca alkaloids with tubulin depolymerizes the microtubules and gives rise to highly regular crystalloid structures (83). The binding site of the vinca alkaloids on the tubulin molecule is different from the colchicine site. The chemical properties of the vinca alkaloids that bind to tubulin and the crystalloids that are formed have been studied in some detail (40). However, it should be cautioned that the vinca alkaloids interact and can precipitate a number of acidic proteins and nucleic acids in addition to tubulin (84). In particular, the vinca alkaloids interact with actin. Thus, the vinca alkaloids appear to be less specific than colchicine. Most of the studies on axoplasmic transport are with vinblastine sulfate and vincristine sulfate, and there is little question that they are potent blocking agents—more so than colchicine—on both the fast and slow types of axoplasmic transport (85, 86), and the retrograde transport as well (87).

The antimitotic activity of several of the vinca alkaloids (mitotic index 50%) is about the same for vinblastine sulfate, vincristine sulfate, and desacetylvinblastine sulfate (7.5×10^{-8} M), while leurosidine is about 100 times less potent. The upper indole moiety of the dimeric alkaloid, catharanthine is a weak antimitotic, while the lower indole moiety, vindoline, is inactive (54). It is noteworthy that the interaction of these derivatives with tubulin parallels the antimitotic activity (54).

5.3 Podophyllotoxin

Another plant aklaloid that arrests mitosis in a similar manner to colchicine is podophyllotoxin. This drug binds to tubulin at the same (or greatly overlapping) site as colchicine, but with somewhat different binding forces (54). Picropodophyllotoxin, an isomer of podophyllotoxin, is reported to have less affinity for tubulin and correspondingly is a weaker antimitotic agent than podophyllotoxin (54). Podophyllotoxin has an inhibitory effect similar to that of vinblastine on the release of iodine from the thyroid stimulated by the thyroid-stimulating hormone (70) and on catecholamine release from the adrenal medulla (71).

5.4 Griseofulvin

Griseofulvin, a product of mold metabolism, is a fungistatic agent that resembles colchicine in its structure and in its antimitotic action. However, its mechanism of action appears to be different since it does not interact directly with tubulin, nor does it block polymerization of MTs in vitro (54). There is evidence that it disrupts the relative position of the microtubules with respect to one another similar to the action of isopropyl N-phenylcarbamate. The possibility has not been tested that it may interact with the "mucopolysaccharide" material ensheathing and connecting the microtubules: the "microtubular network" described in section 4.7 above. Griseofulvin blocks the granule movements in melanocytes (88) and this is rapidly reversible when the drug is removed.

6 CYTOCHALASIN B

The cytochalasins are a group of mold metabolites. One of these, cytochalasin B, (cyto-B) has effects on a variety of cellular activities and has been importantly exploited by Wessels and his colleagues (89). The cytochalasins inhibit a variety of cellular movements (cytoplasmic streaming, cytokinesis, pinocytosis).

The site of action of cytochalasin B seems to be on a class of microfilaments. It does not change the microtubules or neurofilaments in any discernible way. Its effects on axoplasmic transport are not clear-cut. It blocks both the slow (1 mm/day) and a faster (10 mm/day) protein axoplasmic transport in a crayfish ventral cord preparation (90). Also the drug caused a disruption of the "constrainment" of the faster transported protein in the crayfish preparation, which suggests that the cyto-B–sensitive microfilaments may be important to the directionality of the transported materials. On the other hand, there are reports of no effect of cyto-B on axoplasmic transport. For example, it had no effect on the transport of norepinephrine storage granules in adrenergic nerves (60). The drug is poorly soluble in aqueous solutions so the delivery of the drug may account for some of these disagreements. Cytochalasin B inhibits the release of catecholamines and dopamine-β-hydroxylase from adrenergic terminals (69). Further, it inhibits the outward movement of granules in the melanocyte, which colchicine does not; cyto-B does not affect the inward movement of the granules as colchicine and vinca alkaloids do (88).

The intracellular translocation of pigment granules in the dendritic arms toward the cell centers in the chromatophores of the glass shrimp (*Palaemonetes vulgaris*) is not inhibited by colchicine or vinblastine. (Yet the MTs are gone and vinblastine-tubulin crystals appear.) However, this pigment movement is reversibly blocked by cytochalasin B but with no discernible loss of microfilaments (91). Thus centripetal pigment movement in this preparation does not require MTs but some cyto-B-sensitive element. This action is in contrast to the actions of these drugs on the granule movements in the melanocyte described above. Although cyto-B clearly disrupts actin thin filaments in some preparations, there are other preparations that argue against the actin filament as the target molecule. It has been pointed out in a recent discussion of cyto-B actions by Pollard & Weiking that the dose-dependent effects indicate more than one target molecule (34). Indeed, there are reasons to believe that the cyto-B action is at the cell surface and the changes in microfilament structure are secondary (92).

7 ANESTHETICS

The effects of anesthetics on AXT have been valuable in sorting out the immediate relationship of electrical excitability of neurons from AXT.

7.1 Halothane

The effect of the general anesthetic, halothane, on ICM has been studied in several types of preparations. On the strength of the observation that the axopods of *Actinosphaerium* (the axopods are dependent upon MT integrity) retracted during exposure to halothane, Allison & Nunn proposed that the mechanism of the anesthesia is via the disruption of MT (93). More direct studies on halothane anesthesia have shown that this hypothesis is not correct (94). Concentrations of halothane that produce anesthesia do not affect axoplasmic transport (95) nor are the microtubules discernibly affected in vagus nerve axons (94). Much higher concentrations of halothane inhibit axoplasmic transport (95), reduce the number of microtubules, and disrupt their morphology (96).

7.2 Local Anesthetics

The effect of several of the common local anesthetics on axoplasmic transport has been studied. Fink and colleagues examined the effect of lidocaine on the fast axoplasmic transport of protein in rabbit nerves in vitro. Concentrations in the order of 0.2% slowed the transport reversibly, while concentrations in the order of 0.6% completely blocked transport with slight reversibility and also caused a disappearance of axonal microtubules. They later showed that the block of impulse conduction and axoplasmic transport changes did not correlate temporally (97).

Other studies on local anesthetics involving lidocaine topically applied (98), ophthaine c n an optic nerve preparation (99), and procaine (1%) on slow and fast transport of fibers in the sciatic nerve emerging from the ventral horn cells (100) showed no effect. Lidocaine and etidocaine under local anesthetic conditions did not change the rapid transport of catecholamine-synthesizing enzymes in sciatic nerve (101). Thus it appears that local anesthetics at anesthetic concentrations do not directly influence axoplasmic transport. It is worth noting that the electrical excitability of nerves is not directly dependent upon the MTs. That is, vagus nerve fibers treated with colchicine under conditions that extensively reduced the number of MTs did not show any changes in the rates of action potential conduction or amplitude (94). Also, neither the replacement of Na^+ in the medium with an equivalent amount of K^+, which leads to a depolarization of the nerve, nor indeed the replacement of Ringer's solution with an isotonic sucrose solution influences the fast axoplasmic transport (102).

8 NEUROPATHOGENS

A wide variety of agents and diseases have been described as neuropathogens. There are good reasons for believing that some of these that are associated with neurofibrillary pathology have among their effects the disruption of axoplasmic transport.

8.1 Aluminum Salts

Aluminum salts have been used experimentally to induce a neurofibrillary degeneration, and this preparation has been used as an experimental model for neurofibrillary diseases (103). In a study of axoplasmic transport in aluminum-treated rabbits (0.1 ml 1% $AlCl_3$ injected into the cisterna magna) with the neurological signs of the aluminum-induced pathology, the authors concluded that the anterograde protein axoplasmic transport rate was not changed (104). This is a surprising result in view of the rather severe pathology described. However, examination of the data and the methods used make it clear that the experiments were not adequate. That is, as these experiments were designed the axoplasmic transport observed would be that in the remaining normal fibers, and the axoplasmic transport failure in the fibrillary degenerated neurons would not be resolved. The Al-induced neurofibrillary tangles are tangles of 10 nm filaments and do not appear to be associated with alterations in the MTs or the other organelles of the nerve cell body (105). It is an important experimental model because the neurofibrillary tangles induced a state similar to those seen in a number of major neurological diseases.

8.2 Acrylamide and Triorthocresyl Phosphate

Chronic administration of acrylamide induces a type of neuropathy in which one might expect disruption of axoplasmic transport to be implicated. The slow 1 mm/day AXT was reported to be disrupted in cats with acrylamide neuropathy but not in triorthocresyl phosphate neuropathy (106). On the other hand, Bradley and colleagues concluded that both the fast and slow axonal protein transport waves in cats suffering from neuropathies induced with vincristine, acrylamide, and triorthocresyl phosphate were normal (107). They also point out that the complexities involved in transport studies make interpretation of the data difficult. Again, the design of these experiments is such that the transport in unaffected fibers would dominate and poor transport would be revealed only if it were pronounced and not close to the site of precursor injection. It seems evident that a degenerated axon would fail to transport proteins. The question is whether the "causation" site of action of a given neuropathogen is on the transport mechanism. Obviously it would be valuable to study the relationship of axoplasmic transport perturbation to the neuropathogens with better-designed experiments.

8.3 Galactose Neurotoxicity

A galactose neurotoxicity in chicks is associated with tremors and seizures resulting from a general disruption of energy metabolism of the brain. FAXT in the optic nerves was studied in galactose-treated chicks, and the amount of FAXT protein was decreased about 30%. The authors attribute this reduction of transport to an inadequate supply of required energy (108).

9 NEUROTOXINS

9.1 Tetrodotoxin

Tetrodotoxin is a valuable experimental tool that blocks sodium membrane channels and thus arrests the axonal action potential conduction. It does not affect fast axoplasmic transport (100). This might be expected in view of the lack of immediate correlation between electrical excitability and axoplasmic transport (see section 7).

9.2 Batrachotoxin

Batrachotoxin blocks membrane excitability by way of an increased Na^+ permeability (109). It was recently found to block FAXT in micromolar concentrations (110). Increasing Ca^{2+} in the medium had a protective action. The mechanism of action is not known but is unrelated to the increased Na^+ influx because the block occurred in the absence of Na^+ in the medium. Nor was the ATP level sufficiently lowered by the batrachotoxin to account for the inhibition by interruption of available energy supply. A clue to the mechanism may be found in the observation that tetrodotoxin, which blocks the action of batrachotoxin on membrane excitability, also prevented its blockade of axoplasmic transport (110).

10 MONOAMINE OXIDASE INHIBITORS

The monoamine oxidase (MAO) inhibitors pargyline and phenelzine have unusual effects on fast axoplasmic transport (111). Rats were given (75 mg Kg^{-1}) pargyline daily for up to 7 days, and the FAXT in sciatic nerve was studied. The rate of the leading front of the transported protein in the control was about 550 mm/day (in the range of other studies), but the rate of the leading front in the pargyline-treated rats increased almost 4 times (2000 mm/day). The authors related this change in FAXT to a myopathy, which results from the pargyline treatment. Their report is brief but is important enough to deserve comment. The design of the experiments did not permit a discrimination of the following possibilities: (a) an increase in uptake and incorporation of the labeled precursor and hence an earlier release from the cell bodies of the labeled protein; (b) the faster front being composed of proteins other than the control FAXT proteins. Since these findings have a bearing on the trophic actions of neurons and possibily on certain myopathies, they warrant more study.

11 MICROTUBULE-STABILIZING AGENTS

11.1 Dimethyl Sulfoxide

A number of agents that stabilize MTS are known. To date the most powerful is the solvent dimethyl sulfoxide (DMSO). It has been used to isolate a greater number of polymerized MTS from brain (112). In vitro, polymerization of tubulin is more rapid with DMSO present in the medium, and at an optimum concentration of 10% the MTs are stabilized against the depolymerizing actions of cooling and ionic strength (113). The effect of 10% DMSO on FAXT in vagus fibers is a complete blockage which is reversible; at 2% or lower the DMSO does not discernibly affect the FAXT. The ultrastructure of the vagal fibers in 10% reveals a swelling of glial cells and some unmyelinated axons but shrinkage of other unmyelinated axons; the MTs are abundant and prominent. Even these dramatic ultrastructural changes are readily reversible (114). Owing to the wide variety of DMSO's actions, an interpretation of these results is not definitive, but these results are compatible with the idea that stabilizing the MTs (that is, depressing the depolymerization-polymerization dynamics) may render them nonfunctional in ICM.

11.2 Heavy Water

The hypothesis that stabilizing MTs makes them nonfunctional was put forth based on experiments with D_2O on mitotic movements (115). D_2O is known to strengthen the gel state of cytoplasm and also to affect the ionization of weak acids (116). D_2O may also immobilize the filaments extending from the MTs (described in 4.7), which may be important in the motion-generating machinery.

The antimitotic effect of D_2O is well known (117) and it reversibly inhibits melanin granule movement in melanocytes (118). D_2O (50–90%) blocks the FAXT of proteins in frog sciatic nerve (119) and the release of growth hormone and prolactin from the adenohypophysis (74). At least, the idea that the sequential disassembly-reassembly of MTs is necessary for their function (115) is compatible with some of the observations. The subject is complicated in that D_2O facilitates some responses in which the catecholamines are released from the adrenal medulla (71).

12 NERVE GROWTH FACTOR

Nerve growth factor (NGF) is a polypeptide that modifies the maturation and metabolism of adrenergic neurons and is a regulating molecule. It has been intensively studied and its amino acid sequence is known. It is transported retrogradely in specific neurons (see section 3.2). Almon & McClure (120) studied the effects of NGF on AXT in sympathetic neurons and found that NGF increases the rate of the fast-transported protein but decreases the rate of the slow-transported protein, indicating a selective action. They suggest that NGF also has a role in the physiological regulation of axoplasmic transport.

13 CONCLUSION

The intracellular movements of cellular constituents are largely nonrandom, organized events by which molecules and higher order aggregates are relocated within the cell. Pharmacology has an important role in the study of the intracellular movements and in turn, pharmacological research of these events has contributed to the understanding of the mechanism of action of some drugs. The locations of origin or synthesis of cellular constituents are usually not the intracellular locations of function, and ongoing metabolism is associated with continuous translocation. Diffusion as a translocation mechanism is important primarily for small molecules and even with small molecules, diffusion needs to be supplemented with bulk streaming and cytoplasmic stirring. Thus, metabolically generated energy must be available and the chemical form of the energy must be converted to a mechanical event. An additional requirement for intracellular movement is of an informational kind: specific constituents are translocated to specific locations.

Those neurons possessing long axons are useful for the study of intracellular movements of the selective type (the type unrelated to bulk cytoplasmic movement). The neuron has a high degree of segregation of functions and the long axon makes many aspects of transport accessible for study.

Drugs that disrupt the generation or flow of metabolic energy will interfere generally with intracellular movements. The antimitotic drugs (colchicine, vinca alkaloids, etc) have been particularly valuable because they arrest a wide variety of intracellular movements in a large representation of types of cells and there is a compelling correlation between their affinity for tubulin, their disruption of microtubules, and their pharmacological actions. On the strength of such studies, the inescapable conclusion is that the ubiquitous microtubules are directly involved in many intracellular movements. The anesthetics have been useful in resolving questions about the direct relationship between electrical excitability and transport. The basis of anesthetic action does not seem to be a disruption of intracellular movements.

A number of aspects of intracellular movements are promising for future research of practical importance, for example, the trophic functions of neurons, neuropathies, intracellular regulation, and regulation of hormone release.

The long-standing reservations concerning drug specificity, and indirect versus direct actions can be minimized as illustrated in the case of the tubulin-binding drugs. That is, if the correlation between the binding affinities of the drugs to relevant molecules and the pharmacological actions follows a close ranking order, the conclusions about mechanism are strengthened.

Literature Cited

1. Allen, R. 1974. *Symp. Soc. Exp. Biol.* 28:15–26
2. Palay, S. L., Chan-Palay, V. 1972. *Metabolic Compartmentation in the Brain,* 187–207. New York: Macmillan
3. Barondes, S. H., Samson, F. E. 1967. *Neurosci. Res. Program Bull.* 5:307–419
4. Grafstein, B. 1969. In *Advances in Biochemical Neuropharmacology,* 11–25. New York: Raven
5. Lasek, R. J. 1970. *Int. Rev. Neurobiol.* 13:289–324
6. Ochs, S. 1974. *Ann. NY Acad. Sci.* 228:202–23
7. Heslop, J. P. 1974. *Symp. Soc. Exp. Biol.* 28:209–27
8. Lubinska, L. 1964. *Prog. Brain Res.* 13:1–71
9. Weiss, P. 1967. *Neurosci. Res. Program Bull.* 5:371–400
10. McClure, W. O. 1972. *Adv. Pharmacol. Chemother.* 10:185–220
11. Weiss, P., Hiscoe, H. B. 1948. *J. Exp. Zool.* 107:315–95
12. Droz, B., Leblond, C. P. 1963. *J. Comp. Neurol.* 121:325–45
13. Jasinski, A., Gorbman, A., Hara, T. J. 1966. *Science* 154:776–78
14. Albuquerque, E. X., Warnick, J. E., Sansone, F. M., Onur, R. 1974. *Trophic Functions of the Neuron. Ann. NY Acad. Sci.* 228:224–43
15. Fernandez, H. L., Ramirez, B. 1974. *Brain Res.* 49:385–95
16. Jahn, T. L., Bovee, E. C. 1969. *Physiol. Rev.* 49:793–862
17. Allen, R. D., Kamiya, N. 1964. *Primitive Motile Systems in Cell Biology.* New York: Academic
18. *Symp. Soc. Exp. Biol. 1974. Transport at the Cellular Level,* No. 28. Cambridge: Cambridge Univ. Press
19. Kirkpatrick, J. B., Bray, J. J., Palmer, S. M. 1972. *Brain Res.* 43:1–10
20. Cooper, P. O., Smith, R. S. 1974. *J. Physiol.* 242:77–97
21. Forman, D. S., Padjan, A. L., Siggins, G. R. 1974. *Soc. Neurosci. Abstr.* 4:213
22. Price, D. L., Griffin, J., Young, A., Peck, K., Stocks, A. 1975. *Science* 188:945–47
23. Kristensson, K. 1970. *Acta Neuropathol.* 16:293–300
24. Kristensson, K., Olsson, Y. 1971 *Brain Res.* 29:363–65
25. LaVail, J. H., LaVail, M. M. 1974. *J. Comp. Neurol.* 157:303–58
26. LaVail, M. M., LaVail, J. H. 1975. *Brain Res.* 85:273–80
27. Hendry, I. A., Stockel, K., Thoenen, H., Iversen, L. L. 1974. *Brain Res.* 68:103–21
28. Ochs, S. 1971. *Proc. Nat. Acad. Sci. USA* 65:1279–82
29. Ochs, S. 1971. *J. Neurochem.* 18:833–43
30. Ochs, S. 1971. *J. Neurochem.* 18:107–14
31. Edds, K. 1973. *J. Cell Biol.* 59:88a
32. Johnson, G., Smith, R. S., Lock, G. S. 1969. *Am. J. Physiol.* 217:188–91
33. Tani, E., Ametani, T. 1970. *J. Cell Biol.* 46:159–65
34. Pollard, T. O., Weiking, P. R. 1974. *CRC Crit. Rev. Biochem.* 2:1–65
35. Berl, S., Puszkin, S., Nicklas, W. J. 1973. *Science* 179:441–46
36. Fine, R. E., Blitz, A. L., Hitchcock, S. E., Kaminer, B. 1973. *Nature London New Biol.* 245:182–85
37. Davison, P., Winslow, B. 1974. *J. Neurobiol.* 5:119–33
38. Bryan, J. et al 1974. *Fed. Proc.* 33:152–74
39. Olmstead, J. B., Borisy, G. G. 1973. *Ann. Rev. Biochem.* 42:507–40
40. Soifer, D., Chairman. 1975. *Conf. Biol. Cytoplasmic Microtubules, Ann. NY Acad. Sci.* 253:1–848
41. McIntosh, J. R. et al 1974. *J. Supramol. Struct.* 2:385–485
42. Porter, K. R. 1966. In *Principles of Biomolecular Organization. CIBA*

Foundation Symposium, 308–45. London: Churchill
43. Byers, M. R. 1974. *Brain Res.* 75:97–113
44. Troyer, D. 1975. *Nature London* 254:696–98
45. Burton, P. R., Kirkland, W. L. 1972. *Nature London New Biol.* 239:244–46
46. Schmitt, F. O., Samson, F. E. 1968. *Neurosci. Res. Program Bull.* 6:113–219
47. Smith, D. S., Jarlfors, U., Beranek, R. 1970. *J. Cell Biol.* 46:199–219
48. Samson, F. E. 1971. *J. Neurobiol.* 2:347–60
49. Hinkley, R. E. 1973. *J. Cell Sci.* 13:753–61
50. Burton, P. R., Hinkley, R. E. 1974. *J. Submicros. Cytol.* 6:311–26
51. Burton, P. R., Fernandez, H. L. 1973. *J. Cell Sci.* 12:567–83
52. Oosawa, F. 1971. *Polyelectrolytes.* New York: Dekker
53. Taylor, E. W. 1965. *J. Cell Biol.* 25:145–60
54. Wilson, L., Bamburg, J. R., Mizel, S. B., Grisham, L. M., Creswell, K. M. 1947. *Fed. Proc.* 33:158–66
55. Gaskin, F. et al 1974. *FEBS Lett.* 40:281–86
56. Shelanski, M. L., Taylor, E. W. 1967. *J. Cell Biol.* 34:549–54
57. Weisenberg, R. C., Borisy, G. G., Taylor, E. W. 1968. *Biochemistry* 7:4466–78
58. Kreutzberg, G. W. 1969. *Proc. Natl. Acad. Sci. USA* 62:722–28
59. Hökfelt, T., Dahlström, A. 1971. *Acta Physiol. Scand. Suppl.* 357:10–11
60. Banks, P., Mayor, D., Mraz, P. 1973. *Brain Res.* 49:417–21
61. Fernandez, H., Davison, P. F. 1969. *Proc. Natl. Acad. Sci. USA* 64:512–19
62. Boesch, J., Manko, P., Cuenod, M. 1972. *Neurobiology* 2:123–32
63. James, K. A. C., Bray, J. J., Morgan, I. G., Austin, L. 1970. *Biochem. J.* 117:767–71
64. Elam, J. S., Goldberg, J. M., Radin, N. S., Agranoff, B. W. 1970. *Science* 170:458–60
65. Malawista, S. E. 1971. *J. Cell Biol.* 49:848–55
66. Holmes, K. V., Choppin, P. W. 1968. *J. Cell Biol.* 39:526–43
67. Karlsson, J., Sjostrand, J. 1968. *Brain Res.* 11:431–39
68. Lacy, P. E., Howell, S. L., Young, D. A., Fink, C. J. 1968. *Nature London* 219:1177–79
69. Thoa, N. G., Wooten, G. F., Axelrod, J., Kopin, I. J. 1972. *Proc. Natl. Acad. Sci. USA* 69:520–22
70. Williams, J. A., Wolff, J. 1972. *J. Cell Biol.* 54:157–65
71. Poisner, A. M., Bernstein, J. 1971. *J. Pharm. Exp. Ther.* 177:102–8
72. Gillespie, E., Levine, R. J., Malawista, S. E. 1968. *J. Pharmacol. Exp. Ther.* 164:158–65
73. Levy, D. A., Carlton, J. A. 1969. *Proc. Soc. Exp. Biol. Med.* 130:1333–36
74. Labrie, F. et al 1973. *Endocrinology* 93:903–14
75. Kemper, B., Habener, J. F., Rich, A., Potts, J. T. 1975. *Endocrinology* 96:906–12
76. Temple, R., Wolff, J. 1973. *J. Biol. Chem.* 248:2691–98
77. Yin, H., Ukena, T., Berlin, R. 1972. *Science* 178:867–68
78. Edelman, G. 1975. *Functional Linkage in Biomolecular Systems,* 188–201. New York: Raven
79. Trifaro, J. M., Collier, B., Lastoweka, A., Stern, D. 1972. *Mol. Pharmacol.* 8:264–67
80. Zweig, M. H., Chignell, C. F. 1973. *Biochem. Pharmacol.* 22:2141–50
81. Malawista, S. E. 1968. *Arthritis Rheum.* 11:191–97
82. Price, M. T. 1974. *Brain Res.* 77:497–501
83. Bensch, K. G., Malawista, S. E. 1969. *J. Cell Biol.* 40:95–107
84. Wilson, L., Bryan, J., Ruby, A., Mazia, D. 1970. *Proc. Natl. Acad. Sci. USA* 66:807–14
85. Fernandez, H. L., Burton, P. R., Samson, F. E. 1971. *J. Cell Biol.* 51:176–92
86. Karlsson, J. O., Hansson, H. A., Sjostrand, J. 1971. *Z. Zellforsch. Mikrosk. Anat.* 115:265–83
87. Bunt, A. H., Lund, R. D. 1974. *Exp. Neurol.* 45:288–97
88. Malawista, S. E. 1971. *J. Cell Biol.* 49:848–55
89. Wessels, N. K. et al 1971. *Science* 171:135–43
90. Fernandez, H. L., Samson, F. E. 1973. *J. Neurobiol.* 4:201–6
91. Robison, W. G. 1973. *J. Cell Biol.* 59:287a
92. Goldman, R. D., Snipe, D. M. 1972. *Cold Spring Harbor Symp.* 37:523–34
93. Allison, A. C., Nunn, J. F. 1968. *Lancet* ii:1326
94. Hinkley, R. E., Green, L. S. 1971. *J. Neurobiol.* 2:97–106
95. Fink, B. R., Kennedy, R. D. 1972. *Anesthesiology* 36:13–20

96. Hinkley, R. E., Samson, F. E. 1972. *J. Cell Biol.* 53:258–63
97. Fink, B. R., Kennedy, R. D., Hendrickson, A. E., Middaugh, M. E. 1972. *Anesthesiology* 36:422–32
98. Karlsson, J. O., Sjostrand, J. 1969. *Brain Res.* 13:617–19
99. Hendrickson, A. E., Cowan, W. M. 1971. *Exp. Neurol.* 30:403–22
100. Ochs, S., Hollingsworth, D. 1971. *J. Neurochem.* 18:107–14
101. Ngai, S. H., Dairman, W., Marchelle, M. 1974. *Anesthesiology* 41:542–48
102. Ochs, S. 1972. *Soc. Neurosci. Abstr.* 2:255
103. Klatzo, I., Wisniewski, H., Streicher, E. 1965. *J. Neuropathol. Exp. Neurol.* 24:187–99
104. Liwnicz, B. H., Kristensson, K., Wisniewski, H. M., Shelanski, M. L., Terry, R. D. 1974. *Brain Res.* 80:413–20
105. Wisniewski, H. M., Terry, R. D., Hirano, A. 1970. *J. Neuropathol. Exp. Neurol.* 29:163–76
106. Pleasure, D. E., Mishler, K. C., Engel, W. K. 1969. *Science* 166:524–27
107. Bradley, W. G., Williams, M. H. 1973. *Brain* 96:235–46

108. Knull, H. R., Lobert, P. F., Wells, W. W. 1974. *Brain Res.* 79:524–27
109. Albuquerque, E. X., Daly, J. W., Witkop, B. 1971. *Science* 172:995–1002
110. Ochs, S., Worth, R. 1975. *Science* 187:1087–89
111. Boegman, R. S., Wood, P. L., Pinaud, L. 1975. *Nature London* 253:51–52
112. Filner, P., Behnke, O. 1973. *J. Cell Biol.* 59:99a
113. Dulak, L., Crist, R. 1974. *Am. J. Cell Biol.* 63:90a
114. Donoso, J. A., Illanes, J. P., Samson, F. E. 1975. *Soc. Neurosci. Ann. Meet., Abstr.*
115. Tilney, L. G., Gibbins, J. R. 1969. *J. Cell Biol.* 41:227–50
116. Houston, L. L., Odell, J., Lee, Y. C., Himes, R. 1974. *J. Mol. Biol.* 87:141–46
117. Marsland, D., Zimmerman, A. M. 1965. *Exp. Cell Res.* 38:306–13
118. Marsland, D., Meisner, D. O. 1967. *J. Cell. Physiol.* 70:209–16
119. Anderson, K. E., Edström, A., Hanson, M. 1972. *Brain Res.* 43:299–302
120. Almon, R. R., McClure, W. O. 1974. *Brain Res.* 74:255–67

FUNCTIONAL PROPERTIES OF   ✦6643
POSTJUNCTIONAL MEMBRANE

L. G. Magazanik

Sechenov Institute of Evolutionary Physiology and Biochemistry, Academy of Sciences
of the USSR, Leningrad, K–223, USSR

INTRODUCTION

The diverse functions of the postjunctional membrane (PJM) have been associated
with the activity of specific receptors. Synaptic receptors are beginning to be viewed
not as mere abstractions but as macromolecular complexes that can be isolated and
subjected to chemical analysis. In this connection an understanding of how the
various functions of the PJM are carried out is essential. The transduction of a signal
from a chemical into an electrical form consists of several functional stages. In this
study a survey is made of current ideas on the molecular nature, kinetics, and
possible interactions of activation stages of PJM. Because some of these topics have
already been reviewed (1–12), we consider only the most recent or not yet fully
accepted questions. Since the bulk of our knowledge of postsynaptic mechanisms is
gained from the study of effects of acetylcholine (ACh), this review is restricted to
a discussion of the functional organization of cholinoceptive membranes.

ACh-INDUCED CHANGES OF ION PERMEABILITY AND
CLASSIFICATION OF CHOLINORECEPTORS

Ionic mechanisms providing for ACh effects are most diverse. Permeability may
increase selectively for Na^+, K^+, Ca^{++}, or Cl^- and decrease for Na^+ and K^+. Direct
activation of electrogenic ionic pumps is possible but doubtful. Main approaches to
the ionic nature of synaptic potentials have been discussed in detail in the reviews
by Ginsborg (6, 13). Permeability of activated PJM shows selectivity, which means
that molecular devices determining such ion selectivity (ionic channels) are specific.
It is most essential to learn whether these sodium, potassium, and chloride channels
are structural elements of appropriate cholinergic receptors (ChRs) or whether the
functions of PJM are performed by different but interacting macromolecules. There
is no direct answer to this question as yet. We hope, however, that progress in

161

isolating molecular complexes of cholinoceptive membranes will permit identification and localization of the components of PJM (11, 14) and thus elucidate the molecular structure of all elements of the functional chain from the recognition site to the selective ion filter. In any case, these components differ substantially in function.

Pharmacological variations between different ChRs that are likely to reflect peculiarities in the structure of their recognition sites have long been known. However, the biological meaning of these variants is not clear. It would be interesting to know among other things whether there is a correlation between pharmacological properties of ChRs and ionic mechanisms that bring about the ChR activation, that is, whether variants in the combination of the active center of one or another type of ChR with a definite type of the PJM ionic mechanism are random or regular. The evidence presented in Table 1 does not support such a correlation. ChR of the heart, smooth muscle, cortical neurons, and part of ChR of autonomic ganglion neurons are muscarinic. They do not differ pharmacologically, although the ionic effects of their activation vary significantly. Neurons of mollusks were found to contain three different types of ChR controlling three different types of ionic channels (31, 32). In this case, however, a nicotinic-like ChR operates the chloride channel, and its activation leads to hyperpolarization of the neuron. The solution of the important problem of correspondence between types of ChR and ionic effects of their activation is, among other things, limited by imperfect pharmacological classification of ChR. Their division into nicotinic and muscarinic receptors provides only a basic classification. Nicotinic ChRs, for example, differ in their ability to interact with various bisquaternary compounds (41).

Differences between ChRs can be revealed not only with the aid of classical cholinergic drugs but also with the action of α-bungarotoxin or dithiothreitol. It is known that α-bungarotoxin and other postsynaptically acting neurotoxins (NT) block the effect of ACh on skeletal muscles of vertebrates and their derivatives (electroplax). They are inefficient on muscarinic ChR (21) and not all nicotinic Ch-receptors are susceptible to the action of NT. Although the lamprey heart and somatic muscle contain pharmacologically identical nicotinic ChR (42, 43), neurotoxins block only ChR of the muscle without affecting the heart (44). NT does not block ACh effects in neurons of the rabbit sympathetic ganglia (25). NT produces a peculiar effect on ChR in leech. Responses of the dorsal muscle to such compounds as succinyldicholine and decamethonium are blocked selectively (45–47). NT exerts no influence on ChR of neurons (Retzius cells) in leech ganglia (58).

The effect of dithiothreitol is inverse; only the depolarizing action of ACh on the neurons in leech is blocked (58) while the response of the dorsal muscle is not affected (45). Muscles of lamellibranchs, gastropods and cephalopods, mollusk hearts, muscles of polychaetes, sipunculoids, echinoderms, and ascidians are insensitive to NT, but in most cases dithiothreitol blocks ACh effects (39).

Further work is needed to classify ChR and to interpret the biological significance of variation in their pharmacological properties and ionic mechanisms controlled by ChR.

Table 1 Effects of ACh on different cells[a]

Cells	Effect of ACh	Changes of ionic conductance	Type of ChR	Effect of α-bungaro-toxin	References
Skeletal muscle	d	↑ Na, K	n	+	15–17
Electroplax	d	↑ Na, K	n	+	18, 19
Heart of vertebrates	h	↑ K	m	–	20, 21
Smooth muscle of vertebrates	d	↑ Na (K, Ca)	m	–	21, 22
Sympathetic ganglion:					
Fast EPSP	d	↑ Na, K	n	–	23–25
Slow EPSP	d	↓ K	m	–	25–26
		or ↑ Na, Ca			27
		or including the electrogenic pump			28
Slow IPSP	h	↓ Na			120
Cortical neurons	d	↓ K	m		7
Snail neurons:					
Fast EPSP	d	↑ Na, K	n	–	29–32, 121
	d	↑ Cl			33
Fast IPSP	h	↑ Cl	n	+	30, 34, 35, 121
Slow IPSP	h	↑ K		–	31, 32, 121
Leech neurons	d	↑ Na	n	–	36, 58
	h	↑ Cl	m	–	58
Leech muscle	d		n	– +	45–47
Insect neurons	d	↑ Na	n	–	40
Mytilus muscle	d	↑ Na, K	n	–	37–39

[a] d = depolarization; h = hyperpolarization; ↑ = increase of conductance; ↓ = decrease of conductance; n = nicotinic ChR; m = muscarinic ChR; + = block; – = no block.

SOME PECULIARITIES OF PJM IONIC CHANNELS

Takeuchi & Takeuchi (15, 48) describe some important features in ion permeability of the activated end-plate: 1. Permeability increases only for cations (Na, K, and to a small extent, Ca). 2. The ratio between shifts of Na and K conductance is constant ($\Delta G_{Na}/\Delta G_K = 1.29$) and does not change in any time phase of activation, that is, the Na and K currents are completely synchronous. 3. The PJM conductance is not affected by changes in the electrical field and the ionic content.

In the last few years these postulates (2 and 3 in particular) have been revised many times. For instance the influence of the increase of $[K]_o$ had been already shown by Takeuchi (48). Takeuchi also described the influence of the membrane potential on the time course of the end-plate current (e.p.c.) (15). Further analysis of this fact required the revision of the postulate that conductance is independent of the potential (see next section). However, the striking electrochemical behavior of the activated PJM detected by these studies remains irrefutable. Ionic currents of the PJM cannot be described quantitatively by equations commonly used to define resting and action potentials (49). Thus some requirements of the Goldman constant field theory are not fulfilled in the activated PJM. There is a convenient experimental approach for revealing "non-Goldman" behavior of the PJM—a considerable shift of the equilibrium potential by 18–20 mv when $[K]_o$ decreases fivefold. Using this criterion of K = sensitivity we can demonstrate the electrochemical identity of responses to ACh, carbacholine, decamethonium, and succinyldicholine (50). On the other hand, it has been found that the equilibrium potential of responses to suberyldicholine and sebacinyldicholine does not change on lowering of $[K]_o$ (50–52). K = sensitivity disappears as the temperature decreases to 2–3°C (53). These results fit reasonably well with the hypothesis that the peculiar electrochemical behavior of the PJM is due to a very short life span of an open channel during which the concentration profile of a passing ion does not alter significantly (54). Were the time prolonged in some way (by decrease of temperature, action of suberyldicholine) the K = sensitivity as a sign of "non-Goldman" behavior of the PJM would disappear.

The assumption about the longer lifetime of open channels under suberyldicholine and low temperature was later confirmed in experiments analyzing voltage fluctuations induced in the end-plate by cholinomimetics (55, 56). The lifetime of the open state of ionic channels defined by the investigation of membrane noise (msec) substantially exceeds the time (μsec) consistent with the proposed hypothesis of transitional processes. According to this hypothesis the time course should have been determined not by the kinetics of ionic channels but by some other process [changes in ACh concentration in the synaptic cleft or time of existence of the ACh–ChR complex (for details, see section below)].

The independence of K and Na currents is the critical point of the hypothesis of transitional processes. The unitary channel, however, must not show electrochemical anomaly when the life span is short (50). The strict synchronism of changes in Na-K conductance makes it difficult to ascertain whether the cations Na^+ and K^+ move in through the same channel or whether there are selective channels for each of the permeant cations. The ability of the membrane equilibrium potential to alter under the action of some drugs (see Table 2) testifies in favor of separate channels (57). One ChR may control the state of the both Na and K channels so that the kinetics of changes in their conductance depends on the behavior of the common gating mechanism. From this point of view synchronous changes in the Na and K currents upon alteration of the membrane potential level would be more easily comprehended. A shift in the equilibrium potential by the action of certain drugs might be a direct selective effect on one of the channels. The existing facts are not sufficient to advance such a hypothesis.

TIME COURSE OF POSTSYNAPTIC CURRENTS

The use of the voltage clamp technique in the end-plate zone makes it possible to record the time course of changes in the synaptic current (e.p.c.). When the holding potential is −80 mv the maximum rise time for the e.p.c. of frog muscles is 0.5–0.6 msec, and the half-time of the decay is 1.1–1.2 msec.

The course of the decay curve is exponential, but first and last portions of the curve deviate from the exponential (60–63). The time course of the e.p.c. seems to reflect the kinetics of PJM activation. Because it may be assumed that there are differences in the rates of successive reactions constituting the activation process, a search for a rate-limiting factor or factors seems to be the best approach. Of the sequence of PJM activation stages (release of ACh, approach of a molecule to ChR, formation of an ACh-ChR complex, activation of the complex, appearance of ionic conductance, passing of ionic currents, elimination of ACh molecules through diffusion and enzyme hydrolysis, decrease of conductance) not all contribute directly to the postsynaptic current but any one may happen to be rate limiting.

In the 35–40 years since the end-plate potential was first recorded, the interpretation of its time course has undergone considerable change. The enzymic hydrolysis by cholinesterase (ChE) initially appeared to be a main factor (64), because the inhibition of ACh prolongs the e.p.c. Later, ACh diffusion in the synaptic cleft was shown to proceed so rapidly that the enzymic hydrolysis could not be regarded as the only limiting factor (65). It was then supposed that the formation and dissociation of the ACh–ChR complex is the slowest process. This hypothesis accounts for changes in the time course of e.p.c. under the influence of some drugs and altered temperature (63, 112), but it is difficult to use it for interpreting a relationship between the time course of the e.p.c. and the level of muscle fiber polarization. The first studies of the e.p.c. showed that hyperpolarization prolongs while depolarization shortens the e.p.c. (15), and this was confirmed repeatedly (60–63, 66–68). Takeuchi & Takeuchi (15) attempted to explain these findings by suggesting that the postsynaptic current affects the effective concentration of ACh in the vicinity of ChR in end-plate zone by iontophoresis. A thorough experimental analysis of this hypothesis by Stevens and collaborators indicated that this explanation was inappropriate (60, 61, 69, 70). The existence of separate ionic channels was hypothesized (57, 66, 71). Simultaneously it was postulated that the kinetics of these two channels are different and that the sodium channels are open for a longer time than the potassium channels. Kordas (72) checked one of the inevitable consequences of this hypothesis, suggesting different time courses for Na and K currents, i.e. a biphasic total current in the equilibrium potential region, and detected no such phenomenon. Against this interpretation, however, is evidence that the time course can be lengthened progressively on increase of hyperpolarization outside E_k zone to 150–200 mv and that the e.p.c. declines exponentially at any holding potential (60). It is clear now that the concept of potential independence of PJM conductance (15) is not valid, though the main principle of electrical inexcitability of PJM (109) still stands.

Table 2 Effects of modifiers of postjunctional membrane

Drug (references)	Time course of e.p.c.			ACh-noise (life span of channels)	Dependence of e.p.c. amplitude on MP level	Influence on reversal potential	Influence on desensitization kinetics
	Character of decay	Effect on exponential form of e.p.c.	Potential dependence of decay				
Procaine (57, 66, 68, 71, 72, 87, 98, 122)	biphasic decay: initial phase faster, final phase slower than normal			complicated	nonlinear	absent	accelerate
Lidocaine (71, 98, 112)	biphasic decay, but small slow phase					absent	accelerate
Diisopropyl-fluorophosphate (76, 77)	biphasic decay		lost			shift to E_K	
Edrophonium (103)	prolonged	hold	hold		normal		
Scopolamine (67, 81)	biphasic decay	only slow phase	only slow phase		nonlinear	absent	
Atropine (67, 91, 113–116)	shortened	hold	hold	shortened	normal	shift to E_{Na}	absent

Table 2 *(Continued)*

Drug (references)	Time course of e.p.c.		Potential dependence of decay	ACh-noise (life span of channels)	Dependence of e.p.c. amplitude on MP level	Influence on reversal potential	Influence on desensitization kinetics
	Character of decay	Effect on exponential form of e.p.c.					
Serotonin (109, 118)	slightly shortened	hold	lost		nonlinear	shift to E_K	absent
Morphine (118)	slightly shortened	hold	lost		nonlinear		
Amobarbital (52, 98, 104)	shortened	hold				absent	accelerate
Pentobarbital (98, 111)	shortened	hold	hold		normal	absent	accelerate
Chlorpromazine (52, 98)	slightly shortened					absent	accelerate
SKF–525A (119)	shortened	hold				absent	accelerate
Histrionicotoxin (102)	shortened	hold	decrease		nonlinear	absent	accelerate
N–butanol (78, 52, 98)	prolonged			prolonged			accelerate
Hexanol (78)	biphasic						

A valuable suggestion concerning the kinetics of the PJM activation mechanism was made by Magleby & Stevens (60, 61). Using as the basis a scheme proposed earlier (117)

$$ACh + ChR \underset{K_{-1}}{\overset{K_1}{\rightleftharpoons}} AChR \underset{\alpha}{\overset{\beta}{\rightleftharpoons}} AChR^*$$

they suggested that the initial stages, i.e. ACh diffusion within the synaptic cleft and formation of the ACh-receptor complex, proceed faster than the activation of this complex. Hence the process of opening and closing ionic channels was chosen as the time limiting factor. The channel may exist only in one of the two states, open or closed. The transition from one state into another takes almost no time, that is, the form of an elementary impulse of the postsynaptic current approaches the rectangular. The constants β and α reflect the mean probability of these transitions for each of a host of channels. These ideas were applied to the analysis of acetylcholine-induced noise (55). The improvement of the recording technique upon clamping of voltage (69) allowed a study of the conductance kinetics of the PJM comparing the simultaneous action of a large number of ACh molecules making up an integral number of quanta (the e.p.c. and m.e.p.c.) to the effects of asynchronous action of single ACh molecules. Good agreement was observed between the time parameters of the e.p.c. and m.e.p.c. on one hand, and elementary ACh-currents, on the other. The kinetics of macro and micro phenomena were similarly dependent on the membrane potential level and the temperature (55, 60, 69), which permits us to consider in more detail the nature of the e.p.c. time course. The formation of the complex results in opening of ionic channels. Since under given assumptions this is a probability process to be described exponentially, the greatest number of channels may open immediately after formation of the ACh-ChR complex. Distribution of the number of channels opening per unit of time depends on the membrane potential level and temperature; with hyperpolarization or decrease of temperature the rate of increase of the number of open channels declines. The duration time of the open state of the channels obeys the exponential law as well. Should all channels making up a population open synchronously, the rise instantaneously to maximum and purely exponential decay of the e.p.c. will reflect the distribution curve of the number of open channels; however, there is a period when the ACh-ChR formation is not completed, the opening of channels is proceeding, and the closing has already started. This period should probably comply with an experimentally measurable period consisting of the rise time and the initial declining portion of the current. Subsequent exponential decay of current depends only on the process of closing the ionic channel, since the average life span of channels can be measured with a good deal of accuracy by determining a time constant of the e.p.c. decline. This parameter also depends on the membrane potential level and the temperature. Such models of the PJM ionic channel kinetics adequately explain experimental evidence obtained earlier, among other things, variations in the nonlinearity displayed by the dependence of the e.p.c. maximum and ACh-induced potential upon the membrane potential as the latter grows more negative (70). This model may be employed to interpret changes of the e.p.c. time course caused by the action of pharmacological agents such as serotonin (59) and atropine (81), which render the e.p.c. declining phase more rapid without disturbing its exponential form (see Table 2).

The kinetic model of Stevens and collaborators permits a reasonable physical interpretation (61). It suggests a gating molecule that controls a selective ionic channel. The interaction of ACh and ChR decreases the energy barrier of transition of the gating molecule from a state when it bars the passage of ions through the channel into a state admitting them. The electrical field may affect the level of energy barriers if the gating molecule has a dipole. In light of this model the effect of various factors on the kinetics of the PJM conductance changes can be easily explained by the influence on the local surface membrane charge, by direct influence on the gating molecule, or by the influence on its hydrophobic environment. Any of these factors may determine the level of energy barriers of the transition from one state to another.

There are facts, however, that cannot be explained by the two-state model, or that require additional assumptions:

1. The effect of one or another of the agonists is accounted for not only by the affinity of the agonist to ChR but also by the ability, which is different for various agonists, to activate the ChR. In modern molecular pharmacology this ability is defined as *efficacy* (73) or *intrinsic activity* (74). The investigation of membrane noise induced by different cholinomimetics has shown that these drugs vary not only in their different affinities to ChR (judging by effective concentrations) but also by different ways in which the ChR is activated. To date the mean conductance of each channel (γ) and the mean time of open state (τ) have been determined for only a small number of cholinomimetics. In measurements of the noise voltage (56) the mean time of the open state varies from 0.12 msec on activation with acetylthiocholine to 1.65 msec with suberyldicholine. Although the variation of γ is smaller (75) (from 12.8 pmho for phenylpropyltrimethylammonium to 28.6 pmho for suberyldicholine) the authors believe it is great enough to contradict the earlier model (61) according to which the conductance of all channels is identical and invariant once they are opened by different activator agents.

2. The tail of the e.p.c. decay deviates from an exponential time course. This is best seen in the case of hyperpolarization (60–63). A qualitatively identical, but more strongly pronounced, phenomenon may be observed in the presence of some drugs: procaine (57, 68, 71), scopolamine (67, 81), DFP (76, 77), and hexanol (78). There is a biphasic decline of the e.p.c. with different time constants for the initial portion (fast decline) and the tail (slow decline). This phenomenon is difficult to interpret on the basis of the two-state hypothesis (122). If we assume that the relaxation of individual channels obeys the Poisson distribution, only one time constant of the e.p.c. decline should be observed. Biphasic decline could be expected, however, if only a portion of the channels is modified by these agents and if they acquire a longer time constant of relaxation. The biphasic decline may be explained by the fact that both normal and modified channels take part in its formation. In

the presence of procaine and similar substances, however, the initial portion of the e.p.c. decay is faster than normal, but it is difficult to suggest that procaine modifies some of the channels so that they become faster, while others become slower.

3. E. Neher and B. Sakmann (personal communication) compared cholinomimetic-induced current fluctuations on chronically denervated muscle fibers with those on normal end-plates and found the average lifetime of open channels on denervated membrane to be five times longer. At the former end-plate of denervated muscle fibers a response with two components was outlined for which the τ-values correspond to those of the end-plate and extrasynaptic membrane. This could be due to two receptor populations at denervated end-plates.

4. If diffusion of ACh from the synaptic cleft is exceedingly fast and if ChE does not affect the duration of elementary conductance reactions (55, 69) the role of enzymic hydrolysis should be relatively insignificant. Lengthening of the decline phase of e.p.c. and persistence of its potential dependence when ChE is inhibited appears to be certain (60–63). The consistency of this finding with the two-state kinetic model is based on these additional assumptions: (a) the proper effect of anticholinesterase drugs on the time course of e.p.c. independent of the inhibition of enzymic hydrolysis (60); (b) the repeated binding of ACh molecules to ChR (79); (c) a different degree of cooperativity of the effect of ACh in the presence and absence of ChE (80).

5. The non-Goldman behavior of the activated PJM, which cannot be explained by the two-state hypothesis, is a controversial point. It has been suggested, however, that the elementary reaction measured by analysis of ACh noise consists of a great number of short bursts of conductance of a cluster of ionic channels (55, 75). With such an assumption, the above-mentioned hypothesis would agree with the existing evidence. If these channels are separate and open only for microseconds, then a different efficacy of cholinomimetics and a non-Goldman behavior of the PJM becomes explicable.

The nature of the time-limiting factor is not yet fully known. We can only hope that some day true rates of conformational changes will be measured directly in experiments with isolated molecular complexes of the PJM.

PROCESSES OF PJM INACTIVATION

The presence of some peculiar mechanism of slow inactivation in the PJM is beyond doubt. The phenomenon reflecting the existence of this mechanism is known as desensitization. It arises after prolonged action of ACh or cholinomimetics. A reversible inactivation of a great number of functional units of the PJM occurs, which is a sign of a decrease of its sensitivity (82, 83). To interpret the functional properties of the PJM it is necessary to understand the desensitization mechanism. Most hypotheses of desensitization mechanisms suggest either specific changes of a ChR—its transition into an inactive form (82, 84) or blockage of active centers by endogenous inhibitors (85). The question as to which link in the chain of postsynaptic phenomena is subject to inactivation is still open to argument.

A wide variety of effects and factors have been found that can affect desensitization kinetics. The rate of desensitization rises with an increase of $[Ca]_o$ and declines with its decrease (86–91, 97). Some other multivalent ions are able to produce a similar or even stronger effect: Sr^{2+} (90–92), Mn^{2+} (93), UO_2^{2+} (94), AI^{3+} (90), La^{3+} (90, 95). The increase in tonicity of a Ringer solution accelerates desensitization (93). The rate of desensitization declines with the increase of $[K]_o$ but the initial level may be restored by polarization of the fiber. The artificial shift of the membrane potential level results in increase of the rate of desensitization upon hyperpolarization (90), and decrease upon depolarization. The decrease of $[Na]_o$ in the solution also accelerates desensitization (86, 87). An analogous effect is observed when Na^+ is replaced by Li^+ (96). We found a great number of drugs varying in their chemical structure that significantly increased the rate of desensitization. They are local anesthetics [procaine and lidocaine (87, 98)], barbiturates [amobarbital and pentobarbital (98)], some derivatives of diphenylacetic acid [adiphenin (99, 100), mesphenal (91, 99), SKF-525A (117), tropazin (99)] chlorpromazine (98), diphenhydramine (98), promethazine (98), and long-chain alcohols (98). Since all these substances are characterized by an ability to diminish the amplitude of responses to iontophoretic application of ACh at lower concentrations than in the case of m.e.p.p.s., drugs such as hexafluorenium (101), chistrionicotoxin (102), DFP (76, 77), edrophonium (103), and thiopental (104) may accelerate the desensitization. At present it is difficult to conclude whether a common mechanism affecting desensitization exists for such a wide variety of substances. Many of these drugs may be classed with membrane stabilizers (98, 105), and they have similar chemical features: one part of the molecule is a cationic head or an ionizable group while the other is hydrophobic. These drugs probably accelerate the transition of functional units of the postjunctional membrane into an inactive state. To determine the true chemical mechanism of this effect it is essential that these drugs affect only the rate of desensitization without influencing the rate of recovery of the former sensitivity level, i.e. the reactivation kinetics of the PJM functional units. Also important is their ability to affect the rate of desensitization not only when they are added to the bathing fluid but also after intracellular iontophoretic injection inside the muscle fiber in the end-plate zone (106). With the decrease of temperature the rate of onset of desensitization declines considerably more than the rate of recovery of the former sensitivity (107).

The above evidence has led us to advance a hypothesis that the activation of the PJM ion permeability is a limiting factor rather than the reaction of ACh and the recognition site of ChR (87). It was suggested that activation of ionic channels involves changes in the state of Ca in the PJM. If ACh acts for a long time or frequently, Ca ions accumulate near the gates of synaptic ionic channels and disturb the activation mechanism (12, 90–92). Following the physical model proposed by Stevens and collaborators (61) it may be assumed that the state of dipoles controlling changes in the membrane conductance for permeant cations alters. The question whether these changes are "receptory" or "nonreceptory" is open until we know whether a mechanism controlling the state of ionic channels is a part of the protein molecule interacting with ACh or whether these are different but closely interrelated molecules.

The affinity to ACh of "desensitized receptor" may be higher than normal, as was assumed by Katz & Thesleff (82). Changeux and co-workers (110) recently found an increase of ACh binding by fragments of membrane of electroplax treated by local anesthetics, SKF-525A or high $[Ca]_o$. But this phenomenon was not reproducible with purified receptor protein.

Nastuk & Parsons suppose that Ca acts on the inner side of the PJM. This assumption is supported by the observations that caffeine is able to accelerate desensitization (108). Some metabolic inhibitors promoting the increase of $[Ca]_i$ also accelerate desensitization (F. Vyskočil, personal communication). The blockade of Ca channels by manganese, however, increases desensitization (93).

MODIFIERS OF THE POSTJUNCTIONAL MEMBRANE

Since the discovery of the chemical nature of synaptic transmission, understanding of its intimate mechanisms has progressed through the utilization of new and more perfect chemical tools. Initially, these were so-called cholinergic compounds, i.e. drugs imitating ACh effects (cholinomimetics) and playing the part of competing antagonists (cholinolytics) or drugs inhibiting ChE. Now there is a new class of compounds vital to the consideration of the problem of the PJM modifiers. Possibly these drugs do not affect the reaction of ACh with the recognition site of ChR, or the effect they exert is not the main one in their mechanism of action. They rather affect subsequent links in the activation mechanism of ionic conductance.

Table 2 contains available evidence of the phenomenology of modifying effects of some drugs from this vast class. Comparison of the data reveals that the common feature of these drugs is the ability to influence the activation and inactivation kinetics of the PJM ion channels.

Some drugs shorten the open time of channels or prolong it by inducing a biphasic decay of the e.p.c. They influence by different mechanisms the potential dependence of the time course of the e.p.c. Many of these drugs may also affect desensitization by accelerating its onset. No correlation has been found between the effect of these compounds on the activation and inactivation of the PJM. Amobarbital, pentobarbital, chlorpromazine, histrionicotoxin, for example, shorten the time course of the e.p.c. whereas n-butanol prolongs it, but all these drugs potentiate desensitization. On the other hand, atropine substantially shortens the time course of the e.p.c. and exerts no influence on desensitization kinetics. Moreover, there is a distinct difference in the concentration of drugs affecting desensitization and the time course of the e.p.c. Only a small number of drugs can alter the PJM equilibrium potential. Nor is there a correlation between this ability and the effect of the compounds on the time course of the e.p.c. It is sufficient here to compare atropine and histrionicotoxin. Both shorten appreciably the time of the e.p.c. decay, but only atropine affects the equilibrium potential of the e.p.c. Among congeners of atropine there are compounds that produce the same effect on the time course of e.p.c., but they are not able to shift the equilibrium potential. Differences in the behavior of the equilibrium potential of natural responses and responses to ionophoretic application of ACh in the presence of atropine are still puzzling (67).

The molecular mechanisms of the modifying actions of these drugs are still unknown in every detail but they may serve as useful tools for elucidating the important functional properties of the PJM.

CONCLUSION

There are many gaps in the general scheme of the functional organization of the cholinoceptive PJM. So far, attempts have been made to construct a single scheme for the end-plate of vertebrate skeletal muscles despite a great variety of cholinergic membranes. It is not clear, however, which of these functional devices (recognition site of a Ch-receptor, gating mechanism, selective ion channel, mechanism of recovery of the initial state, etc) is of major importance in determining the functional properties of the entire PJM. Possibly the diversity of cholinoreceptive membranes is accounted for by various combinations of these functional "bricks." The unabated growth of potentialities of technique and the use of new approaches, for example, elaboration of mathematical models of the basic synaptic processes, enables us to anticipate further gains in this important field of research.

ACKNOWLEDGMENTS

The author is greatly indebted to Professor H. Grundfest and Professor B. Khodorov for reading the manuscript and for helpful criticism.

Literature Cited

1. Waud, D. R. 1968. *Pharmacol. Rev.* 20:49–88
2. Ehrenpreis, S., Fleisch, J. H., Mittag, T. W. 1969. *Pharmacol. Rev.* 21:131–81
3. Triggle, D. J. 1971. *Neurotransmitter-Receptor Interactions.* London & New York: Academic
4. Rang, H. P. 1974. *Q. Rev. Biophys.* 7:283–399
5. Gershenfeld, H. M. 1973. *Physiol. Rev.* 53:1–119
6. Ginsborg, B. L. 1973. *Biochim. Biophys. Acta* 300:289–317
7. Krnjevic, K. 1974. *Physiol. Rev.* 54: 418–540
8. Hubbard, J. I. 1973. *Physiol. Rev.* 53:674–723
9. Hubbard, J. I., Quastel, D. M. J. 1973. *Ann. Rev. Pharmacol.* 13:199–216
10. Narahashi, T. 1974. *Physiol. Rev.* 54:813–89
11. Cohen, J. B., Changeux, J-P. 1975. *Ann. Rev. Pharmacol.* 15:83–103
12. Magazanik, L. G. 1975. In *Structure and Function of Biomembranes,* ed. A. S. Troshin, 240–65. Moskva: Nauka
13. Ginsborg, B. L. 1967. *Pharmacol. Rev.* 19:289–316
14. De Robertis, E. 1971. *Science* 171: 963–71
15. Takeuchi, A., Takeuchi, N. 1959. *J. Neurophysiol.* 22:395–411
16. Magazanik, L. G., Vyskočil, F. 1969. *Experientia* 25:606–7
17. Barnard, E. A., Wieckowski, J., Chiu, T. H. 1971. *Nature London* 234:207–9
18. Miledi, R., Molinoff, P., Potter, L. T. 1971. *Nature London* 229:554–57
19. Ruiz-Manresa, F., Grundfest, H. 1971. *J. Gen. Physiol.* 57:71–92
20. Trautwein, W., Dudel, J. 1958. *Pfluegers Arch.* 266:324–34
21. Lester, H. A. 1971. *J. Gen. Physiol.* 57:255
22. Bolton, T. B. 1973. In *Drug Receptors,* ed. H. P. Rang, 87–104. London: Macmillan
23. Koketsu, K. 1969. *Fed. Proc.* 28:101–12
24. Nishi, S. 1974. In *The Peripheral Nervous System,* ed. J. I. Hubbard, 225–55. New York: Plenum

25. Magazanik, L. G., Ivanov, A. Ya., Lukomskaya, N. Ya. 1974. *Neurophysiology USSR* 6:652–54
26. Weight, F. F., Votava, J. 1970. *Science* 170:755–58
27. Kuba, K., Koketsu, K. 1974. *Brain Res.* 81:338–42
28. Kobayashi, H., Libet, B. 1974. *Life Sci.* 14:1871–83
29. Sato, M., Austin, G., Yai, H., Murahashi, J. 1968. *J. Gen. Physiol.* 51:312–45
30. Blankenship, J. E., Wachtel, H., Kandel, E. R. 1971. *J. Neurophysiol.* 34:76–92
31. Kehoe, J. S. 1972. *J. Physiol. London* 225:85–114
32. Kehoe, J. S. 1972. *J. Physiol. London* 225:115–46
33. Chiarandini, D. J., Stefani, E., Gershenfeld, H. M. 1967. *Science* 156:1597–99
34. Chiarandini, D. J., Gershenfeld, H. M. 1967. *Science* 156:1595–96
35. Levitan, H., Tauc, L. 1972. *J. Physiol. London* 222:537–58
36. Woodruff, G. N., Walker, R. J., Newton, L. C. 1971. *Gen. Comp. Pharmacol.* 2:106–17
37. Magazanik, L. G., Michelson, M. Ya. 1963. *Fiziol. Zh. SSSR* 49:725–35
38. Hidaka, T., Twarog, B. M. In preparation
39. Magazanik, L. G., Lukomskaya, N. Ya., Fedorov, V. V., Potap'eva, N. N., Snetkov, V. A. 1974. *Zh. Evol. Biokhim. Fiziol.* 10:411–12
40. Pitman, R. M., Kerkut, G. A. 1970. *Comp. Gen. Pharmacol.* 1:221–30
41. Khromov-Borisov, N. V., Michelson, M. Ya. 1966. *Pharmacol. Rev.* 18:1051–90
42. Lukomskaya, N. Ya., Michelson, M. Ya. 1972. *Comp. Gen. Pharmacol.* 3:213–25
43. Rozhkova, E. K. 1972. *Comp. Gen. Physiol.* 3:410–22
44. Lukomskaya, N. Ya., Magazanik, L. G. 1974. *Zh. Evol. Biokhim. Fiziol.* 10:524–26
45. Ross, D. H., Triggle, D. J. 1972. *Biochem. Pharmacol.* 21:2533–34
46. Magazanik, L. G., Vyskočil, F., Lukomskaya, N. Ya. 1973. In *Biofisika Membran. Kaunas,* pp. 424–29
47. Magazanik, L. G., Potapjeva, N. N. 1975. *Bull. Exp. Biol. Med. USSR* 74:39–41
48. Takeuchi, N. 1963. *J. Physiol. London* 167:128–40
49. Katz, B. 1966. *Nerve, Muscle and Synapse.* New York: McGraw-Hill
50. Dunin-Barkovskii, V. L., Kovalev, S. A., Magazanik, L. G., Potapova, T. V., Chailakhyan, L. M. 1969. *Biofisika* 14:485–94
51. Magazanik, L. G., Potapova, T. V. 1969. *Biofisika* 14:658–62
52. Magazanik, L. G. 1970. *Mechanisms of activation of the postsynaptic muscle membrane.* ScD thesis. Pavlov Inst. of Physiol., Leningrad
53. Bregestovski, P. D., Chailakhyan, L. M., Dunin-Barkovskii, V. L., Potapova, T. V., Veprintsev, B. N. 1972. *Nature London* 236:453
54. Dunin-Barkovskii, V. L., Kovalev, S. A., Potapova, T. V., Chailakhyan, L. M. 1967. *Proc. 5th Symp. Neurophysiol. Vilnus,* pp. 9–10
55. Katz, B., Miledi, R. 1972. *J. Physiol. London* 224:665–99
56. Katz, B., Miledi, R. 1973. *J. Physiol. London* 230:707–17
57. Maeno, T. 1966. *J. Physiol. London* 183:592–606
58. Magazanik, L. G., Potapjeva, N. N. In preparation
59. Magazanik, L. G., Illes, P., Snetkov, V. A. 1975. *Doklady Acad. Nauk USSR.* In press
60. Magleby, K. L., Stevens, C. F. 1972. *J. Physiol. London* 223:151–71
61. Magleby, K. L., Stevens, C. F. 1972. *J. Physiol. London* 223:173–97
62. Kordas, M. 1972. *J. Physiol. London* 224:317–32
63. Kordas, M. 1972. *J. Physiol. London* 224:333–48
64. Eccles, J. C., MacFarlane, W. V. 1949. *J. Neurophysiol.* 12:50–80
65. Eccles, J. C., Jaeger, J. C. 1958. *Proc. R. Soc. London Ser. B* 148:38–56
66. Gage, P. W., Armstrong, C. M. 1968. *Nature London* 218:363–65
67. Magazanik, L. G., Vyskočil, F. 1969. *Experientia* 25:618–19
68. Deguchi, T., Narahashi, T. 1971. *J. Pharmacol. Exp. Ther.* 176:423–33
69. Anderson, C. R., Stevens, C. F. 1973. *J. Physiol. London* 235:655–91
70. Dionne, V. E., Stevens, C. F. 1976. *J. Physiol. London* 251:245–70
71. Maeno, T., Edwards, C., Hashimura, S. 1971. *J. Neurophysiol.* 34:32–46
72. Kordas, M. 1970. *J. Physiol. London* 209:689–99
73. Stephenson, R. P. 1956. *Br. J. Pharmacol.* 11:379–93
74. Ariens, E. J. 1964. *Molecular Pharmacology.* New York: Academic
75. Colquhoun, D., Dionne, V. E., Stein-

bach, J. H., Stevens, C. F. 1975. *Nature London* 253:204–6
76. Kuba, K., Albuquerque, E. X., Barnard, E. A. 1973. *Science* 181:853–56
77. Kuba, K., Albuquerque, E. X., Daly, J., Barnard, E. A. 1974. *J. Pharmacol. Exp. Ther.* 189:499–512
78. Gage, P. W., McBurney, R. N., Schneider, G. T. 1975. *J. Physiol. London* 244:409–29
79. Katz, B., Miledi, R. 1973. *J. Physiol. London* 231:549–74
80. Magleby, K. L., Terrar, D. A. 1975. *J. Physiol. London* 244:467–95
81. Magazanik, L. G., Snetkov, V. A. In preparation
82. Katz, B., Thesleff, S. 1957. *J. Physiol. London* 138:63–80
83. Thesleff, S. 1960. *Physiol. Rev.* 40:734–52
84. Rang, H. P., Ritter, J. M. 1970. *Mol. Pharmacol.* 6:357–82
85. Turpaev, T. M., Putintseva, T. G. 1974. *Usp. Fiziol. Nauk.* 5:17–47
86. Manthey, A. A. 1966. *J. Gen. Physiol.* 49:963–76
87. Magazanik, L. G. 1968. *Biofisika* 13:199–203
88. Parsons, R. L. 1969. *Am. J. Physiol.* 217:805–11
89. Magazanik, L. G., Shekhirev, N. N. 1970. *Fiziol. Zh. SSSR* 56:582–88
90. Magazanik, L. G., Vyskočil, F. 1970. *J. Physiol. London* 210:507–18
91. Magazanik, L. G., Vyskočil, F. 1973. In *Drug Receptors*, ed. H. P. Rang, 105–19. London: Macmillan
92. Magazanik, L. G. 1969. See Ref. 46, pp. 94–96
93. Nastuk, W. L., Parsons, R. L. 1970. *J. Gen. Physiol.* 56:218–49
94. Nastuk, W. L. 1967. *Fed. Proc.* 26:1639–46
95. Lambert, D. H., Parsons, R. L. 1970. *J. Gen. Physiol.* 56:309–21
96. Parsons, R. L., Cochrane, D. E., Schnitzler, R. M. 1973. *J. Gen. Physiol.* 61:263
97. Magazanik, L. G. 1969. *Fiziol. Zh. SSSR* 55:1147–55

98. Magazanik, L. G. 1971. *Fiziol. Zh. SSSR* 57:1313–21
99. Magazanik, L. G. 1971. *Farmakol. Toksikol. Moscow* 34(3):292–97
100. Terrar, D. A. 1974. *Br. J. Pharmacol.* 51:259–68
101. Nastuk, W. L., Karis, J. H. 1964. *J. Pharmacol. Exp. Ther.* 144:236–52
102. Albuquerque, E. X. et al 1973. *Proc. Nat. Acad. Sci. USA* 70:949–53
103. Goldner, M. M., Narahashi, T. 1974. *Eur. J. Pharmacol.* 25:362–71
104. Adams, P. R. 1974. *J. Physiol. London* 241:41–42P
105. Seeman, P. 1972. *Pharmacol. Rev.* 24:583–655
106. Vyskočil, F., Magazanik, L. G. 1973. *Brain Res.* 48:417–19
107. Magazanik, L. G., Vyskočil, F. 1975. *J. Physiol. London* 249:285–300
108. Cochrane, D. E., Parsons, R. L. 1972. *J. Gen. Physiol.* 59:437–61
109. Grundfest, H. 1957. *Physiol. Rev.* 37:337–61
110. Cohen, J. B., Weber, M., Changeux, J-P. 1974. *Mol. Pharmacol.* 10:904–32
111. Seyama, J., Narahashi, T. 1975. *J. Pharmacol. Exp. Ther.* 192:95–104
112. Steinbach, A. B. 1968. *J. Gen. Physiol.* 52:144–61
113. Beranek, R., Vyskočil, F. 1968. *J. Physiol. London* 195:493–503
114. Potapova, T. V. 1969. *Biofisica* 14:757–58
115. Kordas, M. 1968. *Int. J. Neuropharmacol.* 7:523–30
116. Katz, B., Miledi, R. 1973. *Proc. R. Soc. London Ser. B* 184:221–26
117. Del Castillo, J., Katz, B. 1957. *Proc. R. Soc. London Ser. B* 146:369–81
118. Magazanik, L. G. 1973. See Ref. 46, pp. 430–35
119. Magazanik, L. G. 1970. *Bull. Exp. Biol. Med.* 69:(I)10–14
120. Weight, F. F., Padjen, A. 1973. *Brain Res.* 55:219–24
121. Kehoe, JS., Sealock, R., Bon C. 1975. *Brain Res.* Submitted for publication
122. Katz, B., Miledi, R. 1975. *J. Physiol. London* 249:269–84

EVALUATION OF THROMBOGENIC EFFECTS OF DRUGS

❖6644

Gerhard Zbinden

Institute of Toxicology, Federal Institute of Technology and University of Zurich, Schwerzenbach, Switzerland

GENERAL CONCEPTS

More than 100 years ago the German pathologist Rudolf Virchow recognized that pathological changes of blood vessel walls, thrombotic diathesis, and altered blood flow were the major causes of thrombosis (1). It is remarkable that no fundamentally new pathogenetic factors have since been added to what is now known as *Virchow's triad.* In recent years biochemical and morphological studies have unraveled many of the processes taking place during hemostasis. As a result, we have also gained a better understanding of the mechanisms contributing to thrombus formation.

The notion that drugs play an important role in the development of thrombosis has gained widespread attention. Extensive investigations undertaken in an effort to explain the apparent thrombogenic effect of steroidal oral contraceptives (OC) have revealed a number of unusual toxicological problems:

1. Few chemical substances are known to cause outright thrombosis. However, many agents seem to increase the risk of thrombosis, that is, they create a state of impending thrombosis or thrombophilia, an ill-defined pharmacological endpoint.

2. Drugs may influence several factors involved in thrombus formation.

3. There are at least three fundamentally different forms of thrombosis, arterial and venous thrombosis, and disseminated microcirculatory thrombosis. Drugs may promote one or more of these forms to a variable degree.

4. Most laboratory methods were originally designed to measure defective blood clotting and platelet function. They are not well suited for the demonstration of impending thrombosis.

5. In man, the recognition of a thrombogenic drug effect often rests on epidemiological data. Serious problems of diagnosis, and the existence of disease-related and environmental factors that influence the incidence of thrombosis, render such studies difficult.

177

Mechanisms of Thrombogenic Drug Actions

It is generally acknowledged that all processes involved in normal hemostasis are also operative in thrombus formation. The physiological and pathological events most likely to be set in motion by thrombogenic substances are listed in Table 1. Remember, however, that the hemostatic equilibrium is maintained by many checks and balances. In some cases a drug-induced shift in a direction favoring coagulation invariably results in thrombosis. In other instances it may merely indicate that the statistical risk of developing thrombosis, however small, is higher than in the absence of the drug. In order to emphasize these differences, a somewhat arbitrary classification that recognizes *thrombogenic substances of the first, second, and third order* was proposed (2): 1. The principal biological action of a thrombogenic substance of the first order is a distinct activation of the hemostatic system, which is usually followed by thrombus formation. Such substances are not used as drugs, but serve as experimental tools to study mechanisms of thrombosis. 2. Thrombogenic substances of the second order also activate hemostatic mechanisms, but thrombosis is only caused at excessively high doses. 3. Thrombogenic substances of the third order include all compounds that shift the hemostatic equilibrium in the direction of thrombus formation without causing outright thrombosis, even at very high doses.

Table 1 Possible mechanisms of thrombogenic substances

Vessel wall	Platelets	Coagulation
Cytotoxic and irritant effect	Symptomatic thrombocythemia	Release of tissue thromboplastin
Generalized deendothelialization	Aggregation	Increased concentration of clotting factors
	Sensitization against ADP and serotonin	Activation of clotting factors
	Increased adhesiveness	Decreased antithrombin III
Blood flow	Reduction of surface charge	Inhibition of fibrinolysis
Vasoconstriction	Reduction of cAMP	
Stasis and hypotension	Induction of release reaction	
Turbulence		
Distension of vessels		

THROMBOGENIC SUBSTANCES ACTING ON THE VESSEL WALL

Cytotoxic and Irritant Effects

Perhaps the most frequent form of iatrogenic thrombosis is that occurring at injection sites. Prerequisites are localized vascular lesions where blood can interact with subendothelial extracellular structures (3), and inflammatory reactions stemming from perivascular deposition of cytotoxic agents.

In order to test for thrombus induction, drugs are injected into a blood vessel that is temporarily occluded to permit the chemical to interact with the endothelium. Blood flow is then restored, and thrombus formation is assessed by visual inspection and histological evaluation. Chemicals may also be applied on the outer layers of a blood vessel. The rate of thrombus formation may then be measured by direct microscopic observation. York, Rogers & Kensler (4) have used this method on blood vessels of the hamster cheek pouch for an evaluation of new anticancer drugs of the phthalanilide series. The thrombogenic potency of three derivatives correlated well with incidence of thrombophlebitis observed in patients.

Generalized Endothelial Damage

That chemical substances may be responsible for widespread endothelial defects was learned from the study of homocystinuria, an inborn error of metabolism. These patients experience frequent episodes of arterial thromboembolism that result from parietal thromboses at the site of patchy deendothelializations. The same lesions were produced in baboons by intravenous (iv) infusion of homocystine (5). This could be diagnosed intravitam by demonstration of circulating endothelial cells. Such cells were also found after injection of endotoxin in rabbits (6), indicating that the potent thrombogenic effect of this agent is, at least in part, a result of endothelial damage.

Another method was used for the demonstration of endothelial lesions induced by polyanethol sulfonate (Liquoid ®, Roche). Rats were treated with this potent thrombogen; the aortas were then incubated in a medium containing tritiated thymidine. Areas of intensive endothelial repair could be demonstrated by autoradiography (7). An uncommon form of endothelial damage was found with sodium acetriozate, a radiocontrast agent. This compound caused disseminated thrombosis in veins and capillaries, even in the absence of platelets and all coagulation factors except fibrinogen. This was explained by the ability of acetriozate to extract a glycoprotein from the endothelium and to form an insoluble fibrinogen derivative (8).

THROMBOGENIC SUBSTANCES ACTING ON THE PLATELETS

Increased Platelet Count

Frequent thrombosis and bleeding is a well-known syndrome in patients whose platelet count exceeds 10^6 per mm^2. Testosterone, progesterone, somatotropic hormone, serotonin, and pantetine (a combination of pantothenic acid and cysteamine) caused a marked increase in platelet count in experimental animals (9). This indicates that drugs can induce symptomatic thrombocythemia. The effect was also seen in man, quite unexpectedly, with vinblastine and vincristine (10, 11).

Platelet Aggregation

Aggregation of platelets is a key step in the process of hemostasis and thrombus formation. It is readily induced by several naturally occurring substances, thrombin, adenosine diphosphate (ADP), collagen, epinephrine, serotonin, fatty acids, and a cyclic endoperoxide formed from arachidonic acid during prostaglandin biosynthesis (12–14). The crucial alterations of platelets that make them aggregable are not known, but the kinetics of the process and the morphological changes of the cells are well studied (15).

Other chemical substances act less specifically, perhaps by direct binding to cell membranes (16), cell damage, or change in surface charge. Some compounds cause loose, reversible aggregates without impairment of platelet function. With others, aggregates are irreversible and associated with loss of function or platelet destruction (17). This qualitative difference is often overlooked, although it appears to be of considerable importance. Irreversible platelet aggregates are retained in the capillaries of the lungs as microemboli, leading rapidly to thrombocytopenia, often also pulmonary hypertension and death (18–20). Induction of reversible aggregates is usually not associated with a drop in platelet count. This indicates that most of the platelets are not sequestered in the capillary bed.

Many methods are available for in vitro testing of platelet aggregation, including turbidimetric measurements (21), microscopic observation of platelets in suspension (18, 22) or on plastic slides (23), and counting of unaggregated platelets in platelet-rich plasma (PRP) or blood before and after contact with the test substance (24, 25).

A drug found to aggregate platelets in vitro must be tested in vivo. Circulating aggregates may be seen as white bodies in exposed and illuminated blood vessels (26, 27) or in a glass tube bypass (28). The blood may also be passed through a filter where aggregates are retained and lead to an increase in filter pressure (29). Determinations of platelet survival give useful indirect information about the rate of platelet destruction following administration of aggregating agents.

A simple method consists of counting aggregates in blood samples suspended in buffered EDTA solutions (18, 30). It was used to demonstrate circulating platelet aggregates developing after iv injection of 2 azo dyes, Evans blue and Congo red, into guinea pigs.

The blood concentration necessary to cause formation of aggregates was determined and compared with blood levels reached during use of the agents in man. From these determinations a satisfactory "safety factor" was calculated for Evans blue, and a marginal one for Congo red (18, 31). It is noteworthy that several cases of shock and disseminated thrombosis have occurred after iv use of Congo red in man (32). These reactions were most likely due to drug-induced microembolization.

The antibiotic ristocetin also aggregates human platelets in vitro and causes dose-dependent thrombocytopenia in rabbits and man (33). It is interesting that this compound does not aggregate platelets of many von Willebrand patients. It thus needs a plasma factor, a property not shared by other aggregating agents (34–36).

As a further mechanism of thrombogenic action the possibility that drugs may sensitize platelets against endogenous aggregators must be considered. For example, platelets of women taking OC exhibit an enhanced response to ADP (37). A significantly increased aggregation response with serotonin was observed in psychiatric patients treated chronically with chlorpromazine (38). In vitro this drug reduces rather than promotes platelet aggregation. From these findings it is concluded that potential drug-induced enhancement of platelet aggregation must not only be investigated in vitro but also during chronic administration.

Increased Platelet Adhesiveness

The major factor responsible for adhesion of platelets to vessel walls is endothelial damage with exposure of collagen fibers and other subendothelial structures (3). The belief that increased stickiness of platelets also promotes this process is based on the finding that platelets of certain thrombosis-prone patient populations have a higher tendency to adhere to foreign surfaces. (39–42). Many test methods have been proposed, using glass slides (39), or beads (43), latex particles (44), traumatized rat omentum (45), and tannic acid–treated human red cells (46) as structures for the platelets to stick on. Strong platelet aggregators, ADP, epinephrine, thrombin, and Evans blue, promote platelet stickiness. One could thus conclude that aggregation and adhesion are manifestations of the same process, so that there would be no need to use the cumbersome adhesiveness tests. There is, however, evidence that the two reactions are not identical: platelets of patients with Glanzmann's thrombasthenia fail to aggregate but adhere normally to subendothelial structures (47). Moreover, serotonin, a potent aggregating agent, did not enhance platelet adhesiveness to tanned red cells (46).

In order to test platelet adhesiveness in vivo, discrete vascular lesions must be induced, for example, with electric current (48), biolaser (49), or iontophoresis of ADP (50). Thrombus formation and embolization are assessed by direct observation. A drug that increases platelet adhesiveness is expected to produce larger thrombi earlier and to prolong microembolization. In a rat experiment in which venous thrombus formation was initiated by a mechanical lesion, urethane, in anesthetic concentrations, was indeed shown to prolong production of microemboli significantly (51).

Changed Platelet Surface Charge

From studies of pH-mobility relationship of platelets in vitro we are well informed about their electrical surface charges and the chemical groups with which they are associated (17). Normally there is a net negative surface charge that keeps platelets separated from each other. Positively charged macromolecules such as polylysine, polyornithine, protamine sulfate (17) were shown to bind to platelets and to cause aggregation when the electrophoretic mobility reached zero. Polyquaternary, a long-chain detergent increased adhesiveness to electrically stimulated blood vessels (52).

Reduced Cyclic AMP

A new concept of platelet function is based on the observation that prostaglandins stimulate adenylcyclase and increase cAMP content of platelets. The aggregation response of these platelets with ADP, arachidonic and other agents is reduced, and this effect is further enhanced by inhibitors of phosphodiesterase, for example, theophylline (14, 53, 54). In vitro ADP and epinephrine cause a rapid drop in platelet cAMP content. This has led to the suggestion that the aggregation response was directly related to the cyclic nucleotide level. If this were the case any influence leading to a reduction of platelet cAMP might be expected to facilitate aggregation.

Release of Platelet Content

The release reaction (55), a liberation of ADP, serotonin, histamine, and enzymes, is set in motion under the influence of several endogenous platelet-aggregating substances, for example, thrombin and epinephrine (56). Of particular importance is the release of ADP which is probably the common effector agent responsible for the aggregating effect of long-chain free fatty acids (57), the cephalin preparation Thrombofax® (58), immune complexes (57), heparin (16), and vasopressin (59). The release reaction is of considerable toxicological importance, since it promotes further growth of platelet aggregates lodged in small blood vessels or deposited on vascular lesions.

Induction of release reaction is conventionally studied in vitro: PRP and test drug are stirred, and the released substances are determined in the plasma fraction (60). Platelets may also be labeled with ^{14}C-serotonin, which they release promptly under the influence of aggregating agents (61). In vivo studies of the release reaction are more difficult, because of the rapid metabolic disposition of the released substances.

THROMBOGENIC SUBSTANCES ACTING ON THE COAGULATION SYSTEM

A description of the intricate biochemical reactions taking place during blood clotting is outside the scope of this review. In the following paragraphs experimental and clinical evidence is presented that demonstrates that chemical substances can create a state of hypercoagulability which may progress to thrombosis. It will also become evident from the examples cited that not every shift in the biological equilibrium of the clotting system represents a significant thrombosis hazard.

Release of Tissue Thromboplastin

Thromboplastic substances, also called *tissue damage factors,* are present in most tissues. They are important as activators of the extrinsic clotting system. It is conceivable that irritant drugs injected into adipose and muscle tissue may cause enough cell damage to make appreciable amounts of such thromboplastic substances available.

Increased Concentration of Clotting Factors

The plasma level of many clotting factors is increased in women taking OC (37), but the significance of this finding is not well understood (62, 63). For the toxicological evaluation it is permissible to assume that increased levels of one or more clotting factors must not be regarded as indicating a state of hypercoagulability. After all, even under normal circumstances these are substances present in excess. Still, a drug causing marked and consistent elevation of one or several clotting factors must be subjected to careful scrutiny.

Acceleration of Clotting Reactions

Epinephrine is a typical example of a thrombogenic substance of the second order, causing fibrin thrombi in rabbits, but only at excessively high doses (64). It accelerates blood clotting in vitro (65) and in vivo (66) and causes an increase in Factors VIII and IX levels (66). Since it promotes clotting also in patients with hemophilia A (67) and in Factor IX–deficient dogs (66) it was suggested that it acted by a generalized catalytic influence on enzymatic processes (66). Several drugs release epinephrine from its body stores. It is conceivable that they also accelerate the clotting process. In rabbits the two hypotensives guanethidine and debrisoquin, known to release epinephrine, caused a transient state of hypercoagulability. The same effect was seen with tyramine, a pressor substance that also acted through epinephrine release (68).

Activation of Contact Factors

The generation of intrinsic thromboplastin is set in motion by activated Hageman factor and Factor XI (PTA). The presence of activated contact factors in the blood is demonstrated by shortened clotting time in siliconized glass tubes, decrease in partial thromboplastin time, acceleration of the thromboplastin generation test, and shortened thrombus formation time as measured with the Chandler loop technique (2, 69). It represents a state of hypercoagulability, but does not necessarily lead to thrombosis (70, 71). An important reason thrombosis does not always develop is probably related to the ability of the reticuloendothelial system of the liver to eliminate thromboplastin from the circulation (72). If this protective mechanism is impaired, the risk for thrombosis through activation of contact factors is increased.

Prolonged and intensive activation of contact factors may produce thrombosis without a contribution of other factors. For example, iv infusion of lactic acid into rats caused complete activation of Hageman factor, arterial thrombosis, and micro-embolization in the lungs (73). Similarly, polyinosinic-polycytidylic acid, a potent activator of contact factors (2), caused severe thrombosis when injected at high doses into dogs and monkeys (H. Levy, personal communication). Long-chain FFA are potent activators of contact factors (74, 75). This may be one of the reasons they cause thrombosis after iv injection (19, 24, 76, 77). Elevated FFA levels may also be produced by drugs, for example, catecholamines, anorexigenic phenethylamines (78), thymoleptics (78), ACTH (79), and nicotine (80). Fortunately, released FFA are bound by serum albumin, so that only very high levels, exceeding the binding capacity of the available serum albumin, may become hazardous. That such high FFA levels can cause thrombosis was demonstrated in experiments with rabbits that were given large doses of ACTH and died from pulmonary thrombosis (79).

Decreased Antithrombin

In 1965 Egeberg (81) described the occurrence of low antithrombin III levels in members of a family. The patients attracted attention because of frequent venous thrombosis, thrombophlebitis, and pulmonary embolism. This was confirmed in other families so that no doubt exists at present that antithrombin III is a very important protective factor against intravascular clotting. It is understandable, therefore, that the finding of low antithrombin III levels in women taking OC attracted great attention (82, 83). It was also reported that the effect seemed to be due to the estrogen component of these drugs (84). There is some indication in the literature that women with the lowest antithrombin III levels are most likely to develop thromboembolic complications (84). However, the available data are not sufficient to permit a final evaluation of this remarkable observation. But of all changes induced by the OC, the effect on antithrombin III appears to be one of the most logical explanations of their suspected thrombogenic effects.

Inhibition of Fibrinolysis

The fibrinolytic system is the ultimate weapon against the consequences of intravascular coagulation. There is much experimental and clinical evidence that drug-induced inhibition of fibrinolysis represents a considerable hazard: just about every experimentally induced form of thrombosis takes a much more serious course if the animal was pretreated with a plasminogen antiactivator, e.g. ϵ-amino caproic acid and tranexamic acid, or a proteinase inhibitor, e.g. aprotinine and iniprol (85). In man such compounds were occasionally associated with thrombosis, particularly in patients with kidney disease (86–88). Corticosteroids, long suspected to increase the incidence of thrombosis, also inhibit fibrinolysis. The detrimental consequences of prednisolone pretreatment were shown in rabbits with thrombin-induced intravascular coagulation (89). Another group of compounds inhibiting fibrinolysis comprises mercurial derivatives, e.g. mercuric chloride (90) and the diuretic Novurit® (91).

THROMBOGENIC SUBSTANCES INDUCING CHANGES IN BLOOD FLOW

Vasoconstriction

Arterial thrombosis as a consequence of prolonged vasoconstriction is found in patients with ergotamine tartrate overdosage (92). It is probable that a lesion of the vessel wall develops as a consequence of the compression of the vasa vasorum during spastic contraction of the artery (93). Another example of thrombosis in a spastic blood vessel is that reported to occur after infusion of pitressin into the superior mesenteric artery (94).

Stasis and Hypotension

The importance of venous stasis as a contributing factor in venous thrombosis is generally accepted, but more on circumstantial evidence than on hard, experimental facts. It is proven experimentally that stasis alone does not produce thrombosis (95, 96). But if a state of hypercoagulability exists, thrombosis will develop preferentially in blood vessels with slow blood circulation (95). Drugs that cause venous stasis must therefore be considered as accessories to such an event. As an example, the OCs must again be cited. They are known to cause venous stasis in the lower extremities (97), an effect that may contribute to their thrombogenic potential.

A sudden lowering of arterial blood pressure, a possible side effect of autonomic blocking drugs, also reduces the blood flow in the periphery. It is noteworthy that formation of platelet aggregates and intravascular coagulation are well recognized consequences of hypovolemic hypotension (98). Further experiments in dogs proved that circulatory failure due to hypercapnia was associated with thrombosis in various organs (99). It is thus quite clear that various disturbances of the peripheral circulation must be considered as potential triggers for a thrombotic process.

Turbulence and Distension of Blood Vessels

Experimental evidence shows that platelet adhesion develops preferentially in regions of disturbed arterial flow, and that the size of the platelet deposits is related to the intensity of the turbulence (100). This indicates that a sudden elevation in blood pressure, which might occur after the injection of a sympathomimetic drug, could create a hazardous situation by increasing turbulence in areas of disturbed arterial flow (bifurcations, atherosclerotic plaques). Moreover, acute hypertension leads to hyperextension of blood vessel. This may damage the endothelial layer of the arteries and facilitate platelet deposition (101).

CONCLUSIONS

The investigation of the pathogenesis of thrombosis was greatly facilitated by the availability of chemical substances with which various forms of intravascular coagulation and thrombosis could readily be induced. Using these *Thrombogenic Substances of the First Order* as experimental tools, it was possible to identify various mechanisms of chemical thrombosis and to develop in vitro and in vivo methods for detection and quantitative assessment of thrombogenic effects. The mechanisms found to be most important for induction of experimental thrombosis included endothelial lesions, platelet aggregation, changes in platelet surface charge, activation of certain clotting reactions, and inhibition of fibrinolysis. Several other factors such as increased platelet counts and platelet adhesiveness, reduction in cAMP content of platelets, induction of platelet release reaction, increased sensitivity of platelets for aggregating action of ADP and serotonin, release of tissue thromboplastin, decreased antithrombin levels, increased concentration of clotting factors, and various changes in blood flow were also identified as being involved in thrombus formation. Most of these processes were shown to be susceptible to changes induced by chemical substances.

A second group of chemical compounds, *Thrombogenic Substances of the Second Order*, caused changes of hemostatic mechanisms similar to those described above. In most instances the compounds only produced a prethrombotic state, a change in the hemostatic equilibrium sometimes also referred to as hypercoagulability, impending thrombosis, thrombotic diathesis, or thrombophilia. But the fact that administration of excessively high doses of these agents was often followed by thrombosis represents a good argument that the changes of hemostatic functions are indeed valid indicators for an increased tendency to develop thrombosis and thromboembolism.

Finally, a sizable group of chemicals including many drugs were recognized as having some influence on hemostatic mechanisms, shifting the balance in the direction of thrombosis. Even at excessively high doses these compounds do not by themselves induce thrombosis. But it is possible that they represent a risk factor whose clinical significance must be determined by epidemiological investigations.

The OC may be mentioned as a prototype of these *Thrombogenic Substances of the Third Order.* Their varied effects on vasculature, platelet function, and clotting mechanisms indicate a distinct tendency to shift the hemostatic equilibrium in favor of thrombosis (37). But the actual occurrence of thrombotic episodes under the influence of these drugs is still a rare event. The evaluation of drugs with methods described in this review thus serves the purpose of identifying potential, however weak, thrombogenic properties of new and commonly used drugs. This knowledge should not discourage the therapeutic use of these compounds. But it must caution the clinician against potential hazards and provide him with useful directions on the methods to be used for monitoring of patients.

ACKNOWLEDGMENTS

Much helpful advice was received from Dr. H. R. Baumgartner, Basel.

Literature Cited

1. Virchow, R. 1856. *Gesammelte Abhandlungen zur wissenschaftlichen Medizin. IV. Thrombose und Embolie. Gefässentzündung und septische Infektion.* Frankfurt: Meidinger
2. Zbinden, G. 1973. *Bull. Schweiz. Akad. Med. Wiss.* 29:191–200
3. Baumgartner, H. R. 1974. *Platelets, Thrombosis and Inhibitors,* ed. P. Didisheim, T. Shimamoto, H. Yamazaki, 39–49. Stuttgart and New York: Schattauer
4. York, I. M., Rogers, W. I., Kensler, C. J. 1963. *J. Pharmacol. Exp. Ther.* 141:36–49
5. Harker, L. A., Slichter, S. J., Scott, C. R., Ross, R. 1974 *N. Engl. J. Med.* 291:537–43
6. Spaet, T., Gaynor, E. 1970. *Adv. Cardiol.* 4:47–66
7. Evensen, S. A., Shepro, D. 1973. *Thromb. Diath. Haemorrh.* 30:347–51
8. Mariscal, I., Moffat, C., Huebner, B., Seaman, A. J. 1973. *Scand. J. Haematol.* 10:390–400
9. DeNicola, P. 1959. *Thromb. Diath. Haemorrh.* 3:615–24
10. Robertson, J. H., McCarthy, G. M. 1969. *Lancet* 2:353–55
11. Hwang, Y. F., Hamilton, H. E., Sheets, R. F. 1969. *Lancet* 2:1075–76
12. Born, G. V. R. 1962. *J. Physiol. London* 162:67P–68P
13. Haslam, R. J. 1967. *Physiology of Hemostasis and Thrombosis,* ed. S. A. Johnson, W. A. Seegers, 88–112. Springfield, Ill.: Thomas
14. Vargaftig, B. B., Zirinis, P. 1973, *Nature London New Biol.* 244:114–16
15. Born, G. V. R. 1974. *Platelet Aggregation and Drugs,* ed. L. Caprino, E. C. Rossi, 1–19. London, New York and San Francisco: Academic
16. Eika, C. 1972. *Scand. J. Haematol.* 9:248–57
17. Zbinden, G., Mehrishi, J. N., Tomlin, S. 1970. *Thromb. Diath. Haemorrh.* 23:261–75
18. Giger, M., Baumgartner, H. R., Zbinden, G. 1974. *Agents Actions* 4:173–180
19. Zbinden, G. 1967. *Thromb. Diath. Haemorrh.* 18:57–65
20. Silver, M. J., Hoch, W., Kocsis, J. J., Ingerman, C. M. Smith, J. B. 1974. *Science* 138:1085–86
21. Born, G. V. R., Cross, M. J. 1963. *J. Physiol. London* 168:178–95
22. Maca, R. D., Fry, G. L., Hoak, J. C. 1972. *Microvasc. Res.* 4:453–57
23. Breddin, K., Bauke, K. J. 1965. *Blut* 11:144–64
24. Zbinden, G., Grimm, L., Muheim, M. 1971. *Thromb. Diath. Haemorrh.* 25:517–23
25. Gordon, J. L., Gresham, G. A. 1972. *Atherosclerosis* 15:383–86

26. Fulton, G. P., Ackers, R. P., Lutz, B. R. 1953. *Blood* 8:140–52
27. Jorgensen, L., Hovig, T., Rowsell, H. C., Mustard, J. F. 1970. *Am. J. Pathol.* 61:161–74
28. Benner, K. U., Frede, K. E., Lauterjung, K. L. 1970, *Pfluegers Arch.* 320:142–51
29. Broersma, R. J., Dickerson, G. D., Sullivan, M. S. 1973. *Thromb. Diath. Haemorrh.* 29:201–10
30. Wu, K. K., Hoak, J. C. 1974, *Fed. Proc.* 33: 243 (Abstr.)
31. Giger, M., Zbinden, G. 1974, *Schweiz. Med. Wochenschr.* 104:1376–77
32. Hörstenmeyer, O. 1964. *Dtsch. Med. Wochenschr.* 89:1845–48
33. Gangarosa, E. J., Johnson, R. R., Ramos, H. S. 1960. *Arch. Intern. Med.* 105:83–89
34. Howard, M. A., Firkin, B. G. 1971. *Thromb. Diath. Haemorrh.* 26:362–69
35. Weiss, H. J., Rogers, J., Brand, H. 1973. *J. Clin. Invest.* 52:2697–2707
36. Meyer, D., Jenkins, C.S.P., Dreyfus, M., Larrieu, M. J. 1973 *Nature London* 243:293–94
37. Dugdale, M., Masi, A. T. 1973. *J. Chronic Dis.* 23:775–90
38. Boullin, D. J. et al 1975. *Br. J. Clin. Pharmacol.* 2:29–35
39. Wright, H. P. 1942. *J. Pathol. Bacteriol.* 54:461–68
40. Murphy, E. A., Mustard, J. F. 1962. *Circulation* 25:114–25
41. Bridges, J. M., Dalby, A. M., Millar, J. H. D., Weaver, J. A. 1965. *Lancet* 1:75–77
42. Bouvier, C. A. et al 1967. *Cardiologia* 50:232–38
43. Hellem, A. J. 1960. *Scand. J. Clin. Lab. Invest.* 12: Suppl. 51, 1–117
44. Glynn, M. F., Movat, H. Z., Murphy, E. A., Mustard, J. F. 1965. *J. Lab. Clin. Med.* 65:179–201
45. Spaet, T. H., Zucker, M. B. 1964. *Am. J. Physiol.* 206:1267–74
46. Zbinden, G., Tomlin, S. 1968. *Thromb. Diath. Haemorrh.* 20:384–96
47. Tschopp, T. B., Weiss, H. J., Baumgartner, H. R. 1975. *Experientia* 31:113–16
48. French, J. E., Macfarlane, R. G., Sanders, A. G. 1964. *Br. J. Exp. Pathol.* 45:467–74
49. Hovig, T., McKenzie, F. N., Arefos, K. E. 1974. *Thromb. Diath. Haemorrh.* 32:695–703
50. Begent, N., Born, G. V. R. 1970. *Br. J. Pharmacol.* 40:592P–93P
51. Born, G. V. R., Philp, R. B. 1965. *Nature London* 205:398–99
52. Aaron, R. K., Srinivasan, S., Burrowes, C. B., Sawyer, P. N. 1970. *Thromb. Diath. Haemorrh.* 23:621–26
53. Salzman, E. W., Levine, L. 1971, *J. Clin. Invest.* 50:131–41
54. Cole, B., Robison, G. A., Hartmann, R. C. 1971. *Ann. NY Acad. Sci.* 185: 477–78
55. Grette, K., 1962. *Acta Physiol. Scand. Suppl.* 56:1–93
56. Zucker, M. B. 1975. *Platelets, Drugs and Thrombosis,* ed. J. Hirsh, J. F. Cade, A. S. Gallus, E. Schönbaum, 27–34. Basel: Karger
57. Haslam, R. J. 1946. *Nature London* 202:765–68
58. DeGaetano, G., Bottecchia, D., Donati, M. B., Vermylen, J. 1974. See Ref. 15, 269–82
59. Haslam, R. J., Rosson, G. M., 1971. *J. Physiol. London* 219:36P–38P
60. Shore, P. A., Alpers, H. S. 1963. *Am. J. Physiol.* 205:348–50
61. Mills, D. C. B., Robb, I. A., Roberts, G. C. K. 1968. *J. Physiol. London* 195: 915–29
62. Hougie, C., Rutherford, R. N., Banks, A. L., Coburn, W. A. 1965. *Metabolism* 14:411–17
63. Donayre, J., Pincus, G. 1965. *Metabolism* 14:418–21
64. Whitaker, A. N., McKay, D. G. 1968. *Fed. Proc.* 27:569 (Abstr.)
65. Waldron, J. M. 1951, *J. Appl. Physiol.* 3:554–58
66. Ozge, A. H., Rowsell, H. C., Downie, H. G., Mustard, J. F. 1966. *Thromb. Diath. Haemorrh.* 15:349–64
67. Egeberg, O. 1963. *Scand. J. Clin. Lab. Invest.* 15:539–49
68. Zbinden, G., Tomlin, S. 1969. *Arch. Int. Pharmacodyn.* 181:152–69
69. Girolami, A., Brunetti, A., Cella, G., Pedrazzoli, S., Bernardi, R. 1973. *Thromb. Diath. Haemorrh.* 29:384–92
70. McKay, D. G., Latour, J. G., Lopez, A. M. 1971. *Thromb. Diath. Haemorrh.* 26:71–82
71. Marbet, G. A., Duckert, F. C. 1973, *Thromb. Diath. Haemorrh.* 29:619–32
72. Spaet, T., Horowitz, H. I., Zucker-Franklin, D., Cintron, J., Biezenski, J. J. 1961. *Blood* 17:196–205
73. Tomikawa, M., Ogawa, H., Abiko, Y. 1974. *Thromb. Diath. Haemorrh.* 31: 86–102
74. Margolis, J. 1962. *Aust. J. Exp. Biol.* 40:505–13
75. Botti, R. E., Ratnoff, O. D. 1963. *J. Clin. Invest.* 42:1569–77

76. Connor, W. E., Hoak, J. C., Warner, E. D. 1963. *J. Clin. Invest.* 42:860–66
77. Zbinden, G. 1964. *J. Lipid Res.* 5:378–84
78. Santi, R., Fassana, G. 1965. *J. Pharm. Pharmacol.* 17:596–97
79. Hoak, J. C., Poole, J. C. F., Robinson, D. S. 1963. *Am. J. Pathol.* 43:987–95
80. Bizzi, A., Tacconi, M. T., Medea, A., Garattini, S. 1972. *Pharmacology* 7:216–24
81. Egeberg, O. 1965. *Thromb. Diath. Haemorrh.* 13:516–30
82. von Kaulla, E., von Kaulla, K. N. 1970. *Lancet* 1: 36
83. Peterson, R. A., Krull, P. E., Finley, P., Ettinger, M. G. 1970. *Am. J. Clin. Pathol.* 53:468–73
84. Conrad, J., Samama, M., Salomon, Y. 1972. *Lancet* 2:1148–49
85. Moriau, M., Rodhain, J., Noel, H., De Beys-Col, C., Masure, R. 1974. *Thromb. Diath. Haemorrh.* 32:171–88
86. Charytan, C., Purtilo, D. 1969. *N. Engl. J. Med.* 280:1102–4
87. Naeye, R. L. 1962. *Blood* 19:694–701
88. Gralnick, H. R., Greipp, P. 1971. *Am. J. Clin. Pathol.* 56:151–54
89. Gerrits, W. B. J., Prakke, E. M., Van der Meer, J., Feltkamp-Vroon, T. M., Vreeken, J. 1974. *Scand. J. Haematol.* 13:5–10
90. Niewiarowski, S., Prokopowicz, J., Poplawski, A., Worowski, K. 1964. *Experientia* 20:101–3
91. Worowski, K., Gabryelewicz, A., Prokopowicz, J., Poplawski, A. 1970. *Thromb. Diath. Haemorrh.* 23:500–503
92. Herlache, J., Hoskins, P., Schmidt, C. M., 1973. *Angiology* 24:369–73
93. Kramer, R. A., Hecker, S. P., Lewis, B. I., 1965. *Radiology* 84:308–10
94. Berardi, R. S., 1974. *Am. J. Surg.* 127:757–61
95. Wessler, S. 1962. *Am. J. Med.* 33:648–66
96. Baumgartner, H. R. 1974. *Thromb. Diath. Haemorrh. Suppl.* 59:91–105
97. Goodrich, S. M., Wood, J. E. 1964. *Am. J. Obstet. Gynecol.* 90:740–44
98. Lauterjung, K. L., Isselhard, W. 1973. *Angiology* 24:107–13
99. Arroyave, R., Vizcaino, C., Mac-Donald, R., Murga, F. 1960. *Surgery* 47:430–35
100. Stein, P. D., Sabbah, H. N. 1974. *Circ. Res.* 35:608–14
101. Baumgartner, H. R. 1963. *Z. Gesamte Exp. Med.* 137:277–47

CURRENT CONCEPTS ABOUT THE TREATMENT OF SELECTED POISONINGS:
Nitrite, Cyanide, Sulfide, Barium, and Quinidine

❖6645

Roger P. Smith and R. E. Gosselin

Department of Pharmacology and Toxicology, Dartmouth Medical School, Hanover, New Hampshire 03755

The hospital and the research laboratory are both important sources of information in clinical toxicology. New knowledge based on recent observations has important implications in treating poisoning by barium, quinidine, methemoglobin-generating chemicals, and inhibitors of cytochrome oxidase. Based on this knowledge, suggestions are offered for the clinical management of these kinds of intoxications. This review emphasizes departures from established forms of therapy. For information about other aspects of the clinical management, a comprehensive treatise such as that by Gosselin et al (1) should be consulted.

Because methemoglobinemia and cytochrome oxidase inhibition cause defects in oxygen transport and utilization respectively, the role of pure oxygen in treating these disorders has long attracted attention. Recent experimental data indicate that hyperbaric oxygen is useful in treating some kinds of toxic methemoglobinemias and is dangerous in other kinds. Similarly, oxygen therapy may have some value against some cytochrome oxidase inhibitors (cyanide) and not others (sulfide). Of the many exogenous chemicals known or suspected to interfere with potassium metabolism, barium and quinidine have been selected for review. Current evidence indicates that the administration of K^+ can be life saving in barium poisoning. In quinidine poisoning K^+ plays a more limited and selective role.

NEW ROLES FOR OXYGEN

Management of Nitrite Poisoning

Until recently no important distinctions were recognized between techniques for the management of methemoglobinemia induced by nitrite salts on the one hand or

189

aniline and its congeners on the other. There has been rather limited experience with exchange transfusion as a general approach to the management of toxic methemoglobinemias (2). The potential advantage of reducing the blood concentration of both the offending chemical and the inert blood pigment simultaneously must be weighed against the risks of multiple transfusions. Alternative recommendations for treating methemoglobinemias have included the administration of ascorbic acid, oxygen at normal and hyperbaric pressures, and methylene blue (3).

The administration of ascorbic acid is attractive because of its extremely low toxicity; human poisonings are unknown (1). Unhappily, its safety is equaled by a lack of efficacy. In otherwise normal human erythrocytes made methemoglobinemic by in vitro exposure to chemicals, concentrations of ascorbate much higher than one could reasonably expect to achieve in the blood of patients did not significantly accelerate methemoglobin reduction (4). Thus, in normal individuals ascorbate offers no advantage over spontaneous methemoglobin reduction. In rare individuals born with an inherited deficiency of methemoglobin reductase, ascorbate administration is accompanied by a slow reversal of the congenital methemoglobinemia. In these and normal patients, however, ascorbate would be a poor choice for a life-threatening exposure to a methemoglobin-generating chemical.

Pure oxygen at atmospheric pressure is often mentioned as a therapeutic adjuvant to the management of acquired methemoglobinemia. Hyperbaric oxygen has been recommended on empirical grounds; we have not encountered published accounts of its use with human patients. Rats given lethal doses of sodium nitrite and exposed to 4 atm of pure oxygen had significantly lower blood methemoglobin concentrations and a lower mortality than groups exposed to air at 1 atm (5). Surprisingly, when the methemoglobinemia was induced by p-aminopropiophenone (PAPP), exposure to 4 atm of oxygen increased both blood methemoglobin and PAPP concentrations over that in animals maintained under air at 1 atm (6).

The above observations suggest that the effect of high pressure oxygen (HPO) in potentiating the methemoglobinemia after PAPP is mediated through an interference with the detoxication of PAPP by conjugation reactions such as acetylation of the amino group (6). If that hypothesis is true, HPO may generally potentiate methemoglobinemias due to aniline-like compounds. At least one other example is known. The avicidal compound, 3-chloro-4-methylaniline (3-CPT), generated significantly higher levels of methemoglobin in mice exposed to HPO than in mice exposed to air at 1 atm (7). This potentiation of the methemoglobinemic response, however, was not accompanied by an increase in mortality. Perhaps mortality was not increased because, like many aniline congeners, 3-CPT lethality in rodents appears to be unrelated to methemoglobinemia (7, 8). The oxygen pressures used in the experiment described above are higher than can be tolerated safely by human subjects, but pending further investigation it would appear prudent to avoid HPO in acute poisonings by aromatic amines (and nitro compounds?). In human nitrite poisoning HPO appears to deserve a clinical trial. No adverse effects of oxygen at 1 atm on either type of methemoglobinemia have been recognized in the laboratory or in the clinic to date.

At present the most widely accepted treatment of toxic methemoglobinemia is the administration of methylene blue. Its efficacy is firmly established, and a broad base of clinical experience exists. It has been suggested, however, that a similar compound, toluidine blue, may have some advantages in terms of greater potency, more rapid onset of action, and fewer side effects (9).

In certain rare circumstances methylene blue has failed as an antidote against a chemically induced methemoglobinemia. One such case involved methemoglobinemia in an individual with an inherited deficiency of glucose-6-phosphate dehydrogenase (10). In this case the dye was without effect on the rate of methemoglobin reduction. It is effective, however, in red cells deficient in methemoglobin reductase (see above). Under some conditions methylene blue can attenuate the methemoglobinemic response of mice to 3-CPT but can significantly increase the mortality (7). It is not clear whether 3-CPT is unique among aniline derivatives in this respect or whether this type of interaction occurs only in rodents.

As tested in mice against nitrite poisoning, the combination of oxygen and methylene blue had at least additive effects in reducing mortality. At a low dose of methylene blue, oxygen at 2 atm was superior to oxygen at 1 atm, which in turn was superior to air at 1 atm. When the dose of methylene blue was increased, the advantage of HPO was lost, but oxygen at 1 atm was still superior to air at 1 atm (11).

Management of Cyanide, Sulfide, and Azide Poisonings

For many years it has been generally accepted that all of the toxic effects of cyanide are due directly or indirectly to an inhibition of cytochrome oxidase. The principles underlying the management of cyanide poisoning are well known (e.g. reference 1) and are directed toward increasing the rate of biological inactivation of cyanide. A moderate dose of sodium nitrite is injected intravenously to convert a tolerable fraction of the circulating blood pigment to methemoglobin. The latter traps and inactivates free cyanide by forming the stable complex, cyanmethemoglobin. Nitrite administration is followed by an intravenous injection of sodium thiosulfate. Thiosulfate furnishes sulfur for a reaction mediated by the enzyme rhodanese, which converts cyanide to the much less toxic thiocyanate.

The rhodanese reaction is insensitive to oxygen (12), and, as noted above, HPO acts to decrease methemoglobin levels after nitrite. The biochemical lesion in cyanide poisoning is one that prevents oxygen utilization instead of impairing its transport. For all these reasons, the administration of oxygen would appear to be superfluous in cyanide poisoning as long as the circulation is not compromised.

In accord with the above expectation even HPO failed to protect mice against death after cyanide or to reverse the course of cyanide poisoning. Moreover, HPO failed to have a significant effect on the anti-cyanide activity of either nitrite or thiosulfate (13). Both HPO and oxygen at 1 atm, however, significantly potentiated the anti-cyanide activity of the nitrite-thiosulfate combination (13–15). The magnitude of the potentiation was the same for oxygen at 1 and 4 atm, i.e. there was no advantage to HPO.

Extensive studies on respiratory, cardiovascular, and other physiological parameters in cyanide-poisoned dogs given nitrite, thiosulfate, and oxygen in various combinations failed to reveal a basis for the potentiating effect of oxygen. Oxygen alone was able to reduce the length of the period of electrical silence of the EEG after cyanide. Although nitrite alone had a similar effect, thiosulfate alone appeared to prolong this period. In each case when oxygen was added (to nitrite, thiosulfate, or the combination), a decrease in the period of electrical silence was observed relative to that in air. No combination of treatments, however, was superior to oxygen alone (16). Clearly, these effects on the EEG do not match the pattern observed in the mortality of mice. However, the potentiating effect of oxygen on the antidotal action of the nitrite-thiosulfate combination has not been demonstrated in dogs as it has been in mice.

When mice were given large but sublethal doses of cyanide, a decrease in the respiratory excretion of $^{14}CO_2$ derived from previously administered uniformly labeled ^{14}C-glucose was observed. This response was identical in mice exposed to air or to oxygen at 1 atm, nor did the addition of either nitrite or thiosulfate result in significant changes in this response. The combination of oxygen with nitrite and thiosulfate, however, did result in a striking enhancement of cyanide-inhibited glucose metabolism (17). These effects of oxygen on glucose metabolism closely match the pattern of the effects on mortality, but they may represent a result of the oxygen effect rather than its cause.

Isom & Way believe that the synergistic effect of oxygen on the nitrite-thiosulfate combination cannot be due to an enhancement of cyanide detoxification because the measured blood cyanide levels in treated animals were several times higher than those in control groups (17). Exception must be taken to that conclusion, however, since the method used to determine blood cyanide concentrations almost certainly measures the total blood cyanide, including a large fraction that is bound in the biologically inactive form of cyanmethemoglobin (18). Thus, it remains to be established whether the free and biologically active fraction of the blood cyanide in treated animals is higher, lower, or substantially the same as in untreated animals.

It has been suggested that the mechanism of acute sulfide poisoning (whether inhaled as hydrogen sulfide or injected as sodium sulfide) also involves an inhibition of cytochrome oxidase. Thus, sulfide poisoning would be expected to resemble cyanide poisoning in many important respects. Accordingly, sodium nitrite protects a variety of animal species against death in acute sulfide poisoning presumably by trapping sulfide as sulfmethemoglobin (19–23). Sulfmethemoglobin is a dissociable complex in which the hydrosulfide anion is attached to ferric heme groups on methemoglobin. It seems to have no relationship to so-called sulfhemoglobin, which is a poorly characterized, irreversible, abnormal blood pigment sometimes seen in association with methemoglobin.

An antidotal effect of intravenous nitrite has been demonstrated in mice after their exposure to otherwise lethal concentrations of hydrogen sulfide in air (24) and of intraperitoneal nitrite in rats after injection of sodium sulfide (24a).

Possible interactions between oxygen, nitrite, and thiosulfate in acute sulfide poisoning have been explored (24a) using an experimental protocol that closely follows the one that uncovered the potentiating effect of oxygen as a cyanide antagonist (14). In accord with the findings for cyanide, oxygen at 1 atm did not protect mice against acute sulfide poisoning when compared with animals maintained in air at 1 atm. Thiosulfate alone given to mice maintained in oxygen or air produced a small but statistically significant protective effect against death due to sulfide. A much larger protective effect was observed with nitrite, which was equally efficacious in animals exposed in air or oxygen. In marked contrast to the findings with cyanide, oxygen failed to potentiate the protective effects of the nitrite-thiosulfate combination.

Thus, it may be inferred that the potentiating effects of oxygen as a cyanide antagonist cannot be mediated through any mechanism that is also common to sulfide poisoning. For example, oxygen cannot be acting to increase methemoglobin levels by some unknown mechanism because such an effect would also be reflected in a change in the mortality after sulfide. Similarly, if oxygen in some way enhanced the pulmonary excretion of hydrogen cyanide gas, it would be expected to have a similar effect with volatile hydrogen sulfide. If indeed the mechanisms for acute poisoning are the same for cyanide and for sulfide, the effect of oxygen in the case of cyanide would most likely be manifested through some metabolic inactivation mechanism that is not available to sulfide. If this were a sluggish pathway in which a fivefold difference in oxygen tension could result in significant differences in rate, the role of nitrite and thiosulfate might simply represent a delaying action such that this pathway might find expression.

For a given circulating level of methemoglobin, a greater protective effect is seen against cyanide than against sulfide, a result that correlates with estimates of the relative stability of the respective anion-methemoglobin complexes (20). Nevertheless, the protective effect of nitrite in acute sulfide poisoning is significant, and this agent deserves a trial in an acute human poisoning. Oxygen can do no harm as an adjuvant, and in the case of cyanide poisoning treated with nitrite-thiosulfate it may significantly increase the antidotal effect.

A very small but statistically significant protective effect of nitrite against acute azide poisoning was also observed in mice (25). Again the magnitude of this effect correlated with the stability of the azide-methemoglobin complex relative to that of the cyanide and sulfide complexes (20). Because no other antidotes to azide poisoning are known and because azide has a high toxicity, a clinical trial with nitrite was recommended. A single remarkable case has now been reported (26). A woman ingested an unknown amount of sodium azide, and after 90 minutes fainted with complaints of loss of vision and nausea. Within a few hours the clinical picture was dominated by pulmonary edema, lactic acidosis, and hypothermia. Among other measures she was given amyl nitrite by inhalation, sodium nitrite by vein, and intranasal oxygen. A clear-cut elevation of methemoglobin levels was documented, but the patient died in shock in 12 hours. Thus, in its only clinical trial, nitrite failed to produce obvious clinical benefit in acute azide poisoning, and a search for more effective antidotes is indicated. Two points might be made, however, the first being that the procedure did no obvious harm and the second being that the patient survived 12 hours. Mice given lethal doses of azide parenterally often expire within 5 minutes; it is conceivable that nitrite might have delayed death in this case.

THE ROLE OF POTASSIUM

Management of Barium Poisoning

Whereas human poisonings by soluble barium salts are uncommon, isolated accidental and suicidal ingestions are reported with surprising frequency (e.g. 27–29). Epidemics have also been described. In the early 1940s an endemic state of barium intoxication arose in a Chinese province due to the contamination of table salt with barium chloride (30, 31). Flour containing barium carbonate poisoned 85 British soldiers in India (32). An outbreak of severe food poisoning involving 100 individuals in Israel was traced to sausage contaminated with barium carbonate (33).

Barium ion stimulates smooth, striated, and cardiac muscle; the result is violent peristalsis, arterial hypertension, muscle twitching, and disturbances in cardiac action. Motor disorders include stiffness and immobility of the limbs and sometimes of the trunk, leg cramps, twitching of facial muscles, and paralysis of the tongue and pharynx with attendant loss or impairment of speech and deglutition (34). The central nervous system may be first stimulated and then depressed (32). Small amounts in cerebrospinal fluid induce convulsions (35). Ventricular tachyarrhythmias (including ventricular fibrillation) and transient asystole have been observed (36). Kidney damage has been described as a late complication, presumably a result of circulatory insufficiency (37). Probably the most distinctive effect of barium in large doses, however, is skeletal muscle weakness and eventually flaccid paralysis involving extremities and respiratory muscles (30–32, 38).

In an experimental study in rats, Schott & McArdle (39) demonstrated that barium-induced paralysis was due to a defect in muscle itself. During intravenous infusions of $BaCl_2$ (cumulative doses of about 20 mg/kg), curarized rat leg muscles stimulated electrically produced twitches with amplitudes that were transiently increased and then greatly attenuated. At the same time the plasma level of potassium fell rapidly to about 2 meq/liter. The partial paralysis correlated with the hypokalemia much better than with the plasma barium concentration. The plasma sodium level was unaffected.

Hypokalemia in barium-poisoned humans was probably first described by Diengott et al (40). Two severely poisoned patients, one of whom had experienced no vomiting or diarrhea, were found to have plasma K^+ levels of 2.0 and 2.4 meq/liter. Both responded clinically to intravenous KCl, although one eventually died from severe pulmonary edema and hemorrhagic gastritis and duodenitis. This episode confirms the dramatic relief of symptoms described by Huang (38) in two victims of barium poisoning treated with intravenous potassium citrate. Huang was impressed with similarities between barium intoxication and the rare disorder known as familial periodic paralysis. Features of the two states have been compared (39).

The mechanism of barium-induced hypokalemia has not been completely clarified. Enhanced renal excretion does not appear to be responsible (41). The rapidity of the fall in plasma potassium suggests that K^+ migrates into tissue cells. Presumably muscle cells are involved, but the phenomenon has been demonstrated in vivo only with dog red blood cells (41). Whereas epinephrine secretion from the adrenal medulla is provoked by barium (42) and this hormone can promote an accumulation of K^+ in cells (43), barium-induced hypokalemia cannot be ascribed to epinephrine because it cannot be prevented by adrenergic blockers such as phentolamine (41) or propranolol (39). A direct action of barium on muscle is inferred. Perhaps it activates Na^+-K^+-stimulated ATPase at cell surfaces to promote K^+ entry at the expense of the extracellular stores (44). In isolated frog muscle, however, it did not modify the K^+ content, but it did decrease inward and outward K^+ permeability constants equally (45).

In poisoned rats, infusions of K^+ (but not of Ca^{2+}) corrected promptly both the hypokalemia and muscle weakness (39). In dogs (41), all signs and symptoms of barium poisoning except hypertension were responsive to the administration of K^+; specifically, muscle weakness, diarrhea, and cardiac arrhythmias were alleviated. Whatever the mechanism of the hypertension, neither K^+ nor adrenergic blocking drugs suppressed it. As noted above, clinical experience with potassium therapy has also been favorable (33, 38), and at times the benefits have been spectacular. Large parenteral doses, however, may be required; in recent reports of acute barium poisoning in three adults (28, 29, 36), the cumulative dose of K^+ administered over the first 24 hr was 420, 260, and 250 meq, respectively.

Thus, potassium administration is judged to be a rational and effective form of treatment for barium poisoning. Although the recommendation is over 30 years old, it apparently is not widely recognized by clinical toxicologists. In any case barium's ability to induce hypokalemia and paralysis is not shared by strontium or any other alkaline earth element (1).

Management of Quinidine Poisoning

Quinidine also induces derangements of K^+ metabolism, as do several other antifibrillatory drugs. The cellular actions of quinidine on ion fluxes are better defined than those of barium, but they also appear to be more complex. Even with little or no change in the resting transmembrane potential, quinidine reduces myocardial sodium influx and potassium efflux during systole, diastole, or both (46–48). At the same time the K^+ influx may be enhanced (46, 49). In several experimental preparations (e.g. isolated atria, excised papillary muscles, perfused hearts), these permeability changes have led to significant increases in the myocardial content of potassium (48, 50), although this is not a universal finding (51).

Presumably other organs and tissues also extract K^+ from the extracellular fluid under the influence of quinidine. At least mild hypokalemia that cannot be accounted for by K^+ losses in vomitus or feces has been described in several cases of poisoning by quinidine (52, 53) and quinine (54). A low plasma K^+ level, however, has not been reported often in these conditions; perhaps the tendency to hypokalemia is masked by extraneous factors commonly associated with quinidine usage, such as the chronic intake of digitalis, poor circulatory reserve, defective renal excretion, and respiratory acidosis. In any case the clinical toxicity of quinidine, unlike that of barium, cannot be explained by any simple defect in K^+ metabolism.

Signs and symptoms of quinidine poisoning are referable to the central nervous system, gastrointestinal tract, blood vessels, and heart (1). In clinical poisonings the most dangerous effects are usually those on the heart. It is important for the therapist to recognize that the cardiotoxicity of quinidine can assume two distinct forms. The first pattern (Type I) involves a failure of cardiac stimulus formation or propagation, terminating in ventricular standstill. The second pattern (Type II) is one of abnormal stimulus formation, leading to ventricular tachyarrhythmias and terminating in ventricular fibrillation. Although the terminology used here is not well established, the distinction is believed to be important because the two situations demand entirely different programs of therapy. The two patterns of toxicity also have different implications with respect to potassium.

Stimulus failure (Type I) can be regarded as a progressive state involving a weakening of impulse formation (pacemaker failure) and a gradual impairment of conduction, particularly through the specialized conducting system of the atrioventricular (AV) junction and ventricles. A lengthening of the QRS interval by 50% or more (120 to 140 msec or longer) is sometimes regarded as a sign that vigorous measures may be required to sustain the cardiac beat (55). Perhaps an infusion of 1 molar sodium lactate is useful under these circumstances (56), but probably one of the catecholamine drugs is preferable. Epinephrine, norepinephrine (levarterenol), and isoproterenol are all capable of stimulating atrial pacemakers and of narrowing a wide QRS complex or of accelerating a slow idioventricular pacemaker in the presence of complete heart block. They also increase the stroke volume and cardiac output by stimulating the quinidine-depressed myocardium (57). At least in rats the lethality of quinidine is distinctly reduced (58). It has been asserted without proof that isoproterenol accomplishes these changes with a smaller risk of inducing ventricular tachycardia or fibrillation than does epinephrine (59). Because isoproterenol is a vasodilator and norepinephrine a vasoconstrictor, the latter would appear to be preferable in the hypotensive patient. In quinidine-poisoned dogs, however, norepinephrine did not increase peripheral vascular resistance (57); the elevation in blood pressure was due entirely to cardiac stimulation.

If an infusion of isoproterenol or norepinephrine fails to sustain an adequate heart rate and stroke volume in Type I poisoning, electrical pacing of the ventricles may be indicated, but the attempt is apt to be unsuccessful because of the high threshold of the quinidine-poisoned heart (52). Certainly all antifibrillatory drugs should be avoided. Except in cases of severe hypokalemia (see above), even potassium should be withheld. Thus, quinidine and potassium induce similar aberrations of the ECG, and mild hypokalemia protects dogs against quinidine-induced intraventricular conduction failure and raises the lethal dose of quinidine (60). Survival of a 42-year-old woman who ingested 100 coated (long-acting) tablets of quinidine sulfate (total dose 20 g) was ascribed (perhaps wrongly) to hypokalemia produced by hemodialysis (61).

In contrast, the abnormal mechanism of ventricular activation in Type II poisoning usually involves a rapid heart rate. The therapist's aim is to moderate and control the ventricular tachycardia and to prevent its deterioration into ventricular fibrillation. Under these circumstances potassium may be a useful agent, and it has been infused in victims of quinidine poisoning (52, 53). Except when used to correct preexisting hypokalemia, however, potassium should probably be discarded in favor of an antifibrillatory drug that is less apt to compromise AV conduction. Both propranolol (62) and lidocaine (63) have been used successfully to terminate ventricular rhythms in quinidine poisoning and to restore a supraventricular mechanism. Diphenylhydantoin sodium would probably be superior to propranolol and perhaps to lidocaine under these circumstances. Ventricular fibrillation may necessitate defibrillation by direct current electroshocks (64), but ventricular contractions may resume spontaneously after brief, recurring periods of fibrillation (65).

To employ these therapeutic regimens correctly, it is necessary of course to recognize both types of poisoning and to distinguish between them. In practice it is sometimes difficult to differentiate between ventricular tachycardia (Type II) and a supraventricular mechanism with bundle branch block or other conduction defect (Type I) (66). Furthermore, clinical signs of both patterns can sometimes be found in a single person. For example, Type I patients occasionally exhibit ventricular premature beats (52, 53), and Type II patients often show widening of the QRS complex before a ventricular mechanism becomes established (65). To predict the ultimate or definitive pattern, one notes that persons with chronic heart disease, especially in congestive failure, usually exhibit a Type II reaction to quinidine overdoses (66). In persons with structurally sound hearts, Type I is thought to be the more common pattern (52, 61). Even when quinidine caused ventricular tachycardia in otherwise healthy hearts, the disorder was well tolerated and fibrillation did not occur (53, 66).

CONCLUSIONS

In certain types of uncommon human poisonings, the therapist must be prepared to act on the basis of experimental findings in animals. Recent laboratory evidence suggests that hyperbaric oxygen is an effective antidote to nitrite poisoning but that it should be avoided in poisonings with aniline and its derivatives. Pure oxygen at atmospheric pressures potentiates the antidotal activity of a nitrite-thiosulfate combination against cyanide. Although oxygen appears to do no harm in acute hydrogen sulfide poisoning, it is not useful, but nitrite has significant protective and antidotal effects. Despite a marginal protective effect of nitrite against azide poisoning in mice, it was not efficacious in a single human intoxication. Both experimental and clinical evidence indicates that barium modifies the cellular distribution of potassium and that K^+ is a valuable agent in the management of barium poisoning. Quinidine also influences the metabolism of potassium, but more observations are required to clarify the roles of K^+ in the pathogenesis and treatment of quinidine poisoning.

ACKNOWLEDGMENTS

Original studies in the authors' laboratories were supported by USPHS Grant HL-14127 from the National Heart and Lung Institute. The literature compilation was supported partially by FD 00010 from the Food and Drug Administration and RR 05392 from NIH.

Literature Cited

1. Gosselin, R. E., Hodge, H. C., Smith, R. P., Gleason, M. N. 1976. *Clinical Toxicology of Commercial Products.* Baltimore: Williams & Wilkins. 4th ed.
2. Lubash, G. D., Phillips, R. E., Shields, J. D., Bonsnes, R. W. 1964. *Arch. Intern. Med.* 114:530–32
3. Smith, R. P., Olson, M. V. 1973. *Semin. Hematol.* 10:253–68
4. Bolyai, J. Z., Smith, R. P., Gray, C. T. 1972. *Toxicol. Appl. Pharmacol.* 21: 176–85
5. Goldstein, G. M., Doull, J. 1971. *Proc. Soc. Exp. Biol. Med.* 138:137–39
6. Goldstein, G. M., Doull, J. 1973. *Toxicol. Appl. Pharmacol.* 26:247–52
7. Felsenstein, W. C., Smith, R. P., Gosselin, R. E. 1974. *Toxicol. Appl. Pharmacol.* 28:110–25
8. Borison, H. L., Snow, S. R., Longnecker, D. S., Smith, R. P. 1975. *Toxicol. Appl. Pharmacol.* 31:403–12
9. Kiese, M., Lörcher, W., Weger, N., Zierer, A. 1972. *Eur. J. Clin. Pharmacol.* 4:115–18
10. Rosen, P. J., Johnson, C., McGehee, W. G., Beutler, E. 1971. *Ann. Intern. Med.* 75:83–86
11. Sheehy, M. H., Way, J. L. 1974. *Toxicol. Appl. Pharmacol.* 30:221–26
12. Sorbo, B. H. 1962. *Acta Chem. Scand.* 16:2455–56
13. Way, J. L., End, E., Sheehy, M. H., de Miranda, P., Feitknecht, U. F., Bachand, R., Gibbon, S. L., Burrows, G. E. 1972. *Toxicol. Appl. Pharmacol.* 22: 415–21
14. Way, J. L., Gibbon, S. L., Sheehy, M. 1966. *J. Pharmacol. Exp. Ther.* 153: 381–85
15. Sheehy, M., Way, J. L. 1968. *J. Pharmacol. Exp. Ther.* 161:163–68
16. Burrows, G. E., Liu, D. H. W., Way, J. L. 1973. *J. Pharmacol. Exp. Ther.* 184:739–48
17. Isom, G. E., Way, J. L. 1974. *J. Pharmacol. Exp. Ther.* 189:235–43
18. Smith, R. P., Kruszyna, H. 1974. *J. Pharmacol. Exp. Ther.* 191:557–63
19. Smith, R. P., Gosselin, R. E. 1964. *Toxicol. Appl. Pharmacol.* 6:584–92
20. Smith, R. P., Gosselin, R. E. 1966. *Toxicol. Appl. Pharmacol.* 8:159–72
21. Smith, R. P., Abbanat, R. A. 1966. *Toxicol. Appl. Pharmacol.* 9:209–17
22. Smith, R. P. 1967. *Mol. Pharmacol.* 3:378–85
23. Smith, R. P. 1969. *Toxicol. Appl. Pharmacol.* 15:505–16
24. Scheler, W., Kabisch, R. 1963. *Acta Biol. Med. Ger.* 11:194–99
24a. Smith, R. P., Kruszyna, R., Kruszyna, H. 1976. *Arch. Environ. Health.* In press
25. Abbanat, R. A., Smith, R. P. 1964. *Toxicol. Appl. Pharmacol.* 6:576–83
26. Emmett, E. A., Ricking, J. A. 1975. *Ann. Intern. Med.* 83:224–26
27. Jacobziner, H., Raybin, H. W. 1959. *NY State J. Med.* 59:3460–64
28. Gould, D. B., Sorrell, M. R., Lupariello, A. D. 1973. *Arch. Int. Med.* 132:891–94
29. Berning, J. 1975. *Lancet* 1:110
30. Allen, A. S. 1943. *Chin. Med. J.* 61:296–301
31. Du, K. T., Dung, C. L. 1943. *Chin. Med. J.* 61:302
32. Morton, W. 1945. *Lancet* 2:738–39
33. Lewi, Z., Bar-Khayim, Y. 1964. *Lancet* 2:342–43
34. Witthaus, R. A. 1911. *Manual of Toxicology.* New York: William Wood
35. Chou, C., Chin, Y. C. 1943. *Chin. Med. J.* 61:313–22
36. Habicht, W., Smekal, P. V., Etzrodt, H. 1970. *Med. Welt* 28:1292–95
37. McNally, W. D. 1925. *J. Am. Med. Assoc.* 84:1805–7
38. Huang, K. 1943. *Chin. Med. J.* 61: 305–12
39. Schott, G. D., McArdle, B. 1974. *J. Neurol. Neurosurg. Psychiatry* 37:32–39
40. Diengott, D., Rozsa, O., Levy, N., Maummar, S. 1964. *Lancet* 2:343–44
41. Roza, O., Berman, L. B. 1971. *J. Pharmacol. Exp. Ther.* 177:433–39
42. Douglas, W. W., Rubin, R. P. 1964. *Nature London* 203:305–7
43. Vick, R. L., Todd, E. P., Leudke, D. W. 1972. *J. Pharmacol. Exp. Ther.* 181: 139–46
44. Henn, F. A., Sperelakis, N. 1968. *Biochim. Biophys. Acta* 163:415–17
45. Henderson, E. G., Volle, R. L. 1972. *J. Pharmacol. Exp. Ther.* 183:356–69
46. Holland, W., Klein, R. L. 1958. *Circ. Res.* 6:516–21
47. Klein, R. L., Holland, W. C., Tinsley, B. 1960. *Circ. Res.* 8:246–52
48. Choi, S. J., Roberts, J., Kelliher, G. J. 1972. *Eur. J. Pharmacol.* 20:10–21
49. Choi, S. J., Roberts, J., Kelliher, G. J. 1972. *Eur. J. Pharmacol.* 20:22–33
50. Conn, H. L., Wood, J. C. 1960. *Am. J. Physiol.* 199:151–56
51. Brown, T. E., Grupp, G., Acheson,

G. H. 1961. *J. Pharmacol. Exp. Ther.* 133:84–89

52. Kerr, F., Kenoyer, G., Bilitch, M. 1971. *Br. Heart J.* 33:629–31

53. Reimold, E. W., Reynolds, W. J., Fixler, D. E., McElroy, L. 1973. *Pediatrics* 52:95–99

54. Reimold, W. V., Larbig, D., Kochsiek, K. 1970. *Dtsch. Med. Wochenschr.* 95:517–21

55. Bellet, S. 1963. *Clinical Disorders of the Heart Beat.* Philadelphia: Lea & Febiger

56. Wasserman, F., Brodsky, L., Dick, M. M., Kathe, J. H., Rodensky, P. L. 1958. *N. Engl. J. Med.* 259:797–802

57. Luchi, R. J., Helwig, J., Conn, H. L. 1963. *Am. Heart J.* 65:340–48

58. Gottsegen, G., Östör, E. 1963. *Am. Heart J.* 65:102–9

59. Nickel, S. N., Thibaudeau, Y. 1961. *Can. Med. Assoc. J.* 85:81–83

60. Brandfonbrener, M., Kronholm, J., Jones, H. R. 1966. *J. Pharmacol. Exp. Ther.* 154:250–54

61. Woie, L., Oyri, A. 1974. *Acta Med. Scand.* 195:237–39

62. Seaton, A. 1966. *Br. Med. J.* 1:1522–23

63. Kaplinsky, E., Yahini, J. H., Barzilai, J., Neufeld, H. N. 1972. *Chest* 62: 764–66

64. Ranier-Pope, C. R., Schrire, V., Beck, W., Barnard, C. N. 1962. *Am. Heart J.* 63:582–90

65. Selzer, A., Wray, H. W. 1964. *Circulation* 30:17–26

66. Rivers, R. P. A., Boyd, R. D. H. 1973. *Acta Paediatr. Scand.* 62:391–95

67. Thomson, G. M. 1956. *Circulation* 14:757–65

DIURETICS: SITES AND MECHANISMS OF ACTION

♦6646

Harry R. Jacobson and Juha P. Kokko

University of Texas Health Science Center at Dallas, Southwestern Medical School, Dallas, Texas 75235

INTRODUCTION

One of the most powerful and frequently used clinical tools in the physician's pharmaceutical armamentarium is the class of diuretic drugs. The list of available and currently investigated agents is quite long. This review examines the renal pharmacology of these drugs with respect to their sites and mechanisms of action. First we outline normal renal physiology with respect to the major locations and mechanisms of salt and water transport along the nephron as determined largely by micropuncture and in vitro microperfusion. Then we examine each class of diuretic agents with respect to what is presently known about their specific alteration of the normal renal physiology that results in their beneficial and, at times, adverse effects.

NORMAL TRANSPORT PHENOMENA

The mechanisms and sites of action of the various diuretics have been studied with multiple experimental techniques: clearance studies, stop-flow technique, in vitro enzyme analysis, toad bladder studies, micropuncture, and most recently in vitro microperfusion of isolated tubules. These techniques have also contributed in a major way to our understanding of normal renal physiology.

In Figure 1 is depicted a schematic representation of salt and water transport along the nephron. Under normal circumstances 50–60% of salt and water reabsorption occurs in the proximal tubule. The early segment of the proximal convoluted tubule actively and electrogenically reabsorbs sodium coupled to organic solute transport (1). This segment also reabsorbs most of the bicarbonate resulting in a commensurate increase in luminal chloride concentration (2–4). Bicarbonate reabsorption is dependent on intracellular and brush border carbonic anhydrase (3, 5, 6). This alteration in luminal fluid constituents by the early proximal convolution establishes several potential passive driving forces for further salt and water reabsorption in the latter proximal tubule: chloride diffusion gradient, chloride diffusion

201

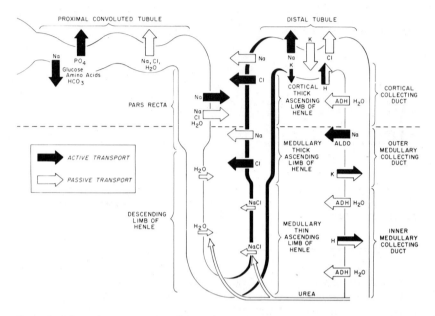

Figure 1   Schematic representation of the major transport processes in the nephron that may be affected by diuretics.

potential (lumen positive), and osmotic effects of higher peritubular concentrations of bicarbonate, glucose, acetate, and amino acids (7, 8). The majority of phosphate reabsorption also occurs in the proximal convolution and appears to be partially mediated by the effects of intraluminal pH on the relative concentrations of the mono- and dihydrogen phosphates (9–18). The presence of phosphate in the urine has been classically used as a marker for proximal tubular inhibition (10). Although its significance with respect to the diuretic agents is unknown, the pars recta of the proximal tubule has recently been shown to exhibit active electrogenic transport of sodium independent of organic solute transport (19). Thus, under normal circumstances approximately 40% of the glomerular filtrate, isosmotic to plasma but with major changes in composition, enters the thin descending limb of Henle's loop.

The thin descending limb of Henle has been shown to lack active sodium chloride transport and to have a low permeability to sodium and a high osmotic water permeability (20). These characteristics enable it to play an important passive role in the countercurrent system by allowing water abstraction and osmotic equilibration with the hypertonic interstitium (21). Hypertonic (mostly due to sodium chloride) fluid thus enters the thin ascending limb of Henle.

The thin ascending limb is relatively impermeable to water, highly permeable to sodium and chloride, and less permeable to urea (22). This segment appears to passively reabsorb sodium chloride along its concentration gradient from lumen to interstitium (21, 22) although this issue is still controversial (23, 24). Both the absolute quantity and concentration of sodium chloride thus gradually decreases as the fluid enters the thick ascending limb.

It now appears that the thick ascending limb of Henle actively reabsorbs sodium chloride by active electrogenic chloride reabsorption (25, 26). This segment has been shown to develop a lumen positive transepithelial potential difference secondary to active chloride transport and to be relatively impermeable to water even in the presence of antidiuretic hormone (25–27). These characteristics, active chloride reabsorption with subsequent passive sodium reabsorption and water impermeability enable the thick limb to complete two most important functions: generate hypotonic luminal fluid that moves into the distal convoluted tubule, and add osmotically active sodium chloride to the medullary interstitium (21). It must be remembered that the thick ascending limb is a long segment with a medullary and cortical component. The medullary segment is the active force behind the generation of the sodium chloride component of the hypertonic medullary interstitium. The cortical segment, by virtue of its water impermeability and active transport of sodium chloride into an interstitium isosmotic to normal plasma, is the major diluting portion of the nephron (21).

The distal convoluted tubule exhibits active electrogenic sodium reabsorption (28, 29). Potassium secretion in this segment is basically passive and dependent on the transepithelial potential difference, luminal membrane permeability, tubular fluid flow rate and sodium content, intracellular potassium stores, and intracellular pH (28, 30, 35). Although potassium secretion is the usual circumstance in mammalian distal tubules, this segment appears to be capable of active potassium reabsorption under conditions of potassium depletion (36). Although previous micropuncture studies have shown that the distal convoluted tubule has a small amount of net volume reabsorptive capacity (37–39) recent evidence from in vitro microperfusion suggests that this segment is impermeable to water even in the presence of antidiuretic hormone (29). It has been recently shown that the microscopic morphology of surface tubules that have been micropunctured as distal tubules have included segments from both cortical thick ascending limb and cortical collecting duct (40).

Fluid leaves the distal convoluted tubule and enters the collecting duct system including the cortical, medullary, and papillary collecting duct. The collecting duct also exhibits active electrogenic sodium reabsorption (29, 41, 42) that appears to depend on the presence of mineralocorticoid (29). Potassium secretion in this segment appears to be secondary to the same passive driving forces as in the distal convoluted tubule (34, 43) although active secretion has been postulated (41). This segment is impermeable to water in the absence of antidiuretic hormone, but in its presence is the important segment responsible for free water reabsorption and final concentration of the urine (29, 44–46). The papillary portion of the collecting duct is also important with respect to recirculation of urea. It appears to be the only segment distal to the thin ascending limb with any degree of urea permeability (27). Under hydropenia this property enables urea to diffuse out of the papillary duct and into the interstitium and thin ascending limb (27). Urea is thus recirculated and kept in the papillary interstitium where it can exert its osmotic effect.

Although this brief discussion of salt and water transport does not touch upon possible differences between superficial and juxtamedullary nephrons or address itself to the transport characteristics for the other major ions, it serves as a useful foundation for discussion of the renal pharmacology of the various diuretics. However, before discussing diuretics, two important concepts about clearance studies require definition. Free water clearance, or C_{H_2O}, is that solute free water that can be removed from the final urine and leave the remaining urinary solutes isosmotic to plasma. Free water clearance will be positive if final urine is hypoosmotic and negative if it is hyperosmotic to plasma. Since free water is formed in those nephron segments that reabsorb sodium chloride but not water, it can be seen that the medullary and cortical thick ascending limbs and, to a small degree, the distal convoluted tubule are the segments responsible for free water formation or clearance. Free water reabsorption, $T^C_{H_2O}$, is the amount of water that needs to be added to hyperosmotic urine to make the solute concentration isosmotic to plasma. Thus, with urine hyperosmotic to plasma, free water reabsorption is positive and with hypoosmotic urine it is negative. For any given delivery of fluid out of the distal convoluted tubule, the collecting duct, depending on the presence or absence of antidiuretic hormone and the degree of hypertonicity of the medullary interstitium, is responsible for changes in free water reabsorption.

For the purpose of convenience, the diuretic compounds are divided into six groups: (a) osmotic diuretics, (b) carbonic anhydrase inhibitors, (c) organomercurials, (d) sulfonamide diuretics including both thiazide and nonthiazide sulfonamides, (e) high ceiling or loop diuretics, and (f) potassium sparing diuretics. These agents can exert their diuretic effect via several different mechanisms. They can specifically inhibit an active transport process, alter the epithelial permeability to various ions, inhibit energy-producing processes within cells and thus indirectly effect active transport, alter intrarenal hemodynamics and peritubular physical forces, and antagonize the effects of endogenous hormones. Keeping these mechanisms in mind and using the previously outlined model of the nephron and the concepts of free water reabsorption and clearance, we discuss the six groups of diuretic agents.

OSMOTIC DIURETICS

Mannitol is the prototype of the osmotic diuretics. Although previous explanations for its action have centered around a pure osmotic effect in the proximal convoluted tubule (47), it is clear that there are several important mechanisms of action. Mannitol has been found to increase renal plasma flow and glomerular hydrostatic pressure secondary to vasodilatation of the afferent arteriole (48, 49).

There is also suggestive evidence that mannitol affects renin release in hypoperfused kidneys and thus may decrease local angiotensin effects in the afferent arteriole (50–52). Mannitol diuresis also has a profound effect on the composition of the renal medulla. Goldberg & Ramirez (53) found that mannitol diuresis in hydropenic dogs caused a significant decrease in medullary and papillary sodium and urea concentration and an increase in water content of the medulla. Goodman & Levitan (54) have similarly found a decrease in sodium content of the medulla and papilla in osmotic diuresis. Seely & Dirks (55), using micropuncture in dogs, found a significant effect of hypertonic mannitol infusion on net fluid reabsorption in the proximal tubule but an even greater effect in the loop of Henle, which was attributed to both the osmotic effect of mannitol and to the dissipation of the medullary osmotic gradient. In a recent micropuncture study Blantz (56) using the hydropenic rat found an increase in renal plasma flow, an increase in superficial single nephron glomerular filtration rate, an increase in glomerular hydrostatic pressure that was offset by an increase in intratubular pressure of the proximal tubule so that net transglomerular hydrostatic pressure was unchanged, and a significant decrease in afferent arteriolar oncotic pressure. This last effect, a decrease in afferent arteriolar oncotic pressure due to dilution of plasma proteins, appeared to play the largest role in increasing the effective filtration pressure and thus glomerular filtration rate.

It thus appears that mannitol and similar osmotic agents have multiple sites and mechanisms of action; their major component probably is a decrease in medullary solute content resulting in less water reabsorption from the thin descending limb of Henle and collecting duct and less sodium chloride reabsorption in the ascending limb of Henle.

CARBONIC ANHYDRASE INHIBITORS

Acetazolamide is the major representative of this class of diuretics. Inhibition of carbonic anhydrase has been shown to decrease bicarbonate reabsorption in the proximal convoluted tubule (57–59). However, direct proof of an effect on salt and water reabsorption in the proximal tubule was provided by Kunau (60) who demonstrated, via micropuncture in rats, decreased sodium chloride and volume reabsorption with the carbonic anhydrase inhibitor benzolamide. Low doses of this agent did not affect glomerular filtration rate whereas high doses produced a significant decrease (6). A similar effect on sodium and water reabsorption in the proximal tubule of the rat was observed by Radtke et al (61). These investigators also postulated that acetazolamide directly inhibited hydrogen ion secretion when glycodiazine instead of bicarbonate was used as a buffer.

Two major questions about the mechanism of action of the carbonic anhydrase inhibitors have recently been partially answered. Through what mechanisms do carbonic anhydrase inhibitors inhibit the enzyme and how is this translated into the diuretic effect? Several investigators have shown that parathyroid hormone increases renal excretion of bicarbonate, phosphate, sodium, and water (16, 62–64). Rodriguez et al (65) recognized the similarity in urinary excretion patterns of parathyroid hormone and carbonic anhydrase inhibitor administration. These investigators showed that acetazolamide increased the urinary excretion of cAMP in normal and parathyroidectomized rats, and that in vitro acetazolamide stimulated renal cortical adenyl cyclase activity (65). This observation, along with recent studies by Beck et al (66) that demonstrated in vitro inhibition of carbonic anhydrase in rat renal cortex by parathyroid hormone and cAMP, led to the conclusion that carbonic anhydrase inhibitors inhibit the enzyme via the intermediary step of adenyl cyclase stimulation.

With respect to the resultant diuretic effect of these agents, recent evidence from in vitro microperfusion suggests that in addition to the small amount of sodium reabsorption that directly accompanies bicarbonate reabsorption in the proximal convolution, the inhibition of bicarbonate reabsorption might negate the osmotic effect of having an increased peritubular bicarbonate concentration (8) and might prevent the development of a chloride concentration gradient in the later proximal convolution, thus decreasing the passive forces for net reabsorption (7). Although carbonic anhydrase inhibitors have been shown to affect distal tubule and collecting duct hydrogen ion secretion (42, 67) there have been no studies demonstrating a direct distal diuretic effect. Rosin et al (68) have shown in clearance studies on dogs that for a given delivery of salt and water out of the proximal tubule, C_{H_2O} increases less with acetazolamide than hypotonic saline volume expansion. This discrepancy, which may well represent the major diuretic expression of carbonic anhydrase inhibitors, was attributed to the greater amount of nonreabsorbable anion presented to the diluting segment with acetazolamide diuresis. This principle of increased distal delivery of nonreabsorbable anion has recently been reemphasized by Seldin, Rosin & Rector (69). Carbonic anhydrase inhibitors cause a significant kaliuresis, which can be attributed to passive forces in the distal nephron—increased lumen negativity and increased flow rate of luminal fluid (28, 30–35).

In summary, carbonic anhydrase inhibitors decrease bicarbonate reabsorption in the proximal convolution via the intermediate step of adenyl cyclase stimulation. However, they also inhibit net volume reabsorption in the proximal tubule possibly through indirect inhibition of passive forces favoring sodium chloride reabsorption. Their major effect on electrolyte and water excretion may be explained by increased delivery of nonreabsorbable sodium bicarbonate to the cortical thick ascending limb and distal tubule.

ORGANOMERCURIALS

Before the development of the loop diuretics, the organomercurials were the most potent diuretic available. However, investigative efforts aimed at defining their renal pharmacology have not been extensive. Early clearance studies have shown conflicting results partially due to the use of different agents and the presence of theophylline in some of the preparations (70–75). A stop-flow study by Schmitt & Sullivan (76) disclosed a distal site of action on sodium transport. These investigators also found that organomercurials decrease potassium secretion in the chronic potassium-loaded animal and increase secretion in potassium depletion. Giebisch (77) found that mercurials decrease the transepithelial potential difference in the proximal tubule of the necturus. However, the mercurial concentration used was 10^{-3} M which has been shown by Burg & Green to have an irreversible, probably toxic, effect in the thick ascending limb of Henle (78).

More recent studies have consistently found that the major effect of organomercurials appears to be in the ascending limb of Henle and specifically, the thick ascending limb. Initially Berliner, Dirks & Cirksena (79) found no proximal effect of the mercurials. Clapp & Robinson (80) found, utilizing micropuncture in dogs, an increase in early distal tubular fluid osmolality with chlormerodrin diuresis. Evanson, Lockhart & Dirks (81) later confirmed the absence of a proximal effect and the increased delivery of sodium chloride out of the ascending limb to the distal tubule. These investigators also confirmed that chlormerodrin decreased distal tubular potassium secretion in chronic potassium loaded dogs given an acute potassium load. A recent in vitro microperfusion study by Burg & Green (78) has shown that mersalyl inhibits active chloride transport in the cortical thick ascending limb of Henle. These authors found a reversible decrease in net chloride flux and transepithelial potential difference (lumen positive) when the thick limb was perfused with a solution containing mersalyl. In this study p-chloromercuribenzoate, which in vivo antagonizes the diuretic effect of mercurials, reversed the potential difference effect of mersalyl.

Although the site of action of organomercurials is reasonably well established, the mechanism of action has generated some controversy. Early experience suggested that the diuretic effect of organomercurials was in part dependent on intraluminal pH and its effect on either the binding of the intact organomercurial to its receptor, or on making available the free mercuric ion (82–85). However, the recent study of Burg & Green (78) found no difference in the effect of mersalyl from pH 6.0 to 7.4. They also discovered significant differences between the effect of mercuric chloride and mersalyl. The mercuric chloride took longer to have an effect which was then not reversed by p-chloromercuribenzoate. It thus still needs to be established specifically how pH affects the response to organomercurials and whether the diuretic response requires in vivo release of mercuric ion.

Another unresolved controversy with respect to these agents is whether the diuresis is dependent on in vivo inhibition of Na-K-dependent ATPase. Jones, Lockett & Landon (86) found that organomercurials inhibit the activity of Na-K-dependent ATPase in kidney membranes and the ability of the membrane-bound enzyme to stimulate glycolysis in the cytoplasm. Similarly, Tulloch, Gibson & Harris (87) found inhibition of the enzyme by high concentrations of mercaptomerin. However, Nechay et al (88) failed to find a correlation between diuretic effect and Na-K ATPase activity. As discussed subsequently, a similar problem exists with respect to the molecular mechanism of other diuretic agents.

In summary then, the organomercurials inhibit active chloride reabsorption in the thick ascending limb of Henle and under appropriate circumstances inhibit or enhance distal potassium secretion. The molecular basis of this effect and the precise role of pH on the degree of diuretic response are unresolved.

SULFONAMIDE DIURETICS

In contrast to the organomercurials, studies on the sulfonamide diuretics, including the thiazides and nonthiazides such as chlorthalidone and the newer agent metholazone, have generally been in agreement about sites and mechanisms of action.

Early clearance studies in animals showed a decrease in C_{H_2O} with no effect on renal concentrating ability (89–91). Clearance studies in man have found an effect both in the cortical diluting segment (thick ascending limb) and a proximal effect (92–94) based on changes in C_{H_2O}.

Subsequent micropuncture studies have demonstrated both decreased proximal reabsorption and increased osmolality and sodium content of early distal tubular fluid (80, 95–98). To date there have been no published studies on this class of diuretics using in vitro microperfusion.

With respect to mechanism of action, most of the sulfonamide diuretics are capable of inhibiting carbonic anhydrase (99, 100). If one can extrapolate from acetazolamide, then the acute phosphaturia and increased bicarbonate excretion seen with the sulfonamides is probably secondary to their capacity to inhibit carbonic anhydrase. The kaliuresis seen with these agents is most likely a passive phenomenon similar to that discussed previously with the other diuretics. Since it is generally considered that these agents must exert their major action on the cortical thick ascending limb, the sulfonamides must be included with the organomercurials and as we see later, the loop diuretics as inhibitors of active chloride reabsorption in this segment. The specific means by which chloride transport is inhibited is unknown. However, although conclusive studies are lacking, inhibition of Na-K ATPase and inhibition of glycolysis and energy supply for transport have been suggested (87, 101, 102).

In summary, the sulfonamides have as their major site of action the cortical thick ascending limb of Henle where they inhibit active chloride transport. Proximal tubular effects are probably secondary to their ability to inhibit carbonic anhydrase. The kaliuresis seen with these agents is secondary to passive phenomena in the distal nephron. Although beyond the scope of the present review, the major impact of the sulfonamides on decreasing calcium excretion with chronic administration and their utility in diabetes insipidus are well documented (103–109).

LOOP DIURETICS

The "high-ceiling" or loop diuretics currently are the most potent available agents and include furosemide, ethacrynic acid, and two newer agents triflocin and bumetanide. Although differences exist between these agents, they are alike in the most important aspect underlying their potency, in their site of action in the medullary and cortical thick ascending limb of Henle.

Initial clearance studies have shown that these agents decrease C_{H_2O} during water diuresis (ethacrynic acid more so than furosemide) and $T^c_{H_2O}$ during hydropenia (91, 110–113). These two properties would localize their site of action to the medullary and cortical thick ascending limb. However, because of greater phosphate and bicarbonate loss in the urine as well as lesser degrees of inhibition of C_{H_2O}, furosemide and bumetanide are thought to have proximal tubular effects also (113–118).

Although no distal tubule micropuncture studies of ethacrynic acid diuresis have been published, micropuncture studies of its proximal tubular action are available but conflicting. Wilczewski, Olson & Carrasquer (124) as well as Berliner, Dirks & Cirksena (79) have found no effect in rats and dogs, while Clapp, Nottebohm & Robinson (125) and Meng & O'Dea (97) have found a decrease in proximal reabsorption in the same species. A recent micropuncture study of triflocin has confirmed an ascending limb site for its action (126).

As with the organomercurials, in vitro microperfusion of rabbit nephrons has confirmed the principal site of action of both furosemide and ethacrynic acid (25, 127). Burg & Green found no effect of furosemide on proximal convoluted tubules and collecting ducts. However, 10^{-5} M furosemide in the lumen of the thick ascending limb reversibly inhibited the lumen positive potential difference and the active transport of chloride out of the lumen. An identical result was obtained with ethacrynic acid (127), although a higher concentration was required. When an ethacrynic acid cysteine adduct (as occurs in vivo) was used, a much lower concentration was required. In addition to the thick ascending limb effect, ethacrynic acid was found to be an antagonist to vasopressin at the level of the receptor site of the hormone in the isolated perfused rabbit collecting tubule by Abramow (128).

These observations of the effects of furosemide and ethacrynic acid were not without precedent since similar effects on active chloride transport have been found in frog cornea, frog skin, and frog gastric mucosa (129–131).

Although the major site of action of loop diuretics is in the medullary and cortical thick ascending limb via inhibition of active chloride reabsorption, several investigators have attributed significant diurectic effects to the alteration of intrarenal hemodynamics that these agents produce (132–134). In spite of reasonable evidence for redistribution of renal blood flow, it has, as of yet, been difficult to translate these changes directly into the diuresis observed with these agents. However, washout of medullary solute as with the osmotic diurectic may be a factor.

A molecular basis of action of these diuretics has been actively sought. This search has centered about three basic process: (a) inhibition of Na-K ATPase; (b) inhibition or displacement of cAMP; (c) inhibition of glycolysis (87, 135–146). Although the majority of these studies did not find a correlation of diuretic action with Na-K ATPase inhibition (135–139, 143), a definitive answer awaits indentification of what role this enzyme actually plays in baseline salt and water reabsorption. Similarly, although profound degrees of inhibition of glycolysis would be expected to affect transport nonspecifically, the degree of inhibition of glycolysis with these agents does not appear to affect transport (145). With respect to inhibition of cAMP genesis or displacement of cAMP from its receptor, further studies are required before any conclusion can be reached.

In summary, loop diuretics inhibit active chloride transport over the entire length of the thick ascending limb of Henle. Whereas, furosemide, bumetanide, and possibly ethacrynic acid have a proximal effect, the clinical importance of this is probably minimal because of the known capacity of the loop to increase reabsorption as delivery increases. The kaliuresis seen with these agents can again be explained by increased distal delivery of fluid and sodium. Although intrarenal hemodynamic changes occur, and multiple studies suggest possible molecular mechanisms of action, the exact significance of these findings requires further study.

POTASSIUM SPARING DIURETICS

The final family of diuretics to be considered are the potassium sparing agents represented by spironolactone, triamterene, and amiloride. The effects on urinary electrolyte composition with these agents are similar in that they cause a mild natriuresis and decrease potassium and hydrogen ion excretion (147–153). In spite of this similarity, these agents actually compose two groups with respect to mechanism of action.

Spironolactone has been adequately shown to be a specific competitive inhibitor of aldosterone at the receptor site level and to have an effect only when aldosterone is present (148, 154–156). Aldosterone has been shown to bind initially to a specific receptor protein in the cytoplasm (157–159). The aldosterone antagonists have been shown to inhibit competitively the initial binding step (160–161). The other two potassium sparing diuretics, triamterene and amiloride, exert their effect independent of the presence or absence of mineralocorticoid (147, 149, 162).

Recently Gross, Imai & Kokko (29) using in vitro microperfusion have localized the site of action of aldosterone to the collecting duct. These investigators have found that the lumen negative potential difference in the cortical collecting duct is dependent on mineralocorticoid activity while the negative potential difference in the distal convoluted tubule appears to be independent of mineralocorticoid. They have also shown that triamterene, on the peritubular side, inhibits the potential in the collecting duct and not the distal tubule while amiloride in the lumen inhibits the potential in both segments (163). Another in vitro microperfusion study of the cortical collecting tubule (41) shows that amiloride significantly decreased the net sodium reabsorption and potential difference as well as the secretion of potassium. These investigators found no effect of amiloride on the lumen positive potential or active chloride transport in the thick ascending limb. The collecting duct thus appears to be the principal site of action of the aldosterone agonists and antagonists as well as of triamterene. Amiloride, however, in addition to its collecting duct site, appears to have an effect in the distal convoluted tubule as shown by Gross & Kokko (163) and a previous micropuncture study (122). In addition, two recent micropuncture studies have shown that amiloride decreases sodium transport in the proximal tubule (124, 164). Although the clinical significance of this finding is probably not significant because of the previously discussed capacity of more distal sites to reabsorb proximally rejected sodium, both of these studies provided insight into the probable mechanism of action of amiloride—alteration of the luminal membrane permeability to sodium. Previous studies on toad bladder and frog skin have suggested that amiloride decreases cell membrane permeability to sodium and thus decreases the amount of sodium available to any active sodium pump (165, 166).

With respect to the decreased potassium and hydrogen secretion seen with these agents, their ability to decrease the negativity of the lumen negative potential difference would decrease the passive force influencing potassium and hydrogen secretion. However, a direct effect on possible active potassium and hydrogen secretion is conceivable but has not been directly examined.

To summarize this last group of diuretic agents, the potassium sparing diuretics are only moderately potent and cause similar electrolyte excretion patterns whether or not they antagonize endogenous mineralocorticoids. Their site of action is in the collecting duct with the exception of amiloride, which decreases sodium reabsorption in the proximal and distal convoluted tubules. Their effect on potassium and hydrogen secretion is, as with the majority of the previously discussed diuretics, basically due to alteration of passive forces controlling the movement of these ions.

ACKNOWLEDGMENTS

This work was supported in part by NIH Program Project Grant 1 P01 HL 11662 and NIH Research Grant 1 R01 AM 14677.

Literature Cited

1. Kokko, J. P. 1973. *J. Clin. Invest.* 52:1362–67
2. Gottschalk, C. W., Lassiter, W. E., Mylle, M. 1960. *Am. J. Physiol.* 198:581–85
3. Rector, F. C. Jr., Carter, N. W., Seldin, D. W. 1965. *J. Clin. Invest.* 44:278–90
4. Kokko, J. P., Rector, F. C. Jr., Seldin, D. W. 1970. *Am. Soc. Nephol.* 4:42 (Abstr.)
5. Walser, M., Mudge, G. H. 1960. *Renal Excreting Mechanisms in Mineral Metabolism*, ed. C. L. Comar, F. Bronner, p. 288. New York: Academic
6. Rector, F. C. Jr., Seldin, D. W., Roberts, A. D. Jr., Smith, J. S. 1960. *J. Clin. Invest.* 39:1706–21
7. Kokko, J. P. 1976. *Renal Pathophysiology*, ed. M. Martinez-Maldonado, N. Kurtzman. Springfield, Ill.: Thomas
8. Hierholzer, K., Kawamura, S., Kokko, J. P. 1976. Submitted for publication
9. Bank, N., Aynedjian, H. S., Weinstein, S. W. 1974. *J. Clin. Invest.* 54:1040–48
10. Strickler, J. C., Thompson, D. D., Klose, R. M., Giebisch, G. 1964. *J. Clin. Invest.* 43:1596–1607
11. Amiel, C., Kuntziger, H., Richet, G. 1970 *Pfluegers Arch.* 317:92–109
12. Agus, Z. S., Puschett, J. B., Senesky, D., Goldberg, M. 1971. *J. Clin. Invest.* 50:617–26
13. Staum, B. B., Hamburger, R. J., Goldberg, M. 1972. *J. Clin. Invest.* 51: 2271–76
14. Frick, A. 1972. *Am. J. Physiol.* 223: 1034–40
15. Kuntziger, H., Amiel, C., Gaudebout, C. 1972. *Kidney Int.* 2:318–23
16. Agus, Z. S., Gardner, L. B., Beck, L. H., Goldberg, M. 1973. *Am. J. Physiol.* 224:1143–48
17. Beck, L. H., Goldberg, M. 1972. *Am. J. Physiol.* 224:1136–42
18. Wen, S. F. 1974. *J. Clin. Invest.* 53:143–53
19. Kawamura, S., Imai, M., Seldin, D. W., Kokko, J. P. 1975. *J. Clin. Invest.* 1269–77
20. Kokko, J. P. 1970. *J. Clin. Invest.* 1838–46
21. Kokko, J. P., Rector, F. C. Jr. 1972. *Kidney Int.* 2:214–23
22. Imai, M., Kokko, J. P. 1974. *J. Clin. Invest.* 53:393–402
23. Jamison, R. L., Bennett, C. M., Berliner, R. W. 1967. *Am. J. Physiol.* 212:357–66
24. Marsh, D. J., Azen, S. P. 1975. *Am. J. Physiol.* 228:71–79
25. Burg, M., Stoner, L., Cardinal, J. Green, N. 1973. *Am. J. Physiol.* 225:119–24
26. Rocha, A. S., Kokko, J. P. 1973. *J. Clin. Invest.* 52:612–23
27. Rocha, A. S., Kokko, J. P. 1974. *Kidney Int.* 6:379–87
28. Malnic, G., Klose, R. M., Giebisch, G. 1966. *Am. J. Physiol.* 211:529–47
29. Gross, J. B., Imai, M., Kokko, J. P. 1975. *J. Clin. Invest.* 55:1284–94
30. Khuri, R. N., Weiderholt, M., Strieder, N., Giebisch, G. 1975. *Am. J. Physiol.* 228:1249–61
31. Kunau, R. 1973. *Am. Soc. Nephrol.* 6:62 (Abstr.)
32. Giebisch, G., Malnic, G., Klose, R. M., Windhager, E. E. 1966. *Am. J. Physiol.* 211:560–68
33. Hierholzer, K., Wiederholt, M., Holzgreve, H., Giebisch, G., Klose, R. M., Windhager, E. E. 1965. *Arch. Ges. Physiol.* 285:193–210
34. Bank, N., Aynedjian, H. S. 1973. *J. Clin. Invest.* 52:1480–90
35. Wright, F. S. 1971. *Am. J. Physiol.* 220:624–38
36. Klose, R. M., Giebisch, G. 1964. *Am. J. Physiol.* 206:674–86

37. Gertz, K. H. 1963. *Arch. Ges. Physiol.* 276:336–56
38. Hayslett, J. P., Kashgarian, M., Epstein, F. H. 1967. *J. Clin. Invest.* 46:1254–63
39. Hierholzer, K. M., Wiederholt, M., Stolte, H. 1966. *Arch. Ges. Physiol.* 291:43–63
40. Woodhall, P. B., Tisher, C. C. 1973. *J. Clin. Invest.* 52:3095–3108
41. Grantham, J. J., Burg, M. B., Orloff, J. 1970. *J. Clin. Invest.* 49:1815–26
42. Stoner, L. C., Burg, M. B., Orloff, J. 1974. *Am. J. Physiol.* 227:453–59
43. Hierholzer, K. 1961. *Am. J. Physiol.* 201:318–24
44. Schafer, J. A., Andreoli, T. E. 1972. *J. Clin. Invest.* 51:1264–78
45. Grantham, J. J., Orloff, J. 1968. *J. Clin. Invest.* 47:1154–61
46. Grantham, J. J., Burg, M. B. 1966. *Am. J. Physiol.* 211:255–59
47. Wesson, L. G., Anslow, W. P. 1948. *Am. J. Physiol.* 153:465–74
48. Goldberg, A. H., Lillienfield, L. S. 1965. *Proc. Soc. Exp. Biol. Med.* 119:635–42
49. Flores, J., DiBona, D. R., Beck, C. H., Leaf, A. 1972. *J. Clin. Invest.* 51:118–26
50. Morris, C. R., Alexander, E. A., Burns, F. J., Levinsky, M. G. 1972. *J. Clin. Invest.* 51:1555–64
51. Vander, A. J., Miller, R. 1964. *Am. J. Physiol.* 207:537–46
52. Fojas, J. E., Schmid, H. E. 1970. *Am. J. Physiol.* 219:464–68
53. Goldberg, M., Ramirez, M. A. 1967. *Clin. Sci.* 32:475–93
54. Goodman, A., Levitan, H. 1964. *Yale J. Biol. Med.* 36:306–7
55. Seely, J. F., Dirks, J. H. 1969. *J. Clin. Invest.* 48:2330–40
56. Blantz, R. C. 1974. *J. Clin. Invest.* 54:1135–43
57. Clapp, J. R., Watson, J. F., Berliner, R. W. 1963. *Am. J. Physiol.* 205:693–96
58. Bernstein, B. A., Clapp, J. R. 1968. *Am. J. Physiol.* 214:251–57
59. Rector, J. C. Jr., Carter, N., Seldin, D. W. 1965. *J. Clin. Invest.* 44:278–90
60. Kunau, R. T. Jr. 1972. *J. Clin. Invest.* 51:294–306
61. Radtke, H. W., Rumrich, G., Kinne-Saffran, E., Ullrich, K. J. 1972. *Kidney Int.* 1:100–105
62. Hellman, D. E., Au, W. Y. W., Bartter, F. C. 1965. *Am. J. Physiol.* 209:643–50
63. Ellsworth, R., Nicholson, W. M. 1935. *J. Clin. Invest.* 14:823–27
64. Agus, Z. S., Puschett, J. B., Senesky, D.,

Goldberg, M. 1971. *J. Clin. Invest.* 50:617–26
65. Rodriguez, H. J., Wallss, J., Yates, J., Klahr, S. 1974. *J. Clin. Invest.* 53:122–30
66. Beck, N., Kim, K. S., Wolak, M., Davis, B. B. 1975. *J. Clin. Invest.* 55:149–56
67. Weinstein, S. W. 1968. *Am. J. Physiol.* 214:222–27
68. Rosin, J. M., Katz, M. A., Rector, F. C. Jr., Seldin, D. W. 1970. *Am. J. Physiol.* 219:1731–38
69. Seldin, D. W., Rosin, J. M., Rector, F. C. Jr. *Yale J. Biol. Med.* 48:337–47
70. Levitt, M. F. 1966. *Ann. NY Acad. Sci.* 139:375–87
71. Goldstein, M. H., Levitt, M. F., Hauser, A. D., Polemeios, D. 1961. *J. Clin. Invest.* 40:731–42
72. Dale, R. A., Sanderson, P. H. 1954. *J. Clin. Invest.* 33:1008–14
73. Grossman, J., Weston, R. E., Borun, E. R., Leiter, L. 1955. *J. Clin. Invest.* 34:1611–24
74. Lambie, A. T., Robson, J. S. 1961. *Clin. Sci.* 20:123–29
75. Kessler, R. H., Hierholzer, K., Gurd, R. S., Pitts, R. F. 1958. *Am. J. Physiol.* 194:540–46
76. Schmitt, R. W., Sullivan, L. P. 1966. *J. Pharmacol. Exp. Ther.* 151:180–88
77. Giebisch, G. 1958. *J. Cell. Comp. Physiol.* 51:221–39
78. Burg, M., Green, N. 1973. *Kidney Int.* 4:245–51
79. Berliner, R. W., Dirks, J. H., Cirksena, W. J. 1966. *Ann. NY Acad. Sci.* 139:424–32
80. Clapp, J. R., Robinson, R. R. 1968. *Am. J. Physiol.* 215:228–35
81. Evanson, R. L., Lockhart, E. A., Dirks, J. H. 1972. *Am. J. Physiol.* 222:282–89
82. Levy, R. I., Weiner, I. M., Mudge, G. H. 1958. *J. Clin. Invest.* 37:1016–23
83. Kessler, R. H., Lozano, R., Pitts, R. F. 1957. *J. Clin. Invest.* 36:656–68
84. Mudge, G. H., Weiner, I. M. 1958. *Ann. NY Acad. Sci.* 71:344–54
85. Weiner, I. M., Levy, R. I., Mudge, G. H. 1962. *J. Pharmacol. Exp. Ther.* 138:96–112
86. Jones, V. D., Lockett, G., Landon, E. J. 1965. *J. Pharmacol. Exp. Ther.* 147:23–31
87. Tulloch, B. R., Gibson, K., Harris, P. 1971. *Clin. Sci.* 40:4p–5p (Abstr.)
88. Nechay, B. R., Palmer, R. F., Chinoy, D. A., Posey, V. A. 1967. *J. Pharmacol. Exp. Ther.* 157:599–617

89. Earley, L. E., Kahn, M., Orloff, J. 1961. *J. Clin. Invest.* 40:857–66
90. Au, W. Y. W., Raisz, L. G. 1960. *J. Clin. Invest.* 39:1302–11
91. Suki, W., Rector, F. C. Jr., Seldin, D. W. 1965. *J. Clin. Invest.* 44:1458–69
92. Heinemann, H. O., Demartini, F. E., Laragh, J. H. 1959. *Am. J. Med.* 26: 853–61
93. Buckalew, V. M. Jr., Walker, B. R., Puschett, J. B., Goldberg, M. 1970. *J. Clin. Invest.* 49:2336–44
94. Materson, B. J. et al 1972. *Curr. Ther. Res.* 14:545–560
95. Fernandez, P. D., Puschett, J. B. 1973. *Am. J. Physiol.* 225:954–61
96. Ullrich, K. J. et al 1966. *Ann. NY Acad. Sci.* 139:416–23
97. Meng, K., O'Dea, K. 1973. *Pharmacology* 9:193–200
98. Holzgreve, H. 1968. *Renal Transport Diuretic Int. Symp.*, pp. 229–34. Berlin, Geidelberg & New York: Springer
99. Beyer, K. H. 1958. *Ann. NY Acad. Sci.* 71:363–79
100. Maren, T. H. 1967. *Physiol. Rev.* 47:597–781
101. Janata, V., Lege, K. 1972. *Int. J. Clin. Pharmacol.* 6:125–29
102. Janata, V., Lege, K. 1972. *Int. J. Clin. Pharmacol.* 6:214–17
103. Costanzo, L. S., Weiner, I. M. 1974. *J. Clin. Invest.* 54:628–37
104. Edwards, B. R., Baer, P. G., Sulton, R. A. L., Dirks, J. H. 1973. *J. Clin. Invest.* 52:2418–27
105. Suki, W. N., Hull, A. R., Rector, F. C. Jr., Seldin, D. W. 1967. *J. Clin. Invest.* 46:1121 (Abstr.)
106. Earley, L. E., Orloff, J. 1962. *J. Clin. Invest.* 41:1988–97
107. Kennedy, G. C., Crawford, J. D. 1959. *Lancet* 1:866–67
108. Lant, A. F., Wilson, G. M. 1971. *Clin. Sci.* 40:497–511
109. Robson, J. S., Lambri, A. T. 1962. *Metabolism* 11:1041–53
110. Goldberg, M., McCurdy, D. K., Foltz, E. L., Bluemle, L. W. Jr. 1964. *J. Clin. Invest.* 43:201–16
111. Seldin, D. W., Eknoyan, G., Suki, W. N., Rector, F. C. Jr. 1966. *Ann. NY Acad. Sci.* 139:328–43
112. Karlander, S. G., Henning, R., Lundvall, O. 1973. *Eur. J. Clin. Pharmacol.* 6:220–23
113. Puschett, J. B., Goldberg, M. 1968. *J. Lab. Clin. Med.* 71:666–77
114. Duarte, C. G. 1974. *Clin. Sci. Mol. Med.* 46:671–78
115. Alguire, P. C., Barlio, M. D., Weaver, W. J., Taylor, D. G., Hook, J. B. 1974. *J. Pharmacol. Exp. Ther.* 190:515–22
116. LeZotte, L. A., MacGaffey, K. M., Moore, E. W., Jick, H. 1966. *Clin. Sci.* 31:371–82
117. Eknoyan, G., Suki, W. N., Martinez-Maldonado, M. 1970. *J. Lab. Clin. Med.* 76:257–66
118. Davies, D. L. et al 1973. *Clin. Pharmacol. Ther.* 15:141–55
119. Knox, F. G., Wright, F. S., Howards, S. S., Berliner, R. W. 1969. *Am. J. Physiol.* 217:192–98
120. Burkee, T. J., Robinson, R. R., Clapp, J. R. 1972. *Kidney Int.* 1:12–18
121. Morgan, T., Tadokov, M., Martin, D., Berliner, R. W. 1970. *Am. J. Physiol.* 218:292–97
122. Duarte, C. G., Chamety, F., Giebisch, G. 1971. *Am. J. Physiol.* 221:632–40
123. Morgan, T. O. 1974. *Prog. Biochem. Pharmacol.* 9:13–20
124. Wilczewski, T. W., Olson, A. K., Carrasquer, G. 1974. *Proc. Soc. Exp. Biol. Med.* 145:1301–05
125. Clapp, J. R., Nottebohm, G. A., Robinson, R. R. 1971. *Am. J. Physiol.* 220:1355–60
126. Kauker, M. L. 1973. *J. Pharmacol. Exp. Ther.* 184:472–80
127. Burg, M., Green, N. 1973. *Kidney Int.* 4:301–8
128. Abramow, M. 1974. *J. Clin. Invest.* 53:796–804
129. Dinno, M. A., Schwartz, M., Olson, A. K., Carrasquer, G. 1974. *Can. J. Pharmacol.* 52:166–73
130. Lote, C. J. 1974. *J. Physiol.* 241:27P–28P (Abstr.)
131. Candia, O. A. 1973. *Biochim. Biophys. Acta* 298:1011–14
132. Epstein, M. et al 1971. *Am. J. Physiol.* 220:482–87
133. Stowe, N. T., Wolterink, L. F., Lewis, A. E., Hook, J. B. 1973. *Arch. Pharmacol.* 277:13–26
134. Birtch, A. G., Zakheim, R. M., James, L. G., Barger, A. C. 1967. *Circ. Res.* 21:869–79
135. Martinez-Maldonado, M., Tsaparas, N. T., Inagaki, C., Schwartz, A. 1974. *J. Pharmacol. Exp. Ther.* 188:605–14
136. Landon, E. J., Fitz, D. F. 1972. *Biochem. Pharmacol.* 21:1561–68
137. Williamson, H. E. 1969. *Proc. 4th Int. Congr. of Nephrol. Stockholm* 2:144–52
138. Ebel, H., Ehrich, J., DeSanto, N. G. Doerken, U. 1972. *Pfluegers Arch. Eur. J. Physiol.* 335:224–34

214   JACOBSON & KOKKO

139. Inagaki, C., Martinez-Maldonado, M., Schwartz, A. 1973. *Arch. Biochem. Biophys.* 158:421–34
140. Nechay, B. R., Contreras, R. R. 1972. *J. Pharmacol. Exp. Ther.* 183:127–36
141. Ferguson, D. R., Twite, B. R. 1973. *Br. J. Pharmacol.* 49:288–92
142. Ferguson, D. R., Twite, B. R. 1974. *Arch. Pharmacol.* 281:295–300
143. Ebel, H. 1974. *Arch. Pharmacol.* 281:307–14
144. Barnes, L. D., Hui, Y. S. F., Dousa, T. P. 1975. *Life Sci.* 16:255–62
145. Bowman, R. H., Dolgin, J., Coulson, R. 1973. *Am. J. Physiol.* 224:416–24
146. Epstein, R. W. 1972. *Biochim. Biophys. Acta* 274:128–39
147. Kagawa, C. M. 1960. *Endocrinology* 67:125–32
148. Liddle, G. W. 1957. *Science* 126:1016–18
149. Baba, W. I., Tudhope, G. R., Wilson, G. M. *Br. Med. J.* 1962. 2:756–64
150. Baba, W. I., Lant, A. F., Smith, A. J., Townshend, M. M., Wilson, G. M. 1968. *Clin. Pharmacol. Ther.* 9:318–27
151. Wiebelhaus, V. D. et al 1965. *J. Pharmacol. Exp. Ther.* 149:397–403
152. Guignard, J. P., Peters, G. 1970. *Eur. J. Pharmacol.* 10:255–67

153. Crosley, A. P. et al 1962. *Ann. Int. Med.* 56:241–51
154. Liddle, G. W. 1966. *Ann. NY Acad. Sci.* 139:466–70
155. Kagawa, C. M., Cella, J. A., van Arman, C. G. 1957. *Science* 126:1015–16
156. Liddle, G. W. 1961. *Metabolism* 10:1021–30
157. Edelman, I. S. 1972. *J. Steroid Biochem.* 3:167–72
158. Funder, J. W., Feldman, D., Edelman, I. S. 1972. *J. Steroid Biochem.* 3:209–18
159. Feldman, D., Funder, J. W., Edelman, I. S. 1972. *Am. J. Med.* 53:545–60
160. Henson, T. S., Fimognari, G. M., Edelman, I. S. 1968. *J. Biol. Chem.* 243:3849–56
161. Forte, L. R. 1972. *Life Sci.* 11:461–73
162. Bull, M., Laragh, J. H. 1968. *Circulation* 37:45–53
163. Gross, J. B., Kokko, J. P. 1975. *Clin. Res.* 23:363A (Abstr.)
164. Carrasquer, G., Fravert, D. G., Olson, A. K. 1974. *Proc. Soc. Exp. Biol. Med.* 146:478–80
165. Salako, L. A., Smith, A. J. 1969. *J. Physiol.* 206:37P–38P (Abstr.)
166. Gatzy, J. T. 1971. *J. Pharmacol. Exp. Ther.* 176:580–94

USE OF DRUGS IN MYOPATHIES

❖6647

David Grob
Department of Medicine, Maimonides Medical Center, Brooklyn, New York 11219 and
Department of Medicine, State University of New York, Downstate Medical Center,
Brooklyn, New York 11203

The most important recent advances in understanding and managing myopathies have occurred in relation to diseases associated with alterations in the immune mechanism: polymyositis and myasthenia gravis. Some progress has also been made in the management of diseases associated with abnormal movement of potassium ions, and in understanding the effects of neuromuscular blocking drugs. Unfortunately, there has been less progress in understanding or managing the muscular dystrophies.

DISEASES OF MUSCLE ASSOCIATED WITH ALTERATIONS IN THE IMMUNE MECHANISM

Polymyositis and Dermatomyositis

DIAGNOSIS *Polymyositis* is an inflammatory myopathy of unknown cause, to which the term *dermatomyositis* is applied when a skin rash is present. These disorders constitute the commonest myopathy of adults, and in children are second in frequency to muscular dystrophy. They are characterized by symmetrical weakness of the limb-girdle muscles and neck flexors, progressing over weeks to months; muscle-biopsy evidence of necrosis of type I and II fibers, diffuse atrophy, and a mononuclear inflammatory exudate, often perivascular; elevation in serum of skeletal muscle enzymes, particularly creatine phosphokinase (CPK); polyphasic motor unit potentials of reduced amplitude and duration; and often heliotrope discoloration and edema of the eyelids and face, and erythematous dermatitis over the dorsum of the hands, knees, elbows, face, neck, and upper trunk (1, 2). Occasionally, the diagnosis may be made in the absence of elevated muscle enzymes in serum or of electromyographic changes, and more than one muscle biopsy may have to be obtained. Some patients have features of one or more of the connective tissue disorders, including scleroderma, systemic lupus erythematosus, rheumatoid arthri-

215

tis, polyarteritis, and Sjögren's syndrome. Approximately 15% of adult patients have or develop a neoplasm. In these patients, the polymyositis tends to be more resistant to therapy.

PATHOGENESIS   There is some evidence that a cellular immune mechanism may be responsible for the muscle injury that characterizes the disease. In guinea pigs repeated injection of heterologous muscle homogenates in Freund's complete adjuvant produces myositis with lymphocytic infiltrates (3). Lymphocytes from patients with active polymyositis produce cytotoxic effects on human fetal muscle-cell cultures by releasing a mediator of delayed hypersensitivity, lymphotoxin (4). Lymphocytes of patients receiving high-dosage prednisone or azathioprine show little cytotoxicity (5). The nature of the hypothetical antigen involved in the postulated cellular immune response is unknown. A role for humoral antibodies has not been established, although deposition of IgG, IgM, and C3 in muscle-vessel walls has been reported (6). In a few patients polymyositis has followed viral infection due to influenza, herpes zoster, rubella, Coxsackie virus, and cytoplasmic inclusion bodies resembling viral particles have been found in some (7). Polymyositis also occurs in trichinosis, which in the acute stage is invariably accompanied by eosinophilia and which can then be treated with corticosteroid and thiabendazole (Mintezol®) (25 mg/kg orally twice daily), and in toxoplasmosis, which can be treated with sulfadiazine (1 g orally four times a day) and pyrimethamine (Daraprine®) (50 mg orally daily for 2 weeks and then 25 mg daily for 2 weeks) (8). Pyrimethamine is a folic acid antagonist that may produce leukopenia and thrombocytopenia, so that blood counts should be obtained twice weekly and folinic acid (leucovorin), 6 mg orally three times a day, administered simultaneously.

TREATMENT   *Corticosteroids* are generally considered beneficial in most patients with polymyositis or dermatomyositis, particularly during the acute stage and during exacerbations of the disease (2, 9). In the absence of any controlled study, their long-range effect on the course of the disease is impossible to document. Most (2), but not all (10), studies have indicated a favorable effect. Prolonged administration of relatively high doses of corticosteroid is usually required before muscle strength improves (9). The initial dose should be from 80 to 120 mg of prednisone, or its equivalent, daily by mouth, although occasionally higher doses may be necessary. In patients who are more severely ill, it is preferable to administer this in divided daily doses, but in patients who are only moderately ill a single morning dose or every-other-morning dose may be tried, in an effort to reduce the severity of steroid side effects and suppression of adrenal cortical function. After one to four weeks of corticosteroid administration, the level of serum enzymes derived from muscle, particularly CPK, will begin to fall and will gradually decline over a period of months. The enzymes usually begin to decrease three to four weeks before improvement in muscle strength begins, and the improvement may not be manifest until high doses of corticosteroid have been administered for one to two months. The dose of steroid should not be reduced until there is good evidence of improvement, as indicated by increased muscle strength, decreased muscle tenderness, decreased serum enzymes derived from muscle, and decreased creatinuria (11). When improvement is manifest, the dose of steroid should be reduced by about 10% every one to two weeks. Too rapid reduction in steroid dose may result in clinical relapse, which usually necessitates an increase in dose. A rise in the level of serum enzymes derived from muscle, or in creatinuria, usually precedes clinical relapse by three to six weeks and may be a helpful sign. Unfortunately, there is not always a good correlation between these laboratory tests and the clinical condition of the patient, which is a more important guide to management (12). Occasionally, the serum enzymes are within normal range despite active myositis, particularly when muscle atrophy is extensive in long-standing disease. If the disease goes into remission, it may be possible to discontinue steroid, but if not, steroid administration is continued at the lowest dose that suppresses active manifestations. Since most patients require long-term administration of steroid, it is necessary that precautions be taken to observe for and attempt to prevent complications of steroid therapy, including steroid myopathy. Decrease in strength accompanied by a rise in serum enzymes derived from muscle is usually due to exacerbation of the disease and warrants an increase in steroid dose. In patients who are receiving high doses of steroid for prolonged periods, decrease in strength without a rise in serum enzymes may be due to steroid myopathy. Unfortunately, there is no laboratory test for steroid myopathy, which can be diagnosed only if reduction in dose of steroid, or gradual discontinuation, is followed by improvement in strength.

The other synthetic analogs of cortisol have no advantage over prednisone in the management of polymyositis, although they differ in potency and duration of action. One mg of cortisol (biologic half-life 8 to 12 hr) has the same anti-inflammatory potency as 0.25 mg prednisolone, methylprednisolone, or triamcinolone (half-life 12 to 36 hr), 0.1 mg paramethasone, or 0.04 mg betamethasone or dexamethasone (half-life 36 to 54 hr) (13). The mechanism of the anti-inflammatory, anti-allergic, and anti-immunologic actions of the corticosteroids is not known. They inhibit the inflammatory reaction to nearly any type of injury by blocking increased permeability of cell membranes, including capillary endothelium, and of lysosomal membranes. They exert a suppressive effect at each stage of the immune response, including phagocytosis of antigens, migration of cells to areas of inflammation, metabolism of lymphocytes, and cell-mediated hypersensitivity reactions. Thymus-derived (T) lymphocytes, which are required for cell-mediated immunity, are more susceptible to the effects of corticosteroids than the bursa-derived (B) lymphocytes that elaborate humoral antibody. Hence humoral antibody production is rarely reduced significantly, except with very large doses of corticosteroids, whereas cell-mediated immunity is modified at lower corticosteroid concentration (13).

The complications of corticosteroid therapy vary with the dose, anti-inflammatory potency, and duration of administration of corticosteroid. The more serious effects include peptic ulceration (often gastric), osteoporosis with vertebral compression fractures and aseptic necrosis of bone, glaucoma and posterior subcapsular cataracts, cerebral edema, and superimposition of bacterial, fungus, and viral infections. Less serious effects include myopathy, psychiatric disorders, edema, elevation of blood pressure, hypokalemic alkalosis, hyperlipidemia, centripetal obesity,

growth retardation, impaired wound healing, acne, and suppression of the hypo-
thalamic-pituitary-adrenal system. Most of these effects appear to be reduced when
corticosteroid can be administered on alternate days (13). Steroid myopathy is more
likely to occur following fluorinated steroid and prolonged physical inactivity. Cerebral edema (pseudotumor cerebri) is seen mainly in children undergoing withdrawal
from corticosteroid treatment, and is manifested by headache, nausea, vomiting,
drowsiness, stupor, convulsions, papilledema, and increased intracranial pressure
(14). It requires restoring corticosteroid dosage, and then attempting more gradual
reduction. Acute adrenocortical insufficiency may occur during or after withdrawal
from corticosteroid treatment in the event of physiologic stress, and requires immediate parenteral administration of hydrocortisone and saline.

Immunosuppressant therapy is employed in patients whose strength does not
improve following the administration of at least 60 mg prednisone daily for at least
two to four months, and in patients who are unable to tolerate the large doses of
steroid that may be required to suppress the disease (15). In the latter, it is usually
possible to reduce the dose of steroid if supplemented by immunosuppressive medication. Methotrexate (Amethopterin®), a folic acid antagonist, has been used most
(15, 16). In a group of patients who failed to respond to prednisone, intravenous
weekly injections of methotrexate normalized serum CPK in 77% of the group in
a mean of 10 weeks, and improved strength in a mean of 13 weeks (16). The initial
dose was 10 to 15 mg, which was increased if well tolerated to 0.5 to 0.8 mg/kg
(30–50 mg) at weekly intervals. After several weeks, methotrexate administration
was decreased to biweekly, triweekly, or monthly intervals. It is necessary to perform preinjection blood counts and serum alkaline phosphatase activity, and to
check for the occurrence of stomatitis, sore throat, skin rash, purpura, fever, or
gastrointestinal complaints. Although the reported beneficial effects of methotrexate
in polymyositis have been with weekly intravenous administration, weekly, or semi-
weekly intramuscular or oral administration may also prove to be effective (15).
Other immunosuppressive drugs that have been employed with variable success
include azathioprine (17), cyclophosphamide, 6-mercaptopurine, and chlorambucil
(15, 16). Thoracic duct drainage of lymph to remove lymphocytes has also been
employed, but without benefit (16).

Azathioprine (Imuran®) is inactive until it is converted, primarily in the liver, into
its active metabolite, 6-mercaptopurine, a purine analog that inhibits purine synthesis and disrupts both RNA and DNA function. It is administered orally in dosages
of 2 to 3 mg per kg daily. Toxic effects requiring decrease in dose or discontinuation
include leukopenia, granulocytopenia, pancytopenia, gastrointestinal distress, and
superimposed infection. Patients should have weekly blood counts for the first four
weeks and at least every two or three weeks thereafter. Since azathioprine and
6-mercaptopurine are metabolized by xanthine oxidase, the dosage of azathioprine,
and perhaps of other cytotoxic drugs as well, should be decreased by one half to two
thirds in patients receiving the xanthine oxidase inhibitor, allopurinol (18).

Cyclophosphamide (Cytoxan®) is converted by the liver into several alkylating
agents that bind guanine nucleotides on the DNA helix and have cytotoxic effects,
including on T and B lymphocytes. The initial oral dose is 50 mg daily. If after four

weeks there have been no therapeutic or toxic effects, the dose is increased to 100 mg daily, and if no effects after another four weeks, to 150 mg daily. Complete blood counts are obtained weekly, and the drug is withheld when the white blood count falls below 2500 per mm^3. Other toxic effects include nausea, vomiting, diarrhea, reversible hair loss, thrombocytopenia, hemorrhagic cystitis, and amenorrhea or azoospermia (19).

Antilymphocyte and antithymocyte globulins have been used as immunosuppressive agents on an experimental basis, but their clinical application is not yet clear (20, 21).

Levamisole, an antihelminth that has been found to stimulate the immune response and to restore impaired cutaneous hypersensitivity, is receiving clinical trial in some diseases associated with abnormal immune response, including rheumatoid arthritis (22).

Drug-Induced Polymyositis

Weakness, elevation of serum enzymes derived from muscle, including CPK, and histologic changes in muscle, resembling those of polymyositis, have been reported following the administration of clofibrate (Atromid-S®) (23) or penicillamine (Cupramine®) (24), and in severe alcoholism (25). Administration of penicillamine has also been reported to be followed by a lupus-like syndrome (26), glomerulonephritis, and myasthenia gravis (27). Penicillamine has been reported either to accelerate or suppress the antibody response to serum albumin, depending on the timing of the doses (28), and it has been suggested that the drug may affect the immune mechanism by acting as, or forming a haptene.

Myasthenia Gravis

DIAGNOSIS   Myasthenia gravis is a chronic disease characterized by weakness and abnormal fatigability of skeletal muscle. The muscles innervated by the cranial nerves are particularly affected, and usually those of the neck, trunk, and extremities. In severe cases, weakness of the muscles of respiration occurs. Smooth and cardiac muscles are not involved. The disease usually becomes generalized, but in a minority of cases it remains localized to the extraocular muscles. The weakness is due to deficient action of the transmitter (acetylcholine) on the motor end-plates of involved muscles, probably owing to a competitive (acetylcholine-inhibitory) block, similar to that produced by *d*-tubocurarine in normal subjects (29). The weakness is usually ameliorated, although to a variable degree, by anticholinesterase compounds, which enhance the action of transmitter by inhibiting muscle cholinesterase. This response serves as the basis for diagnosis and management of the disease (30).

PATHOGENESIS   There is increasing evidence that myasthenia gravis is associated with alterations in the immune mechanism. The IgG fraction of the serum of 19 to 68% of patients binds with complement, cross striations of skeletal muscle, saline extract and ribonucleoprotein of skeletal muscle, cytoplasm of thymic epithelial cells, thyroglobulin, and nuclei of various cells (31). In 50% of myasthenic patients the thymus is hyperplastic, in 75% it contains numerous germinal centers, and in 15% there is a thymoma. The number of binding sites for acetylcholine in biopsied nerve-muscle junctions is reported to be decreased (32). Serum globulins from one third of patients competed with α-bungarotoxin for the acetylcholine binding sites on rat muscle acetylcholine receptor protein (33). The sera of 72 of 74 patients were found to contain antibody to human acetylcholine receptor protein (34). Immunization of guinea pigs with subcellular fractions of calf thymus and skeletal muscle homogenates produced thymitis and a partial neuromuscular block (35). Immunization of rats, guinea pigs, or rabbits with acetylcholine receptor protein from the electric organs of *Electrophorus electricus* and *Torpedo californica* resulted in weakness and neuromuscular block which improved following the administration of anticholinesterase compounds (34).

TREATMENT   *Anticholinesterase compounds* are administered for the amelioration of weakness in day-to-day management. The most useful of these are pyridostigmine (Mestinon®, 60–180 mg orally every 4 hr), neostigmine (Prostigmin®, 15–30 mg orally every 3 hr or 0.5–1 mg intramuscularly every 2–3 hr), and ambenonium (Mytelase®, 5–10 mg orally every 4 hr). Another and shorter acting anticholinesterase compound, edrophonium (Tensilon®) is useful in diagnosis (10 mg intravenously) and in evaluation of adequacy of dose of the longer-acting compounds (2 mg intravenously). The maximum strength obtained after optimal doses of any of these compounds is approximately the same. The compounds differ mainly in their duration of action (ambenomium > pyridostigmine > neostigmine > edrophonium), and in the severity of their parasympathomimetic side effects (neostigmine > ambenomium > pyridostigmine > edrophonium). The administration of graded doses of any of these compounds results in an increase in strength in muscles affected by the disease, but the maximal strength obtained is usually below normal, and may be far below normal (30).

Corticosteroids and corticotropin are administered to patients who are responding poorly to anticholinesterase medication. If the patient is severely ill, treatment should be initiated in an intensive care unit with methylprednisolone (60 mg intramuscularly) or prednisone (100 mg) or dexamethasone (12 mg) orally, in divided doses, or corticotropin (100 units) intramuscularly, daily for 10 days (36–39). Exacerbation of weakness occurs in about half the patients during the first week, and may require intubation or assisted respiration. Improvement occurs in most patients, to a marked degree in about half, usually beginning during the second week. If improvement does not occur, repeated courses of hormones should be reinstituted within one or two weeks until improvement begins, following which smaller doses of oral prednisone (35 mg) or dexamethasone (4 mg) should be administered every other day. On this regimen improvement persists for three to six months in about one half the patients, and over a year in one fourth. If exacerbation of the disease recurs, higher doses of steroid should be reinstituted. In patients who are less severely ill, prednisone can be administered orally in smaller doses [100 mg on alternate days (40), or 25 mg daily and gradually increased (41)]. This results in slower improvement, but also in a lower incidence of initial exacerbation, which may nevertheless be severe (42).

It has been suggested that the initial exacerbation may be due to adverse interaction between corticosteroid and anticholinesterase medication (43), and that withholding anticholinesterase medication during prednisone administration may be advantageous (40). Evidence has been presented in experimental animals that prolonged administration of anticholinesterase compounds produces impairment of neuromuscular structure and function (44) and myopathy (45). While excessive doses of anticholinesterase medication should be avoided, as this may not only precipitate cholinergic crisis but may also accelerate the development of drug resistance (acetylcholine refractoriness) (46), there is no good evidence that withholding anticholinesterase medication improves the response to steroid or the rate of remission (36, 37, 47). In the severely ill patient, withholding such medication may be hazardous, and it is preferable to administer the smallest dose needed to improve respiration, cough, and deglutition.

The complications of steroid treatment have included, in addition to initial exacerbation of the disease, those described under the treatment of polymyositis. Because of these complications, steroid should be reduced in dose as improvement occurs, and discontinued whenever possible. Most physicians have limited the prolonged use of steroid to patients with generalized myasthenia gravis, but administration of corticotropin or prednisone may also be helpful in refractory ocular myasthenia gravis (48).

Thymectomy is followed by improvement in most myasthenic patients, sometimes over a period of months, but more often over many years (49–51). While the natural history of the disease is that of gradual improvement after the first one to three years, patients who have had thymectomy early in the disease do appear to have a more benign course. Therefore, thymectomy is recommended in patients with generalized myasthenia gravis who are not able to carry out normal activity on anticholinesterase medication. If there is no radiologic evidence of thyoma, thymectomy can be performed through a transverse neck incision, with the aid of a mediastinoscope (49).

Immunosuppressant drugs (azathioprine, methotrexate, and 6-mercaptopurine) have been administered to patients with severe generalized myasthenia gravis who have become unresponsive to anticholinesterase medication and corticosteroids (52). The doses, precautions, and complications are the same as described for the treatment of polymyositis. Improvement is reported to have occurred in a majority of patients after periods ranging from weeks to months. Removal of lymphocytes by drainage of thoracic duct lymph has been reported to produce improvement within 48 hr (53).

Other drugs that may produce slight improvement in strength in a minority of patients include potassium chloride (2 g orally in dilute solution three times a day), ephedrine sulfate (25 mg orally three times a day), calcium gluconate (1 g orally four times a day), aldosterone antagonists [spironolactone, 50–100 mg orally, or triamterin 100–200 mg orally (54)], oxtriphylline [Choledyl®, a choline salt of theophylline, 0.3–2.4 g orally daily in divided doses (55)], and germine diacetate. Certain drugs may increase neuromuscular block and should be avoided. These include certain antibiotics [streptomycin, neomycin, kanamycin, vancomycin, novobiacin, polymixin, rolitetracycline, colistin, and colistimethate (56)], d-tubocurarine, succinylcholine, quinine, quinidine, magnesium sulfate, sodium lactate (57), and drugs that may produce a lupus-like syndrome, including procainamide, penicillamine (24), and trimethadione (58).

Myasthenic Syndrome

The Eaton-Lambert syndrome is manifested by weakness and fatigue, usually most marked in the extremities and sometimes accompanied by aching (59). It is usually, but not always, associated with neoplasm, particularly small-cell bronchogenic carcinoma, and may have an immunologic basis (60). The syndrome resembles myasthenia gravis in symptomatology, and usually in increased reactivity to d-tubocurarine and abnormal reactivity to decamethonium and succinylcholine. It differs from myasthenia gravis in that the muscle action potentials evoked by nerve stimulation are much smaller than normal, and increase markedly in amplitude following repetitive stimulation or voluntary contraction. Only a minority of patients with the Eaton-Lambert syndrome improve following administration of anticholinesterase compounds, but most improve following administration of guanidine sulfate (125–250 mg orally four times a day). The syndrome is due to deficient release of transmitter from the nerve endings (59). Guanidine increases release of transmitter. The drug is seldom helpful in myasthenia gravis and may aggravate weakness in some patients with lower motor neuron disease (61). The defect in the Eaton-Lambert syndrome is also partially corrected by epinephrine, methylxanthines, calcium, and caffeine, which has led to the suggestion that it may be due to impairment of cAMP and calcium-activated acetylcholine release (60).

DISEASES ASSOCIATED WITH ELECTROLYTE DISTURBANCE

Potassium

HYPOKALEMIA   Reduction in body and serum potassium may develop when there is deficient intake or absorption of potassium, or excessive loss in vomitus, stool, or urine. Approximately half of patients who receive 50 mg hydrochlorothiazide twice daily, as in the control of hypertension, develop a decrease in serum potassium concentration of at least 0.5 meq/liter for more than two months. Hypokalemia may also occur as a result of excessive movement of potassium into cells of the liver following the administration of large amounts of glucose and insulin in the treatment of diabetic acidosis, into cells throughout the body in alkalosis, or into muscle in hypokalemic periodic paralysis. There is sufficient reduction in wholebody potassium in most diabetic patients, particularly in those who are poorly controlled, to require daily replacement even in the presence of normal serum potassium (62).

Hypokalemia due to any cause, if severe, may impair the function of skeletal, cardiac, and smooth muscle. Weakness may involve the muscles of one or all extremities, and the neck, trunk, and respiration, but seldom the muscles innervated by the cranial nerves. Severe loss of potassium, whether in the gastrointestinal tract as a result of steatorrhea, malabsorption, or cathartics (63), or in the urine as a result of diuretics or renal tubular injury from disease or drugs such as amphotericin B (64), may result in profound weakness, elevation of serum enzymes derived from muscle, and muscle degeneration, necrosis, and infiltration by macrophages (hypokalemic myopathy) (65). Hypokalemia may also produce broadening and lowering of the T wave of the electrocardiogram, depression of the ST segment, extrasystoles and other arrhythmias, and increased sensitivity to the arrhythmic effects of digitalis.

Treatment of potassium deficiency is accomplished by supplying potassium, either orally or parenterally if necessary. For mild deficiency, at least 60 meq of potassium chloride is required daily. Potassium-containing foods, such as orange juice (5 meq per 100 ml) or bananas (10 meq per 100 g), are seldom ingested in sufficient amount to provide adequate replacement. For severe deficiency, several times this amount may be required. In the presence of normal renal function, the only practical limit to the amount of potassium given orally is the development of abdominal cramps or diarrhea, which usually occur at doses greater than 150 meq of potassium per day. Potassium salts in tablet form may cause stenosis of the esophagus (66) and small bowel (67), with or without ulceration, even when enteric-coated, and should never be used. A wax-coated, slow-release tablet (Slow-K) has been introduced (68), but has been reported to produce esophageal ulceration and stricture (69). The organic anion compounds of potassium are more palatable than the chloride, but are somewhat less suitable, since most of the organic anions, such as gluconate or citrate, are converted to bicarbonate, and may aggravate the metabolic alkalosis accompanying hypokalemia. For intravenous treatment, potassium chloride (40 meq/L) is administered at a rate of 20 meq per hour, or more rapidly if necessary, with electrocardiographic monitoring.

Hypokalemic periodic paralysis is managed by the daily oral administration of potassium (40 to 80 meq), spironolactone (100 mg), or acetazolamide (500 mg), in an attempt to prevent attacks of weakness (70), which usually occur during sleep, and administration of two or three times these amounts to treat attacks (71). Spironolactone probably acts by reducing kaliuresis, and acetazolamide by producing metabolic acidosis, which retards the entry of potassium into muscle (71). The vacuoles that occur in the muscles of some patients are not visibly altered during attacks or by treatment (72), nor does treatment affect the chronic myopathy that may ensue. In the hypokalemic periodic paralysis that occurs in a few patients with thyrotoxicosis, and which may occur in previously euthyroid patients following the ingestion of thyroid extract (73), attacks of weakness have been prevented and treated with propanolol (40 mg orally four times a day) (74, 75).

HYPERKALEMIA Hyperkalemia results mainly from renal insufficiency, usually with oliguria or anuria, from muscle necrosis due to paroxysmal myoglobinuria or trauma, or from excessively rapid administration of potassium. Hyperkalemia, if severe, results in impairment of skeletal, cardiac, and smooth muscle, with weakness, peaked T waves in the electrocardiogram, heart block, and asystole. Emergency treatment consists of infusion of glucose (100 g), insulin (25 units), and sodium bicarbonate (50 meq every 20 min), to produce an intracellular shift of potassium, and of calcium gluconate (1 g) to antagonize the cardiac toxicity of hyperkalemia. If the patient was previously digitalized, calcium should be omitted, since it increases digitalis toxicity. For longer-lasting treatment the patient can be hemodialyzed and given Kayexalate® cation exchange resin (20–40 g four times a day) orally or by enema.

In *hyperkalemic periodic paralysis,* potassium moves out of the muscle during attacks of weakness, which usually occur after exercise or exposure to cold and which may be accompanied by myotonic contractions. Attacks of weakness can sometimes be prevented by the prior administration of diuretics such as acetazolamide or chlorothiazide, which increase excretion of potassium, or by the intravenous administration of calcium, glucagon, or epinephrine (76).

Calcium

HYPOCALCEMIA   Hypocalcemia may occur in rickets, osteomalacia, hypoparathyroidism, steatorrhea, and uremic phosphate retention. Hypocalcemia, or reduced ionization of calcium without change in concentration, which occurs in alkalosis due to hyperventilation or sodium bicarbonate ingestion, results in increased irritability and spontaneous discharge of sensory and motor nerves and muscle, producing paresthesias, twitching, and muscular spasms (tetany). Most patients are not weak, but some with osteomalacia (77–79) or hypoparathyroidism (80) develop proximal muscle weakness and histologic changes compatible with myopathy, and one patient (79) developed increased serum enzymes derived from muscle. Improvement occurred following treatment with calcium and vitamin D, or, in one patient (77), phosphate.

HYPERCALCEMIA   Hypercalcemia may occur in primary or secondary hyperparathyroidism, sarcoidosis, administration of calcium and alkali or of vitamin D, and in malignant disease with or without bony metastasis. Hypercalcemia results in a moderate decrease in muscle strength and tone, decreased intestinal motility, drowsiness and nephrocalcinosis. Some patients with primary (81) or secondary (79) hyperparathyroidism had more pronounced proximal weakness and wasting, myopathic potentials, and atrophy of type I and type II muscle fibers. Improvement occurred following removal of a parathyroid adenoma or alleviation of the cause of parathormone stimulation.

Sodium

Hyponatremia results from loss of sodium in the urine, gastrointestinal glands, or sweat, or from inappropriate secretion of antidiuretic hormone. *Hypernatremia* may result from restriction of water intake, dehydration, hyperaldosteronism, or certain lesions of the brain. Either hyponatremia or hypernatremia may result in lassitude or weakness, which, in severe hypernatremia, may progress to paralysis (82).

DISORDERS ASSOCIATED WITH ABNORMAL RESPONSE TO DRUGS

Malignant hyperthermia is a potentially lethal, autosomal-dominant syndrome characterized by an abnormal response of muscle to certain inhalational anesthetic agents such as halothane, and skeletal-muscle relaxants such as succinylcholine or *d*-tubocurarine (83–85). Some members of many, but not all susceptible families have increased muscle bulk, cramps, local or general weakness, ptosis, myopathic potentials, elevated serum enzymes derived from muscle, and histologic changes in muscle. Susceptible patients develop during anesthesia fulminant hypermetabolism of muscle, which may be induced by a sudden rise in myoplasmic calcium released from the sarcoplasmic reticulum. This results in a vast rise in heat production, fever, release of potassium, enzymes, and myoglobin from muscle, muscle rigidity, flushing, cyanosis, tachycardia, hypotension, hypoxia, tachypnea, and respiratory and metabolic (lactic) acidosis. Late complications include muscle and pulmonary edema, consumption coagulopathy, decerebration, and acute renal shutdown. Management relies on prompt cessation of all anesthetics and muscle relaxants, hyperventilation with oxygen, cooling, and the intravenous administration of sodium bicarbonate to correct the lactic acidosis; procaine or procainamide (0.5–1 mg/kg per min) under electrocardiographic control to correct arrhythmias and restore calcium to the sarcoplasmic reticulum; glucose and insulin to correct hyperkalemia; and mannitol and furosemide to flush myoglobin out of the renal tubules. If renal failure persists, dialysis may be necessary. The mortality of recognized cases has been over 50%. Members of affected families should avoid inhalational anesthetic agents (except nitrous oxide), all muscle relaxants, lidocaine, mepivacaine and cardiac glycosides, but they may receive barbituates, tranquilizers, narcotics, and procaine or tetracaine.

Plasma cholinesterase deficiency may occur as a genetic disorder, or as a result of liver disease, acute febrile illness, or the administration of anticholinesterase compounds. The only resulting abnormality is delay in the breakdown of esters such as succinylcholine, which are hydrolyzed by this enzyme. Persistence of succinylcholine results in prolonged and increased neuromuscular block, with persistence of paralysis and apnea. Respiration must be sustained mechanically until the effect of the drug wears off, which may take hours. Patients with the deficiency should be identified so that anesthetists may be duly warned, and, if no cause is found, family members should be examined (86).

Burns, trauma, upper and lower motor neuron lesions, and tetanus increase the sensitivity of muscle to depolarizing agents, including succinylcholine, which cause efflux of potassium from muscle during depolarization. Following the administration of succinylcholine to patients with these disorders, the serum potassium may rise to toxic levels and may cause cardiac arrest (87).

OTHER METABOLIC MYOPATHIES

Hyperthyroidism results in mild to moderate weakness and wasting in 70% of patients, and marked weakness and wasting, termed *chronic thyrotoxic myopathy*, in a small number. Rarely, patients with severe hyperthyroidism may develop acute myopathy or encephalomyopathy, characterized by the acute development of severe weakness, marked tremor, delerium, and sometimes dysphagia, dysarthria, and coma. Concomitant myasthenia gravis should be excluded by the edrophonium test. Management of thyroid "storm," with or without encephalomyopathy, relies on rapid institution of antithyroid treatment with potassium iodide and propylthiouracil, supplemented by propanolol, reserpine, and corticosteroid (88).

Hypothyroidism results in mild weakness of proximal muscles, increased muscle bulk, slowness of movement and of muscle contraction and relaxation in response to percussion of the muscle or its tendon, and sometimes muscle stiffness, aching, and cramps. The serum enzymes derived from muscle, including CPK, are elevated. Treatment with thyroid hormone reverses all these changes (88).

Mitochondrial myopathy is characterized by proximal limb-girdle weakness and wasting, a hypermetabolic state despite normal thyroid function, and muscle mitochondria that are structurally abnormal and are associated with partial uncoupling of oxidative phosphorylation. The heart may also be affected. Elevated plasma levels of lactic and pyruvic acids and of alanine may occur, especially after exercise. No definitive therapy is available, but heavy exercise should be avoided, and sodium bicarbonate may be administered for the acidosis (89).

McArdle's syndrome is characterized by muscle stiffness and cramps after exercise. Glycogen accumulates in the muscle because of deficiency of amylophosphorylase. Ingestion of 100 to 200 g of glucose or fructose prior to exertion is reported to be helpful (90).

Paroxysmal myoglobinuria is characterized by muscle pain, cramps, and weakness, and myoglobinuria after exercise. Limitation of exercise is essential. If hyperkalemia and renal failure occur, these must be treated.

Type-IV hyperlipoproteinemia may result in muscle stiffness and aching, as well as arthralgias (91). It is treated by diet and clofibrate administration.

Vitamin E ingestion, 800 IU daily for 3 weeks, was reported to result in fatigue, weakness, creatinuria, and elevated serum CPK (92).

Allopurinol administration to patients with gout resulted in deposition of crystals of hypoxanthine, xanthine, and oxipurinol in skeletal muscle, but no clinical manifestations of muscle disease (93).

Chronic renal failure may produce not only neuropathy, but also proximal weakness and wasting attributable to myopathy. Maintenance dialysis or renal transplantation resulted in dramatic improvement (94).

MUSCULAR DYSTROPHIES

DUCHENNE MUSCULAR DYSTROPHY   Prednisone administration was reported to produce in 13 of 14 patients improvement in motor power, which was maintained for up to 28 months in 8 patients (95). Serum CPK fell in 9 patients by more than 45%, but subsequently returned to pretreatment levels. However, other studies have indicated no significant clinical effect of prednisone, despite reduction in serum CPK (96). α-Tocopherol, Vitamin E, anabolic steroids, amino acids, and mixtures of nucleotides were at one time proposed for management, but have been found to be ineffective (90). Management is limited to physical therapy, avoidance of obesity, and careful attention to respiratory complications.

MYOTONIC DYSTROPHY   There is no treatment for the weakness, which is the main problem in this disease. However, the myotonia can be improved by administration of quinine (0.6 g), procainamide (250–500 mg), or diphenylhydantoin (100–200 mg) orally four times a day (90).

CONGENITAL MYOTONIA   These patients have myotonia, but little or no weakness or wasting, so that management with the above drugs is satisfactory.

CENTRAL CORE DISEASE, NEMALINE MYOPATHY, MYOTUBULAR MYOPATHY   There is no drug treatment for these diseases. Management is limited to physical therapy.

SUMMARY

Some progress has been made in understanding the pathogenesis of muscle diseases that are associated with alterations in the immune mechanism, and in treating them with corticosteroids and immunosuppressant drugs. The diseases associated with electrolyte disturbances, abnormal response to drugs, and endocrine and metabolic changes are also usually amenable to management. The challenge for the future lies in learning the pathogenesis and treatment of the muscular dystrophies.

Literature Cited

1. Medsger, T. A. Jr., Dawson, W. N. Jr., Masi, A. T. 1970. *Am. J. Med.* 48:715–23
2. Bohan, A., Peter, J. B. 1975. *N. Engl. J. Med.* 292:344–47, 403–7
3. Dawkins, R. L. 1965. *J. Pathol. Bacteriol.* 90:619–25
4. Johnson, R. L., Fink, C. W., Ziff, M. 1972. *J. Clin. Invest.* 51:2435–49
5. Dawkins, R. L., Mastaglia, F. L. 1973. *N. Engl. J. Med.* 288:434–38
6. Whitaker, J. N., Engel, W. K. 1972. *N. Engl. J. Med.* 286:333–38
7. Tang, T. T., Sedmak, G. V., Siegesmund, K. A., McCreadie, S. R. 1975. *N. Engl. J. Med.* 292:608–11
8. Greenlee, J. E., Johnson, W. D. Jr., Campa, J. F., Adelman, L. S., Sande, M. A. 1975. *Ann. Int. Med.* 82:367–71
9. Pearson, C. M. 1963. *Ann. Int. Med.* 59:827–38
10. Winkelmann, R. K., Mulder, D. W., Lambert, E. H. 1968. *Mayo Clin. Proc.* 43:545–56
11. Vignos, P. J., Goldwyn, J. 1972. *Am. J. Med. Sci.* 263:291–308
12. Rose, A. L. 1974. *Am. J. Dis. Child.* 127:518–22
13. Melby, J. C. 1974. *Ann. Int. Med.* 81:505–12
14. Sita, J. A. 1974. *Postgrad. Med.* 55:111–20
15. Haas, D. 1973. *Neurology* 23:55–62
16. Metzger, A. L., Bohan, A., Goldberg, L. S., Bluestone, R., Pearson, C. M. 1974. *Ann. Int. Med.* 81:182–89
17. Benson, M. D., Aldo, M. A. 1973. *Arch. Int. Med.* 132:547–51
18. Boston Collaborative Drug Surveillance Program. 1974. *J. Am. Med. Assoc.* 227:1036–40
19. Decker, I. L., Bertino, I. R., Hurd, K. R., Steinberg, A. D. 1973. *Arthritis Rheum.* 16:78–85
20. Simmons, R. L., Moberg, A. W., Gewurz, H., Sold, R., Tallent, M. B., Najarian, J. S. 1970. *Surgery* 68:62–68
21. Cosimi, A. B., Skamene, E., Bonney, W. W., Russell, P. S. 1970. *Surgery* 68:54–61
22. Schuermans, Y. 1975. *Lancet* 1:111
23. Katsilambros, N., Braaten, J., Ferguson, D., Bradley, R. F. 1972. *N. Engl. J. Med.* 286:1110–11
24. Schraeder, P. L., Peters, H. A., Dahl, D. S. 1972. *Arch. Neurol.* 27:456–57

25. Perkoff, G. T., Dioso, M. M., Bleisch, V., Klinkerfuss, G. 1967. *Ann. Int. Med.* 67:481–93
26. Harpey, J. P., Caille, B., Moulias, P. 1971. *Lancet* 1:292–94
27. Bucknall, R. C., Dixon, A. St. J., Glick, E. N., Woodland, J., Zutski, D. W. 1975. *Br. Med. J.* 1:600–602
28. Altman, K., Tobin, M. 1965. *Proc. Soc. Exp. Biol. Med.* 118:554–57
29. Grob, D. 1971. *Ann. NY Acad. Sci.* 183:248–69
30. Grob, D. 1976. *Current Therapy,* ed. H. F. Conn. Philadelphia: Saunders. In press
31. Namba, T., Himei, H., Grob, D. 1967. *J. Lab. Clin. Med.* 70:258–72
32. Fambrough, D. M., Drachman, D. B., Satyamurti, S. 1973. *Science* 182:293
33. Almon, R. R., Andrew, C. G., Appel, S. H. 1974. *Science* 186:55
34. Lennon, V. A., Lindstrom, J. M., Seybold, M. E. 1975. *J. Exp. Med.* 141:1365–75
35. Kalden, J. R., Williamson, W. G., Irvine, W. J. 1973. *Clin. Exp. Immunol.* 13:79–88
36. Namba, T., Brunner, N. G., Shapiro, M. S., Grob, D. 1971. *Neurology* 21:1008–18
37. Brunner, N. G., Namba, T., Grob, D. 1972. *Neurology* 22:603–10
38. Liversedge, L. A., Yiull, G. M., Wilkinson, I. M. S., Hughes, J. A. 1974. *J. Neurol. Neurosurg. Psychiatry* 37:412–15
39. Engel, W. K. et al 1974. *Ann. Int. Med.* 81:225–46
40. Warmolts, J. R., Engel, W. K. 1972. *N. Engl. J. Med.* 286:17–20
41. Seybold, M. E., Drachman, D. B. 1974. *N. Engl. J. Med.* 290:81–84
42. McQuillan, M. P. 1974. *N. Engl. J. Med.* 290:631
43. Patten, B. M., Oliver, K. L., Engel, W. K. 1974. *Neurology* 24:442–49
44. Engel, A. G., Lambert, E. H., Santa, T. 1973. *Neurology* 23:1273–81
45. Fenichel, G. M., Kibler, W. B., Olson, W. H., Dettbarn, W. D. 1972. *Neurology* 22:1026–33
46. Grob, D., Namba, T., Feldman, D. S. 1966. *Ann. NY Acad. Sci.* 135:247–75
47. Brunner, N. G., Berger, C. L., Namba, T., Grob, D. 1976. *Ann. NY Acad. Sci.* In press
48. Cape, C. A. 1973. *Arch. Ophthalmol.* 90:292–93
49. Papatestas, A. E., Genkins, G., Kornfeld, P., Horowitz, S., Kark, A. E. 1975. *Surg. Gynecol. Obstet.* 140:535–40
50. Thomas, T. V. 1972. *Ann. Thorac. Surg.* 13:499–512
51. Cohn, H. E., Solit, R. W., Schatz, N. J., Schlezinger, N. 1974. *J. Thorac. Cardiovasc. Surg.* 68:876–85
52. Mertens, H. G., Balzereit, F., Leipert, M. 1969. *Eur. Neurol.* 2:321–39
53. Bergström, K., Frankson, C., Matell, G., Nilsson, B. Y., Persson, A., von Reis, G., Stensman, R. 1975. *Eur. Neurol.* 13:19–30
54. Özdemir, C., Hatemi, H., Yardimci, B. 1974. *Panminerva Med.* 16:190–94
55. Brumlik, J., Jacobs, R., Karczmar, A. G. 1973. *Clin. Pharmacol. Ther.* 14:380–84
56. Decker, D. A., Fincham, R. W. 1971. *Arch. Neurol.* 25:141–44
57. Patten, B. M., Oliver, K. L., Engel, W. K. 1974. *Neurology* 24:986–90
58. Booker, H. E., Chun, R. W. M., Sanguino, M. 1970. *J. Am. Med. Assoc.* 212:2262–63
59. Lambert, E. H., Elmquist, D. 1971. *Ann NY Acad. Sci.* 183:183–99
60. Takamori, M., Mori, M. 1973. *Arch. Neurol.* 29:420–24
61. Norris, F. H. Jr., Fallet, R. J., Calenchini, P. R. 1974. *Neurology.* 24:135–37
62. Walsh, C. H., Soler, N. G., James, H., Fitzgerald, M. G., Malius, J. M. 1974. *Br. Med. J.* 4:738–40
63. Coers, C., Telerman-Toppet, N., Cremer, M. 1972. *Am. J. Med.* 52:849–56
64. Drutz, D. J., Fan, J. H., Tai, T. Y., Cheng, J. T., Hsieh, W. C. 1970. *J. Am. Med. Assoc.* 211:824–26
65. Van Horn, G., Drori, J. B., Schwartz, F. D. 1970. *Arch. Neurol.* 22:335–41
66. Boley, S. J., Allen, A. C., Schultz, L., Schwartz, S. 1965. *J. Am. Med. Assoc.* 193:997–1000
67. Pemberton, J. 1970. *Br. Heart J.* 32:267–68
68. Ben-Ishay, D., Engelman, K. 1973. *Clin. Pharmacol. Ther.* 14:250–58
69. Howie, A. D., Strachan, R. W. 1975. *Br. Med. J.* 1:176
70. Resnick, J. S., Engel, W. K., Griggs, R. C., Stam, A. C. 1968. *N. Engl. J. Med.* 278:582–86
71. Vroom, F. W., Jarrell, M. A., Maren, T. H. 1975. *Arch. Neurol.* 32:385–92
72. Gordon, A. M., Green, J. R., Lagunoff, D. 1970. *Am. J. Med.* 48:185–95
73. Layzer, R. B., Goldfield, E. 1974. *Neurology* 24:949–52
74. Conway, M. J., Seibel, J. A., Eaton, R. P. 1974. *Ann. Int. Med.* 81:332–36
75. Yeung, R. T. T., Tse, T. F. 1974. *Am. J. Med.* 57:584–90

76. Brillman, J., Pincus, J. H. 1973. *Arch. Neurol.* 29:67–69
77. Baker, L. R. I., Ackrill, P., Cattell, W. R., Stamp, T. C. B., Watson, L. 1974. *Br. Med. J.* 3:150–52
78. Skaria, J., Katiyar, B. C., Srivastava, T. P., Dube, B. 1975. *Acta Neurol. Scand.* 51:37–58
79. Mallette, L. E., Patten, B. M., Engel, W. K. 1975. *Ann. Int. Med.* 82:474–83
80. Hower, J., Stuck, H., Tackmann, W., Bohlmann, H. G. 1974. *Z. Kinderheilk.* 116:193–96
81. Patten, B. M. et al 1974. *Ann. Int. Med.* 80:182–93
82. Maddy, J. A., Winternitz, W. W. 1971. *Am. J. Med.* 51:394–402
83. Harriman, D. G. F., Sumner, D. W., Ellis, F. R. 1973. *Q. J. Med.* 42:639–74
84. Britt, B. A. 1974. *N. Engl. J. Med.* 290:1140–42
85. Britt, B. A., Webb, G. E., LeDuc, C. 1974. *Can. Anaesth. Soc. J.* 21:371–75
86. Cherington, M., Lasater, G. 1973. *Arch. Neurol.* 73:274–75
87. Grovert, G. A., Theye, R. A. 1975. *Anesthesiology* 43:89–97
88. Grob, D. 1963. *NY State J. Med.* 63:218–28
89. Sengers, R. C. A. et al 1975. *J. Pediatr.* 86:873–80
90. Satoyoshi, E., Kinoshita, M. 1972. *Int. J. Neurol.* 9:54–60
91. Goldwan, J. A. et al 1972. *Lancet* 2:449–52
92. Briggs, M. H. 1974. *Lancet* 1:220
93. Watts, R. W. E. et al 1971. *Q. J. Med.* 40:1–14
94. Floyd, M. et al 1974. *Q. J. Med.* 43:509–24
95. Drachman, D. B., Toyka, K. V., Myer, E. 1974. *Lancet* 2:1409–12
96. Munsat, T. L., Walton, J. N. 1975. *Lancet* 1:276–77

PHARMACOLOGY AND TOXICOLOGY OF LITHIUM

♦6648

Mogens Schou

The Psychopharmacology Research Unit, Aarhus University Institute of Psychiatry, Risskov, Denmark

INTRODUCTION

Interest in the biology and pharmacology of lithium (lithium ions, lithium salts) is at present very keen. During the five years since lithium was last reviewed in this series (1) the literature has increased from about 2000 to about 4000 references. The present review can deal with only selected aspects of the pharmacology and toxicology of lithium. Additional information may be found in a basic review (2), in recent reviews and bibliographies (3–7), and in two multi-author books about lithium therapy and research (8, 9).

Although the therapeutic applications of lithium are outside the scope of this review, its pharmacology and toxicology must be viewed in the light of its clinical uses (10). Only two of these are fully established: the therapeutic use in mania and the prophylactic use against relapses of mania and depression in recurrent manic-depressive disorder of the bipolar and monopolar type. There is fairly good evidence that lithium may be of use also in recurrent schizo-affective disorder, some cases of depression, pathological emotional instability, periodic pathological aggressiveness, thyrotoxicosis, and, in combination with radioactive iodine, thyroid cancer. Other psychiatric and nonpsychiatric uses are based on less solid evidence.

Lithium occurs in trace amounts in plants and animal tissues, but it is not known whether the lithium naturally present in the organism plays any physiological role. The idea has been advanced that lithium ingested with drinking water might protect against illness, and inverse correlations have been found between the lithium content of water from various districts and the frequency of mental or cardiovascular disease. However, correlation is very far from being the same as causation, and even the mineral waters richest in lithium contain so little that many gallons would have to be consumed daily to provide a lithium intake comparable to that used for lithium therapy and prophylaxis.

231

EXPERIMENTAL CONDITIONS

Lithium is one of the alkali metals, and many experimental studies deal with the results of partial or complete substitution of lithium for sodium in the medium or perfusion fluid. Such studies have provided information about effects of lithium on nerve impulse generation and conduction, neuromuscular transmission, transport of amino acids, amines and electrolytes, metabolic events in tissue preparations and purified enzymes, etc (reviews: 3, 11, 12). It should be noted, however, that in such studies lithium has usually been present in the medium in concentrations of 50–150 mmol per liter, levels far above those involved when lithium is used as a drug. During treatment of patients, the lithium concentration in blood serum is about 0.5–1 mmol per liter and in tissues about 0.5–5 mmol per kg wet weight. During lithium poisoning one may encounter serum lithium concentrations of 2–10 mmol per liter and tissue concentrations of up to about 10 mmol per kg wet weight. Studies carried out with much higher lithium concentrations are hardly of relevance to the pharmacology and toxicology of lithium and are not dealt with in this review.

Pharmacological lithium studies have involved in vitro experiments as well as investigations on animals, patients, and healthy human volunteers. Many of the studies have been concerned with the effects of a single or a few lithium doses, fewer with the effects of long-term administration. Acute and chronic lithium administration may produce entirely different effects as shown by studies on brain amine concentration and turnover (13–15), liver glycogen concentration (16, 17), thyroid iodide transport and metabolism (18), and thirst and urine flow (19).

Lithium may be administered to animals by intraperitoneal or subcutaneous injection, usually given once or twice daily, with the drinking water, by gavage, or mixed with the food (20, 21). After injection there is a rise of the serum lithium concentration to a peak value followed by a fall to a low value before the next injection. The procedure should therefore be used only in experiments where large variations of the serum concentration are acceptable. Administration of lithium with the drinking fluid is not practical, because the animals may develop lithium-induced polyuria and polydipsia and hence increase lithium consumption. Administration with the food ensures a fairly constant serum lithium level throughout the 24 hours of the day (21). The serum level can therefore be used as a quantitative measure of the exposure to lithium. Administration with food is time and labor saving.

For a number of years it was difficult to maintain rats at serum lithium concentrations higher than 0.6–0.8 mmol per liter; if the lithium concentration in the food was raised, the animals lost weight and were apt to develop intoxication. The difficulty was overcome by increasing the sodium content of the food or by giving rats a free choice between water and a hypertonic (0.46 M) sodium chloride solution (22–24). With this procedure rats can be maintained at serum levels up to about 1.5 mmol per liter; this is the same as the upper level tolerated by patients. When offered hypertonic sodium chloride, the rats seem to consume just enough sodium to prevent lithium poisoning, and it has been suggested that the intake of salt solution be used as a measure of the minimum sodium requirement of the organism (J. Jensen, K. Thomsen, and O. V. Olesen, submitted for publication).

Also, the potassium content of the food plays a role in maintaining health and normal growth during long-term administration of lithium (25). It would be useful if publications reported the electrolyte composition of the fodder. For studies on rats with lithium-induced polyuria it may be difficult to know whether differences observed between these and control rats are due to the lithium administration as such or to the high urine flow. It may then be practical to use Brattleboro rats with hereditary hypothalamic diabetes insipidus as controls (24).

PHARMACOKINETICS

Pharmacokinetic studies in patients have led to safer and more effective lithium treatment through monitoring of serum levels under standardized conditions (26).

Absorption

Lithium is not metabolized; its pharmacokinetics are therefore determined solely by absorption, distribution, and excretion. Absorption of lithium by animals has already been dealt with. Lithium may be administered to patients as conventional or as sustained-release preparations. Use of the latter leads to reduction of certain side effects through attenuation of variations in the serum lithium concentration (27). It is not clear whether concentration maxima or concentration changes are more important for the intensity of the side effects.

Lithium aspartate and lithium orotate have been reported therapeutically superior to the more commonly used lithium carbonate because of alleged ionophore properties of the anions (28, 29). The clinical evidence is not convincing, and the claims for special cell affinities of these salts have been refuted in experiments with rats (D. F. Smith, submitted for publication) and healthy human volunteers (30).

Distribution

Lithium is distributed differently from both sodium and potassium (review: 31). Intracellular: extracellular concentration ratios in some tissues are below unity and in others above, but they never approach those of sodium and potassium. Lithium seems to be transported out of nerve and muscle cells by the active sodium pump, although inefficiently. It is carried into erythrocytes by the carrier usually transporting potassium.

The lithium concentration in whole brain is of the same order as that in blood serum, whereas the concentration in spinal fluid is only about one fourth of that. The lithium concentration in various brain regions has been determined in patients who died during lithium treatment and in lithium-treated rats. Findings differ among the authors, but differences in concentration between brain regions have been small in all studies (man: 32; rat: 33, 34). In brain homogenates lithium is bound to particle fractions (35); the subcellular distribution can be altered by changing the housing conditions of the experimental animals (36). Studies of lithium distribution in brain seem often based on the assumption that if a particular region or particle fraction could be shown to have an especially high lithium concentration, that would also be the place where lithium exerts its action. This reasoning is predicated on the assumption of an unproved and indeed unlikely equal sensitivity of various brain structures to lithium.

In view of the high sodium content in bone and the existence of sodium fractions with different turnover rates, it is hardly astonishing that lithium concentration in bone rises to a level several times higher than the concentration in extracellular fluid (37), or that disappearance of lithium after discontinuation indicates one rapidly lost fraction and another and larger one that is lost very slowly (38).

Lithium concentration in the thyroid gland is 2–5 times the concentration in serum (18). A substantial fraction of thyroid lithium may be located extracellularly, for example in the follicular lumen.

It has been suggested that the lithium concentration in erythrocytes, or the erythrocyte:serum concentration ratio, may be correlated with clinical state and treatment outcome in affective disorders (39–42). Evidence has also been presented suggesting that the concentration ratio may be genetically determined and may be an indicator of a more generalized membrane defect in patients suffering from manic-depressive disorder (43–45). Even when one refrains from comparing studies in which lithium was administered to patients with studies in which lithium was added in vitro, there are striking differences between the findings of various authors (cf 30, 46). This conflict of data indicates that the kinetics of lithium transport across the erythrocyte membrane and the factors governing steady state concentrations are still insufficiently known and that experimental conditions are inadequately standardized to give generally reproducible results.

Lithium passes freely through the placental membrane (47) and is excreted in low concentration in the milk (48).

Although subjected to only few systematic studies it is a frequently made observation that patients on lithium maintenance treatment with constant dosage tend to show a lowering of the serum lithium concentration when a manic relapse occurs and sometimes an increase when the patient suffers a depressive relapse. Comparison of the renal lithium clearance of manic patients, depressed patients, and patients after recovery from mania or depression failed to show any significant difference between the groups when values were corrected for age and body surface (49). This does not exclude the possibility that shortlasting changes of the renal lithium clearance may have occurred early in the manic and depressive episodes. An alternative explanation of the changes in serum levels might be that manias or depressions are associated with alterations in the distribution volume of lithium. Hormone-induced changes in lithium distribution have been described (50).

Elimination and its Significance for the Development of Intoxication

Lithium elimination takes place almost exclusively through the kidneys. After filtration through the glomerular membrane, lithium is reabsorbed with sodium and water in the proximal kidney tubules; little or no lithium is reabsorbed in the distal parts of the nephron (51). The renal lithium clearance is therefore identical with the proximal clearance of sodium, about 20% of the glomerular filtration rate. It increases slightly with increasing sodium clearance but is unaffected by procedures that influence only distal sodium reabsorption.

The sodium balance plays a major, although not a solitary, role in renal lithium clearance. The latter falls under conditions of severe sodium deficiency resulting from, for example, administration of a low-sodium diet or long-term administration of thiazides (52, 53). This fall may to a large extent be accounted for by an increase in the fractional proximal reabsorption of sodium and hence of lithium.

Lithium administration may in itself lower the capacity of the kidneys to conserve sodium (23). Lithium lowers the response of the kidneys to mineralocorticoids (K. Thomsen, J. Jensen, and O. V. Olesen, submitted for publication), but other factors must also be at work since the sodium requirement of adrenalectomized lithium-treated rats is higher than that of adrenalectomized control rats. The lower capacity for conserving sodium leads to a rise of the requirement for sodium. If the requirement exceeds the intake, sodium deficiency develops. This leads to a fall of the renal lithium clearance, resulting in further rise of the serum lithium concentration and additional increase of the minimum sodium requirement, so that a vicious circle is started (54). It may be broken by the administration of sodium in appropriate dosage.

In man, lithium poisoning affects primarily the CNS and the kidneys. Death may occur during protracted coma, anuria, or circulatory failure. The capacity for eliminating sodium may be lowered. Lithium intoxication is treated symptomatically and by accelerating elimination of lithium, most efficiently through hemodialysis (55; H. E. Hansen and A. Amdisen, submitted for publication).

Renal lithium elimination is influenced by factors other than sodium balance. Among these are pregnancy, the time of day, physical exercise, exposure to cold, and the administration of epinephrine (56–60). During the latter half of pregnancy the glomerular filtration rate, and hence the amount of lithium filtered through the glomerular membrane, is increased. The mechanism underlying the effect of the other factors is not known.

EFFECTS AND PHARMACODYNAMICS

Behavior and Mental Functions

Administered to animals lithium does not exhibit marked sedative or excitatory actions (although severely intoxicated rats are jumpy and irritable), but with sophisticated recording equipment it has been possible to demonstrate effects of lithium on spontaneous behavior, learned behavior, and abnormal behavior induced by drugs (reviews: 61, 62; selected recent references: 63–68). The studies have all been carried out on rats and mice.

Many of the studies aim at correlating behavioral changes with changes in brain amine concentration and metabolism. Two general lines of research have been followed. Studies concerned with the antimanic action of lithium have used the decreased spontaneous and exploratory activity of lithium-treated animals as their starting point and have attempted to restore activities to normal levels by administering drugs that alter brain amines. Amphetamine, morphine, parachlorophenylalanine, and monamine oxidase (MAO) inhibitors can reverse the effects of lithium on locomotor activity (69–72). Lithium has also been used to prevent hyperactivity induced by drugs in order to investigate the antimanic activity of lithium (69, 73). On the other hand, studies concerned with the antidepressant action of lithium have used the changes in behavior seen after administration of lithium to animals given MAO inhibitors or reserpine. Under these circumstances lithium leads to an increase in the activity level that seems to be related to an increase in the availability of biogenic amines in the brain (74–76).

In spite of its striking effects on the pathological mood changes of manic-depressive patients, lithium affects normal mood to an astonishingly small degree. Only subtle mental changes have been observed in healthy human volunteers and in manic-depressive patients who started prophylactic treatment during an interval between episodes: slight indifference, altered response to environmental stimuli, impaired concentration, slowing of mentation, and reduced intellectual initiative (77, 78). These changes occur early in the treatment; they disappear under long-term lithium administration. Studies on healthy volunteers have shown impairment of choice reaction performance after lithium administration for two weeks (79). Lithium ingestion for six months did not interfere with driving skill as tested in a car simulator (80). An effect on cognitive functions has been observed in lithium-treated patients suffering from Huntington's chorea with preexisting dementia (81). Narrowing of the emotional range and loss of initiative and inspiration during lithium treatment have occasionally been reported by business executives and artists, but these changes may be the result of removal of slight manic features (82–84). Occasionally lithium alters the taste of certain foods (85).

Amines

Current amine hypotheses on the biochemistry of manic-depressive disorder suggest that mania is associated with a surplus and depression with a lack of neurotransmitters at the cerebral synapses. Many lithium effects on brain amines are compatible with this concept as long as lithium is considered only as an antimanic drug. But treatment with lithium prevents depressive recurrences as effectively as it does manic recurrences, and hypotheses should therefore include a stabilizing action of lithium on the—hypothetical—metabolic processes that underlie pathological mood changes: attenuation of a positive feedback mechanism or stimulation of a negative one.

Findings based on experiments with lithium administration in vivo, or on in vitro experiments with lithium concentrations below 10 mmol per liter, include the following: stimulation of norepinephrine turnover, inhibition or stimulation of serotonin turnover, alteration of catecholamine breakdown, inhibition of stimulus-induced amine release, stimulation or inhibition of amine re-uptake, changes in brain or spinal fluid concentrations of amine precursors, amines, and amine metabolites, inhibition of platelet serotonin uptake, and increase of platelet MAO activity (reviews: 1, 86; selected references: 15, 87–92). Differences between the findings of different authors are often due to different modes of administering lithium. Short-term lithium administration typically leads to an increase in serotonin synthesis, norepinephrine re-uptake, and MAO activity, while these effects are observed less consistently or reversed during prolonged lithium administration. In addition to its effects on catecholamines and indoleamines, lithium may influence other established or putative neurotransmitters: acetylcholine (93) and the γ-aminobutyric acid (GABA) glutamate system (94).

Electrophysiology

Studies on human volunteers, patients, and experimental animals have revealed lithium-induced alterations of electroencephalogram (EEG) and cortical-evoked potentials (reviews: 95, 96). In patients the changes seem related to the occurrence of toxic effects rather than to therapeutic outcome. One study found better correlation with the lithium concentration in red blood cells than in serum (97). In some cases EEG changes during lithium treatment seem to represent accentuation of previous abnormalities rather than a specific effect on the normal EEG (98).

Electromyographic changes during lithium treatment include partial reversible block of the response to tetanic stimulation (99) and reduction of motor nerve conduction velocity (100). Symptoms of fatigue and muscular weakness occasionally experienced by patients might be related to such changes in peripheral neuromuscular function. Lithium-induced hand tremor is not accompanied by electromyogram (EMG) synchronization (P. Juul-Jensen and M. Schou, unpublished). It responds to treatment with β-receptor blocking agents (101, 102). Since practolol, which supposedly does not enter the CNS, is active, a peripheral site of action is likely. ECG changes may occur during lithium treatment even when serum potassium is normal, for example, T-wave depression possibly due to interference with myocardial repolarization (103, 104). In lithium-treated patients there is an increase of the transmucosal potential difference in rectum, possibly caused by lowered response to vasopressin (105, 106).

Electrolytes

Although undoubtedly having specific effects of its own, lithium resembles sodium, potassium, magnesium, and calcium in many respects. This partial similarity of lithium with each of the four biologically important cations may account for some of its effects.

Lithium administration to animals and man leads to initial transient changes in fluid and electrolyte balance and also to later changes that are more long-lasting but disappear when lithium is discontinued (reviews: 107, 108). Among relatively consistent findings during long-term lithium administration to animals and man are the following: decrease of brain magnesium (34, 109), decrease of urinary calcium excretion in man (110, 111), and increase in rats (17, 112). There is an increase of plasma magnesium (34, 109, 113, 114), and it has been suggested (115) that an early rise (within the first five days) predicts good response to lithium treatment of depression. Lithium treatment of patients leads to a slight but statistically significant decrease of bone calcium as assessed by X radiography (108) and by photonabsorptiometry (C. Christiansen, P. C. Baastrup, and I. Transbøl, submitted for publication).

Thyroid Function

Since the discovery in 1968 that lithium-treated patients may develop goiter (116) or show lowering of protein-bound iodine in serum (117) the effects of lithium on thyroid function have been subjected to extensive research (reviews: 18, 118). One of the antithyroid properties of lithium, its inhibition of thyroid hormone release from the gland, has even been put to therapeutic use in the treatment of thyrotoxicosis, especially thyrotoxic crises, and, in combination with radioactive iodine, of thyroid cancer (119–123).

Three forms of thyroid dysfunction have been seen during lithium treatment of patients: transitory biochemical changes such as elevated thyroid stimulating hormone (TSH) levels and decreased levels of triiodothyronine and thyroxine in serum without clinical changes; compensated dysfunction in the form of goiter with euthyroidism; and hypothyroidism with or without goiter. The frequency with which they occur varies considerably from one report to another. Lithium affection of thyroid function seems to be less frequent in countries where table salt is iodinated (Switzerland, Czechoslovakia), indicating that a marginal iodine intake may be a predisposing factor. Among other such factors may be mentioned previous thyroid disease such as Hashimoto thyroiditis.

Animal experiments provide further information about the effects of lithium on the thyroid. Chronic experiments have often provided different results from acute experiments and are probably of more clinical relevance. Under controlled conditions iodide transport, clearance, and overall uptake are unchanged or increased. Where such measurements are low, they tend to reflect toxic doses or damaged thyroid parenchyma. Formation of triiodothyronine and thyroxine may be normal or inhibited. Lithium consistently inhibits TSH-stimulated thyroid adenyl cyclase, but Berens & Wolff (18) regard it as unlikely that the effect of lithium is primarily on the TSH receptor. They consider secretion of hormone from the gland to be the major locus of the lithium effect and have succeeded in showing that the inhibition is exerted on the first step of the secretion mechanism, the engulfment of colloid droplets by pseudopods at the apical cell border protruding into the follicular lumen. Lithium prolongs the biological half-life of ^{131}I-labeled thyroxine (120, 124), an effect contrary to its other effects. It is noteworthy that lithium treatment of pregnant rats may affect thyroid function and iodine metabolism of the young and that these effects can persist even into adult life (125).

Thirst and Urine Flow

Lithium may produce primary polyuria with secondary polydipsia. It may also produce primary polydipsia. A direct stimulating effect on thirst has been demonstrated in rats after administration of a single intragastric or subcutaneous dose of lithium (126); this occurs in the absence of polyuria. The effect seems to be directly on the CNS since lateral hypothalamic lesions abolish the induction of primary polydipsia (127).

Primary polyuria with secondary polydipsia develops more gradually during lithium treatment and may be seen as a side effect during the clinical use of lithium. It can also be produced consistently in experimental animals (reviews: 128, 129). Lithium inhibits the response of the kidney to the antidiuretic hormone (19). Studies with addition of lithium in vitro (130) and, more significantly, studies in which lithium was administered to rats for some time before the kidneys were removed for enzyme assay (131) have demonstrated that there is inhibition of the vasopressin-induced rise of renal adenyl cyclase activity. The lithium effect seems to be an indirect one, because the inhibition occurs long after achievement of steady state lithium concentrations in kidney tissue, and because the lithium-induced inhibition is found after all measurable traces of lithium are washed away during preparation of the kidney particle fraction (132). Independence of the presence and concentration of lithium in the system has also been demonstrated in experiments dealing with vasopressin effects on toad bladder (133). Lithium also may inhibit at a site distal to the generation of cAMP, and which effect is the more important for the development of polyuria is being debated.

Lithium-induced polyuria is accompanied by histological changes in the distal nephron (134), but the glomerular filtration rate and lithium clearance remain unaltered (19). The condition seems to be fully reversible, but urine flow may not return to normal values until some time after discontinuation of lithium. Experiments with rats have shown that lithium-induced polyuria varies inversely with the potassium content of the food (25).

Cyclic AMP and Hormone Responses

Lithium inhibition of hormone-stimulated adenyl cyclase activity is not restricted to thyroid and kidney. Similar inhibitions have been demonstrated with norepinephrine in brain, ACTH in fat cells, luteinizing hormone in ovary, vasopressin in toad bladder, and prostaglandin E_1 in human platelets (review: 135). Most of the experiments were carried out in vitro and with high lithium concentrations, but in some studies lithium was administered to the animals before removal of the tissue for enzyme assay.

It does not seem a farfetched idea that lithium might produce a general lowering of all hormone responses that are mediated via cAMP. However, this assumption has not stood up to experimental testing. Lithium administration does not lower the renal response to parathyroid hormone, nor does it decrease the response to glucagon administration as measured by liver glycogen breakdown (17, 21). Lithium in fact enhances glucagon-stimulated excretion of cAMP (136).

Carbohydrate Metabolism

Lithium affects carbohydrate metabolism at several points: hexokinase activity, activation of liver adenyl cyclase and protein kinase, glycogen synthesis, pyruvate kinase activity (review: 137). Connection with lithium-induced weight gain as seen in some patients is possible.

Teratogenic Effects

Teratogenic effects of lithium have been demonstrated in mice and rats: cleft palate, external ear and eye defects. An increased frequency of malformations has been reported among children born of mothers who were given lithium during the first three months of the pregnancy: out of 150 such children 16 had malformations (138, 139; M.R. Weinstein, personal communication). This could be the result of more conscientious reporting of malformed children than of children without malformations, or it could be due to lithium teratogenicity. The latter assumption is supported by the observation that in 12 out of the 16 reported cases the malformations involved the heart and the great vessels. This increased relative frequency is unlikely to be due to biased information collection.

Interaction with Other Drugs

It has already been mentioned that prolonged administration of diuretics leads to lowering of the renal lithium clearance, that lithium lowers the responses to vasopressin and aldosterone, and that it interferes with a number of drug-induced changes of animal behavior. Lithium administration to rats and mice may alter the analgesic effects of codeine, dextropropoxyphene, glafenine, and morphine (71, 140–142); the effects of morphine and reserpine on body temperature (71, 141, 143); and amphetamine-induced euphoria in man (144, 145). Lithium administration to rats may induce drug-metabolizing enzyme activity (N-dealkylation) in liver (146). Combination treatment with haloperidol has led to neurotoxicity after administration of rather high haloperidol doses (147, 148). It may be inadvisable to combine lithium and methyldopa (149, 150).

CONCLUSIONS

The mode of action of lithium in manic-depressive disorder is as yet unknown, and it is difficult to decide which, if any, of the many known lithium effects are relevant to the clinical actions of the drug. Animal models of the endogenous psychoses do not exist, and information about alterations of brain metabolism in manic-depressive patients must be obtained indirectly. Lithium research has given a number of clues, but hypotheses have not always taken the dual action of lithium in manic-depressive disorder into account, and speculation about the biochemical mode of action often suffers from too ready incorporation of data that fit one's favorite hypothesis, regardless of the experimental conditions used to collect them. Selection of appropriate doses and concentrations, routes of administration, and duration of experiments are important for the provision of relevant information.

ACKNOWLEDGMENTS

The author thanks Drs. A. Amdisen, O. V. Olesen, D. F. Smith, and K. Thomsen for critical comments on the manuscript.

Literature Cited

1. Davis, J. M., Fann, W. E. 1971. *Ann. Rev. Pharmacol.* 11:285–302
2. Schou, M. 1957. *Pharmacol. Rev.* 9:17–58
3. Schou, M. 1973. *Biochem. Soc. Trans.* 1:81–87
4. Shopsin, B., Gershon, S. 1974. *Am. J. Med. Sci.* 268:306–23
5. Schou, M. 1969. *Psychopharmacol. Bull.* 5:33–62
6. Schou, M. 1972. *Psychopharmacol. Bull.* 8:36–62
7. Schou, M. 1975. *Psychopharmacol. Bull.* In press
8. Gershon, S., Shopsin, B., ed. 1973. *Lithium. Its Role in Psychiatric Research and Treatment.* New York: Plenum. 358 pp.
9. Johnson, F. N., ed. 1975. *Lithium Research and Therapy.* London: Academic. 569 pp.
10. Schou, M. 1976. In *Lithium in Psychiatry. A Synopsis,* ed. A. Villeneuve. Quebec: Presse Univ. Laval. In press
11. Mellerup, E. T., Jørgensen, O. S. 1975. See Ref. 9, 353–58
12. Johnson, S. 1975. See Ref. 9, 533–56
13. Corrodi, H., Fuxe, K., Hökfelt, T., Schou, M. 1967. *Psychopharmacologia* 11:345–53
14. Corrodi, H., Fuxe, K., Schou, M. 1969. *Life Sci.* 8:643–52
15. Genefke, I. K. 1972. *Acta Psychiatr. Scand.* 48:400–404
16. Plenge, P., Mellerup, E. T., Rafaelsen, O. J. 1970. *J. Psychiatr. Res.* 8:29–36
17. Olesen, O. V., Thomsen, K. 1974. *Acta Pharmacol. Toxicol.* 34:225–31
18. Berens, S. C., Wolff, J. 1975. See Ref. 9, 443–72
19. Thomsen, K. 1970. *Int. Pharmacopsychiatry* 5:233–41
20. Morrison, J. M., Pritchard, H. D., Braude, M. C., d'Aguanno, W. 1971. *Proc. Soc. Exp. Biol. Med.* 137:889–92
21. Olesen, O. V. 1975. In *Proc. IX Coll. Int. Neuro-Psychopharmacol.,* ed. J. R. Boissier, H. Hippius, P. Pichot, 629–32. Amsterdam: Excerpta Med.
22. Thomsen, K. 1973. *Acta Pharmacol. Toxicol.* 33:92–102
23. Thomsen, K., Jensen, J., Olesen, O. V. 1974. *Acta Pharmacol. Toxicol.* 35: 337–46
24. Thomsen, K., Olesen, O. V. 1974. *Int. Pharmacopsychiatry* 9:118–24
25. Olesen, O. V., Jensen, J., Thomsen, K. 1975. *Acta Pharmacol. Toxicol.* 36: 161–71
26. Amdisen, A. 1975. *Dan. Med. Bull.* 22:277–91
27. Amdisen, A. 1975. See Ref. 9, 197–210
28. Consbruch, U., Orth, M., Degkwitz, R. 1974. *Arzneim. Forsch.* 24:1077–79
29. Nieper, H. -A. 1973. *Agressologie* 14: 404–11
30. Greil, W., Schnelle, K., Seibold, S. 1974. *Arzneim. Forsch.* 24:1079–84
31. Greenspan, K. 1975. See Ref. 9, 281–86
32. Francis, R. I., Traill, M. A. 1970. *Lancet* II:523–24
33. Ebadi, M. S., Simmons, V. J., Hendrickson, M. J., Lacy, P. S. 1974. *Eur. J. Pharmacol.* 27:324–29
34. Bond, P. A., Brooks, B. A., Judd, A. 1975. *Br. J. Pharmacol.* 53:235–39
35. Christensen, S. 1974. *J. Neurochem.* 23:1299–1301
36. DeFeudis, F. V. 1972. *Brain Res.* 43:686–89
37. Birch, N. J., Hullin, R. P. 1972. *Life Sci.* 11:1095–99
38. Birch, N. J. 1974. *Clin. Sci. Mol. Med.* 46:409–13
39. Elizur, A., Shopsin, B., Gershon, S., Ehlenberger, A. 1972. *Clin. Pharmacol. Ther.* 13:947–52
40. Souček, K. et al 1974. *Act. Nerv. Super.* 16:193–94
41. Cazzullo, C. L., Smeraldi, E., Sacchetti, E., Bottinelli, S. 1975. *Br. J. Psychiatry* 126:298–300
42. Mendels, J. 1975. See Ref. 9, 43–62
43. Mendels, J., Frazer, A. 1974. *Am. J. Psychiatry* 131:1240–46
44. Dorus, E., Pandey, G. N., Frazer, A., Mendels, J. 1974. *Arch. Gen. Psychiatry* 31:463–65
45. Schless, A. P., Frazer, A., Mendels, J., Pandey, G. N., Theodorides, V. J. 1975. *Arch. Gen. Psychiatry* 32:337–40
46. Rybakowski, J. et al 1974. *Int. Pharmacopsychiatry* 9:166–71
47. Schou, M., Amdisen, A. 1975. *Am. J. Obstet. Gynecol.* 122:541
48. Schou, M., Amdisen, A. 1973. *Br. Med. J.* 2:138
49. Geisler, A., Schou, M., Thomsen, K. 1971. *Pharmakopsychiatrie* 4:149–55
50. Söderberg, U. 1974. *Nord. Psykiatr. Tidsskr.* 28:473–75
51. Thomsen, K., Schou, M. 1968. *Am. J. Physiol.* 215:823–27
52. Thomsen, K., Schou, M. 1973. *Pharmakopsychiatrie* 6:264–69
53. Petersen, V., Hvidt, S., Thomsen, K., Schou, M. 1974. *Br. Med. J.* 3:143–45

242   SCHOU

54. Thomsen, K., Olesen, O. V., Jensen, J., Schou, M. 1976. In *Current Developments in Psychopharmacology,* ed. L. Valzelli, W. B. Essman. New York: Spectrum. In press
55. Thomsen, K., Schou, M. 1975. See Ref. 9, 227–36
56. Schou, M., Amdisen, A., Steenstrup, O. R. 1973. *Br. Med. J.* 2:137–38
57. Zvolsky, P., Krulík, R. 1972. *Act. Ner. Super.* 14:207–9
58. Smith, D. F. 1973. *Int. Pharmacopsychiatry* 8:99–103
59. Smith, D. F. 1973. *Int. Pharmacopsychiatry* 8:217–20
60. Smith, D. F., de Jong, W. 1975. *Pharmakopsychiatrie* 8:132–35
61. Johnson, F. N. 1975. See Ref. 9, 315–37
62. Johnson, F. N. 1975. See Ref. 9, 339–50
63. Smith, D. F., Smith, H. B. 1973. *Psychopharmacologia* 30:83–88
64. Sanger, D. J., Steinberg, H. 1974. *Eur. J. Pharmacol.* 28:344–49
65. Tomkiewicz, M., Steinberg, H. 1974. *Nature London* 252:227–29
66. Furukawa, T., Ushizima, I., Ono, N. 1975. *Psychopharmacologia* 42:243–48
67. Judd, A., Parker, J., Jenner, F. A. 1975. *Psychopharmacologia* 42:73–77
68. Segal, D. S., Callaghan, M., Mandell, A. J. 1975. *Nature London* 254:58–59
69. Matussek, N., Linsmayer, M. 1968. *Life Sci.* 7:371–76
70. Lal, S., Sourkes, T. L. 1972. *Arch. Int. Pharmacodyn.* 199:289–301
71. Jensen, J. 1974. *Acta Pharmacol. Toxicol.* 35:395–402
72. Smith, D. F. 1975. *Psychopharmacologia* 41:295–300
73. Davies, C., Sanger, D. J., Steinberg, H., Tomkiewicz, M., U'Prichard, D. C. 1974. *Psychopharmacologia* 36:263–74
74. Matussek, N. 1971. *Int. Pharmacopsychiatry* 6:170–86
75. Grahame-Smith, D. G., Green, A. R. 1974. *Br. J. Pharmacol.* 52:19–26
76. Segawa, T., Nakano, M. 1974. *Jpn. J. Pharmacol.* 24:319–24
77. Schou, M., Amdisen, A., Thomsen, K. 1968. In *De Psychiatria Progrediente,* ed. P. Baudiš, E. Peterová, V. Šedivec, II: 712–21. Plzen
78. Small, J. G., Milstein, V., Perez, H. C., Small, I. F., Moore, D. F. 1972. *Biol. Psychiatry* 5:65–77
79. Linnoila, M., Saario, I., Maki, M. 1974. *Eur. J. Clin. Pharmacol.* 7:337–43
80. Bech, P. Rafaelsen, O. J., Thomsen, J., Theilgaard, A. March 1975. Simuleret bilkørsel: Virkning af phenemal, phenytoin og lithium efter langtidsdosering. Presented at Meet. Scand. Psychopharmacol. Soc., Copenhagen
81. Aminoff, M. J., Marshall, J., Smith, E., Wyke, M. 1974. *Br. J. Psychiatry* 125:109–10
82. Marshall, M. H., Neumann, C. P., Robinson, M. 1970. *Psychosomatics* 11:406–8
83. Polatin, P., Fieve, R. R. 1971. *J. Am. Med. Assoc.* 218:864–66
84. Schou, M., Baastrup, P. C. 1973. In *Psychopharmacology, Sexual Disorders and Drug Abuse,* ed. T. A. Ban et al, 65–68. Prague: Avicenum
85. Himmelhoch, J. M., Hanin, I. 1974. *Br. Med. J.* 4:233
86. Shaw, D. M. 1975. See Ref. 9, 411–23
87. Genefke, I. K. 1972. *Acta Psychiatr. Scand.* 48:394–99
88. Schubert, J. 1973. *Psychopharmacologia* 32:301–11
89. Bockar, J., Roth, R., Heninger, G. 1974. *Life Sci.* 15:2109–18
90. Iwata, H., Okamoto, H., Kuramoto, I. 1974. *Jpn. J. Pharmacol.* 24:235–40
91. Beckmann, H., St.-Laurent, J., Goodwin, F. K. 1975. *Psychopharmacologia* 42:277–82
92. Knapp, S., Mandell, A. J. 1975. *J. Pharmacol. Exp. Ther.* 193:812–23
93. Vizi, E. S. 1975. See Ref. 9, 391–410
94. Gottesfeld, Z., Samuel, D., Icekson, I. 1973. *Experientia* 29:68–69
95. Small, J. G., Small, I. F. 1973. See Ref. 8, 83–106
96. Dimitrakoudi, M., Jenner, F. A. 1975. See Ref. 9, 507–18
97. Zabrowska-Dabrowska, T., Rybakowski, J. 1973. *Acta Psychiatr. Scand.* 49:457–65
98. Reilly, E., Halmi, K. A., Noyes, R. Jr. 1973. *Int. Pharmacopsychiatry* 8:208–13
99. Pinelli, P., Tonali, P., Scoppetta, C. 1972. *Arch. Psicol. Neurol. Psichiatr.* 33:497–508
100. Girke, W., Krebs, F. -A., Müller-Oerlinghausen, B. 1975. *Int. Pharmacopsychiatr.* 10:24–36
101. Kirk, L., Baastrup, P. C., Schou, M. 1973. *Lancet* II:1086–87
102. Floru, L., Floru, L., Tegeler, J. 1974. *Arzneim. Forsch.* 24:1122–25
103. Schou, M. 1962. *Acta Psychiatr. Scand.* 38:331–36
104. Demers, R. G., Heninger, G. 1970. *Dis. Nerv. Syst.* 31:674–79
105. Rask-Madsen, J., Baastrup, P. C., Schwartz, M. 1972. *Br. Med. J.* 2:496–98

106. Peet, M. 1975. *Br. J. Psychiatr.* 127:144–48
107. Baer, L. 1973. See Ref. 8, 33–49
108. Hullin, R. P. 1975. See Ref. 9, 359–79
109. Birch, N. J., Jenner, F. A. 1973. *Br. J. Pharmacol.* 47:586–95
110. Bjørum, N., Hornum, I., Mellerup, E. T., Plenge, P. K., Rafaelsen, O. J. 1975. *Lancet* I:1243
111. Crammer, J. 1975. *Lancet* I:215–16
112. Andreoli, V. M., Villani, F., Brambilla, G. 1972. *Psychopharmacologia* 25:77–85
113. Nielsen, J. 1964. *Acta Psychiatr. Scand.* 40:190–96
114. Vendsborg, P. B., Mellerup, E. T., Rafaelsen, O. J. 1973. *Acta Psychiatr. Scand.* 49:97–103
115. Carman, J. S., Post, R. M., Teplitz, T. A., Goodwin, F. K. 1974. *Lancet* II:1454
116. Schou, M., Amdisen, A., Jensen, S. E., Olsen, T. 1968. *Br. Med. J.* 3:710–13
117. Sedvall, G., Jönsson, B., Pettersson, U., Levin, K. 1968. *Life Sci.* 7:1257–64
118. Wolff, J. 1975. See Ref. 21, 621–28
119. Spaulding, S. W., Burrow, G. N., Bermudez, F., Himmelhoch, J. M. 1972. *J. Clin. Endocrinol.* 35:905–11
120. Temple, R., Berman, M., Robbins, J., Wolff, J. 1972. *J. Clin. Invest.* 51:2746–56
121. Gerdes, H., Littmann, K. -P., Joseph, K., Mahlstedt, J. 1973. *Dtsch. Med. Wochenschr.* 98:1551–54
122. Brière, J., Pousset, G., Darsy, P., Guinet, P. 1974. *Ann. Endocrinol.* 35:281–82
123. Lazarus, J. H., Richards, A. R., Addison, G. M., Owen, G. M. 1974. *Lancet* II:1160–63
124. Ohlin, G., Söderberg, U. 1970. *Acta Physiol. Scand.* 79:24A–25A
125. Söderberg, U. 1973. *Nord. Psykiatr. Tidsskr.* 27:414–19
126. Smith, D. F., Balagura, S., Lubran, M. 1970. *Science* 167:297–98
127. Smith, D. F., Balagura, S., Lubran, M. 1971. *Physiol. Behav.* 6:209–14
128. Singer, I., Rotenberg, D. 1973. *N. Engl. J. Med.* 289:254–60
129. MacNeil, S., Jenner, F. A. 1975. See Ref. 9, 473–84
130. Douša, T., Hechter, O. 1970. *Life Sci.* 9:765–70
131. Geisler, A., Wraae, O., Olesen, O. V. 1972. *Acta Pharmacol. Toxicol.* 31:203–8
132. Wraae, O., Geisler, A., Olesen, O. V. 1972. *Acta Pharmacol. Toxicol.* 31:314–17
133. Harris, C. A., Jenner, F. A. 1972. *Br. J. Pharmacol.* 44:223–32
134. Lindop, G. B. M., Padfield, P. L. 1975. *J. Clin. Pathol.* 28:472–75
135. Forn, J. 1975. See Ref.9, 485–97
136. Olesen, O. V., Jensen, J., Thomsen, K. 1974. *Acta Pharmacol. Toxicol.* 35:403–11
137. Mellerup, E. T., Rafaelsen, O. J. 1975. See Ref. 9, 381–89
138. Schou, M., Goldfield, M. D., Weinstein, M. R., Villeneuve, A. 1973. *Br. Med. J.* 2:135–36
139. Weinstein, M. R., Goldfield, M. D. 1975. *Am. J. Psychiatry* 132:529–31
140. Weischer, M.-L., Opitz, K. 1970. *Arzneim. Forsch.* 20:1046–48
141. Tulunay, F. C., Kiran, B. K., Kaymakcalan, S. 1971. *Acta Med. Turc.* 8:51–60
142. Männistö, P. T., Saarnivaara, L. 1973. *Pharmacology* 8:329–35
143. Perkinson, E., Ruckart, R., DaVanzo, J. P. 1969. *Proc. Soc. Exp. Biol. Med.* 131:685–89
144. Flemenbaum, A. 1974. *Am. J. Psychiatry* 131:820–21
145. Kammen, D. P., van, Murphy, D. L. 1974. *Am. J. Psychiatry* 131:1414
146. Parmar, S. S., Ali, B., Spencer, H. W., Auyong, T. K. 1974. *Res. Commun. Chem. Pathol. Pharmacol.* 7:633–36
147. Marhold, J., Zimanová, J., Lachman, M., Král, J., Vojtechovsky, M. 1974. *Act. Nerv. Super.* 16:199–200
148. Cohen, W. J., Cohen, N. H. 1974. *J. Am. Med. Assoc.* 230:1283–87
149. Byrd, G. J. 1975. *J. Am. Med. Assoc.* 233:320
150. Gershon, S. 1975. *Drug Ther.* 5:141–43

IDENTIFICATION AND EFFECTS ❖6649
OF NEURAL TRANSMITTERS
IN INVERTEBRATES

JacSue Kehoe and Eve Marder
Laboratoire de Neurobiologie, Ecole Normale Supérieure, Paris 5, France

INTRODUCTION

This review treats almost exclusively of investigations that have been published over the last three years (for work prior to that period see 1). Preference is given to data obtained from identified neurons, in particular, from neurons for which the transmitter has been evaluated biochemically as well as electrophysiologically and pharmacologically. Finally, only those synaptic studies that deal directly with the problems of transmitter pharmacology have been considered.

The first half of this review deals with recent advances in single-cell neurochemistry. Biochemical and histochemical work concerned with the identification of transmitters in identified neurons is summarized in Table 1, and is followed by a brief consideration of some issues raised by the table and by other recent work in this field. The second half of this review covers electrophysiological and pharmacological studies that clarify the role of transmitters or putative transmitters at some identified junctions, giving preferential treatment to experimental preparations and problems that have received rather extensive attention.

NEUROCHEMISTRY

One of the major advances in the field of invertebrate neurochemistry is the development of sophisticated techniques for the measurement of putative transmitter substances in single identified neurons. These techniques have been used for two main purposes: (a) to identify transmitter candidates, and (b) to study the dynamic aspects of transmitter synthesis, mobilization, storage, and release in identified neurons. These techniques have been used to determine endogenous levels (in picomole quantities) of γ-aminobutyric acid (GABA) (2), dopamine (3), acetylcholine (ACh) (4), octopamine (5), histamine (6, 7), glutamate (2, 8), and serotonin (5-HT)

245

(3, 7). In addition, the enzymes responsible for the biosynthesis of putative transmitters can be assayed, either directly [(choline acetyltransferase (9–12), aromatic amino acid decarboxylase (13–15), or glutamic acid decarboxylase (16–19)] or indirectly by measuring the incorporation of radioactive precursors into putative transmitters, using uptake from the bath (20, 21), or by injecting radioactively labeled precursors into neuronal somata (22, 23) or axons (24).

Much recent work has been done on the characterization of transmitter biosynthetic enzymes in invertebrate nervous tissue (9, 11–13, 17, 25–27) and on the measurement of endogenous levels of putative transmitters in ganglia and connectives of many animals (3, 4, 6, 11, 28–32). The emphasis of this review is on single cells, and Table 1 is a summary of presently available biochemical and histochemical evidence on identified neurons.

In the past, biochemical analyses have focused on finding neurons that contain considerably higher concentrations of a putative transmitter than do other neurons (1, 2, 4, 61). This approach remains valuable for suggesting new transmitter candidates and has brought histamine and octopamine into consideration as possible transmitters in invertebrate neurons. Weinreich, Weiner & McCaman (6) assayed histamine in single *Aplysia* neurons and found that although there were low levels of histamine in several of the neurons they assayed, two cerebral ganglia neurons contained considerably higher histamine concentrations. These neurons are promising candidates for histamine-releasing neurons, and this information facilitates a physiological search for a histamine-mediated monosynaptic connection. Likewise, octopamine-containing neurons have been found in *Aplysia* ganglia (5) and in the second root of the thoracic connective in *Homarus* (66) (see last section of this paper for a discussion of the currently available literature concerning octopamine function in arthropod systems).

Examination of Table 1 shows that in single neurons whose transmitter is known or suspected low quantities of many other putative transmitters can be detected. For example, R2 in *Aplysia* contains about 25 pmol of ACh (4) (thought to be its transmitter) but also contains about 0.15 pmol of histamine (6) and 0.43 pmol of octopamine (5). This is no new phenomenon. For example, Kravitz & Potter (61) found low levels of GABA in sensory and excitatory axons in *Homarus*. In this and other similar cases the concentration of the putative transmitter substance in the neurons thought to employ it as a transmitter was about 100-fold higher than in the neurons not thought to use it as transmitter.

Two recent studies have sought to refocus our attention on these low levels of multiple transmitter molecules. Hanley et al (58) report that the metacerebral giant cell in *Helix*, which uses 5-HT as a transmitter, also contains significant choline acetyltransferase activity. Hanley & Cottrell (57) found 0.1 ng of ACh in the soma of the metacerebral cell, which also contains about 1.0 ng of 5-HT. Brownstein et al (7) present measurements of many transmitter substances in several *Aplysia* neurons.

Two questions can be raised about these low levels of multiple putative transmitter substances. First, are they possibly experimental artifacts? Virtually all of this work has been done on hand-dissected neurons, which certainly contain an un-

Table 1 Single cell transmitter chemistry[a, b]

Animal	Cell	Suspected transmitter	Substance assayed	Amount per cell	Concentration	Biosynthetic capability	Physiological corroboration
Leech	retzius	5-HT	5-HT	3.8×10^{-10} g (34)	6.0 mM (34)	AAD—25.6 pmol DA/cell/hr (14)	(35)
			5-HT	2.5 pmol (3)		incorporation of ^{14}C-trp and ^{14}C-5-HTP into ^{14}C-5-HT (20)	
Aplysia	R2	ACh	ACh	25.7 pmol (4)	0.39 mM (4)	ChAc—2.11 nmol ACh/cell/hr (4)	
			choline	11.0 pmol (4)		ChAc—3.0 nmol ACh/cell/hr (9)	
						~ 80% conversion of injected ^{3}H-choline to ^{3}H-ACh (22–24, 36)	
			oct	0.43 pmol (5)	0.0025 mM (5)	AAD—440 pmol DA/cell/hr (13)	
			5-HT		0.018 mM (7)	1.4% conversion of injected ^{3}H-5-HTP to ^{3}H-5-HT (37)	
			HA	0.15 pmol (6)	0.002 mM (6)		
					0.003 mM (7)		
			asp	1746 pmol (38)	25.0 mM (38)		
			glu	86 μmol/gprot (8)			
			gln	39 μmol/gprot (8)			
Aplysia	R14	?	oct	3.66 pmol (5)	0.15 mM (5)	AAD—144.7 pmol DA/cell/hr (13)	
			HA	0.12 pmol (6)	0.005 mM (6)		
			HA		0.007 mM (7)		
			5-HT		0.034 mM (7)		
			asp	586 pmol (38)	27.0 mM (38)		
			glu	34 μmol/gprot (8)			
			gln	21 μmol/gprot (8)			
Aplysia	R15	?	asp	833 pmol (38)	47.0 mM (38)	AAD—520 pmol DA/cell/hr (13)	
			glu	64 μmol/gprot (8)			
			gln	24 μmol/gprot (8)			

Table 1 *(Continued)*

Animal	Cell	Suspected transmitter	Substance assayed	Amount per cell	Concentration	Biosynthetic capability	Physiological corroboration
Aplysia	L2-L6	?	oct asp glu gln	1.04 pmol (5) 1152 pmol (38) 44 μmol/gprot (8) 24 μmol/gprot (8)	0.046 mM (5) 28.0 mM (38)	AAD—152-369 pmol DA/cell/hr (13)	
Aplysia	L7	?	oct asp glu gln	1.46 pmol (5) 771 pmol (38) 94 μmol/gprot (8) 32 μmol/gprot (8)	0.065 mM (5) 34.0 mM (38)	AAD—135.8 pmol DA/cell/hr (13)	(39)
Aplysia	L10	ACh	ACh choline oct	3.8 pmol (4) 9.9 pmol (4) 0.11 pmol (5)	0.35 mM (4) 0.014 mM (5)	ChAc—2.16 nmol ACh/cell/hr (4) ChAc—1.8 nmol ACh/cell/hr (9) 85% conversion of injected ^{3}H-choline to ^{3}H-ACh (23, 41) firing-dependent, Ca^{2+} dependent release of radioactivity after ^{3}H-choline (41) AAD—218 pmol DA/cell/hr (13)	(42-44)
Aplysia	L11	ACh	ACh choline oct 5-HT HA asp glu gln	6.2 pmol (4) 13.3 pmol (4) 1.6 pmol (5) 1237 pmol (38) 65 μmol/gprot (8) 23 μmol/gprot (8)	0.33 mM (4) 0.009 mM (5) 0.011 mM (7) 0.005 mM (7) 44.0 mM (38)	ChAc—1.8 nmol ACh/cell/hr (4) ChAc—2.0 nmol ACh/cell/hr (9) 71% conversion of injected ^{3}H-choline to ^{3}H-ACh (23) AAD—279 pmol DA/cell/hr (13)	

Table 1 *(Continued)*

Aplysia	L13	?	oct	0.19 pmol (5)	0.023 mM (5)		
Aplysia	LD	ACh				84% conversion of injected ^{3}H-choline to ^{3}H-ACh (23)	
Aplysia	LDG$_1$	ACh				ChAc—630 pmol ACh/cell/hr (39) 86% conversion of injected ^{3}H-choline to ^{3}H-ACh (39)	(39)
Aplysia	LD$_{HI}$	ACh				82.5% conversion of injected ^{3}H-choline to ^{3}H-ACh (45)	(45, 46)
Aplysia	LB$_{VC}$	ACh				78% conversion of injected ^{3}H-choline to ^{3}H-ACh (45)	(45, 46)
Aplysia	RB	5-HT				9.7% conversion of injected ^{3}H-trp to ^{3}H-5-HT (23) 18.6% conversion of injected ^{3}H-5-HTP to ^{3}H-5-HT (37)	
Aplysia	RB$_{HE}$	5-HT				7.8% conversion of injected ^{3}H-trp to ^{3}H-5-HT (45)	(45, 46)
Aplysia	LPGC (left pleural giant)	ACh	ACh choline asp glu gln	30 pmol (4) 10.2 pmol (4) 2597 pmol (38) 66 μmol/gprot (8) 42 μmol/gprot (8)	0.34 mM (4) 0.34 mM (38)	ChAc—1.7 nmol ACh/cell/hr (4) ChAc—2.8 nmol ACh/cell/hr (9) AAD—180 pmol DA/cell/hr (13)	

Table 1 *(Continued)*

Animal	Cell	Suspected transmitter	Substance assayed	Amount per cell	Concentration	Biosynthetic capability	Physiological corroboration
Aplysia	LC2	?	HA	1.68 pmol (6)	0.476 mM (6)		
Aplysia	RC2	?	HA	0.99 pmol (6)	0.309 mM (6)		
Aplysia	C-1 (GCN)	5-HT	5-HT	6.2 pmol (47)	0.94 mM (7)	AAD—2.3 nmol DA/cell/hr (47)	(48)
			5-HT			2.3% conversion of injected ^{3}H-trp to ^{3}H-5-HT (23)	
						24.7% conversion of injected ^{3}H-5-HTP to ^{3}H-5-HT (37)	
			HA	0.18 pmol (6)	0.012 mM (6)		
			HA		0.014 mM (7)		
			asp	365 pmol (38)	34 mM (38)		
			glu	36 µmol/gprot (8)			
			gln	25 µmol/gprot (8)			
Aplysia	buccal cells	?	oct	0.09–1.3 pmol (5)	0.012–0.39 mM (5)		
			asp	300–520 pmol (38)	49–90 mM (38)		
Tritonia	C-1	5-HT	5-HT	4.0 pmol (47)		AAD—620 pmol DA/cell/hr (47)	
Tritonia	PD-1	5-HT	5-HT	4.2 pmol (47)		AAD—377 pmol DA/cell/hr (47)	
Planorbis	left pedal giant neuron	DA	DA	5.4 pmol (49) fluorescence histochemistry (50)		synthesis of ^{3}H-DA from ^{3}H-tyr (51)	(52)
Planorbis	GSC	5-HT	5-HT	fluorescence histochemistry (50)			

Table 1 *(Continued)*

						(54)
Helix	GSC (metacerebral giant)	5-HT	5-HT	fluorescence histochemistry (53); 1.1 ng (56)	AAD—21 pmol DA/cell/hr (15); synthesis of ^{14}C-5-HT from ^{14}C-5-HTP (56); AAD—26 pmol DA/cell/hr (58); ChAc—20-22 pmol ACh/cell/hr (58)	
			ACh	0.1 ng (57)		
Helix	buccal 0–6	?			ChAc—18-31 pmol ACh/cell/hr (15)	
Helix	buccal 1, 2				AAD—11 pmol DA/cell/hr (15)	
Helix	cerebral 7–12	?			ChAc—9-26 pmol ACh/cell/hr (15)	
Helix	p. visceral 13–26	?			ChAc—22-99 pmol/ ACh/cell/hr (15)	
Helix	p. visceral 5–14				AAD—9-52 pmol DA/cell/hr (15)	
Helix	pedal 27–36	?			ChAc—11-127 pmol ACh/cell/hr (15)	
Helix	pedal 15–20				AAD—8-24 pmol DA/cell/hr (15)	
Schistocerca	common inhibitor	GABA			GAD—12.9 pmol GABA/cell/hr (19)	
Chortoicetes	common inhibitor	GABA			GAD—14.4 pmol GABA/cell/hr (19)	
Chortoicetes	anterior inhibitor	GABA			GAD—19.3 pmol GABA/cell/hr (19)	
Chortoicetes	posterior inhibitor	GABA			GAD—22.5 pmol GABA/cell/hr (19)	

Table 1 *(Continued)*

Animal	Cell	Suspected transmitter	Substance assayed	Amount per cell	Concentration	Biosynthetic capability	Physiological corroboration
Romalae	DUMETI	oct				synthesis of ³H-oct from ³H-tyr (59)	(60)
Homarus	12	GABA	GABA	79 pmol (2)	13.4 mM (2)	¹⁴C-GABA synthesized from ¹⁴C-glu (20)	
			glu	103 pmol (2)	14.9 mM (2)		
Homarus	11	GABA	GABA	27 pmol (2)			(110) stimulation-produced release of GABA (40)
Homarus	13	GABA	GABA	44 pmol (2)	14.6 mM (2)		
			glu	96 pmol (2)	20.6 mM (2)		
Homarus	inhibitor, opener crusher claw	GABA					stimulation-produced release of GABA (40)
Homarus	inhibitor, opener cutter claw	GABA					stimulation-produced release of GABA (40)
Homarus	inhibitor, walking leg opener	GABA	GABA	1.4 nmol/cm axon (61)	99 mM (61)		
Homarus	inhibitor, walking leg closer	GABA	GABA GABA glu asp	1.5 nmol/cm axon (61)	110 mM (61) 49.5 mM (55) 31.5 mM (55) 149.5 mM (55)	GAD—90 pmol GABA/cm axon/hr (18)	
Homarus	inhibitor, walking leg flexor	GABA	GABA	0.22 nmol/cm axon (61)	108 mM (61)		

Table 1 *(Continued)*

Homarus	M6/M7	glu	glu	85 pmol (2)	18.3 mM (2)	
Homarus	excitor, walking leg opener	glu	GABA glu asp	90 pmol/cm axon (61)	0.64 mM (61) 41.6 mM (55) 131.9 mM (55)	
Homarus	large excitor, closer walking leg	glu	GABA	20 pmol/cm axon (61)	0.83 mM (61)	
Homarus	small excitor, closer walking leg	glu	GABA	6.9 pmol/cm axon (61)	0.58 mM (61)	
Homarus	large excitor, walking leg bender	glu	GABA	14 pmol/cm axon (61)	1.0 mM (61)	
Homarus	small excitor, walking leg bender	glu	GABA	9.5 pmol/cm axon (61)	0.88 mM (61)	
Homarus	abdominal stretch receptors	ACh	ACh	1.9 pmol/μg prot (11) 2.9 pmol/cm axon (11)	0.4–0.6 mM (11)	ACh synthesis (20) ChAc—17.1 pmol ACh/cm axon/hr (21, 11) (21)
Homarus	medial giant fibers	?	GABA	40 pmol/cm axon (61)	0.68 mM (61)	
Homarus	lateral giant fibers	?	GABA	50 pmol/cm axon (61)	0.59 mM (61)	
Homarus	thoracic ganglion 2nd root cells	oct	oct	~10 pmol (66)	~0.1 mM (66)	biosynthesis from 3H-tyrosine and 3H-tyramine (66), high K+ induced 3H-oct efflux (67)

Table 1 *(Continued)*

Animal	Cell	Suspected transmitter	Substance assayed	Amount per cell	Concentration	Biosynthetic capability	Physiological corroboration
Panulirus	large commissural ganglion cell	DA	DA	fluorescence histochemistry (63)	³H-DA synthesis from ³H-tyr (63)		
Panulirus	stomatogastric motor neurons PD, VD, GM, LPG	ACh				ChAc—5-30 pmol ACh/cell/hr (65)	(64, 65)
Carcinus	large commissural ganglion cell	DA	DA	fluorescence histochemistry (62)			
Cancer	pooled walking leg excitors	glu	glu asp GABA		53 mM (31) 196 mM (31) 3.1 mM (31)		
Cancer	pooled walking leg inhibitors	GABA	GABA glu asp		46 mM (31) 47 mM (31) 168 mM (31)		

[a] In the interests of brevity, results of assays that were negative were omitted, although they would in some cases have added interesting information.
[b] Abbreviations used in this table: AAD, aromatic amino acid decarboxylase; ACh, acetylcholine; asp, aspartate; ChAc, choline acetyltransferase; DA, dopamine; GABA, γ-aminobutyric acid; GAD, glutamic acid decarboxylase; gln, glutamine; glu, glutamate; HA, histamine; 5-HTP, 5-hydroxytryptophan; oct, octopamine; tyr, tyrosine; trp, tryptophan. Abbreviations used in the name of cell column are those used by the quoted authors.

known amount of glial and likely even neuronal contamination. With increasingly sensitive assays, the small amounts of substances contributed by contaminating tissue become more significant. In injection studies, leakage could be a problem. Second, even if low levels of substances are actually present in the neurons involved, are they physiologically significant? Phrased differently, this question asks, how useful are biochemical techniques alone for transmitter identification? In reference to the work of Hanley et al (57, 58) the transmitter function of 5-HT has been confirmed by physiological studies (54) (see later section of this paper) whereas the ACh reported in this cell has not yet been shown to be utilized in a monosynaptic connection made by this neuron. These data point out the caution that must be exercised when drawing conclusions from biochemical data alone, and stress the importance of combining physiological and biochemical techniques for transmitter identification.

A further examination of Table 1 shows that somata transmitter concentrations vary from about 0.3 mM for the large ACh-containing neurons of *Aplysia* (4) to about 15 mM for the large GABA-containing neurons of *Homarus* (2). The axonal concentrations of GABA in the latter cells are even higher: about 100 mM (61). It is interesting that the axons of the assayed excitatory motor neurons of lobster had GABA concentrations of almost 1 mM (61) i.e. a concentration higher than that of ACh in cholinergic cells [e.g. molluscan somata (4) or the *Homarus* stretch receptor axons (11)]. Thus it appears that the absolute concentration of these substances is not a useful indicator of transmitter function unless extensive data on other cells and other transmitters are available for comparison.

Aromatic amino acid decarboxylase (AAD) is involved in the biosynthesis of dopamine, octopamine, and 5-HT in invertebrate nervous tissue. However, Weinreich, Dewhurst & McCaman (13) showed that all *Aplysia* cells assayed contained significant levels of AAD. This fact was exploited by Goldman & Schwartz (37) in an interesting attempt to study the specificity of transmitter packaging and storage in cholinergic and serotoninergic neurons in *Aplysia*. These authors found that after injecting ^{3}H-5-HTP, the immediate precursor of 5-HT and substrate for aromatic amino acid decarboxylase, they detected significant amounts of 5-HT in the cholinergic neuron R2. However, they found that whereas the ^{3}H-5-HT formed in serotonin-containing neurons was transported into the axon, and was associated with particulate fractions (presumably synaptic vesicles), the ^{3}H-5-HT formed in R2 was apparently not packaged and transported. From these data the authors argued that in addition to specificity in transmitter biosynthetic capability there is also specificity in packaging and transport mechanisms. It would have been interesting to have the results of a similar experiment done on a cholinergic neuron that had been depleted of ACh, by one means or another, to determine whether the cholinergic neuron was capable of storing and transporting 5-HT under conditions where ACh was not present and synthesized.

Biochemical techniques have been used to study two additional processes directly involved in synaptic transmission: (*a*) release of the transmitter, and (*b*) uptake of both transmitter precursors and of the transmitters themselves as a mechanism of terminating the action of a synaptically released transmitter.

Demonstration of release of a given substance by synaptic activity is the most convincing proof that a substance is the neurotransmitter at a given junction, and this proof is most important for synapses where the suspected transmitter is a ubiquitous molecule, such as L-glutamate. Unfortunately, little new evidence has been forthcoming in this area since that reported and reviewed by Kravitz et al (68). The difficulty in obtaining such data is shown by the work of Koike et al (41) who injected ^{3}H-choline into L10, a known cholinergic neuron in *Aplysia* and then attempted to recover ^{3}H-ACh in amounts proportional to synaptic activity. The authors were able to demonstrate that released radioactivity is dependent on firing frequency and external calcium concentration, but were unable to recover the radioactivity as ACh, apparently because the acetylcholinesterase was incompletely blocked.

Thorough and interesting studies of uptake in invertebrate systems in recent years have been those by Evans on L-glutamate uptake in arthropod nervous tissue (69–71) and that by Schwartz et al (33) and Eisenstadt et al (72) on choline uptake and metabolism in *Aplysia* nervous tissue.

Schwartz et al (33) showed that choline uptake has two kinetic components: a high affinity uptake system with a K_m of about 2–8 μM and a low affinity system that does not saturate at 420 μM. Eisenstadt & Schwartz (36) followed this work with a very interesting study of ACh metabolism in R2 of *Aplysia*. They showed that choline concentrations in the soma limit the amount of somatic ACh synthesis, and that the proportion of radioactivity incorporated into ACh from choline is much greater when ^{3}H-choline is injected into the soma rather than taken up from the bath. Furthermore, the authors were able to measure the kinetics of ACh synthesis within the intact neuron, and found that their values were similar to those previously obtained for choline acetyltransferase in homogenates of *Aplysia* nervous tissue. Perhaps most disturbing of all for those who are using incorporation of radioactive precursors from the bath to study transmitter synthesis and mobilization, these authors found that ACh formed from choline in the bath turned over at a different rate from that formed from injected choline, which suggests that there are two pools of ACh within these neurons; one pool preferentially labeled when the choline enters the cell either by high affinity uptake or injection, and the other when the choline enters the cell by low affinity uptake. Under conditions of bath incubation the amount of choline entering the cell by low affinity uptake is considerable; if this situation is general, these considerations complicate the interpretation of experiments using bath-applied precursors.

GANGLIONIC SYNAPTIC TRANSMISSION IN INVERTEBRATES

Gastropod central neurons that, because of their large size, are so amenable to single-cell neurochemistry, have also proven to be a particularly satisfactory preparation for the study of receptor pharmacology and synaptic transmission. This experimental preparation has become even more valuable in recent years because of the identification of pairs of monosynaptically connected neurons, and, in some cases, because of the identification of the transmitter used at the synapses made between these neuron pairs.

Acetylcholine

The analysis of the effects of ACh on gastropod neurons first revealed the complexity that seems to be typical of transmitter receptor systems in invertebrate ganglia (see 1, 77 for detailed and documented accounts). ACh, whether applied iontophoretically or released by activation of cholinergic neurons, was shown to elicit many different types of response. The response variety was shown to be due to the existence of three pharmacologically distinct ACh receptors, each of which mediates a selective change in membrane permeability. One receptor type mediates an increase in membrane permeability to Na (thereby causing an excitatory potential when activated); two others mediate inhibitory responses—one, resulting from an increase in permeability to Cl; the other, to K. These different receptor types have been shown to coexist on the same cell membrane, and, in such cases, ACh (whether applied synaptically or iontophoretically) elicits multicomponent responses.

A pharmacological comparison (see 77, 78) of the three types of ACh receptor on molluscan neurons with cholinergic receptors previously described in other neural tissues suggests that the molluscan receptor that mediates the increase in Na permeability most resembles the vertebrate receptor mediating the rapid excitatory postsynaptic potential (EPSP) of the sympathetic ganglion cells (both are blocked, for example, by hexamethonium as well as by curare). The molluscan receptor mediating the Cl-dependent inhibition, on the other hand, most resembles the receptor of the frog skeletal muscle (which, itself, mediates increases in Na and K permeabilities). These two receptors are much more sensitive to curare than to hexamethonium, this latter compound being completely without effect on the molluscan receptor mediating the Cl response.

The above two comparisons have recently been reinforced by findings with α-bungarotoxin (*B. multicinctus*) (78). This toxin has been shown to block quasi-irreversibly the frog end-plate potential, but to be ineffective in blocking the rapid EPSP (hexamethonium-sensitive) of the sympathetic ganglion. In *Aplysia* the same toxin was found to block the receptor mediating the Cl-dependent response (hexamethonium-insensitive) while having no effect on the receptor mediating the Na-dependent response (hexamethonium-sensitive) or on the receptor mediating the K-dependent response. Similarly selective actions of α-neurotoxins from *Dendroaspis viridis* were observed on the ACh responses in snail neurons (79).

The third cholinergic receptor of *Aplysia* neurons, that mediating an increase in K permeability, resembles no known vertebrate receptor (80), being unaffected by both curare and atropine, as well as by both nicotine and muscarine. It can, however, be selectively blocked by tetraethylammonium (TEA) and can be selectively activated by arecoline (see 77 for further characteristics). This pharmacological picture has recently been extended by the finding that it can also be selectively activated by a compound extracted from the venom of the conus snail (81). From data gathered on clam and *Aplysia* heart (see below) it appears that this same cholinergic receptor mediates inhibition in molluscan atrial cells.

Serotonin

The observation that 5-HT can depolarize and excite some snail neurons and hyperpolarize and inhibit others (see 1 for review) has been extended by the recent work of Gerschenfeld & Paupardin-Tritsch (82), which shows that six types of 5-HT response can be identified. Four of these responses are due to an increase in membrane conductance: Two (one rapid and one slow) are excitatory and result from an increase in Na conductance; two are inhibitory, one rapid, due to an increase in Cl conductance, and one slow, due to an increase in K conductance. In contrast, the last two of the six response types result from a *decrease* in membrane conductance; one is an excitatory response, due to a reduction in K conductance; the other, an inhibitory response due to decreases in both Na and K conductances.

The pharmacological analyses have shown that the responses that reflect increases in membrane conductance are due to the activation of four different types of 5-HT receptors. 7-Methyltryptamine blocks selectively the rapid Na-dependent response; 5-methoxygramine blocks only the K-dependent inhibitory response, whereas neostigmine blocks only the Cl-dependent inhibitory response. Curare blocks both the rapid Na-dependent response and the Cl-dependent inhibitory response, whereas bufotenine blocks the two Na-dependent excitatory responses (fast and slow) as well as the K-dependent inhibitory response (see 82 for further pharmacological characteristics). These results strongly suggest that at least the four responses resulting from an increase in membrane conductance are due to the activation of four distinct 5-HT receptors.

The two responses reflecting conductance decreases are less well understood. No specific antagonists have as yet been found. These responses, as well as another, nonserotoninergic, synaptically activated decrease in K conductance (83) observed in *Aplysia,* have ionic mechanisms that resemble those observed in the sympathetic ganglion by Weight & Votava (84). However, there has as yet been no evidence that these decreases in membrane conductance are associated with increases in either cAMP or cGMP, as are the potentials reflecting conductance decreases in the sympathetic ganglion (85, 86).

The relevance for synaptic transmission of this wide variety of serotonin response types has been revealed by the work of Cottrell & Macon (54) in *Helix pomatia* and by Gerschenfeld & Paupardin-Tritsch (48) in *Aplysia californica* using the biochemically defined serotoninergic neurons of the cerebral ganglia of these animals (see Table 1) and studying the responses to firing of these neurones in monosynaptically connected follower cells of the buccal ganglia. Analyses of the synaptic responses elicited by the serotoninergic neurons of *Aplysia* showed that at least four of the six response types can be elicited synaptically, and that these responses are affected by pharmacological agents in the same way as are the corresponding responses to iontophoretically applied 5-HT. These electrophysiological and pharmacological data show that the 5-HT biochemically detected in these neurons is indeed serving a transmitter function.

One action of 5-HT that is difficult to include in this rather extensive array of 5-HT receptors is that recently described by Shimahara & Tauc (87). These authors were able to cause, by repetitive stimulation of a nerve trunk, a long-lasting facilitation of an EPSP evoked in the *Aplysia* giant cell by an identified, monosynaptically connected presynaptic neuron. This so-called heterosynaptic facilitation could be imitated by an iontophoretic application of 5-HT in the neuropile, with the 5-HT presumably reaching the presynaptic terminals of the EPSP-eliciting neuron. Both the facilitation produced by repetitive stimulation of the nerve trunk, as well as that caused by iontophoretically applied 5-HT, could be blocked by LSD. These authors concluded that afferent nerve stimulation causes a release of 5-HT into the presynaptic terminals and that the 5-HT causes a change in the presynaptic membrane that favors an increase in transmitter release when the presynaptic neuron is fired. This increased release is thus responsible for the long-term facilitation of the EPSP measured in the giant cell.

If such a serotoninergic effect takes place, it seems most probable that, in order to result in an increase in transmitter release, 5-HT would be causing a decrease in conductance of the presynaptic terminal membrane. Such decreases in membrane conductance by 5-HT were observed by Gerschenfeld & Paupardin-Tritsch (82) (see above), and might be a possible mechanism for heterosynaptic facilitation. However, the only responses that Gerschenfeld & Paupardin-Tritsch found that could be blocked by LSD were those mediated by a classical increase in membrane conductance; the two 5-HT elicited increases in membrane resistance that they demonstrated were unaffected by LSD, the drug used by Shimahara & Tauc to eliminate the heterosynaptic facilitation they observed. Thus, one must assume that if 5-HT is truly mediating the facilitatory effect via an increase in release from synaptic terminals, either a new receptor mechanism is involved, or it is in some way mediated via a more classical conductance *increase*.

Dopamine

A similar but somewhat less complex multireceptor system has emerged for the more recently established transmitter dopamine. Two types of dopamine response have been characterized in molluscan neurons (see 1, 77): one, a relatively rapid excitatory response due to an increase in cationic permeability; the other, a slow inhibitory response due to an increase in K permeability. Preliminary data of Carpenter & Gaubatz (88) suggest that certain dopamine responses might reflect an increase in membrane permeability to Cl ions.

In *Aplysia* it has been shown (see 77) that the excitatory dopamine response is much more readily desensitized than is the inhibitory response, and can be selectively blocked by curare and strychnine. The inhibitory response, on the other hand, can be blocked by ergometrine, which at higher doses also blocks the depolarizing response. Berry & Cottrell (52), studying the effects of iontophoretically applied dopamine in the central neurons of *Planorbis corneus,* showed that the excitatory and inhibitory responses they observed had the same pharmacological characteristics as the dopamine responses in *Aplysia.* They further extended the pharmacological analysis of dopamine receptors by finding a more specific blocking agent of the inhibitory response, 6-hydroxydopamine. They then studied the synaptic potentials elicited in monosynaptically connected follower cells in response to firing of the giant dopamine-containing neuron (49, 50), and demonstrated (1) that the response of a given follower cell to presynaptic stimulation was the same as that elicited by iontophoretically applied dopamine, and (2) that the pharmacological effects observed on the synaptic responses were identical with those observed on the responses to iontophoretically applied dopamine. These experiments confirm the transmitter function of histochemically detected dopamine in these neurons.

Octopamine

Octopamine has been detected in individual neurons of *A. californica* (see Table 1) that do not contain dopamine and norepinephrine (5). Little is known of the effects of exogenously applied octopamine on possible target organs. One brief report (89) has been made on the observation that iontophoretically applied octopamine on certain cells of *Aplysia* elicits a hyperpolarization that seems to be due to an increase in K permeability. Until now, no connections have been established between the octopamine-containing neurons and follower cells, and until a battery of antagonists is developed, the confirmation of the transmitter role of octopamine might be delayed.

The above data yield a list of three rather firmly established transmitter substances in molluscan ganglionic synaptic transmission: ACh, 5-HT, and dopamine. In each of these cases it has been possible to study the effects of synaptically released as well as of the exogenously applied transmitter substance. It has been shown that for each of these transmitters, the molluscan neurons have a number of different receptor types, each mediating a different type of postsynaptic response. Thus, the response of a given cell is determined by which and how many of these receptor types are on the membrane of a given follower cell, and, because of such a differential distribution of receptor types on different follower cells, a single presynaptic neuron can cause excitation in some cells, while eliciting inhibition or complex responses in others.

Although other transmitter candidates [e.g. GABA, glutamate, histamine, glycine (see 1 and 77 for documentation), as well as peptides (e.g. 90) and other neuronal extracts] have been demonstrated to have receptors on molluscan neurons, it is not yet clear whether these receptors serve a synaptic function. Even in the cases where these same substances have been detected in differential quantities in different neurons (see Table 1), their transmitter function in such neurons remains to be established.

MOLLUSCAN MUSCLE

The most conclusive recent evidence concerning the identification of transmitter substances at molluscan neuromuscular junctions has been obtained in *Aplysia* heart, vessels, and gills. Although 5-HT and ACh have been assumed for some time to be the excitatory and inhibitory transmitters, respectively, in molluscan hearts (see 91), the recent coupling in *Aplysia* of biochemical and electrophysiological analyses of identified neurons shown to control monosynaptically heart excitation and inhibition, respectively, has provided a very nice confirmation of conclusions drawn from preparations that have not yet lent themselves to such complete analyses.

Role of Serotonin in Heart Excitation

A motor neuron shown biochemically to be serotoninergic (see RB_{HE}, Table 1) was shown (45) to have direct, monosynaptic excitatory effects on the heartbeat and on blood pressure; these effects could be imitated by exogenously applied serotonin. Dopamine, the only agent with a similar excitatory effect, was 45 times less effective. Finally, the synaptically activated acceleration in heartbeat, as well as the synaptically activated increase in blood pressure, could be blocked by the serotonin antagonist, cinanserin.

Role of ACh in Heart Inhibition

The neurons shown electrophysiologically to inhibit heartbeat by presumed monosynaptic connections were demonstrated biochemically to be cholinergic (see Table 1, LD_{HI}) (45). Exogenous ACh imitated the action of heart-inhibitory neurons, both in producing irregularities in heartbeat and in lowering blood pressure. A similar effect was obtained with the cholinomimetic arecoline. The heart-inhibitory action, like that of exogenous ACh, could be blocked by TEA. The imitation of the heart inhibition by arecoline and its block by TEA suggest that the cholinergic receptor mediating this inhibition is the same as that mediating the K-dependent cholinergic inhibition in molluscan ganglia (see above: also 77, 80).

Role of ACh in Vasoconstriction

The transmitter shown to act on the aortic sphincter musculature was shown also to be ACh (45). The vasoconstrictor neurons of *Aplysia* were shown biochemically to be cholinergic (see Table 1, LB_{VC}). The contractions caused by activation of these neurons could be imitated by ACh, and both the synaptically activated constriction and that caused by exogenous ACh could be blocked by hexamethonium and curare. From the available information, one would anticipate that this cholinergic receptor is the same as that mediating Na-dependent cholinergic excitation in the ganglion. In view of that similarity it could be expected that this response (in spite of being a cholinergic excitatory neuromuscular response) would most probably be unaffected by α-bungarotoxin (78).

Two Excitatory Transmitters Acting on the Gill Muscle

In a recent analysis of the innervation of *Aplysia* gill muscle (39), three major motor neurons were shown to innervate, monosynaptically, different combinations of the main muscle groups. Two of the motor neurons were shown biochemically to be cholinergic (see LDG, Table 1), and the excitatory junctional potentials (e.j.p.'s) resulting from their activation were blocked by hexamethonium. On the other hand, the third motor neuron studied (see L7, Table 1) produces contractions that are unaffected by hexamethonium. Furthermore, the effect produced by this motor neuron (antiflaring of the two halves of the gill) is opposite to that produced by either of the two cholinergic neurons or by exogenous ACh. A biochemical analysis confirmed the conclusions from electrophysiological findings, showing that the neuron L7, unlike the other two motor neurons, is unable to convert choline into

ACh, and does not contain choline acetyltransferase. The experiments thus show that motor neurons liberating different transmitters make monosynaptic contacts with the same muscle fibers, and both elicit e.j.p.'s in those target organs. Thus, excitation appears to be mediated in the same fiber by two different excitatory transmitters.

ARTHROPOD MUSCLE

Recent Investigations on the Role of Glutamate at Insect and Crustacean Muscle

Although much work has been done in the last few years to further characterize the glutamate receptors found on many arthropod muscles, few new data have been obtained that strengthen the position that glutamate is the transmitter at any of these junctions. However, except for the special cases treated in the last sections of this review, glutamate remains the most promising candidate for the transmitter at most of the excitatory junctions on these muscles.

EXTRAJUNCTIONAL RECEPTORS MEDIATING AN INCREASE IN Cl PERMEA-BILITY   Recent investigations on the action of glutamate and other agonists have shown that there are probably at least two different types of glutamate receptors on the insect striated muscle. Cull-Candy & Usherwood (92, 93) showed that whereas glutamate applied iontophoretically at the junctional membrane imitated the depolarizing action of the junctional transmitter (presumably glutamate) glutamate applied to the extrajunctional membrane induced either a biphasic response or a pure hyperpolarizing response. The hyperpolarization caused by glutamate was shown to be due to an increase in membrane permeability to Cl ions. Lea & Usherwood (94, 95) had previously shown that, on the same muscle, ibotenic acid selectively elicited an extrajunctional, hyperpolarizing, Cl-dependent response, and had no effect on the junctional membrane. Cross desensitization was demonstrated between ibotenic acid and glutamate, which strongly suggests that the compounds act on the same extrajunctional receptors. When these extrajunctional receptors were blocked, either by a prior desensitization by ibotenic acid, or by the addition of picrotoxin to the bath, the response of the muscle to bath-applied glutamate was enhanced. These conditions did not enhance the amplitude of the iontophoretically applied junctional response to glutamate, suggesting that the shunting effect of Cl conductance on the depolarization by bath-applied glutamate does not interfere with the localized junctional response (since, as has been shown (96), there is no effect on this response of changes in Cl concentration).

The failure to observe cross desensitization between GABA (the inhibitory transmitter at these junctions which, like ibotenic acid, causes an increase in Cl permeability) and ibotenic acid suggests that the ibotenic acid–glutamate extrajunctional receptor is not the same as that acted upon by the inhibitory transmitter. This is further supported by the finding that ibotenic acid causes a hyperpolarization of all fiber types, even of those which do not receive inhibitory innervation and are not responsive to GABA (95).

In the *striated muscle of the crayfish vas deferens* Florey & Murdock (97) obtained evidence for a similar two-receptor glutamate system. They observed that (*a*) contractures produced by L-glutamate were eliminated in Na-free solutions and were enhanced when external Cl was reduced; (*b*) a glutamate contracture could still be obtained in Na-free solutions if external Cl was also reduced; (*c*) picrotoxin enhanced the glutamate-induced contracture in normal sodium solutions, but eliminated it when Cl was low.

These authors concluded that glutamate increases membrane permeability to both Na and Cl ions and that the glutamate-induced Cl permeability change is the result of an interaction of glutamate with the GABA receptor, since increases in Cl permeability, whether activated by glutamate or GABA, are blocked by picrotoxin. However, in view of the data obtained on locust muscle (see above) it appears probable that in the crayfish vas deferens, as in locust muscle, the glutamate-induced Cl permeability change is mediated by extrajunctional glutamate receptors which, though blocked by picrotoxin, are insensitive to GABA. Experiments testing the effects of ibotenic acid (as well as experiments evaluating cross-desensitization between glutamate and ibotenic acid) would be useful for clarifying whether the Na-independent glutamate effect on the vas deferens is mediated by a glutamate-specific (i.e. GABA insensitive) or a nonspecific (i.e. GABA sensitive) receptor.

EFFECTS OF KAINIC ACID: RELATIONSHIP TO EXTRAJUNCTIONAL RECEPTORS   Shinozaki & Shibuya (98) first observed that the depolarization brought about in crayfish muscle by bath-applied L-glutamate was markedly enhanced by adding kainic acid to the bathing medium. In contrast, this compound did not affect the e.j.p.'s which are presumably due to synaptically released glutamate. Takeuchi & Onodera (99), using iontophoretically applied glutamate, have shown that when the application of glutamate is restricted to the junctional membrane, kainic acid causes no enhancement of the response. However, when the application is made over a wider surface, thereby including nonjunctional membrane, kainic acid increases both the amplitude and the duration of the response.

Both groups of authors assume that kainic acid interacts with an extrajunctional glutamate receptor which is assumed to have different pharmacological properties (hence its sensitivity to kainic acid) than does the junctional receptor. That extrajunctional excitatory receptors may exist in arthropod muscle is suggested by the biphasic responses seen in locust extrajunctional membrane (92) and by the spread of glutamate sensitivity seen in denervated locust muscle (100). However, similar efforts to demonstrate an increase in extrajunctional receptors in crayfish muscle (proximal accessory flexor) by denervation have thus far been unsuccessful (101).

FURTHER ANALYSES OF THE IONIC MECHANISMS OF THE JUNCTIONAL GLUTAMATE RESPONSES   A number of investigators have continued and refined the analyses of the ionic mechanisms underlying the junctional responses to synaptic activation and to iontophoretically applied glutamate (e.g. 102–104). Their work has revealed that a wide variation exists in the estimated and observed inversion potential values obtained for these responses, even when studied by the same author in the same preparation. In some cases, the variations were shown to reflect differential contributions of potassium ions to what was otherwise a primarily Na-dependent potential (104). In other instances, it has been suggested that calcium currents make a contribution to the junctional potential (102), accounting presumably for some atypically positive inversion potentials. This conclusion, however, was not reached by other investigators (103). Little seems to be understood as yet about the factors controlling the differential permeabilities of different junctional membranes or of the same type of junctional membrane in different experiments.

FURTHER ANALYSES OF DRUG-RECEPTOR INTERACTIONS BY GLUTAMATE AT THE JUNCTIONAL MEMBRANE   Measuring with voltage clamp techniques the junctional currents elicited by application of glutamate with or without leakage from the micropipettes, Dudel (105, 106) demonstrated that when leakage occurs, the dose-response curve yields a log-log slope of 2. In contrast, when no leakage is permitted (using very high resistance pipettes) the resulting dose-response curve yields a log-log slope of 4–6. Furthermore, when the dose-response curve obtained with the no-leakage pipette is used in conjunction with the observed junctional currents to predict the concentration of glutamate reaching the membrane, this concentration is found to be identical with that predicted by the diffusion equation. The steep-sloped S shape of the dose-response curve might avoid interference from the circulating low doses of glutamate found in this preparation, while rendering more effective the high doses liberated synaptically.

Role of ACh in Arthropod Muscle

Until 1972, all studies performed on crayfish or lobster neuromuscular junctions led to the conclusion that glutamate was the best candidate for a mediator at excitatory junctions. The majority of studies yielding this conclusion were performed on the muscles of the walking legs and the claw. These data remain free from contradiction, although it is perhaps worthwhile to note that another amino acid (quisqualic acid) has recently been shown (107) to be much more effective than glutamic acid on the abductor muscle in the first walking leg of the crayfish.

Although the transmitter role of glutamate is not yet under serious reconsideration, there are clear indications that glutamate is not the only excitatory neuromuscular transmitter in these organisms. Futamachi (108) was the first to obtain evidence that in the slow flexor of the crayfish abdomen ACh might serve this function. He demonstrated that the nerve terminal regions innervated by the motor neuron with the largest extracellularly recorded spike were sensitive to iontophoretically applied ACh. The localization of the sensitive spots was highly correlated with the region of synaptic terminals. Furthermore, the e.j.p.'s of this motor neuron were antagonized by curare. These electrophysiological data have received support recently from light and electron microscopy studies (109) showing that the slow abdominal flexor muscle disclosed staining for acetylcholinesterase, whereas the claw abductor muscle (that was used in many studies of glutamate sensitivity) did not. Electron microscopic examination revealed that the AChE staining was confined to the postjunctional membrane.

Both Evoy & Beranek (110) and Lowagie & Gerschenfeld (111) demonstrated that muscle fibers in the slow flexor system gave localized responses to glutamate. These findings are not necessarily inconsistent with the failure of Futamachi to observe glutamate responses under the same conditions he used for observing ACh responses, because he restricted his analysis to the postjunctional membrane innervated by only one of the five excitatory motor neurons innervating this muscle. Some of these muscle fibers may be similar to those of the *Aplysia* gill muscles, which receive excitatory innervation from two neurons liberating different transmitters (39).

The argument for ACh involvement in excitation of crustacean muscle has received more support from the recent work of Marder (64) in the striated musculature of the lobster stomach, innervated exclusively by neurons of the stomatogastric ganglion. Certain neurons (see Table 1) shown to contain choline acetyltransferase innervate the dorsal dilator muscles that respond to ACh but not to glutamate, and elicit e.j.p.'s that can be blocked by curare (64) and potentiated by edrophonium (65). It was also shown (65) that exogeneously applied ACh blocked the e.j.p.'s in this muscle, and that the reversal potentials estimated by extrapolation for the ionophoretic ACh and junctional responses were the same. In contrast, motor neurons in which no choline acetyltransferase could be detected were shown to innervate muscles that do not respond to ACh. Thus, at least two transmitters are being used by the stomatogastric ganglion motor neurons: one, presumably ACh; the other, presumably glutamate.

Octopamine in Arthropods

Much interesting information about the role of octopamine in arthropod nervous systems is now becoming available. Barker et al (28) first reported a high concentration of octopamine in extracts of *Homarus* thoracic connectives, one root of which was shown by Wallace et al (66) to contain small neurons capable of synthesizing and accumulating octopamine. Evans et al (67) showed that these neurons contained large dense-cored vesicles (67), but were unable to locate any conventional synaptic endings made by these neurons. These authors were able to demonstrate release of octopamine from this piece of tissue by depolarization with high K concentrations, and were also able to produce a long-lasting contracture in the dactyl opener muscle by application of $10^{-5}M$ octopamine.

Barker & Hooper (73) demonstrated octopamine synthesis in parts of the *Panulirus* foregut nervous system which also contain dense-cored vesicles that are likewise uncorrelated with any synaptic terminals (74). Hoyle (60) showed that low (2.5 X $10^{-9}M$) octopamine concentrations mimicked the effects of the dorsal unimpaired medial (DUMETI) neurons of the locust and grasshopper that contain dense-cored vesicles. These neurons were proposed to have a neurosecretory function (60), and were shown (59) to be capable of synthesizing octopamine. Nathanson & Greengard (75) showed an octopamine-sensitive adenyl cyclase in cockroach nervous tissue, and Sullivan & Barker (76) report that concentrations of octopamine that cause physiological changes in lobster and crab ganglia also affect cAMP levels. All of these data are consistent with a neuromodulator role for octopamine in these systems.

ACKNOWLEDGMENT

E. Marder was supported by NIH postdoctoral fellowship 1 F22-NS00751–01.

Literature Cited

1. Gerschenfeld, H. M. 1973. *Physiol. Rev.* 53:1–119
2. Otsuka, M., Kravitz, E. A., Potter, D. D. 1967. *J. Neurophysiol.* 30:725–52
3. McCaman, M. W., Weinreich, D., McCaman, R. E. 1973. *Brain Res.* 53:129–37
4. McCaman, R. E., Weinreich, D., Boyrs, H. 1973. *J. Neurochem.* 21:473–76
5. Saavedra, J. M., Brownstein, M. J., Carpenter, D. O., Axelrod, J. 1974. *Science* 185:364–65
6. Weinreich, D., Weiner, C., McCaman, R. E. 1975. *Brain Res.* 84:341–45
7. Brownstein, M. J., Saavedra, J. M., Axelrod, J., Zeman, G. H., Carpenter, D. O. 1974. *Proc. Natl. Acad. Sci. USA* 71:4662–65
8. Boyrs, H. K. Weinreich, D., McCaman, R. E. 1973. *J. Neurochem.* 21:1349–51
9. Giller, E. Jr., Schwartz, J. H. 1971. *J. Neurophysiol.* 34:93–107
10. McCaman, R. E., Dewhurst, S. A. 1970. *J. Neurochem.* 17:1421–26
11. Hildebrand, J. G., Townsel, J. G., Kravitz, E. A. 1974. *J. Neurochem.* 23:951–63
12. Emson, P. C., Malthe-Sorenssen, D., Fonnum, F. 1974. *J. Neurochem.* 22:1089–98
13. Weinreich, D., Dewhurst, S. A., McCaman, R. E. 1972. *J. Neurochem.* 19:1125–30
14. Coggeshall, R. E., Dewhurst, S. A., Weinreich, D., McCaman, R. E. 1972. *J. Neurobiol.* 3:259–65
15. Emson, P. C., Fonnum, F. 1974. *J. Neurochem.* 22:1079–88
16. Kravitz, E. A., Molinoff, P., Hall, Z. W. 1965. *Proc. Natl. Acad. Sci. USA* 54:778–82
17. Molinoff, P. B., Kravitz, E. A. 1968. *J. Neurochem.* 15:391–409
18. Hall, Z. W., Bownds, M. D., Kravitz, E. A. 1970. *J. Cell Biol.* 46:290–99
19. Emson, P. C., Burrows, M., Fonnum, F. 1974. *J. Neurobiol.* 5:33–42
20. Hildebrand, J., Barker, D. L., Herbert, E., Kravitz, E. A. 1971. *J. Neurobiol.* 2:231–46
21. Barker, D. L., Herbert, E. A., Hildebrand, J. G., Kravitz, E. A. 1972. *J. Physiol.* 225:205–29
22. Koike, H., Eisenstadt, M., Schwartz, J. H. 1972. *Brain Res.* 37:152–59

23. Eisenstadt, M., Goldman, J. E., Kandel, E. R., Koike, H., Koester, J., Schwartz, J. H. 1973. *Proc. Natl. Acad. Sci. USA* 70:3371–75
24. Treistman, S. N., Schwartz, J. H. 1974. *Brain Res.* 68:358–64
25. Donnellan, J. F., Jenner, D. W., Ramsey, A. 1974. *Insect Biochem.* 4:243–65
26. Langcake, P., Clements, A. N. 1974. *Insect Biochem.* 4:225–41
27. Baxter, C. F., Torralba, G. F. 1975. *Brain Res.* 84:383–97
28. Barker, D. L., Molinoff, P. B., Kravitz, E. A. 1972. *Nature London New Biol.* 236:61–62
29. Aprison, M. H., McBride, W. J., Freeman, A. R. 1973. *J. Neurochem.* 21:87–95
30. Juorio, A. V., Molinoff, P. B. 1974. *J. Neurochem.* 22:271–80
31. Sorenson, M. M. 1973. *J. Neurochem.* 20:1231–45
32. Juorio, A. V., Philips, S. R. 1975. *Brain Res.* 83:180–84
33. Schwartz, J. H., Eisenstadt, M. L., Cedar, H. 1975. *J. Gen. Physiol.* 65:255–73
34. Rude, S., Coggeshall, R. E., Van Orden, L. C. 1969. *J. Cell Biol.* 41:832–54
35. Lent, C. M. 1973. *Science* 179:693–95
36. Eisenstadt, M. L., Schwartz, J. H. 1975. *J. Gen. Physiol.* 65:293–313
37. Goldman, J. E., Schwartz, J. H. 1974. *J. Physiol.* 242:61–76
38. Zeman, G. H., Carpenter, D. O. 1976. *Comp. Biochem. Physiol.* In press
39. Carew, T. J., Pinsker, H., Rubinson, K., Kandel, E. R. 1974. *J. Neurophysiol.* 37:1020–40
40. Otsuka, M., Iversen, L. L., Hall, Z. W., Kravitz, E. A. 1966. *Proc. Natl. Acad. Sci. USA* 56:1110–15
41. Koike, H., Kandel, E. R., Schwartz, J. H. 1974. *J. Neurophysiol.* 37:815–27
42. Kandel, E. R., Frazier, W. T., Waziri, R., Coggeshall, R. E. 1967. *J. Neurophysiol.* 30:1352–76
43. Wachtel, H., Kandel, E. R. 1971. *J. Neurophysiol.* 34:56–68
44. Kehoe, J. S. 1972. *J. Physiol.* 225:147–72
45. Liebeswar, G., Goldman, J. E., Koester, J., Mayeri, E. 1975. *J. Neurophysiol.* 38:767–79

46. Mayeri, E., Koester, J., Kupferman, I., Liebeswar, G., Kandel, E. 1974. *J. Neurophysiol.* 37:458–75
47. Weinreich, D., McCaman, M. W., McCaman, R. E., Vaughn, J. E. 1973. *J. Neurochem.* 20:969–76
48. Gerschenfeld, H. M., Paupardin-Tritsch, D. 1974. *J. Physiol.* 243:457–81
49. Powell, B., Cottrell, G. A. 1974. *J. Neurochem.* 22:605–6
50. Marsden, C., Kerkut, G. A. 1970. *Comp. Gen. Pharmacol.* 1:101–16
51. Osborne, N. N., Priggemeier, E., Neuhoff, V. 1975. *Brain Res.* 90:261–71
52. Berry, M. S., Cottrell, G. A. 1975. *J. Physiol.* 244:589–612
53. Cottrell, G. A., Osborne, N. N. 1970. *Nature London* 225:470–72
54. Cottrell, G. A., Macon, J. G. 1974. *J. Physiol.* 236:435–64
55. McBride, W. J., Shank, R. P., Freeman, A. R., Aprison, M. H. 1974. *Life Sci.* 14:1109–20
56. Osborne, N. N. 1972. *Int. J. Neurosci* 3:215–19
57. Hanley, M. R., Cottrell, G. A. 1974. *J. Pharm. Pharmacol.* 26:980
58. Hanley, M. R., Cottrell, G. A., Emson, P. C., Fonnum, F. 1974. *Nature London* 251:631–33
59. Hoyle, G., Barker, D. L. 1975. *J. Exp. Zool.* 193:433–39
60. Hoyle, G. 1975. *J. Exp. Zool.* 193:425–31
61. Kravitz, E. A., Potter, D. D. 1965. *J. Neurochem.* 12:323–28
62. Cooke, I. M., Goldstone, M. W. 1970. *J. Exp. Biol.* 53:651–68
63. Kushner, P. D., Maynard, E. 1975. *Soc. Neurosci. 5th Ann. Meet. (Abstr.)*
64. Marder, E. 1974. *Nature London* 251:730–31
65. Marder, E. 1976. *J. Physiol.* In press
66. Wallace, B. G., Talamo, B. R., Evans, P. D., Kravitz, E. A. 1974. *Brain Res.* 74:349–55
67. Evans, P. D., Talamo, B. R., Kravitz, E. A. 1975. *Brain Res.* 90:340–47
68. Kravitz, E. A., Slater, C. R., Takahashi, M. D. 1970. In *Excitatory Synaptic Mechanisms*, 85–93. Oslo: Scand. Univ. Books
69. Evans, P. D. 1973. *Biochem. Biophysics. Acta* 311:302–13
70. Evans, P. D. 1974. *J. Cell Sci.* 14:351–67
71. Evans, P. D. 1975. *J. Exp. Biol.* 62:55–67
72. Eisenstadt, M. L., Treistman, S. N., Schwartz, J. H. 1975. *J. Gen. Physiol.* 65:275–91
73. Barker, D. L., Hooper, N. K. 1975. *Soc. Neurosci. 5th Ann. Meet.* (Abstr.)
74. Friend, B., Maynard, E. 1975. *Soc. Neurosci. 5th Ann. Meet.* (Abstr.)
75. Nathanson, J. A., Greengard, P. 1973. *Science* 180:308
76. Sullivan, R. E., Barker, D. L. 1975. *Soc. Neurosci. 5th Ann. Meet.* (Abstr.)
77. Ascher, P., Kehoe, J. S. 1975. In *Handbook of Psychopharmacology*, ed. L. L. Iversen, S. Iversen, S. Snyder, 4:265–310. New York Plenum
78. Kehoe, J. S., Sealock, R., Bon, C. 1976. *Brain Res.* In press
79. Szczepaniak, A. C. 1974. *J. Physiol.* 241:55–56P
80. Kehoe, J. S. 1972. *J. Physiol.* 225:115–46
81. Elliott, E. 1975. *Chemical properties and physiological activity of a neuroactive component from the venom of Conus californicus.* PhD thesis. Calif. Inst. Technol., Pasadena. 172 pp.
82. Gerschenfeld, H. M., Paupardin-Tritsch, D. 1974. *J. Physiol.* 243:427–56
83. Kehoe, J. S. 1975. *J. Physiol.* 244:23P
84. Weight, F. F., Votava, J. 1970. *Science* 170:755–58
85. McAfee, D. A., Greengard, P. 1972. *Science* 178:310–12
86. Weight, F., Petzold, G. L., Greengard, P. 1974. *Science* 186:942–44
87. Shimahara, T., Tauc, L. 1975. *J. Physiol.* 247:321–42
88. Carpenter, D., Gaubatz, G. 1974. *Fed. Proc.* 33:541 (Abstr.)
89. Carpenter, D. O., Gaubatz, G. L. 1974. *Nature London* 252:483–85
90. Barker, J. L., Ifshin, M. S., Gainer, N. 1975. *Brain Res.* 84:501–13
91. Martin, A. 1974. *Ann. Rev. Physiol.* 36:171–86
92. Cull-Candy, S. G., Usherwood, P. N. R. 1973. *Nature London New Biol.* 246:62–64
93. Usherwood, P. N. R., Cull-Candy, S. G. 1974. *Neuropharmacology* 13:455–61
94. Lea, T. J., Usherwood, P. N. R., 1973. *Comp. Gen. Pharmacol.* 4:351–63
95. Lea, T. J., Usherwood, P. N. R. 1973. *Comp. Gen. Pharmacol.* 4:333–50
96. Anwyl, R., Usherwood, P. N. R. 1974. *Nature London* 252:591–93
97. Florey, E., Murdock, L. L. 1974. *Comp. Gen. Pharmacol.* 5:91–99
98. Shinozaki, H., Shibuya, I. 1974. *Neuropharmacology* 13:1057–65
99. Takeuchi, A., Onodera, K. 1975. *Neuropharmacology* 14:619–26
100. Usherwood, P. N. R. 1969. *Nature London* 223:411–13

101. Frank, E. 1974. *J. Physiol.* 242:371–82
102. Dudel, J. 1974. *Pfluegers Arch.* 352: 227–41
103. Takeuchi, A., Onodera, K. 1975. *J. Physiol.* 252:295–318
104. Taraskevich, P. S. 1975. *J. Gen. Physiol.* 65:677–91
105. Dudel, J. 1975. *Pfluegers Arch.* 356: 317–28
106. Dudel, J. 1975. *Pfluegers Arch.* 356: 329–46
107. Shinozaki, H., Shibuya, I. 1974. *Neuropharmacology* 13:665–72
108. Futamachi, K. J. 1972. *Science* 172: 1372–75
109. Diliberto, E. J., Davis, R., Koelle, G. B. 1973. *Pharmacologist.* Vol. 15, p. 222
110. Evoy, W., Beranek, R. 1972. *Comp. Gen. Pharmacol.* 3:178–86
111. Lowagie, C., Gerschenfeld, H. M. 1974. *Nature London* 248:533–35

NEUROPHARMACOLOGY OF   ❖6650
THE PANCREATIC ISLETS

Phillip H. Smith and Daniel Porte, Jr.
Department of Medicine, University of Washington School of Medicine,
and Division of Endocrinology and Metabolism, Veterans Administration Hospital,
Seattle, Washington 98108

INTRODUCTION

Following the discovery that insulin and glucagon are produced by the pancreatic islets, a vast literature has accumulated concerning the role of substrates, nonpancreatic hormones, and intracellular factors in the control of islet hormone release. The results of such work are the subject of several reviews (1–4) and therefore are not covered in-depth in this paper. More recently, however, it has been appreciated that the nervous system is also intimately involved in the regulation of endocrine pancreatic secretion. The purpose of this review is to discuss the anatomic, physiologic, and pharmacologic evidence for the role of neural factors in the regulation of insulin and glucagon secretion, and to demonstrate that the endocrine pancreas is an important neuroendocrine organ.

CYTOLOGY AND ORIGIN OF THE PANCREATIC ISLETS

In most species the principal components of the endocrine pancreas are the A, B, and D cells. Although variations of islet cytoarchitecture may have evolutionary and functional implications (5–7), an equally important cytologic consideration is the hormonal content of each of the islet cell types. It has been accepted for some time that the A cells contain glucagon and that the B cells contain insulin (8). However, there is no general agreement as to the hormonal product of the D cell. Some investigators have reported that these cells contain gastrin (7), but subsequent studies have pointed to the absence of this hormone in the islets of a large number of species (9). Renewed interest in the D cell has been sparked by the recent immunocytochemical evidence that this cell type contains somatostatin (10, 11), a hormone originally isolated from the hypothalamus. This cytologic finding is the latest of a series that indicates a close functional relationship between the pancreatic islets and the nervous system. Further, this observation is compatible with the hypothesis that some, if not all, of the islet cells originate from the ectoderm, an embryonic source different from that of the pancreatic exocrine cells. As discussed below, this hypothesis is markedly different from the commonly held view that the pancreatic islet and exocrine parenchyma are both derived from the endoderm.

Within the framework of a common origin of islet and exocrine cells there are a number of theories regarding the genesis of the endocrine pancreas. Some early investigators (see 6) postulated that there might be multiple generations of pancreatic islets formed by the transdifferentiation of exocrine cells into functional endocrine cells. The possibility that islet cells and the adjacent exocrine tissue are in a dynamic state of flux and interconversion has been supported by a few recent studies (12). Several investigators, however, have failed to find evidence that acinar-islet cell transformations play a role in the formation and maintenance of the pancreatic islet mass (see 6, 13). In fact, most studies of islet development suggest that islet formation takes place in regions adjacent to the pancreatic ducts. The process whereby islets might develop from pancreatic ductal cells has been recently reviewed by Pictet & Rutter (6). These workers have shown that during early phases of histogenesis the cells of the pancreatic diverticula undergo a series of divisions forming numerous closed acini. In general, these acini elongate and form the elaborate structure of the adult pancreas by cell divisions that are parallel to the developing duct lumen; each daughter cell thus maintains the same contacts as its parent via junctional complexes with the neighboring cells. Pictet & Rutter also observed, concomitant with acinar development, certain mitoses that were in a plane perpendicular to the axis of the lumen. They have hypothesized that as a result of this type of division, one of the daughter cells is no longer in contact with its former neighbors and begins to differentiate into an endocrine cell, thereby initiating the formation of a pancreatic islet. Pictet & Rutter (6) have additionally shown that pancreatic rudiments (endothelium plus the associated mesenchyme) develop normally in vitro and produce approximately 90% exocrine cells and 10% endocrine cells. However, when the mesenchyme is removed from the rudiment, 90% of the cells develop as endocrine cells, with A cells in the majority. Studies such as these are suggestive of how the pancreatic islets are formed and show that pancreatic rudiments contain all of the cells necessary to form the adult pancreas. Unfortunately, these studies have not clearly defined the precise cellular ancestry of the endocrine pancreas. In their review, Pictet & Rutter (6) suggested several hypothetical mechanisms to account for exact differentiation of islet cells and exocrine tissue from a common endodermal source. In contrast to the view that the pancreatic islets are derived from the endoderm, evidence has been presented by Pearse (14) that suggests that the islets originate from the neuroectoderm. Because various polypeptide-secreting endocrine cells share certain ultrastructural and cytochemical characteristics, Pearse has classified them as the APUD series (Amine Precursor Uptake and Decarboxylation). Pearse has further suggested that all cells having this property arise from the neural crest. While some cells derived from the neural crest are known to produce and secrete amines as their primary function (e.g. adrenal medullary cells), many endocrine cells secrete peptides and retain the ability to convert enzymatically specific precursor molecules [dihydroxyphenylalanine (DOPA) or 5-

hydroxytryptophan (5-HTP)] to the corresponding biogenic amine (dopamine or serotonin, respectively). Such APUD cells have been shown to migrate from the neural crest of the developing embryo to colonize several areas (15, 16) including the foregut and its derivatives (17). In an experiment using fetal mouse pancreas, Pearse et al (13) observed "clear cells" that did not have recognizable secretory granules and displayed no insulin and glucagon immunoreactivity. These cells, however, displayed APUD characteristics. At a later stage of development these same APUD cells had ultrastructurally identifiable secretory granules and im- munocytochemical reactions to insulin and glucagon antibodies. Studies of this type show that presumptive islet cells can be readily identified using specific cytochemical criteria prior to the onset of hormone synthesis and storage. Unfortunately, they do not prove beyond doubt that the islets are of neural crest origin. In fact, recent studies have been performed in which the ectoderm has been removed from chick and mouse embryos prior to the formation of the neural crest; in each case, fully differentiated APUD cells were found in the gut (18) and pancreatic islets (19). Thus, by strict definition the presumptive islet cells may not arise from the neural crest per se. It is possible, however, that some ectodermal cells populate the en- doderm prior to the formation of the neural crests. If so, such cells could migrate with the developing exocrine and ductal cells and be responsible for the formation of the pancreatic islets in the fashion suggested by Pictet & Rutter (6). Although the neuroectodermal origin of the pancreatic islet cells remains to be proven, the validity of this theory is supported by the fact that some polypeptide-secreting endocrine cells of known ectodermal origin (e.g. thyroid C cells) share common cytochemical characteristics with the APUD cells of the endocrine pancreas.

INNERVATION OF THE PANCREATIC ISLETS

There is abundant anatomic and physiologic evidence that the endocrine pancreas of most vertebrates is innervated by both the sympathetic and parasympathetic components of the autonomic nervous system (for reviews see 8, 20, 21). The notable exceptions are cyclostomes (5), certain reptiles (5, 22), and birds (23). The only mammal not known to have innervated islets is the spiny mouse, *Acomys cahirinus* (24).

The nerve supply to the pancreas is derived from the vagal and splanchnic trunks and enters the gland in association with the arteries. Nerves arising from within the pancreas reach the level of the spinal cord via the splanchnic nerves. These latter fibers presumably mediate only pain due to distention (25), but it is not known whether any of them arise within the islets. Nerve fibers that reach the pancreatic islets also accompany the blood vessels (26, 27). Depending upon the species, these fibers are arranged as the so-called peri-insular plexus (28), but may also form an intra-insular plexus at the more central portions of the islet (29). In addition to an extrinsic nerve supply, nerve cell bodies are sometimes observed within the islets (6, 20). These intrinsic neurons are likely to be postganglionic parasympathetic nerves, but their identification as such is yet to be determined. Therefore, the precise function of these nerves is unknown. However, as discussed below, the functional significance of the extrinsic islet nerves is fairly well established.

Cytochemical and ultrastructural studies have shown that nerve endings within the endocrine pancreas can be divided into three types according to their synaptic vesicles. The terminals of cholinergic nerves contain 30–50 nm agranular vesicles, whereas those of adrenergic nerves contain mainly 30–50 nm dense-cored structures (30). Both types of terminals also contain a few 80–100 nm electron-opaque vesicles of unknown function. A third type of islet nerve terminal contains 60–200 nm dense-cored vesicles that are histochemically distinct from those of the other autonomic nerves. Since these endings are structurally similar to the "purinergic" terminals of mammalian smooth muscle recently described by Burnstock (31), it is possible that they might release ATP as a neurotransmitter. This latter type of nerve has not been reported in mammalian islets, but it does appear to be the predominant ending in the endocrine pancreas of certain teleosts (32). While there are different ratios of adrenergic to cholinergic endings in the islets of various species, there seems to be no preferential relationship between one type of ending and any given islet secretory cell. There are, however, important differences in terms of nerve secretory cell structural relationships between the various vertebrate groups. Typical pre- and postsynaptic complexes have been observed between neurons and islet cells in some lower vertebrates (5), but in mammals the islet nerve terminals end blindly at a distance of 20–30 nm from the secretory cells. This suggests that, at least in the case of mammals, neurotransmitters may be released into the islet intercellular space and simultaneously stimulate or inhibit a large number of islet cells. Another means of dispersing a neural signal to the general population of islet cells might occur via a more anatomically direct mechanism. Orci et al (33, 34) have recently shown gap junctions between various cells within the islets, and between nerves and islet B cells. These intercellular junctions are known to be areas of low electrical resistance (e.g. as in cardiac muscle) that also allow the passage of molecules of low molecular weight. It is, therefore, possible that the secretory response of a functionally coupled islet could be rapidly altered by electrical and/or chemical signals from the nerves. Further, such a signal could be markedly amplified because of the numerous gap junctions that presumably exist between the cells of the islet. The possibility that electrical signals play a role in the regulation of islet function is further suggested by electrophysiologic studies demonstrating that islet cells have spontaneous electrical activity, and that their firing pattern is altered when challenged with different glucose concentrations (35, 36).

Other features of the endocrine pancreas are indicative of the close structural and functional coupling of islet cells and nerve endings. For example, the relationship between the Schwann's cells of the intra-islet nerve terminals and the endocrine parenchyma of the pancreatic islets of the dog (37) suggests that the islets of this species are structurally similar to autonomic ganglia. Thus, if the theory of neuroectodermal origin of the islets proves correct, this observation would indicate that the endocrine pancreas is cytologically analogous to the adrenal medulla. The islets, therefore, could be considered as specialized metabolic ganglia having both cholinergic and adrenergic innervation.

INTRACELLULAR MONOAMINES AND ISLET FUNCTION

Fluorescence microscopy, using the technique of Falck and Hillarp, has clearly demonstrated that amines are present not only in the islet nerve endings but also within the A and B cells (38). These amines have been specifically identified as serotonin and dopamine by their spectral characteristics and by extraction and chemical analysis of either whole pancreas or isolated islets. The type and amount of these monoamines vary considerably according to several factors. They are not normally found in albinos but are detectable in the islets of pigmented animals. Further, the amines are far more concentrated in the islets of younger animals, including man (38). Although the A and B cells of the albino mouse do not normally contain monoamines, the administration of DOPA or 5-HTP leads to the appearance of amines within these endocrine cells. This ability of islet cells to concentrate and decarboxylate DOPA to dopamine and 5-HTP to serotonin has been found in all species studied thus far (39, 40) and forms part of the evidence that these APUD cells are of neuroectodermal origin.

Autoradiographic studies have shown that following the injection of radiolabeled DOPA or 5-HTP, the corresponding amine is present within the cytoplasm of the islet cells for several hours. Using quantitative grain-counting techniques at the ultrastructural level, it has been shown that the labeled amines are localized within the halo of the secretory granules of the A and B cells (41; I. Lundquist, personal communication). While it is clear that islet cells incorporate the immediate precursors of dopamine and serotonin, the circulating levels of DOPA and 5-HTP are ordinarily quite low. Therefore, the existence of intracellular amines in the islets of certain species implicates amino acids such as tyrosine and tryptophan as the precursors of dopamine and serotonin, respectively. These amino acids are part of the normal intraneural biosynthetic pathway of dopamine and serotonin. The concept that they may serve as precursors in islets cells is supported by preliminary studies (42) that transplantable islet cell carcinomas of hamsters contain tyrosine hydroxylase and L-aromatic amino acid dicarboxylase, two enzymes necessary for the synthesis of dopamine and serotonin respectively. From the studies using labeled precursors, it is evident that once formed the amines turn over rapidly whether or not insulin is released. Since pretreatment with the monoamine oxidase (MAO) inhibitor, pargyline hydrochloride, increases the grain count over islet cell secretory granules (41), amine degradation is also an important determinant of the functional role of intracellular serotonin and dopamine. Of the two catecholamine degrading enzymes, MAO and catechol-O-methyl transferase (COMT), the former appears primarily responsible for the breakdown of islet cell amines. This is due to the fact that although COMT is important in the degradation of extracellular amines, this enzyme has not been identified in pancreatic islet cells. On the other hand, MAO levels have been found to be approximately three times higher in islet cells than in the surrounding exocrine pancreas (43, 44).

As described in the next section, the administration of serotonin and dopamine alters insulin secretion in vivo and in vitro. However, because of their poor penetration into the islet cells, it has been generally concluded that serotonin and dopamine when applied extracellularly do not necessarily elicit the same effect that they would as intracellular substances. Therefore, the role of intracellular amines as regulators of islet cell secretion has been assessed by either examining the effects upon insulin release produced by the administration of amine precursors, or by inhibiting the breakdown of intracellular serotonin and dopamine.

The in vivo infusion of amine precursors such as 5-HTP or DOPA induces a state of reduced insulin responsiveness to glucose when isolated islets or pieces of pancreas from these animals are subsequently incubated with glucose in vitro (45–47). With this approach, in vivo responses to glibenclamide and isoproterenol are reduced, while glucose-stimulated insulin release remains normal (48). Antagonists known to block the inhibitory effects of extracellular monoamines such as phentolamine and dibenzyline do not block the inhibitory effects of 5-HTP or DOPA (47), suggesting that the intracellular presence of serotonin and dopamine is a critical factor in their inhibitory effects upon insulin release. This concept is supported by in vitro studies of islets from obese hyperglycemic mice that clearly demonstrate the local uptake of 5-HTP and its conversion to serotonin within the islet cells (45). Furthermore, blockade of the decarboxylating enzyme prohibits the inhibitory effect of 5-HTP or DOPA upon pancreatic islet secretion (45, 47, 48).

These inhibitory effects have also been studied using the serotonin antagonist, methysergide. Although some of the inhibitory effects of 5-HTP administration are reversed by pretreatment with methysergide (47), this drug by itself produces roughly the same increase of insulin secretion in controls, leading to results that are difficult to interpret. Further, methysergide also blocks the inhibitory effect of extracellular amines by acting as an α-adrenergic blocking agent (49). Attempts to elucidate the role of intracellular serotonin using other drugs have been conflicting. Parachlorophenylalanine (PCPA), an agent that depletes brain serotonin, has no effect on in vivo glucose-stimulated insulin release from rabbits and fed hamsters (50). However, PCPA does increase the in vitro secretion of insulin from islets of fasted animals (51). Two other serotonin antagonists, cyproheptadine and cinanserin, also increase insulin secretion (50). Again there is complexity, since cyproheptadine stimulates insulin release in the absence of glucose. This latter effect is incompatible with a direct action of cyproheptadine upon serotonin activity because serotonin has been found to inhibit only glucose-induced insulin secretion (50).

There is also conflicting data concerning the in vivo and in vitro effects of MAO inhibitors such as nialamide, pargyline, tranylcypromine, and mebanazine upon insulin secretion. The conflicting data may be related to the ability of these drugs to interact with adrenergic receptors or to interference with enzyme systems other than MAO (see 52–54). Aleyassine & Gardiner (44) have found that the effects of many MAO-inhibiting drugs are concentration dependent. At low doses these agents stimulate insulin secretion, and at high doses they inhibit the release of insulin. All of the MAO inhibitors were found to be effective at relatively low concentrations but neither the stimulation nor inhibition of insulin secretion could be directly correlated with the degree of MAO inhibition. Furthermore, when given in association with 5-HTP some of these drugs elicit hypoglycemia unrelated to insulin secretion (48). Studies using MAO-inhibiting drugs, therefore, cannot be used to support or refute the hypothesis that intracellular monoamines alter insulin secretion.

In summary, pancreatic A and B cells of many species normally contain monoamines, and in all species the islet cell stores of these monoamines can be either increased or induced by the administration of DOPA and 5-HTP. The responsiveness of the insulin-secreting cells is usually reduced when amine precursors are given. However, many of the compounds used to evaluate intracellular monoamines interact in complex ways with extracellular catecholaminergic and serotonergic receptors. Despite these limitations, Lundquist (48) and Lebovitz (39) have proposed attractive theories that suggest an important inhibitory control of insulin secretion by intracellular monoamines. To date, no convincing evidence has been presented that refutes these theories; nevertheless, most of the evidence for them is circumstantial, and many of the studies upon which they are based have been contradictory.

EXTRACELLULAR AMINES AS REGULATORS OF ISLET FUNCTION

Extracellular amines also control islet secretory rates. These amines originate from three primary sources: (a) intra-islet nerve endings secreting acetylcholine or norepinephrine, (b) enterochromaffin cells within the islets that contain serotonin and possibly dopamine, and (c) amine-secreting cells in other areas of the body (i.e. adrenal medulla and extra-islet nerve endings) whose products reach the islets via the blood. The role of various amines has been approached experimentally by stimulation or sectioning of the pancreatic nerves in vivo, or by the administration of amines and their analogs either in vivo or in vitro. In the course of such studies it has been found that certain other substances related to the nervous system, including somatostatin and prostaglandins, also modulate the effects of amines and their control of islet function.

Electrical stimulation of the vagus nerve (54–58) or the ventrolateral hypothalamus (59, 60), a parasympathetic center, has been found to enhance insulin release. Glucagon secretion following vagal stimulation has also been observed in some species (58, 61) but not in others (62). Under these conditions islet hormone secretion is a direct neural effect, and the response is dependent upon the prevailing glucose level (63, 64). Bilateral destruction of the ventrolateral hypothalamic nuclei (VLH) produces a decrease of plasma insulin levels (60, 65). Vagotomy abolishes conditioned insulin secretion in rats (66) and impairs both insulin and glucagon secretion in man (67). Another important role of the parasympathetic system has been recently suggested by the work of Powley & Opsahl (68) who reported that the hypothalamus may regulate the numbers of pancreatic islet cells via the vagus nerves.

Confirming studies using parasympathomimetic drugs have shown that these agents increase both insulin and glucagon (69–72) secretion indicating that these cells are well supplied with muscarinic receptors. Nicotinic acid does not increase insulin secretion in vitro (73), and this finding has been used to suggest that its stimulatory effect in vivo (74) is mediated by postganglionic neurons (73). However, there is no evidence that nicotinic acid stimulates nicotinic receptors, and therefore the role of ganglionic stimulating agents remains unexplored. Atropine blocks the increased secretion of insulin and glucagon produced by cholinergic agents (55, 61, 70, 75, 76) and also blocks conditioned insulin secretion (66). Although gut hormones may be released by vagal stimulation or administration of cholinergic drugs, the increased levels of insulin observed under these conditions has been found to be a direct effect upon the B cell (57, 77) and not related to the known insulinotropic effects of gut hormones.

Sympathetic stimulation of the islet cells initiates a dual effect. Stimulation of the splanchnic nerves (57) or the ventromedial hypothalamus (78) elicits a decline of insulin secretion and a concurrent increase of glucagon levels. This effect is complicated by the differing activities of the α-and β-adrenergic receptors of the islet cells. As reviewed elsewhere (20, 79, 82), norepinephrine or epinephrine inhibits glucose-mediated insulin release both in vivo and in vitro. α-Adrenergic blockers such as phentolamine or phenoxybenzamine have been found to reverse the inhibition of insulin secretion during a catecholamine infusion. No reversal of this inhibition, however, has been observed when propranolol, a β-blocker, is administered. In contrast, β-adrenergic agonists stimulate insulin secretion and are blocked by propranolol. Thus, α-receptor activation inhibits insulin secretion, whereas β-stimulation increases insulin secretion. A number of reports also credit β-adrenergic stimulation as the factor responsible for the elevation of glucagon levels (83, 84). However, in one case α-blockers reportedly abolished this effect (85). At present it would seem that there is clear evidence that β-receptors mediate an increase of both insulin and glucagon secretion and that α-adrenergic stimulation inhibits insulin release.

There is now convincing evidence that the opposing effects of α- and β-receptor stimulation upon insulin secretion can occur simultaneously. This is due to the fact that although glucose is ineffective in stimulating insulin release during a catecholamine infusion because of α-stimulation, insulin levels nonetheless rise over time as a function of β-receptor activation (86). This response indicates that two separate phenomena are occurring. First, there is an abrupt stoppage of insulin release by activation of the α-adrenergic receptor that remains operative even in the face of glucose stimulation. Second, there is a tonic, albeit slow, rise of insulin secretion related to the β-adrenergic receptor. Turtle & Kipnis (87) made the observation that, in the presence of theophylline, islet levels of cyclic AMP were elevated by β-adrenergic stimulation and decreased by α-adrenergic stimulation. It was therefore assumed that the inhibition of insulin release by α-agonists was a function of lowered cyclic AMP within the B cell, and that the β-stimulated elevation of cyclic AMP was responsible for the increase of insulin secretion. Under this concept a simultaneous inhibition and stimulation of insulin release by epinephrine, due to changes of cyclic AMP, would be impossible (81). The evidence for cyclic AMP as the second messenger for β-adrenergic activity remains overwhelming. However, two studies have shown that the insulinotropic effect of exogenous cyclic AMP is blocked by simultaneous incubation with catecholamines (88, 89). Thus it appears the α-adrenergic stimulation initiates a signal that is responsible for the inhibition of insulin secretion independently of its ability to lower cyclic AMP levels. The precise nature of this signal is unknown and warrants further investigation.

The dual effects of catecholamines upon insulin secretion can be illustrated using isoproterenol as a prime example. This amine is a mixed α- and β-agonist that stimulates insulin release in vivo (90), but inhibits insulin secretion in vitro (91). These effects are undoubtedly related to a number of factors including the doses used, which provide different degrees of α- and β-adrenergic receptor stimulation, and interactions, or lack thereof, with other amines. Thus in one system isoproterenol may lead to a net stimulation of insulin secretion, but in the other it would produce a net inhibition. Likewise, other amines including serotonin (92) and histamine (80) have been found to stimulate, inhibit, or have no effect upon insulin secretion. These differences must be viewed in relation to changes of capillary blood flow within the islet as in the case of histamine (80), or the ability of serotonin to enhance the release of catecholamines (93, 94) independently of its direct action upon islet cells. However, the known ability of these amines to activate simultaneously receptors that stimulate (β) and those that inhibit (α) insulin secretion is likely to be the principal factor in these conflicting results.

The molecular configuration of amines is a determinant of their interaction with the islet cells. In a recent review, Lebovitz & Feldman (39) have pointed out that while the ammonium ion (NH_4^+) inhibits glucose-stimulated insulin release, only aromatic amines have the ability to inhibit insulin secretion to other stimuli. This pharmacologic action of monoamines appears to be dependent primarily upon the presence of a terminal amine on the aliphatic portion of the molecule and partially dependent upon the hydroxyl groups of the aromatic ring (91). Insulin secretion is inhibited by serotonin (5-hydroxytryptamine), but its deaminated breakdown product 5-hydroxyindoleacetic acid has no such effect. On the other hand, 5-hydroxytryptophan, an aminated serotonin precursor, does not inhibit insulin release as an extracellular agent, presumably because of the presence of its carboxyl group. The importance of the hydroxyl group is further indicated by the greater potency of dopamine compared to tyramine as an inhibitor of insulin secretion (the former has one additional hydroxyl group). Methylation of the hydroxyl group abolishes the inhibition of insulin release as indicated by the lack of effect of 5-methoxytryptamine or metanephrine. The hydroxyl group is not an absolute requirement for pharmacologic action because β-phenylethylamine and tryptamine both decrease insulin secretion in vitro. The stimulatory properties of β-receptor agonists, however, are more closely related to the hydroxyl groups and can be found almost selectively when the amine group is blocked but not removed (e.g. isopropylnorepinephrine).

There is evidence that many of the monoamines share receptors. The α-receptor antagonist phentolamine blocks the inhibition of insulin secretion produced by serotonin, tryptamine, catecholamines, and histamine. All of these, except histamine, are also blocked by methysergide (39). The blockade of catecholamine and serotonin action by either phentolamine or methysergide strongly supports the concept that these different groups of amines inhibit insulin secretion via the same or similar membrane receptors. Because serotonin also enhances catecholamine release from nerve endings in addition to its direct effect upon the B cell, its properties may be altered by the release of norepinephrine (94). Alternatively, serotonin may stimulate insulin secretion via β-receptors either directly or in conjunction with catecholamines. This kind of modulation probably explains why serotonin inhibits or stimulates insulin secretion depending upon the particular circumstances.

The ability of amines to stimulate insulin secretion by activation of the β-adrenergic receptor is blocked by agents such as propranolol. Using selective agents such as practolol and salbutamol, Loubatieres et al (95) found that amine-induced insulin secretion is dependent upon stimulation of the β_2-receptor and does not require simultaneous activation of the β_1-receptors. Therefore, the differential stimulation of the two kinds of β-receptors is also important.

Recently, the fatty acid derivatives known as prostaglandins (PGs) have attracted wide attention because of their diverse effects in a number of endocrine systems. Of particular interest is their pharmacologic action upon islet hormone release because of their known interaction with catecholamines in other systems (96, 97). Much like serotonin, PGs have been found to stimulate, inhibit, or have no effect upon insulin secretion (98, 99). Robertson et al (100) found that PGE_1 inhibits basal and stimulated insulin secretion of the dog in vivo. This inhibitory response was not blocked by phentolamine, suggesting the PGs act independently of catecholamine receptors. In contrast, Bressler et al (52) observed a stimulation of insulin secretion by PGE_1. In this in vivo system, β-adrenergic blockade reversed the enhanced release of insulin. Both findings were confirmed by Burr & Sharp (101) who reported that insulin secretion in vitro was increased by PGE_1 at low glucose concentrations, but that at high glucose levels PGE_1 produced an inhibitory effect. In the same study, the concurrent administration of epinephrine and PGE_1 at high glucose concentrations resulted in a paradoxical stimulation of insulin secretion (i.e. the drugs alone would have inhibited insulin secretion with these conditions). These authors suggested that this response could be due to a prostaglandin-mediated change of α- or β-receptor activity, or to an alteration of calcium flux by PGs that is modulated by adrenergic stimulation.

Another recently discovered neurohormone, somatostatin, has been found to have pharmacologic actions upon islet hormone secretion. This cyclic polypeptide was originally isolated from the ovine hypothalamus (102) and was found to inhibit somatotropin (growth hormone) release. It thus became known as somatostatin or SRIF (Somatotropin Release Inhibiting Factor), although it also acts upon other pituitary hormones (103). Somatostatin became of interest to islet physiologists when it was observed to induce hypoglycemia in vivo (104). Further investigation has proven that this hormone is a potent inhibitor of both insulin and glucagon secretion (105–110). The islet hormone responses to somatostatin administration are clearly unique when compared to those of the agents previously discussed. First of all, somatostatin is the only naturally occurring hormone known to inhibit the secretion of both islet hormones simultaneously. Further, at appropriate doses, somatostatin obliterates insulin and glucagon release to all known secretagogues and reduces the basal rates of islet hormone secretion to nearly undetectable levels in the plasma. Because of these properties, somatostatin has recently been employed as an experimental tool in many phases of pancreatic islet research.

We have observed that this hormone inhibits basal and glucose-stimulated insulin secretion in the perfused dog pancreas in vivo (82, 105). At a dose of 1.7 μg/min, somatostatin inhibited insulin secretion when infused into the pancreatic artery, portal vein, or femoral vein. Surprisingly, when somatostatin was infused into the pancreatic artery at one tenth of this dose, there was no reliable inhibition of either insulin or glucagon, even though this particular dose was calculated to be approximately twice that reaching the pancreatic artery when a dose of 1.7 μg/min was infused into either the portal or femoral vein. We have therefore postulated that somatostatin may act indirectly. To test this theory, we have compared the effects of somatostatin upon insulin secretion during an infusion of either glucose or phentolamine (111). When somatostatin was infused alone (via the femoral vein) at a rate of 1.7 μg/min, the levels of both plasma insulin and glucose fell and remained depressed over a 30 minute interval. This same dose of somatostatin also inhibited the insulin secretion stimulated by glucose infusions ranging from 1 to 6 mg/kg per min. However, with this same protocol, the elevated levels of plasma insulin observed during a phentolamine infusion were not inhibited by somatostatin. During these experiments the phentolamine and glucose infusions increased basal insulin output to comparable steady state levels and produced no significant changes of pancreatic blood flow. Since the steady state insulin output was inhibited by somatostatin during the glucose infusions but not in the presence of the α-blocker, we conclude that phentolamine was responsible for the lack of somatostatin-mediated inhibition of insulin release. This implicates the α-receptor as a site of interaction between somatostatin and the sympathetic nervous system. In contrast with our findings, Efendic & Luft (112) reported that α-blockade had no effect on the ability of somatostatin to inhibit insulin secretion in humans. Some investigators have found that the in vitro inhibition of insulin secretion by somatostatin is reversed by elevating the levels of extracellular calcium (113, 114). Since calcium uptake by the B cell has been implicated as a trigger for insulin release (115), it is possible that a somatostatin-α-receptor interaction would elicit an alteration of calcium flux leading to an inhibition of insulin secretion.

The recent immunocytochemical localization of somatostatin in the pancreatic islet D cells (10, 11) suggests the possibility that this hormone plays a role in the normal and pathophysiologic regulation of islet hormone secretion. This finding also lends support to the hypothesis that the pancreatic islet cells are derived from the neuroectoderm, since it seems unlikely that cells producing somatostatin in the hypothalamus would be of different embryonic origin from those containing the same hormone in the pancreatic islets.

INTERACTING SYSTEMS IN ISLET FUNCTION: A SUMMARY

The complex nature of insulin and glucagon secretion makes an integrated discussion of the role of amines and other neural factors in the regulation of islet hormone secretion quite speculative at present. Nevertheless, the majority of papers cited in this review can be placed into a coherent framework. The authors offer in Figure 1 a schematic diagram of the potential interactions that have been covered.

We have concentrated on the B cell and have followed the suggestions of Lacy (8, 116) for the fundamental synthesis and storage of insulin. That is, insulin is synthesized in the endoplasmic reticulum and transported to the Golgi complex where it is packaged into granules. These granules are subsequently stored in the cytoplasm and are available for release when the appropriate signal is provided. Insulin is believed to be secreted via two different mechanisms. Some investigators (see 117, 118) have observed that insulin is released simply by the intracytoplasmic breakdown of the secretory granules and the diffusion of the hormone through the plasma membrane of the B cell. However, others (8, 116, 119, 120) have found that the granules are pulled toward the membrane of the B cell by an interaction with the microtubules and microfilaments within the cytoplasm. The membrane of the secretory granules then fuses with the plasma membrane and the insulin granules are thus released into the extracellular space via emiocytosis. Recent studies have shown that during emiocytotic release, the membranes of several granules fuse with one another in a process called *vesicular binesis* (121); thus a single channel can serve as a focal release point for many secretory granules. This fusion of secretory

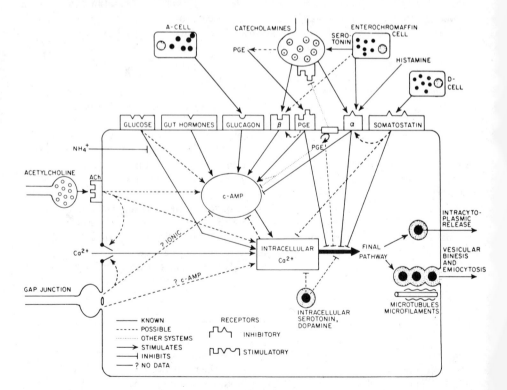

Figure 1 A hypothetical model of interacting systems in insulin secretion.

granules has also been observed during the intracytoplasmic dissolution of the B-cell granules (23, 118) indicating that it may play a wider role in insulin secretion.

Intracellular calcium plays a major regulatory role in the process leading to the triggering of insulin secretion. The availability of intracellular Ca^{2+} is primarily regulated by the concentration of substrates in the blood (particularly glucose and amino acids). Glucagon and gut hormones in conjunction with locally released neural factors may also regulate Ca^{2+} flux of the B cell. Intracellular amines also influence insulin release, and some interaction between them and intracellular calcium seems likely.

One possible interaction is that intracellular amines and Ca^{2+} compete for the same negatively charged ligands within the B-cell granules (122, 123; I. Lundquist, personal communication). This is separate from the regulatory role of extracellular amines, since some blocking agents that effectively alter insulin responses to extracellular serotonin and dopamine are ineffective when the intracellular concentration of these same amines has been elevated.

Extracellular amines, somatostatin, and possibly prostaglandin influence insulin secretion by interactions with cell surface receptors. Although some agents are purely stimulatory (e.g. acetylcholine) and others are purely inhibitory (e.g. somatostatin), the catecholamines, indoleamines, and prostaglandins have been found to be both stimulators and inhibitors. All of these compounds bind to cell surface receptors that in turn interact with the basic secretory processes of the cell to regulate insulin secretion. Some of them bind to more than one receptor. The net effect upon insulin secretion will depend on the receptor stimulated, the pathway regulated, and the endogenous activity of the cell. All of this must be viewed in light of recent evidence (124, 125) indicating that the number of cell surface receptors is not constant, as was previously thought, but varies from time to time as a function of the agonist concentration and the metabolic state of the B cell. Therefore, it is not surprising that different results have been reported for many of the pharmacologic agents used to study insulin secretion. The reader must be wary when a compound is reported to be either stimulatory or inhibitory upon insulin secretion unless a wide range of drug concentrations has been studied over a variety of conditions. Further, there are compounds that interact both with cell surface receptors and with the basic cellular machinery of the islet. Glucose is one such example. Since the net product of B-cell function is insulin secretion, any compound that alters intracellular glycolytic rates, protein synthetic rates, or oxidative metabolism may be expected to change insulin secretion.

Despite these complexities, one can make the following generalizations: 1. Acetylcholine is representative of neurally related compounds that stimulate both insulin and glucagon secretion, have no inhibitory properties, and do not appear to interact with islet metabolism. 2. Somatostatin is representative of a class of compounds that inhibits insulin and glucagon release and neither alters islet cell metabolism nor elicits any stimulatory effect. 3. The other neurally related compounds that influence insulin secretion (indoleamines, catecholamines, and prostaglandins) possess the ability to regulate stimulatory and inhibitory pathways of insulin release simultaneously. Stimulation ∩f insulin secretion by these latter agents appears to involve the activation of adenylcyclase. It is conceivable, therefore, that all of them interact either directly with the β-adrenergic receptor or alter its sensitivity, thereby changing intracellular cyclic AMP levels. Indoleamines and catecholamines inhibit insulin release via activation of the α-adrenergic receptors and primarily affect glucose-stimulated insulin release. Prostaglandins also inhibit glucose-induced insulin secretion, but do so by a mechanism not requiring adrenergic receptor activation. Somatostatin inhibits insulin and glucagon secretion regardless of the stimulus; but even with this agent there are complex interactions because α-adrenergic blockers modulate the ability of somatostatin to inhibit insulin release. While it was originally hypothesized that α-adrenergic inhibition of insulin secretion is due to reduced adenylcyclase activity and a subsequent decrease of cyclic AMP formation, this explanation is now quite unlikely. This is due to the fact that even though α-adrenergic stimulation lowers adenylcyclase activity, insulin release cannot be stimulated by exogenous cyclic AMP in the presence of epinephrine. Whether cyclic GMP will eventually become identified as an inhibitory second messenger for insulin and glucagon secretion, or whether basic electrolyte transport processes involving calcium flux will be shown to be related to α-receptor activation is not clear at the present time.

Interactions between neuropharmacologically active agents occur because so many of them are present within the islet (i.e. acetylcholine and the catecholamines are found within nerve endings, somatostatin and serotonin are stored in islet cells, and prostaglandins are presumably synthesized by the islet cells). The release of autonomic transmitters is known to be sensitive to the concentration of prostaglandins, and transmitter release is also altered by exogenous serotonin and circulating catecholamines. The stimulus for the release of serotonin stored in enterochromaffin cells of the islet is unknown at present. Nevertheless, a complete picture of islet function must consider the possibility that intra-islet serotonin plays a role in the regulation of insulin and glucagon secretion. Somatostatin present in islet D cells may also be expected to regulate insulin and glucagon release, just as intra-islet glucagon alters insulin secretion. Finally, the purinergic nervous system and gap junctions should be mentioned. Purinergic nerves have been observed in the islets of teleosts and are known to exist in the smooth muscles of mammals. This portion of the autonomic nervous system is believed to be an inhibitory system whose transmitter is ATP. The effects of ATP release upon serotonin, somatostatin, catecholamines, acetylcholine, or islet cells themselves are unknown, but the finding of such nerves in one mammalian system suggests their possible presence in others. The physiologic role of gap junctions observed between islet cells and between nerves and islets cells is also unknown at present. However, it is conceivable that such junctions serve to transmit and amplify stimulatory or inhibitory messages throughout the islet parenchyma.

In conclusion, the islet should be looked upon as a metabolic computer that is capable of adjusting the output of insulin and glucagon according to direct substrate levels and that is modulated by a wide variety of hormonal and neural messages. These hormonal and neural signals often arise within the islet and in some cases are directly connected to the central nervous system. This system of hormonal and neural controls provide for both short- and long-term regulation of metabolic processes.

ACKNOWLEDGMENTS

This review was written with the support of funds from the Veterans Administration (MRIS numbers 8007, 7155) and the National Institutes of Health (AM 05498, AM 12829). Dr. Smith is the recipient of a National Institutes of Health Fellowship (F22 AM 03433) and a grant from the Boeing Employees Good Neighbor Fund. We thank S. C. Woods, S. A. Metz, R. P. Robertson, J. D. Brunzell, and I. Lundquist for their helpful suggestions and comments on the manuscript.

Literature Cited

1. Grodsky, G. M. 1970. *Vitam. Horm. NY* 28:37–101
2. Lefebvre, P. J., Unger, R. H., eds. 1972. *Glucagon: Molecular Physiology, Clinical and Therapeutic Implications.* Oxford: Pergamon. 370 pp.
3. Steiner, D. F., Freinkel, N., ed. 1972. *Endocrine Pancreas, Handbook of Physiology,* Sect. 7, Vol 1. Baltimore: Williams & Wilkins. 721 pp.
4. Unger, R. H. 1974. *Metab. Clin. Exp.* 23:581–93
5. Epple, A., Brinn, J. 1975. *Gen. Comp. Endocrinol.* In press
6. Pictet, R., Rutter, W. J. 1972. See Ref. 3, pp. 25–66
7. Falkner, S., Patent, G. J. 1972. See Ref. 3, pp. 1–24
8. Lacy, P. E., Greider, M. H. 1972. See Ref. 3, pp. 77–90
9. Lostra, F., Van der Loo, W., Gepts, W. 1974. *Diabetologia* 10:290–302
10. Dubois, M. P. 1975. *Proc. Natl. Acad. Sci. USA* 72:1340–43
11. Polak, J., Pearse, A. G. E., Grimelius, L., Bloom, S. R., Arimura, A. 1975. *Lancet* 1:1220–22
12. Melmed, R., Benitez, C., Holt, S. J. 1972. *J. Cell Sci.* 11:449–75
13. Pearse, A. G. E., Polak, J., Heath, C. M. 1973. *Diabetologia* 9:120–29
14. Pearse, A. G. E. 1969. *J. Histochem. Cytochem.* 17:303–13
15. Le Douarin, N., Le Lievre, C. 1970. *C. R. Acad. Sci. Ser. D* 270:2857–60
16. Pearse, A. G. E., Polak, J. 1971. *Histochemie* 27:96–102
17. Pearse, A. G. E., Polak, J. 1971. *Gut* 12:783–88
18. Andrew, A. 1974. *J. Embryol. Exp. Morphol.* 31:589–98
19. Pictet, R. L. et al 1976. *Science* 191:191–93
20. Woods, S. C., Porte, D. Jr. 1974. *Physiol. Rev.* 54:596–619
21. Kern, H. F., Grübe, D. 1972. *Proc. Int. Congr. Endocrinol., 4th, Wash. DC,* pp. 224–28
22. Miller, M., Lagios, M. 1970. *Biology of the Reptilia,* ed. C. Gans, 3:319–46. New York: Academic. 413 pp.
23. Smith, P. H. 1974. *Anat. Rec.* 178: 567–86
24. Orci, L. et al 1970. *Acta Diabetol. Lat.* 7:184–222
25. Kurotsu, T., Tabayashi, C., Ban, T. 1953. *Med. J. Osaka Univ.* 3:529–46
26. Coupland, R. E. 1958. *J. Anat.* 92: 143–49
27. Shorr, S. S., Bloom, F. E. 1970. *Z. Zellforsch. Mikrosk. Anat.* 103:12–25
28. Simard, L. C. 1935. *C. R. Soc. Biol.* 119:27–28
29. Morgan, C. R., Lobl, R. T. 1966. *Anat. Rec.* 160:231–38
30. Richardson, K. C. 1964. *Am. J. Anat.* 114:173–205
31. Burnstock, G. 1972. *Pharmacol. Rev.* 24:509–81
32. Brinn, J. E. 1975. *Cell Tissue Res.* 162:357–65
33. Orci, L., Unger, R. H., Renold, A. E. 1973. *Experientia* 29:1015–18
34. Orci, L., Perrelet, A., Ravazzola, M., Malaisse-Lagae, F., Renold, A. E. 1973. *Eur. J. Clin. Invest.* 3:443–45
35. Dean, P. M., Matthews, E. K. 1970. *J. Physiol.* 210:255–64
36. Meissner, H. P., Schmelz, H. 1974. *Pfluegers Arch.* 357:195–206
37. Smith, P. H. 1975. *Am. J. Anat.* 144:513
38. Cegrell, L. 1968. *Acta Physiol. Scand. Suppl.* 314:1–60
39. Lebovitz, H. E., Feldman, J. M. 1973. *Fed. Proc.* 32:1797–1802
40. Omar, C., Hakanson, R., Sundler, F. 1973. *Fed. Proc.* 32:1785–91
41. Ekholm, R., Erickson, L. E., Lundquist, I. 1971. *Diabetologia* 7:339–48
42. Lebovitz, H. E. 1976. *Pancreatic Interactions: A Conference,* ed. S. C. Woods, D. Porte, Jr. In press

43. Feldman, J. M., Chapman, B. 1975. *Metab. Clin. Exp.* 24:581–88
44. Aleyassine, H., Gardiner, R. J. 1975. *Endocrinology* 96:702–10
45. Lernmark, A. 1971. *Horm. Metab. Res.* 3:305–9
46. Rossini, A. A., Buse, M. G. 1973. *Horm. Metab. Res.* 5:26–28
47. Wilson, J. P., Downs, R. W., Feldman, J. M., Lebovitz, H. E. 1974. *Am. J. Physiol.* 227:305–11
48. Lundquist, I., Ekholm, R., Erickson, L. E. 1971. *Diabetologia* 7:414–22
49. Feldman, J. M., Lebovitz, H. E. 1972. *Experientia* 28:433–34
50. Feldman, J. M., Quickel, K. E., Lebovitz, H. E. 1972. *Diabetes* 21:779–88
51. Feldman, J. M., Lebovitz, H. E. 1973. *Endocrinology* 92:1469–74
52. Bressler, R., Vargas-Gordon, M., Lebovitz, H. E. 1968. *Diabetes* 17:617–24
53. Lundquist, I. 1971. *Acta Physiol. Scand. Suppl* 372:1–47
54. Aleyassine, H., Lee, S. H. 1972. *Am. J. Physiol.* 222:565–69
55. Frohman, L. A., Ezdinli, E. Z., Javid, R. 1967 *Diabetes* 16:443–88
56. Kaneto, A., Kosaka, K., Nakao, K. 1967. *Endocrinology* 80:530–36
57. Porte, D. Jr., Girardier, L., Seydoux, J., Kanazawa, Y., Posternak, J. 1973. *J. Clin. Invest.* 52:210–14
58. Kaneto, A., Miki, E., Kosaka, K. 1974. *Endocrinology* 98:1005–10
59. Kuzuya, T. 1962. *J. Jpn. Soc. Int. Med.* 51:65–74
60. Steffens, A. B., Mogenson, G. J., Stevenson, J. A. F. 1972. *Am. J. Physiol.* 222:1446–52
61. Bloom, S. R., Edwards, A. V., Vaughn, N. J. A. 1974. *J. Physiol.* 236:611–23
62. Esterhuizen, A. C., Howell, S. L. 1970. *J. Cell Biol.* 46:593–631
63. Allen, F. M. 1924. *Am. J. Physiol.* 67:275–90
64. Britton, S. W. 1925. *Am. J. Physiol.* 74:291–307
65. Chlouverakis, C., Bernardis, L. L. 1972. *Diabetologia* 8:179–84
66. Woods, S. C. 1972. *Am. J. Physiol.* 223:1424–27
67. Russell, R. C. G., Thomson, J. P. S., Bloom, S. R. 1974. *Br. J. Surg.* 61:821–24
68. Powley, T. L., Opsahl, C. A. 1975. *Hunger: Basic Mechanisms and Clinical Implications,* ed. D. Novin, W. Wyrwicka, G. A. Bray. New York: Raven. In press
69. Malaisse, W. J., Malaisse-Lagae, F.,

Wright, P. H., Ashmore, J. 1967. *Endocrinology* 80:975–78
70. Lundquist, I. 1973. *Proc. Scand. Soc.* 9:18–19
71. Iversen, J. 1973. *Diabetes* 22:381–87
72. Kaneto, A., Kosaka, K. 1974. *Endocrinology* 95:676–81
73. Sharp, R., Culbert, S., Cook, J., Jennings, A., Burr, I. M. 1974. *J. Clin. Invest.* 53:710–16
74. Miettinen, T. A., Taskinen, M. R., Pelkonen, R., Nikkilä, E. A. 1969. *Acta Med. Scand.* 186:247–53
75. Kajinuma, H., Kaneto, A., Kuzuya, T., Nakao, K. 1968. *J. Clin. Invest.* 28:1384–88
76. Bergman, R. N., Miller, R. E. 1973. *Am. J. Physiol* 225:481–86
77. Findlay, J. A., Gill, J. R., Lever, J. D., Randle, P. J., Spriggs, T. L. B. 1969. *J. Anat.* 104:580 (Abstr.)
78. Frohman, L. A., Bernardis, L. L. 1971. *Am. J. Physiol.* 221:1596–1603
79. Porte, D. Jr. 1969. *Arch. Int. Med.* 123:252–60
80. Malaisse, W. J. 1972. See Ref. 3, 237–60
81. Porte, D. Jr., Robertson, R. P. 1973. *Fed. Proc.* 32:1792–96
82. Porte, D. Jr., Woods, S. C., Chen, M., Smith, P. H., Ensinck, J. W. 1975. *Pharmacol. Biochem. Behav.* 3:Suppl. 1, 127–33
83. Iversen, J. 1973. *J. Clin. Invest.* 52:2102–16
84. Gerich, J. E., Langlois, M., Noaxxo, C., Schneider, V., Forsham, P. H. 1974. *J. Clin. Invest.* 53:1441–46
85. Harvey, W. D., Faloona, G. R., Unger, R. H. 1974. *Endocrinology* 94:1254–58
86. Robertson, R. P., Porte, D. Jr. 1973. *Diabetes* 22:1–8
87. Turtle, J. R., Kipnis, D. M. 1967. *Biochem. Biophys. Res. Commun.* 28:797–802
88. Feldman, J. M., Lebovitz, H. E. 1970. *Diabetes* 29:480–86
89. Malaisse, W. J., Brisson, G., Malaisse-Lagae, F. 1970. *J. Lab. Clin. Med.* 76:895–902
90. Porte, D. Jr. 1967. *Diabetes* 16:150–55
91. Feldman, J. M., Boyd, A. E., Lebovitz, H. E. 1971. *J. Pharmacol. Exp. Ther.* 176:611–21
92. Telib, M., Raptis, S., Schröder, K. E., Pfeiffer, E. F. 1968. *Diabetologia* 4:253–56
93. Innes, I. R. 1962. *Br. J. Pharmacol.* 19:427–41
94. Quickel, K. E., Feldman, J. M., Lebovitz, H. E. 1971. *Endocrinology* 89:1295–1302

95. Loubatieres, A., Mariani, M. M., Sorel, G., Savi, L. 1971. *Diabetologia* 7: 127–32
96. Hedqvist, P. 1973. *The Prostaglandins,* ed. P. V. Ramwell, 101–31. New York: Plenum. 400 pp.
97. Robertson, R. P. 1974. *Prostaglandins* 6:501–8
98. Robertson, R. P. 1975. *Metabolic Regulation: Insulin and Diabetes,* ed. R. B. Tobin. New York: Academic. In press
99. Johnson, D. G., Fujimoto, W. Y., Williams, R. H. 1973. *Diabetes* 22:658–63
100. Robertson, R. P., Gavareski, D. J., Porte, D. Jr., Bierman, E. L. 1974. *J. Clin. Invest.* 54:310–15
101. Burr, I. M., Sharp, R. 1974. *Endocrinology* 94:835–39
102. Brazeau, P. et al 1973. *Science* 179:77–79
103. Siler, T. M., Yen, S. S. C., Vale, W., Guillemin, R. 1974. *J. Clin. Endocrinol. Metab.* 38:742–45
104. Koerker, D. J. et al 1974. *Science* 184:482–84
105. Chen, M., Smith, P. H., Woods, S. C., Johnson, D. G., Porte, D. Jr. 1974. *Diabetes* 23:356 (Abstr.)
106. Chideckel, E. W. et al 1975. *J. Clin. Invest.* 55:754–62
107. Johnson, D. G., Ensinck, J. W., Koerker, D. J., Palmer, J. C., Goodner, C. J. 1975. *Endocrinology* 96:370–74
108. Gerich, J. E., Lovinger, R., Grodsky, G. M. 1975. *Endocrinology* 96:749–54
109. Leblanc, H., Anderson, J. R., Sigel, M. B., Yen, S. S. C. 1975. *J. Clin. Endocrinol. Metab.* 40:568–72
110. Sakurai, H., Dobbs, R., Unger, R. H. 1974. *J. Clin. Invest.* 54:1395–1402
111. Smith, P. H., Woods, S. C., Porte, D. Jr. 1975. *Diabetes* 24:408 (Abstr.)
112. Efendic, S., Luft, R. 1975. *Acta Endocrinol.* 78:516–23
113. Curry, D. L., Bennett, L. L. 1974. *Biochem. Biophys. Res. Commun.* 60: 1015–19
114. Bhathena, S. et al 1975. *Diabetes* 24:408 (Abstr.)
115. Malaisse, W. J., Malaisse-Lagae, F. 1970. *Acta Diabetol. Lat.* 7:Suppl 1, 264–75
116. Lacy, P. E. 1975. *Am. J. Pathol.* 79:170–87
117. Petkov, P., Donev, S. 1973. *Acta Diabetol. Lat.* 10:454–77
118. Smith, P. H. 1975. *Gen. Comp. Endocrinol.* 26:310–20
119. Lacy, P. E. 1970. *Diabetes* 19:895–905
120. Malaisse, W. J. 1973. *Diabetologia* 9:167–73
121. Gabbay, K. H., Korff, J., Schneeberger, I. 1975. *Science* 187:177–79
122. Herman, L., Sato, T., Hales, C. N. 1973. *J. Ultrastruct. Res.* 42:298–311
123. Shäfer, H. J., Klöppel, G. 1974. *Virchows Arch. A.* 362:231–45
124. Gavin, J. R., Roth, J., Neville, D. M., De Meyts, P., Buell, D. N. 1974. *Proc. Natl. Acad. Sci. USA* 71:84–88
125. Archer, J. A., Gorden, P., Roth, J. 1975. *J. Clin. Invest.* 55:166–74

RENIN AND THE THERAPY OF HYPERTENSION

♦6651

Gordon P. Guthrie, Jr., Jacques Genest, and Otto Kuchel[1]
Clinical Research Institute of Montreal, Montreal, Quebec, Canada

INTRODUCTION

The measurement of the activity of the circulating proteolytic enzyme, renin, has come to hold a unique place in modern concepts of hypertension. Recognized since its initial discovery by Tigerstedt & Bergman (1) as capable of inducing an elevated blood pressure, the overactivity of renin (and overproduction of the vasoactive octapeptide angiotensin II) is now thought to be directly responsible for high blood pressure in but a minority of humans afflicted with this disease. The implication of renin as a causative factor in this small, but important, subgroup of patients (with predominantly renal, renovascular, and malignant hypertension) belies its current importance, for it has facilitated the classification of hypertension, both primary (essential) and secondary in humans and experimental animals, yielding important new information on the variety of hypertensive states. The purpose of this paper is to summarize recent concepts of the etiology and therapy of hypertension based on knowledge of the activity of the renin-angiotensin system and its modification by therapeutic and diagnostic agents.

FACTORS AFFECTING RENIN RELEASE

Since most agents used in the therapy of hypertension affect plasma renin activity in some way, it is worthwhile to discuss briefly those mechanisms affecting renin release. Several recent reviews (2–5) outline this subject in greater detail.

Renin is a specific enzyme of 40,000 mol wt that is synthesized, stored, and released from specialized granular cells in the arteriole at the vascular pole of the renal glomerulus. Although extrarenal sources of renin or isorenins have been described, notably the brain (6), uterus (7), and adrenal glands (8), the physiologic significance of these enzymes remains undefined. The associated periglomerular grouping of the afferent arteriole, efferent arteriole, lacis cells, and the group of

[1]This work was supported by a group grant from the Medical Research Council of Canada to the multidisciplinary Research Group on Hypertension at the Clinical Research Institute of Montreal.

287

specialized cells at the origin of the nearby distal tubule known as the macula densa form the "juxtaglomerular apparatus" (9), a microstructure involved in the fine control of renin release. Although the specific intracellular mechanisms responsible for renin secretion remain speculative, its modulation by the physiologic variables of vascular volume, blood pressure, sympathetic nervous tone, sodium, and potassium appears to involve the juxtaglomerular apparatus (10, 11).

The baroreceptor hypothesis (that the afferent arteriole responds to a decreased (or increased) mean renal perfusion pressure with an altered stretching or a decreased transmural pressure in this vessel by an increase (or decrease) in renin release) followed from the observation of altered juxtaglomerular cell granularity with varied perfusion pressures (12, 13). Further experiments in the nonfiltering kidney preparation (13), in which an influence on renin release by alterations in intratubular sodium concentration was excluded, specifically in the area of the macula densa, have established strong support for this hypothesized mechanism (14). That an altered sodium concentration in the region of the macula densa can regulate renin release has been suggested by several studies (15–17), although whether the stimulus to renin secretion is an increase (17) or decrease (16) in this concentration is unresolved.

The following illustrate the intimate relation between sympathetic nervous activity and plasma renin activity: observations of the close histologic association of sympathetic nervous fibers with the juxtaglomerular apparatus (17–19a), the induction of renin release by renal nerve stimulation (20), the reduction of resting plasma renin activity in response to volume depletion by renal sympathectomy (21), and the blunting of renin responsiveness after administration of ganglionic blocking agents (22). The closely related stimulation of renin release by circulating catecholamines is further considered under the section on propranolol.

Although β, and not α, receptors (23) are thought to control adrenergic modulation of renin, the cellular mechanisms involved are controversial, but are thought by many to involve β-receptor mediation of the intracellular cyclic adenosine monophosphate (cAMP) system (24–27). Michelakis et al (26) have shown in vitro stimulation of renin release into the incubating medium by both catecholamines and cAMP, and Nolly and co-workers (30) have demonstrated potentiation of catecholamine-stimulated release by the phosphodiesterase inhibitor theophylline. Similarly, Winer and colleagues (24) demonstrated in vivo stimulation of renin release by cAMP, but because propranolol prevented cAMP-induced renin release, also suggested an adrenergic site of action distal to cAMP. Reid (28), however, found that propranolol did not prevent theophylline-stimulated renin secretion in vivo. Also controversial is the observation of Beck et al (29) that lithium pretreatment in vitro and in vivo, which prevented isoproterenol-induced increases in intracellular and excreted cAMP, did not affect isoproterenol-induced renin release. Hence, the precise role of intracellular cAMP in this scheme is at present unclear, since the sequence of activation of a juxtaglomerular cell membrane-bound β-receptor and adenylate cyclase stimulation leading to increased intracellular cAMP and renin release does not conform to several experimental findings.

Of related interest are the demonstrated experimental alterations in renin release by central nervous system interventions, specifically stimulation of medullary and hypothalamic centers (31) and inhibition by intracerebral 6-hydroxydopamine administration (32), which, together with other central mechanisms of blood pressure regulation, appear to be mediated through the peripheral sympathetic nervous system. The demonstration of a central pressor action of the active product of renin activity, angiotensin II, probably via an action at the area postrema and again mediated by the autonomic nervous system (33) highlights the variety of interrelationships of the central nervous system, renin activity, and blood pressure control.

Renin release is affected by changes in serum potassium concentration and excretion, which in turn are often affected by the treatment of hypertension with various types of diuretics and/or necessary potassium supplementation. Administration of potassium to humans tends to reduce plasma renin activity despite an induced natriuresis from this cation (34), directly related to alterations in plasma concentration and urinary excretion. Potassium depletion results in the converse rise in plasma renin activity, despite an induced sodium retention (and lower aldosterone secretion), and both these effects appear mediated through a renal tubular mechanism, possibly at the macula densa (35).

The control mechanisms of renin release are all interrelated, with several feedback cycles. The end product of renin activity, angiotensin II, inhibits renin release directly by an effect presumably at the renin-containing afferent arteriolar cells (36–39) independent of vasoconstrictive activity (37), and indirectly by several mechanisms. First, angiotensin II stimulates aldosterone production by the adrenal zona glomerulosa (40) with consequent increased distal tubular sodium reabsorption, expansion of the extracellular fluid volume, a sensed increased perfusion pressure by the afferent arteriole, and hence a depressed rate of renin release. Second, the direct systemic vasoconstrictor effect of angiotensin II would effect the same sensed increased perfusion pressure and renin inhibition, as would the third indirect step, the mentioned central pressor effect of angiotensin II. Other postulated indirect actions are afferent or efferent arteriolar vasoconstriction in response to locally formed angiotensin II from an increased distal sodium load as sensed by the macula densa and the consequent increased renin secretion (41), or a converse single nephron feedback system with suppression of renin release upon distal sodium delivery (42). Of all these mentioned indirect feedback inhibitory factors upon renin release, that via aldosterone stimulation and vascular volume expansion is thought to be the most physiologically significant.

Before considering the classification of hypertension and the use of such subgrouping, attention should be focused on the variations of the renin activity during antihypertensive therapy, which are related to the above-mentioned control mechanisms of renin release.

EFFECT OF ANTIHYPERTENSIVE DRUGS ON PLASMA RENIN ACTIVITY

Virtually all the drugs currently employed as antihypertensive agents affect plasma renin activity in some manner, although these effects may not necessarily be related to the mechanism of the antihypertensive effect. The effects of single agents on renin activity are discussed below. Because evidence of the relation of the adrenergic nervous system to renin has evolved through study with a multitude of antiadrenergic drugs, each with a unique effect on the sympathetic nervous system, the concepts of this relation are discussed relative to the mechanism of action of each drug.

Diuretics

The mechanism of the antihypertensive action of diuretic agents is unknown, but appears related to an initial negative sodium balance (43), possibly with sustained plasma volume reduction (50). Certain types, such as those of the thiazide and chlorthalidone group and those affecting the loop of Henle, may also act through a direct dilatory action on arteriolar smooth muscle or through alterations in the electrolyte or water content of the arteriolar wall (44, 45). However, whether this latter mechanism is significant is unclear (46), since the blood pressure of normotensive individuals is not reduced by these drugs and the antipressor activity can be nullified by a high sodium diet (47) and can be duplicated by sodium restriction (48) or diuretic agents with no demonstrated direct arteriolar action, such as mercuhydrin (43). A diminished vascular reactivity to sympathetic stimulation possibly via effective chronic sodium depletion after thiazide administration has also been shown (49), which may blunt a compensatory blood pressure rise upon volume depletion, and may also in part account for the well-known potentiation of the antihypertensive effect of other agents by the oral diuretics. With chronic diuretic therapy, the plasma renin activity is usually increased and remains so (50). Although possessing a somewhat lesser chronic antihypertensive effect than the thiazide or chlorthalidone group (51) [although nonetheless effective as single agents for mild hypertension (52)], the loop of Henle diuretics, ethacrynic acid and furosemide, promote a greater initial diuresis with consequent volume depletion, often leading to a rise in plasma renin activity. This phenomenon has been used to stimulate renin release for renin subgroup classification (61). That the mechanism of acute stimulation of renin release is not completely via volume depletion, and may involve an increased sodium delivery to the macula densa, is suggested by the incomplete inhibition of renin release by simultaneous urine reinfusion by uretero-venous anastamosis (53), although effective vascular volume reduction by extrarenal effects, such as an effect on postcapillary capacitance vessels (54), may also occur.

Spironolactone

This drug is a specific competitive antagonist of aldosterone, and competitively inhibits the sodium-retaining and kaliuretic effect of this steroid (and other mineralocorticoids) at the distal tubular site of the nephron. It is devoid of diuretic effect in adrenalectomized subjects (55). A possible mechanism of action of spironolactone may be a competitive inhibition of endogenous mineralocorticoid action on the arteriolar resistance vessels, suggested by findings of a direct extrarenal effect of aldosterone and other mineralocorticoids on the maintenance of vascular tonicity (56, 57). When employed in the treatment of unselected patients with essential hypertension, some workers have reported a therapeutic potency comparable to the thiazide diuretics (58), although others have found a greater hypotensive effect in the subset of patients with low renin essential hypertension (59–61), in contrast to those with normal renin values. Also spironolactone has been shown by Spark and co-workers to restore normal renin responsiveness to posture and furosemide stimulation (62), in contrast to lack of a similar response after chronic thiazide administration. These studies, and others discussed below, have been taken as evidence for an excessive secretion of mineralocorticoid as a cause for low renin essential hypertension, with spironolactone being as effective a specific antagonist as it is for the alleged prototype of such hypertension, primary aldosteronism. Another unusual and unexplained effect of spironolactone in such patients is a prolonged restoration of renin responsiveness for many weeks after discontinuation of the drug, although the hypertensive state itself is soon resumed (63).

Diazoxide

This agent, with a benzothiadiazine (thiazide) structure and antinatriuretic action, is currently used in North America solely by rapid intravenous injection for the treatment of hypertensive emergencies, although it is possibly also effective by oral administration (64). Its action in hypertensive patients is via direct arteriolar smooth muscle relaxation and consequent reduction of total peripheral resistance and blood pressure (65). The hypotensive response is dissociable from the rise in plasma renin activity, the latter occurring maximally two hours after injection in two thirds of patients (66). The remaining one third, although showing a comparable hypotensive response, show no or little change in plasma renin and probably correspond to low renin essential hypertensives as defined by other techniques, such as dietary sodium restriction and upright posture (66). The mechanism of renin release in hypertensive patients responsive to diazoxide is more complex than one would expect. It is dissociable from changes in extracellular fluid volume (67) and may be related to a sensed decreased renal blood flow by the juxtaglomerular apparatus (68) or a compensatory increased adrenergic activity, as adrenergic blocking agents prevent the diazoxide-induced renin release (69). Involvement of an intracellular increase in cAMP with enhanced renin release has also been hypothesized (70), as diazoxide is a phosphodiesterase inhibitor (71) (as are the other thiazide diuretics).

Other Direct Vasodilators

Similar to diazoxide, other vasodilating drugs exert their antihypertensive effect by relaxation of arteriolar smooth muscle and decreased total peripheral resistance. Agents in this group include sodium nitroprusside (72) (used intravenously only for hypertensive emergencies), minoxidil (73), hydralazine (74), and guancydine (75). The vasodilating drugs have similar secondary effects that may limit their usefulness as solitary antihypertensive agents. They promote a reflex increase in sympathetic activity, causing increased heart rate and cardiac output (72–74), and can induce sodium retention with extracellular fluid and volume expansion (76), which may blunt the hypotensive effect. Vasodilating drugs consistently increase the plasma renin activity (73, 77, 79), possibly by a changed renal perfusion pressure and an increased renal sympathetic discharge (69, 77). An enhanced renin release by direct renal vasodilation has been stressed by Kaneko and colleagues (78), as small amounts of a vasodilator infused directly into a renal artery without significant systemic vasodepression produce large increases in plasma renin activity. The combination of vasodilating drugs with adrenergic blocking agents to prevent the reflex cardiac and renal responses, and addition of diuretics to counteract the induced sodium retention caused by these drugs has been shown to result in an effective combination capable of controlling virtually all degrees of hypertension, from mild to severe, without consideration of the baseline renin subgroup of such patients (80–82).

Clonidine

This potent antihypertensive drug, an imidazoladine derivative, differs from most other antihypertensive agents in its mechanism of action. Parenteral administration results in an acute brief hypertensive response from direct vascular adrenergic stimulation not related to catecholamine release (83). This effect is not seen with chronic oral therapy. The antihypertensive action of the drug is due to a long-acting central inhibition of medullary vasomotor and cardiac centers (84), as indicated by the absence of its effect with reserpine pretreatment, and in the spinal animal, and by the vasodepressor response following minute doses injected into the cisterna magna.

The effect of clonidine on plasma renin release is primarily inhibitory. In the anesthetized dog, intravenous injection after the initial pressor response leads to a decreased mean arterial pressure and a parallel drop in plasma renin activity, suggesting that the renin suppression is from central sympathetic inhibition (83). Intracisternal injection effects a similar depression of renin release. That renin activity is suppressed in the face of a decreased renal perfusion pressure, itself a stimulus to renin release via the juxtaglomerular apparatus sensing mechanism, has been taken as evidence that centrally controlled sympathetic tone has a predominant role in controlling renin release. However, other more direct interventions against sympathetic nervous control such as ganglionic blockade have been shown to raise plasma renin under certain conditions in the face of the parallel hypotensive response (85). Thus the relative hierarchy of control over renin release is not clear cut, as discussed below. The administration of clonidine to patients with essential hypertension also lowers the plasma renin activity (83), but as mentioned above this relation to the antihypertensive effect is uncertain.

Guanethidine

This potent drug exerts its antihypertensive action by interfering with neurotransmission at the adrenergic postganglionic nerve terminals by both preventing norepinephrine release and depleting norepinephrine stores at these terminals (86). The sympatholytic effect on cardiac innervation, with decreased heart rate, stroke volume, and hence cardiac output, contributes to the effect on blood pressure as with other agents affecting the sympathetic nervous system. The dependence of the antihypertensive action on upright posture (87) reflects its greater effect in a condition with enhanced sympathetic discharge from the postural reflex, and accounts for the common side effect of orthostatic hypotension. Similar to other drugs that impair adrenergic function, sodium retention and plasma volume expansion may result from its chronic use (88), which would have a depressive influence on the plasma renin activity. However, the net effect of guanethidine on plasma renin is variable. When given to hypertensive patients under conditions of sodium depletion, guanethidine was shown by Jose, Crout & Kaplan to augment renin increase after assumption of upright posture (89), probably via renal detection of the unbuffered blood pressure decline and lessened perfusion pressure. Lowder & Liddle (90) have demonstrated that low-renin hypertensive patients on a normal diet, with suppressed renin values despite oral furosemide (three doses of 40 mg over a 15-hr period) and upright posture, do respond with significant renin elevations to the same maneuvers after concurrent guanethidine therapy. Presumably, furosemide induces an effective sodium-depleted state in this interval. Without sodium depletion, guanethidine diminishes the renin response to upright posture (91), probably reflecting a greater dependence of the sympathetic reflexes on renin release in the sodium replete state.

Reserpine

Reserpine and the other rauwolfia alkaloids exert their antihypertensive action primarily by lowering total peripheral resistance through interference with neurotransmission at the postganglionic adrenergic nerve terminus by norepinephrine depletion, and to a lesser degree by interference with sympathetic discharge by a central action on the hypothalamus and vasomotor centers. The interference with intraneuronal storage of catecholamines appears to be the primary mechanism for impairment of adrenergic neurotransmission (92). As reserpine is thus an effective antiadrenergic drug, it would be expected to blunt reactive rises in renin activity from volume-depleting stimuli, and indeed reserpine pretreatment in rats does lessen the posthemorrhage increase (93) and in man the thiazide-induced saliuretic rise in renin activity (94). However, baseline plasma renin activity after reserpine injection has been reported to increase in dogs with renovascular hypertension (85). Morphologic evidence suggests an increase in renal renin synthesis (with a parallel decrease in plasma renin activity) after reserpine treatment, with the lack of functional sympathetic terminals impairing the release of these increased renin stores (95). Thus, reserpine may dissociate the mechanisms of renin synthesis, which are stimulated by the sensing by the juxtaglomerular apparatus of a decreased perfusion pressure from those of renin release, which are impaired by a functional sympathetic nervous blockade.

α-Methyldopa

Although this widely used drug appears to reduce the blood pressure in patients with essential hypertension by a decrease in peripheral arteriolar resistance (96), the major mechanism of action of α-methyldopa is probably central. Interference with the peripheral biosynthesis of norepinephrine (by dopa decarboxylase inhibition) or conversion to α-methylnorepinephrine with action as a *peripheral* "false" neurotransmitter appears not to account for the chronic antihypertensive effect (97). Recent studies have suggested that the hypotensive action is mediated by an effect on the central nervous system (98–100), primarily from evidence of effect from intravertebral artery and intraventricular injections of systemically suppressor doses of the drug. The mechanism is probably brain entry of the drug and *central* conversion to and accumulation of α-methylnorepinephrine with either displacement of the more potent natural central nervous system neurotransmitter norepinephrine (101) or direct stimulation of inhibitory α-adrenergic neurons in the brainstem (101a). This concept is consistent with the earlier observation by Sjoerdsma and co-workers (102) that administration to a hypertensive patient of the potent peripheral dopa decarboxylase inhibitor MK-485 (which does not cross the blood-brain barrier, but does prevent *peripheral* formation of α-methylnorepinephrine) has no effect on the hypotensive response to α-methyldopa.

Chronic oral administration of α-methyldopa to hypertensive and normotensive humans (103, 111) usually lowers the plasma renin activity in both the supine and upright positions and attenuates renin release from similar maneuvers and renal nerve stimulation in the dog (104). Similarly, a decrease in the renin activity in Bartter's syndrome (105) and the severe hypertension with hyperreninemia in end-stage renal failure (106) have been shown, and Kaplan's (107) demonstration of a blunting of the thiazide-induced rise in plasma renin activity in hypertensive subjects is in accord with the observations by Sweet and co-workers on renal hypertensive dogs (112). The peripheral "false transmitter" hypothesis has been invoked to account for this suppression of renin activity, since infused α-methylnorepinephrine has been demonstrated by Privitera & Mohammed to possess but one third the potency of the natural neurotransmitter in producing renin release (108). However, the convincing evidence for a primarily central effect of the drug and the observed analogous depression of renin activity by the centrally acting drug clonidine (83) make such a mechanism unlikely.

That the antihypertensive effect of α-methyldopa depends upon the suppression of the plasma renin activity (and a lessened production rate of angiotensin II) is also improbable. First, the drug appears to produce a supersensitivity to the pressor effects of exogenous (and by implication endogenous) angiotensin II (109), which would be expected to offset any induced lowering of the renin activity. Second, the hypotensive effect of the drug and its effect on renin, as with certain of the other antiadrenergic drugs, are dissociable. Holuska & Keiser (110) reported that in dogs with unilateral renal vessel ligation and denervation of the contralateral kidney, α-methyldopa infusion consistently lowered the blood pressure without changing the peripheral renin activity. And Lowder & Liddle (90) have recently shown that α-methyldopa therapy, which adequately controlled the blood pressure of low- and normal-renin hypertensive humans, neither lowered the baseline renin activity nor altered the renin subgroup classification by concurrent provocative testing (furosemide and upright posture), again illustrating this dissociation. Observed correlation between the antihypertensive effect of α-methyldopa and decrease in the plasma renin activity in patients with essential hypertension (111) probably reflects simply parallel effects, and not a cause and effect relationship.

Propranolol

In the past 10 years multiple studies have demonstrated the efficacy of the β-receptor blocking agents as antihypertensive drugs, both alone (113–118) and in combination with other medications (79–82). The mechanisms of this antihypertensive effect remain controversial, mostly in relation to the suppression of the plasma renin activity as a primary antihypertensive mechanism.

Propranolol antagonizes endogenous cardiac β-adrenergic stimulation, both from circulating catecholamines and from norepinephrine at the sympathetic nerve terminus. A reduction in myocardial contractility, heart rate, and cardiac output follows with a subsequently reduced blood pressure from but a minimal compensatory rise in total peripheral resistance (117–119) in responsive hypertensive patients. This lack of parallel rise of resistance with chronic propranolol administration appears to differentiate those responding from those not responding to the hypertensive effect, and includes those with both essential and renovascular hypertension (118). Although intravenous propranolol induces a reduction in cardiac output similar to chronic oral therapy, total peripheral resistance rapidly rises (119) and accounts for the usual lack of acute antihypertensive effect (120). The mechanism for a lack of compensatory rise in resistance with chronic therapy is unknown, although an enhanced sensitivity of the baroreceptor reflex has been suggested (119). In addition, little change in plasma volume is seen in most hypertensive patients (123), in contrast to the usual volume expansion with other solitary antiadrenergic drugs, probably deriving from the lack of effect on α-adrenergic-mediated vascular reflexes.

A central antihypertensive effect of propranolol has been proposed (121, 124) but not established for therapeutic antihypertensive levels of the drug in man. Introduction into the carotid or vertebral artery (122) and cerebral ventricles (125) induces hypotension in animals, and brain-tissue entry of the drug from the bloodstream has been demonstrated (126).

That suppression of renin release constitutes a primary mechanism for the antihypertensive effect of the β-blockers has been proposed by Bühler and co-workers (127), and extended as a proposal that β-blockade represents specific therapy for hypertensive patients with high baseline renin values (including high renin essential, malignant, and renovascular hypertension), primarily from observations of correlation of hypotensive effect with both preexisting renin values and lowering of renin activity during treatment. However, subsequent studies by Michelakis & McAllister (133), Stokes et al (134), and others (136, 137) have failed to confirm either correlation with long-term β-blockade, and increasing evidence indicates that the suppression of renin release is not a primary antihypertensive mechanism of the β-adrenergic blockers.

In hypertensive patients, the dissociation between the effect of chronic propranolol therapy on the plasma renin activity and the blood pressure response suggests a separate mechanism for each effect. Suppression of plasma renin is easily attained in most hypertensive and normal subjects, including baseline measurements or stimulation by posture or other agents (69, 133, 134), although total suppression is rarely achieved. Yet, as mentioned, the antihypertensive response is variable. Significantly, the suppression of the plasma renin occurs with relatively lower doses of the drug, and the antihypertensive effect in those so responding occurs only with greater doses and relatively higher plasma levels (133, 134). Analysis of the dose-response relationships between plasma propranolol levels, plasma renin, and degree of blood pressure reduction in hypertensive patients by Leonetti et al (134a) showed a dissociation of the latter two effects with virtually complete renin suppression occurring at propranolol levels having no effect on the blood pressure. Thus, a lack of correlation and a different behavior of the hypotensive and renin-suppressing responses to propranolol appear to suggest different mechanisms of action.

The varying response to acute and chronic propranolol administration under conditions of long-term stimulation of renin synthesis has led to the concept that renal β-receptor stimulation is involved primarily in renin release and not in synthesis. Acute propranolol administration to hypertensive patients with high plasma renin levels from chronic diuretic treatment lowers these levels (153), whereas chronic oxyprenolol (138) or propranolol (154) therapy does not, despite the pronounced antihypertensive effect obtained on addition of the second drug. Analogously, Guthrie and co-workers (154a) have noted that neither renal renin content nor plasma renin activity (nor brain or adrenal gland isorenin activities) is changed in rats after two weeks of propranolol treatment; that is, long-term synthesis is unaltered. The distinction between renin synthesis and release (135) may also in part account for the maintenance of renin elevations during long-term propranolol therapy (154). The antihypertensive effect of propranolol is thus maintained in the face of persistent plasma renin elevation from diuretics, clearly dissociating the antirenin from the antihypertensive effect.

Propranolol inhibits the acute renin release induced by various exogenous [epinephrine (128) or isoproterenol (70, 129–131) infusion] and endogenous adrenergic stimuli [from sympathetic discharge (132) and catecholamine release during upright posture (133), volume depletion (69) or hypoglycemia (139)]. Such inhibition appears to derive from competitive blockade of a renal β-adrenergic receptor (140, 141) by L-propranolol contained in the racemic mixture of the drug.

Distinct subpopulations exist among the various tissue β-receptors, with the cardiac receptor classified as β-1 [stimulating cardiac contractility and rate (142)] and receptors in muscle and liver (stimulating glycogenolysis) and bronchial smooth muscle (stimulating relaxation) classified as β-2 (143). Recent evidence suggests that the renal receptor mediating renin release is of the β-2 type on the basis of studies with selective β-2-agonists (144) and antagonists (144–146, 151). However, this classification has been disputed (147). Propranolol is nonspecific in that it competitively blocks both types of β-receptors, in the same way as do other nonspecific β-blockers such as oxyprenolol and prindolol. But the use of the specific β-1-adrenergic blocking agent, practolol (148), has clarified the relationship of the plasma renin activity to the antihypertensive response from β-blockade. This drug lowers the blood pressure when administered chronically to hypertensive patients (149) without significantly changing baseline plasma renin activity (150, 151). Concurrent isoproterenol infusion, an agonist to both β-1 and β-2 receptors, raises the plasma renin while effecting a markedly lessened increase in the heart rate (151). Propranolol in comparison blunts both responses (70). Intravenous practolol has no acute effect on blood pressure or renin activity (151), whereas intravenous propranolol, again in comparison, may have no effect on blood pressure but usually lowers the plasma renin activity in hypertensive patients (136). A similar potent antihypertensive effect in man without suppression of either recumbent or upright plasma renin activity during treatment with another cardioselective β-1 antagonist (ICI 66,082) has been reported (145). And animal studies using a selective β-2 adrenergic blocker (H35/25) have confirmed the impression that renin release is mediated by the β-2 receptor, as this agent significantly reduced the plasma renin activity without affecting baseline blood pressure (146).

The conclusions suggested by these studies using the selective β-blockers are that the antihypertensive effect of a nonselective blocker such as propranolol derives from β-1-receptor blockade only. The suppression of renin activity by the drug appears to be but a parallel renal β-2 blockade that does not cause the blood pressure response, supporting the view that there are isolated mechanisms for renin and blood pressure reductions.

However, conflicting data suggest that a solitary β-1 cardiac mechanism for the hypotensive effect of propranolol is not conclusively established. A correlation between the hypotensive response to 1-sarcosine 8-alanine angiotensin II and propranolol in hypertensive patients has been reported by Streeten et al (152), supporting an earlier correlation between propranolol response and renin subgroup classification by Bühler et al (127). Recent reports by Pettinger and co-workers (155, 156) have also concluded that lowering of blood pressure following addition of propranolol to antecedent vasodilator drugs is mediated by the former compound's inhibition of vasodilator-induced renin relase, because 1-sar-8-ala angiotensin II infusions potentiated the vasodilator-induced hypotensive response before but not after propranolol therapy in rats and hypertensive humans. Furthermore, the "short feedback" direct inhibition of renin release by angiotensin II was thought to be proximal to the site of propranolol inhibition of renin release in these studies, as propranolol failed to prevent the 1-sar-8-ala–induced rise in plasma renin activity (156).

CLASSIFICATION OF HYPERTENSION BY RENIN VALUES

The use of the plasma renin determination has proved of some value in defining subpopulations of hypertensive patients with characteristic physiologic traits. Patients found to have a plasma renin activity subresponsive or nonresponsive to appropriate stimuli, including upright posture alone or combined with dietary sodium restriction or various drugs stimulatory to renin release, have been classified as low renin hypertensive, and have attracted much recent attention. Variations in methods of definition of this low renin group have proved a source of difficulty in comparison of data from different laboratories. A standardized technique of in-hospital dietary sodium restriction (10 meq per day) for three to five days and subsequent renin determination before and after four hours of upright posture is often inconvenient, whereas outpatient techniques using oral or intravenous furosemide have been used with moderately good agreement with the dietary technique (61, 157–159). However, Drayer et al (160) have noted a poor correlation between the ability of oral furosemide and sodium restriction to identify low renin patients, although five days of oral chlorthalidone did compare well. It appears that when diuretics [or hypotensive agents (66)] are used to stimulate renin release and to identify low renin patients, their administration must be standardized and shown to compare with the results of sodium restriction. The technique of an ad libitum sodium intake with indexation of the plasma renin activity against the measured 24 hr sodium excretion as used by Brunner et al (161) is probably insufficiently discriminating to identify accurately the low renin group, especially with sodium intakes near or above 150 meq per day.

The assumption that low renin hypertension is a stable, well-defined state may not be valid. Crane et al (162) have found that fully 22% of patients they defined as belonging to the low renin group had normal renin responsiveness on retesting. Analysis of the data of Brunner et al (163) by Dunn & Tannen (164) determined that one third of their patients did not have reproducible renin determinations, and Genest et al (165) have noted an inconsistent and variably suppressed plasma renin activity in many subjects. These findings suggest that the phenomenon of renin unresponsiveness may be labile for a given patient. Furthermore, the time when the renin determination is made may influence the value, since prolonged antecedent diuretic therapy may result in the elevation of renin activity, even in patients previously classified as being of the low renin type (158, 166).

Racial idiosyncrasies may affect the classification of hypertension by renin values. Black patients have a greater incidence of low renin hypertension; the frequency has been found to be 42% by Mroczek et al (167), 42% by Brunner (163), and 43% by Gulati et al (168), in contrast to an incidence of 9–30% (165–170) in white populations. The degree of renin stimulation by furosemide also appears lower in normotensive and hypertensive blacks than whites, as shown by Kaplan's group (171), suggesting fundamental racial differences in the renin response.

The age and sex of patients appear to influence the renin classification. Crane and co-workers (162) found twice as many females as males in his hypertensive low renin group; Gulati et al (168) found a male to female ratio of 1:1.2; and Mroczek (167) found 75% of their low renin patients to be female. Several studies have shown that the low renin hypertensive state is correlated with the age of the patient. Gulati (168) reported a significantly higher incidence in his older than 50 group for both races compared to younger groups. Genest et al (169a) and Tuck et al (169) have found that approximately 9% of 20- to 30-year-old essential hypertensives are of the low renin type (compared to age-matched normal controls), compared to about 30% in the 35–65 year age group similarly matched. In addition, Tuck and co-workers (169) demonstrated a correlation of a low renin subgrouping with level of diastolic pressure. An increased frequency of low renin hypertension in older patients may reflect the known decline in renin responsiveness in normotensive humans with advancing age (172) or may relate to a subtle renal or adrenal defect impairing sodium excretion, which some workers (94) feel is established in the hypertensive state over a period of time.

Finally, the inherent lability of the renin-angiotensin system combined with the variability of the renin determination itself can make reproducible values for classification difficult, especially in distinguishing a high from normal renin value. Even indexation against an outpatient timed urinary sodium excretion, which has not been established to accurately reflect average daily sodium intake, leaves much room for uncertainty of classification, especially since Laragh and colleagues (172a) collect the major fraction of urine (21 hr of the 24 hr volume) *after* the corresponding renin determination.

Renin as a Prognostic Factor for Cardiovascular Disease

The pretreatment plasma renin activity has been proposed as a prognostic factor for the development of subsequent morbid cardiovascular events in hypertensive patients by Brunner et al (163). Their study of 219 hypertensive patients observed retrospectively over a ten-year period revealed that 59 low renin patients suffered no heart attacks or strokes in this interval, whereas 11% of the normal renin group and 14% of the high renin group did incur one of these events. This original study has been criticized on several grounds (165, 174). One is a lack of comparability between the normal control group (used to define the boundaries between a normal and abnormal renin profile) and the hypertensive patients. The normal control group contained no blacks, whereas the hypertensive patients were 27% black, and this racial group appears to have a higher incidence of hypertension and its resultant complications despite a greater frequency of suppressed renin activities (175). Furthermore, the high renin group contained patients with higher blood urea nitrogen levels and mean diastolic pressures, implying both established renal (and vascular) disease and increased risk from the level of blood pressure. Other criticisms have pointed out (*a*) that misleading conclusions have been arrived at because of the retrospective nature of the study, because a heart attack (by an alteration in cardiac output and vascular dynamics) or stroke may have altered the plasma renin activity (and subgroup classification) or established renal vascular or glomerular disease at the time of the renin determination may have changed a given patient's past renin profile; (*b*) that low renin essential hypertensive patients respond well to antihypertensive therapy, especially diuretics (176), implying a correlation with blood pressure control; (*c*) that a renin subgroup classification is labile, since renin levels may change unpredictably (162, 165) or decline with age.

More importantly, however, the conclusion that low renin essential hypertensive patients are at lesser risk for a morbid cardiovascular event has not been supported by subsequent independent studies (165, 167, 168, 177–179) save one (180) with major qualifications. Although these studies have employed varying techniques for the renin determination and for provocative testing, and have used differing definitions of a normal, low, or high renin classification for the hypertensive group, their conclusions are surprisingly similar. Most classify approximately 20–30% of hypertensive patients as being of the low renin type, and find a similar incidence of vascular complications in the low and normal renin groups. The speculation that a low plasma renin activity is protective against strokes or heart attacks, allegedly by a lesser degree of vascular damage from circulating renin, is not supported by these reports. Also deemed improbable is the implication that an induced rise in the plasma renin from treatment may be harmful, for Doyle and co-workers (179) have reported that those low renin patients with a plasma renin stimulated into the "normal" range by chronic antihypertensive therapy suffered an incidence of morbid events similar to that suffered by patients whose plasma renin remained suppressed.

That a low renin essential hypertensive patient may be at lesser risk than his normal or high renin counterpart will not be disproved until prospective studies are completed that match age, sex, race, and degree of blood pressure control in the comparison groups; that employ standardized techniques for both renin subgroup classification and the renin determination; and that establish a stable renin profile (if this is possible) during antihypertensive therapy. Until then, all patients with fixed diastolic hypertension, regardless of their renin profile, are best treated to attain maximal practical blood pressure control, since most evidence indicates that the elevated blood pressure itself is the most significant risk factor for mortality (184) and cardiovascular morbidity, including heart attack (185), stroke (186), and congestive heart failure (187), and that effective blood pressure control does lessen the incidence of strokes (184, 185) and possibly myocardial infarctions (183).

Renin as a Guide for Evaluation and Therapy

The plasma renin activity is useful as a guide in several stages of the evaluation of hypertensive patients. A major objective of the modern clinical evaluation of hypertension is to identify currently known curable causes of the hypertensive state, not so much to effect immediate correction of the primary abnormality (although this is usually done), but to provide the physician with information to aid his management of the patient. Virtually all of the secondary hypertensive states can be successfully controlled with currently available drugs, as an alternative to surgical correction of such diverse conditions as renovascular hypertension, an aldosterone-producing adrenal adenoma, or even a pheochromocytoma for a limited period. But if the alternative of life-long pharmacotherapy is deemed too great a burden or risk to the patient, as it most often is, surgical therapy may hold reasonable promise for a permanent cure. Expanded arguments for (188, 189) and against (190, 191) a vigorous search for secondary hypertension may be found elsewhere. The plasma renin activity aids in such an evaluation by the presence of abnormally high or low values.

A low plasma renin activity is seen in a variety of secondary hypertensive states characterized by the production of excessive amounts of adrenal mineralocorticoids, with excessive distal renal tubular sodium retention and sustained expansion of the extracellular fluid volume, thus leading to chronic renin suppression (192, 193). An often associated hypokalemia is from the mineralocorticoid-induced kaliuresis (193). Known causes of mineralocorticoid-induced low renin hypertension include aldosterone overproduction from an adrenal adenoma or bilateral hyperplasia of the adrenal cortex or zona glomerulosa (194), 11-deoxycorticosterone (DOC) overproduction either from a 17α-hydroxylation deficiency (195) with associated elevations of corticosterone (B) and 18-hydroxycorticosterone or as an isolated non-ACTH-dependent overproduction (196), 11β-hydroxylation deficiency in children with

DOC and 11-deoxycortisol overproduction (197), and mixtures of mineralocorticoids with adrenal carcinomas (198) or ectopic ACTH-producing tumors. Overproduction of 18-hydroxy-DOC in some patients with low renin hypertension has been reported by Melby et al (199) and Genest et al (200), and recently Liddle et al (201) have reported increased urinary excretion of the C-19 steroid 16β-hydroxy-dehydroepiandrosterone (16β-OH-DHEA) in some patients with low renin hypertension, shown by them to be a weak mineralocorticoid in adrenalectomized rats, although others report a lack of binding of this compound to the renal mineralocorticoid receptor (201a). However, the elevated secretion of 18-OH-DOC and 16β-OH-DHEA is not yet a firmly established cause of low renin hypertension owing to an as yet incomplete confirmation of their reported oversecretion and to the lack of a demonstrated mineralocorticoid effect of these compounds in man.

The postulated existence of excessive mineralocorticoid activity in patients with low renin essential hypertension is a topic stimulating active current research, as much direct and indirect evidence, reviewed elsewhere (164, 170), suggests such a possibility. Some workers suggest that the secretion of an "abnormal" steroid may be responsible (199, 201–203). Other evidence suggests a disordered regulation of aldosterone metabolism, since plasma levels and secretion rates for aldosterone are not found depressed appropriate to the low renin levels (204–206), or a decreased metabolic clearance rate for aldosterone may be a contributory factor (207), possibly from an altered binding to a plasma globulin fraction as recently shown by Nowaczynski et al (208).

Other mechanisms have been postulated to account for the renin unresponsiveness of low renin essential hypertension. Laragh and colleagues (209) have suggested that an impairment of the ability to normally excrete potassium may be at fault, although little available data support and many studies discount this explanation, as reviewed elsewhere (164). An impaired peripheral β-adrenergic responsiveness has been proposed, with the suppression of renin merely reflecting inadequate adrenergic renin release and the hypertension resulting from an unopposed α-adrenergic activity. An observed blunted rise in urinary norepinephrine excretion in such patients to postural stimuli (210, 211) suggests an adrenergic dysfunction, but further work is needed to explore this proposal. Finally, Schalekamp and co-workers (173) and others (169) argue that low renin essential hypertension may be but a late state of the hypertensive state itself, with a low plasma renin the result of a long-term effect of an elevated blood pressure on the kidney. Evidence supporting this view is a lack of bimodality in the frequency distribution of renin levels in hypertension (212) and the known inverse relation of renin activity to age in normotensive and hypertensive patients. Because individuals with low renin essential hypertension are quite probably a heterogeneous group, several pathogenic mechanisms may be involved.

A suppressed plasma renin activity can guide the evaluation of hypertensive patients first by providing an indication that available steroid measurements ought to be taken, most commonly a 24-hour aldosterone excretion during augmented sodium intake to detect the estimated 0.5% of hypertensive patients with primary aldosteronism (189). Additional steroid determinations such as measurements of DOC or 18-OH-DOC levels may provide evidence that a glucocorticoid-suppressible type of hypertension is present, such as partial or complete 17α-hydroxylase deficiency. And since chronic low dose dexamethasone therapy is generally without side effects and well tolerated, usually much more so than most other antihypertensive therapy, such a search may prove quite rewarding to the patient. Thus, a supressed plasma renin together with other clinical and laboratory data can aid in the detection and treatment of known causes of mineralocorticoid hypertension.

A low plasma renin activity is useful as a guide to the therapy of a patient with essential hypertension primarily as an indication that effective diuretic treatment must be begun. Many groups have observed that diuretics appear to effect a greater antihypertensive response in patients whose renin values are suppressed than in normal or high renin hypertensive patients (176, 213–215). And since such therapy if effective is relatively inexpensive and well tolerated compared to other drugs, the indication to so attempt blood pressure control may prove rewarding.

The reason for the sensitivity of low renin essential hypertensive patients to diuretic treatment is controversial. Some have taken this observation as evidence that such patients possess a volume-expanded type of hypertension and that diuretics correct this primary abnormality by inducing volume depletion. Whereas some types of hypertension such as fluid retention from chronic renal failure (216), primary aldosteronism (217), and 17α-hydroxylase deficiency (195) clearly represent volume-mediated hypertensive states, many reports of direct measurements of plasma and extracellular fluid volumes and exchangeable sodium spaces have not produced convincing evidence that low renin essential hypertension is so mediated. For example, the data of Jose et al (89), Helmer & Judson (218), Birkenhäger and co-workers (219), and Woods et al (202) all show no significant difference between the plasma or blood volumes of low- compared with normal-renin essential hypertensive patients. Measurements of the exchangeable sodium space by Schalekamp and co-workers (216) are not different for the two groups, conflicting with an earlier report by Woods et al (202), that low renin hypertensives possess a larger space than do normal renin patients, although no difference was found between the low renin group and their matched controls. The sum of results from most studies fails to support the presence of an expanded extracellular fluid volume in low renin hypertension, most certainly not of a degree comparable to that of established hypermineralocorticoid states.

The response to spironolactone therapy by low renin essential hypertensive patients is of special interest partly as supporting evidence for an occult hypermineralocorticoid state. Yet several groups (176, 213–215) report comparable efficacy to the more conventional diuretics, which suggests that a nonspecific natriuresis and not an antagonism to occult mineralocorticoids is responsible for the action of the drug. In view of the high doses of spironolactone (200–400 mg per day) necessary for blood pressure control in such patients and the consequent expense and relatively higher incidence of undesirable side effects than with other diuretics, the latter drugs are best tried first.

The presence of a high baseline plasma renin activity in a hypertensive patient usually prompts a search for a correctable renal or renovascular abnormality, and thus may be of aid in detecting the estimated 5% incidence of a renovascular cause among an unselected hypertensive population (189). Yet the absence of a peripheral venous renin elevation does not exclude renovascular disease, since approximately 40% of patients with such hypertension have a normal baseline renin value (220), and up to 15% may remain normal after stimulatory maneuvers (221). Selective renal venous renin determinations and presence of a greater than 1:1.5 ratio of uninvolved to involved side values are the current criteria for detection and operability of renal and renovascular hypertension.

Studies with 1-sar-8-ala angiotensin II by Streeten et al (152) on unselected hypertensive patients have shown that most (13 of 16) reacting with a hypotensive response had an elevated baseline plasma renin activity, and that all had some type of renal or renovascular disorder. Such results suggest that high renin *essential* hypertension may be a misnomer, as a renal abnormality may be common to all such patients, concordant with earlier findings by Hollenberg et al (222) that patients with high renin essential hypertension without overt structural lesions by arteriography possessed renal cortical ischemia by ^{133}xenon washout techniques. Moderately advanced renal disease and hypertension without marked azotemia or fluid retention, such as in some cases of chronic pyelonephritis, may occasionally be associated with a suppressed renin activity (O. Kuchel and J. Genest, unpublished observations) and bilateral renal artery stenosis may also be associated with low or normal peripheral renin values (223). Hypertension from a renin-producing renal tumor has recently been reported by Hollifield and colleagues (224) with a normal peripheral plasma renin value (although previously reported cases of reninomas have noted elevated peripheral renin activities). Such reports illustrate that the peripheral renin value may be an inconsistent marker, and although this fact can be valuable as a piece of diagnostic information, it does not rigidly define subgroups of patients with essential or secondary hypertension.

The presence of an elevated renin value as a guide to the selection of specific antihypertensive drugs has been proposed by some workers in an attempt to direct specific "antirenin" therapy against the presumed pathophysiologic state (225). Such an approach is intellectually appealing but is often not appropriate to our current inadequate knowledge about essential hypertension. As mentioned above, the hypotensive response to the antiadrenergic drugs is quite probably not via their effect on the plasma renin activity. But most importantly, the blood pressure of almost all essential hypertensive patients can be controlled by an empiric approach, as by the initiation of diuretic therapy followed by an antiadrenergic drug, with the later addition of vasodilators if necessary. Such a scheme produced the impressive reduction of morbidity in the Veterans' Administration Cooperative Study (181, 182) and other workers have testified to its efficacy. But since the degree of successful response to antiadrenergic drugs alone has been shown to correlate with an antecedent elevated renin activity, the use of such agents by themselves may be of value for patients with an elevated renin activity who are intolerant of other drugs or not compliant with a multiple drug regimen.

Literature Cited

1. Tigerstedt, R., Bergman, P. G. 1898. *Skand. Arch. Physiol.* 8:223–71
2. Oparil, S., Haber, E. 1974. *N. Engl. J. Med.* 291:389–401, 446–57
3. Peart, W. S. 1975. *N. Engl. J. Med.* 292:302–6
4. Stein, J. H., Ferris, T. F. 1973. *Arch. Intern. Med.* 131:860–72
5. Davis, J. O. 1973. *Am. J. Med.* 55: 333–50
6. Ganten, D., Marquez-Julio, A., Granger, P., Barbeau, A., Genest, J. 1971. *Am. J. Physiol.* 221:1733–37
7. Ferris, T. F., Gorden, D., Mulrow, P. J. 1967. *Am. J. Physiol.* 212:698–706
8. Ryan, J. W. 1967. *Science* 158:1589–90
9. Goormaghtigh, N. 1939. *Proc. Soc. Exp. Biol. Med.* 42:688–89
10. Tobian, L. 1967. *Fed. Proc.* 26:48–54
11. Vander, A. J. 1967. *Physiol. Rev.* 47:359–82
12. Tobian, L., Tomboulian, A., Janecek, J. 1959. *J. Clin. Invest.* 38:605–10
13. Rojo-Ortega, J. M., Boucher, R., Genest, J. 1968. *Clin. Res.* 16:398
14. Blaine, E. H., Davis, J. O., Prewitt, R. L. 1971. *Am. J. Physiol.* 220:1593–97
15. DiBona, G. F. 1971. *Am. J. Physiol.* 221:511–14
16. Vander, A. J., Carlson, J. 1969. *Circ. Res.* 25:145–55
17. Thurau, K., Dahlheim, H., Grüner, A., Mason, J., Granger, P. 1972. *Circ. Res.* 31:Suppl. II, 182–86
18. Nilsson, O. 1965. *Lab. Invest.* 14: 1392–95
19. Wågermark, J., Ungerstedt, U., Ljungqvist, A. 1968. *Circ. Res.* 22:149–53
19a. Rojo-Ortega, J. M., Hatt, P. Y., Genest, J. 1968. *Pathol. Biol.* 16:497–504
20. Vander, A. J. 1965. *Am. J. Physiol.* 209:659–62
21. Mogil, R. A., Iskovitz, H. D., Russell, J. H., Murphy, J. J. 1969. *Am. J. Physiol.* 216:693–97
22. Bunag, R. D., Page, I. H., McCubbin, J. W. 1966. *Circ. Res.* 19:851–58
23. Ganong, W. F. 1973. *Fed. Proc.* 32:1782–84
24. Winer, N., Chokshi, D. S., Walkenhorst, W. G. 1971. *Circ. Res.* 29:239–48
25. Robison, G. A., Butcher, R. W., Sutherland, E. W. 1968. *Ann. Rev. Biochem.* 37:149–74
26. Michelakis, A. M., Caudle, J., Liddle, G. W. 1972. *Proc. Soc. Exp. Biol. Med.* 130:748–53
27. Beck, N., Reed, S. W., Murdaugh, H. V., Davis, B. B. 1972. *J. Clin. Invest.* 51:939–44
28. Reid, I. A., Stockigt, J. R., Goldfien, A., Ganong, W. F. 1972. *Eur. J. Pharmacol.* 17:325–32
29. Beck, N., Kim, K. S., Davis, B. B. 1975. *Circ. Res.* 36:401–5
30. Nolly, H. L., Reid, I. A., Ganong, W. F. 1974. *Circ. Res.* 35:575–79
31. Zehr, J. E., Feigl, E. O. 1973. *Circ. Res.* 32:Suppl. I, 17–27
32. Finch, L., Haeusler, G., Thoenen, H. 1972. *Br. J. Pharmacol.* 44:356–62
33. Ferrario, C. M., Gildenberg, P. L., McCubbin, J. W. 1972. *Circ. Res.* 30:257–62
34. Brunner, H. R., Baer, L., Sealy, J. E., Laragh, J. H. 1970. *J. Clin. Invest.* 49:2129–38
35. Shade, R. E., Davis, J. O., Johnson, J. A., Witty, R. T. 1972. *Circ. Res.* 31:719–27
36. de Champlain, J., Genest, J., Veyratt, R., Boucher, R. 1966. *Arch. Intern. Med.* 117:355–63
37. Blair-West, J. R. et al 1971. *Am. J. Physiol.* 220:1309–15
38. Van Dongen, R., Peart, W. S., Boyd, G. W. 1974. *Am. J. Physiol.* 226:277–82
39. Vander, A. J., Geelhoed, G. W. 1965. *Proc. Soc. Exp. Biol. Med.* 120:399–403
40. Biron, P., Koiw, E., Nowaczynski, W., Brouillet, J., Genest, J. 1961. *J. Clin. Invest.* 40:338–47
41. Thurau, K., Schnermann, J., Nagel, W., Horster, M., Wohl, M. 1967. *Circ. Res.* 20–21:Suppl. II, 79–91
42. Vander, A. J., Luciano, J. R. 1967. *Circ. Res.* 20–21:Suppl. II, 69–75
43. Dustan, H. P., Tarazi, R. C., Bravo, E. L. 1974. *Arch. Intern. Med.* 133: 1007–13
44. Conway, J., Palermo, H. 1963. *Arch. Intern. Med.* 111:203–7
45. Kusumoto, M. et al 1974. *Proc. Soc. Exp. Biol. Med.* 147:767–74
46. Tobian, L. 1967. *Ann. Rev. Pharmacol.* 7:399–408
47. Winer, B. M. 1961. *Circulation* 24: 788–95
48. Parijs, J. et al 1973. *Am. Heart J.* 85:22–34
49. Freis, E. D. et al 1960. *J. Clin. Invest.* 39:1277–81
50. Tarazi, R. C., Dustan, H. P., Frohlich, E. D. 1970. *Circulation* 41:709–17
51. Anderson, J., Godfrey, B. E., Hill, D. M. 1971. *Q. J. Med.* 40:541–60

52. Atkins, L. L. 1973. In *Hypertension: Mechanisms and Management*, ed. G. Onesti, K. E. Kim, J. H. Moyer, 273–81. New York: Grune & Stratton
53. Meyer, P. et al 1968. *Am. J. Physiol.* 215:908–15
54. Dikshit, K. et al 1973. *N. Engl. J. Med.* 288:1087–90
55. Liddle, G. W. 1961. *Metabolism* 10:1021–28
56. Efstratopoulos, A. D., Peart, W. S. 1974. *Clin. Sci.* 48:219–26
57. Abboud, F. M. 1974. *Fed. Proc.* 33:143–49
58. Winer, B. M., Lubbe, W. F., Colton, T. 1968. *J. Am. Med. Assoc.* 204:775–79
59. Crane, M. G., Harris, J. J. 1970. *Am. J. Med. Sci.* 260:311–30
60. Spark, R. F., Melby, J. C. 1971. *Ann. Intern. Med.* 75:831–36
61. Carey, R. M., Douglas, J. G., Schweikert, J. R., Liddle, G. W. 1972. *Arch. Intern. Med.* 130:849–54
62. Spark, R. F., O'Hare, C. M., Regan, R. M. 1974. *Arch. Intern. Med.* 133:205–11
63. Lowder, S. C., Liddle, G. W. 1974. *N. Engl. J. Med.* 291:1243–44
64. Pohl, J. E. F., Thurston, H., Swales, J. D. 1972. *Clin. Sci.* 42:145–52
65. Hamby, W. N., Janowski, G. J., Pouget, J. M., Dunea, G., Gantt, O. 1968. *Circulation* 37:169–75
66. Kuchel, O., Fishman, L. M., Liddle, G. W., Michelakis, A. 1967. *Ann. Intern. Med.* 67:791–99
67. Baer, L., Goodwin, F. J., Laragh, J. H. 1969. *J. Clin. Endocrinol. Metab.* 29:1107–15
68. Kapitola, J., Kuchel, O., Schreiberova, O., Jahoda, I. 1968. *Experientia* 24:242–43
69. Winer, N., Chokshi, D. S., Yoon, M. S., Friedman, A. D. 1969. *J. Clin. Endocrinol. Metab.* 29:1168–75
70. Winer, N., Chokshi, D. S., Walkenhorst, W. G. 1971. *Circ. Res.* 29:239–48
71. Moore, P. F. 1968. *Ann. NY Acad. Sci.* 150:256–66
72. Palmer, R. F., Lasseter, K. C. 1975. *N. Engl. J. Med.* 292:294–96
73. DuCharme, D. W., Freyburger, W. A., Graham, B. E., Carlson, R. G. 1973. *J. Pharmacol. Exp. Ther.* 184:662–70
74. Ablad, B. 1963. *Acta Pharmacol. Toxicol.* 20:Suppl. 1, 1–53
75. Hammer, J., Ulrych, M., Freis, E. D. 1971. *Clin. Pharmacol. Ther.* 12:78–90
76. Finnerty, F. A., Davidov, M., Mroczek, W. J. 1970. *Circ. Res.* 27:Suppl. I, 71–80
77. Ueda, H., Kaneko, Y., Takeda, T., Ikeda, T., Yagi, S. 1970. *Circ. Res.* 27:Suppl. II, 201–6
78. Kaneko, Y., Ikeda, T., Takeda, T., Ueda, H. 1967. *J. Clin. Invest.* 46:705–15
79. Gottlieb, T. B., Katz, F. H., Chidsey, C. A. 1972. *Circulation* 45:571–82
80. Gilmore, E., Weil, J., Chidsey, C. 1970. *N. Engl. J. Med.* 282:521–27
81. Tuckman, J., Messerli, F., Hodler, J. 1973. *Clin. Sci.* 45:Suppl. I, 159–61
82. Zacest, R., Gilmore, E., Koch-Weser, J. 1972. *N. Engl. J. Med.* 286:617–22
83. Onesti, G., Schwartz, A. B., Kim, K. E., Paz-Martinez, V., Swartz, C. 1971. *Circ. Res.* 28:Suppl. II, 53–69
84. Constantine, J. W., McShane, W. K. 1968. *Eur. J. Pharmacol.* 4:109–15
85. Ayers, C. R., Harris, R. H., Lefer, L. G. 1969. *Circ. Res.* 24:Suppl. I, 103–12
86. Twist, C. I. 1967. *Adv. Drug Res.* 4:133–61
87. Cohn, J. N., Liptak, T. E., Freis, E. D. 1963. *Circ. Res.* 12:298–307
88. Weil, J. V., Chidsey, C. A. 1968. *Circulation* 37:54–61
89. Jose, A., Crout, J. K., Kaplan, N. M. 1970. *Ann. Intern. Med.* 72:9–20
90. Lowder, S. C., Liddle, G. W. 1975. *Ann. Intern. Med.* 82:757–60
91. Kuchel, O., Genest, J. 1973. See Ref. 52, pp. 411–27
92. Alper, M. H., Flacke, W., Krayer, O. 1963. *Anesthesiology* 24:524–42
93. Birbari, A. 1971. *Am. J. Physiol.* 220:16–18
94. Slotkoff, L. M., Eisner, G. M., Adamson, W., Lilienfield, L. S. 1971. *Proc. Soc. Exp. Biol. Med.* 132:683–90
95. Silverman, A., Barajas, L. 1974. *Lab. Invest.* 30:723–31
96. Onesti, G. N., Brest, A. N., Novack, P., Kasparian, H., Moyer, J. H. 1964. *Am. Heart J.* 67:32–38
97. Prescott, L. F. et al 1966. *Circulation* 34:308–21
98. Henning, M., Van Zwieten, P. A. 1968. *J. Pharm. Pharmacol.* 20:409–17
99. Ingenito, A. J., Barrett, J. P., Procita, L. 1970. *J. Pharmacol. Exp. Ther.* 175:593–99
100. Heise, A., Kroneberg, G. 1972. *Eur. J. Pharmacol.* 17:315–17
101. Henning, M., Rubenson, A. 1971. *J. Pharm. Pharmacol.* 23:407–12
101a. Henning, M. 1975. *Clin. Sci.* 48:Suppl. 2, pp. 195–203
102. Sjoerdsma, A., Vendsalu, A., Engelman, K. 1963. *Circulation* 28:492–99

103. Mohammed, S. et al 1969. *Circ. Res.* 25:543–48
104. Mohammed, S., Privitera, P. J. 1971. *Clin. Res.* 19:329
105. Strauss, R. G. et al 1970. *J. Pediatr.* 77:1071–75
106. Weidmann, P., Maxwell, M. H., Lupu, A. N., Lewin, A. J., Massry, R. G. 1971. *N. Engl. J. Med.* 285:757–63
107. Kaplan, N. M. 1975. *Arch. Intern. Med.* 135:660–63
108. Privitera, P. J., Mohammed, S. 1972. In *Control of Renin Secretion*, ed. T. A. Assaykeen, 93–101. New York: Plenum
109. Privitera, P. J., Mohammed, S. 1970. *Proc. Soc. Exp. Biol. Med.* 133:1358–62
110. Holuska, P. V., Keiser, H. R. 1974. *Circ. Res.* 35:458–63
111. Weidmann, P., Hirsch, P., Maxwell, M. H., Okun, R. 1974. *Am. J. Cardiol.* 34:671–76
112. Sweet, C. S., Wanger, H. C., O'Malley, T. A. 1974. *Can. J. Physiol. Pharmacol.* 52:1036–40
113. Hansson, L., Zweifler, A. J. 1974. *Acta Med. Scand.* 195:397–401
114. Prichard, B. N. C., Gillam, P. M. S. 1969. *Br. Med. J.* 1:7–16
115. Zacharias, F. J., Cowen, K. J., Prestt, J., Vickers, J., Wall, B. C. 1972. *Am. Heart J.* 83:755–61
116. Lydtin, H. et al 1972. *Am. J. Cardiol.* 83:589–95
117. Frohlich, E. D., Tarazi, R. C., Dustan, H. P., Page, I. H. 1968. *Circulation* 37:417–23
118. Tarazi, R. C., Dustan, H. P. 1972. *Am. J. Cardiol.* 29:633–40
119. Hansson, L., Zweifler, A. J., Julius, S., Hunyor, S. N. 1974. *Acta Med. Scand.* 196:27–34
120. Ulrych, M., Frohlich, E. D., Dustan, H. P., Page, I. H. 1968. *Circulation* 37:411–20
121. Murmann, W., Almirante, L., Saccani-Guelfi, M. 1966. *J. Pharm. Pharmacol.* 18:317–19
122. Stern, S., Hoffman, M., Braun, K. 1971. *Cardiovasc. Res.* 5:425–30
123. Tarazi, R. C., Frohlich, E. D., Dustan, H. P. 1971. *Am. Heart J.* 82:770–76
124. Dollery, C. T., Lewis, P. J., Myers, M. G., Reid, J. L. 1973. *Br. J. Pharmacol.* 48:343P
125. Day, M. D., Roach, A. G. 1973. *Fed. Proc.* 32:724–28
126. Masuoka, D., Hansson, E. 1967. *Acta Pharmacol. Toxicol.* 25:447–52
127. Bühler, F. R., Laragh, J. H., Baer, L., Vaughn, E. D., Brunner, H. R. 1972. *N. Engl. J. Med.* 287:1209–14
128. Assaykeen, T. A., Clayton, R. L., Goldfien, A., Ganong, W. F. 1970. *Endocrinology* 87:1318–22
129. Reid, I. A., Schrier, R. W., Earley, L. E. 1972. *J. Clin. Invest.* 51:1861–69
130. Wallace, J. M., Anderson, F. G., Sheppard, J. A. Jr. 1970. *Clin. Res.* 18:28
131. Assaykeen, T. A., Tanigawa, H., Allison, D. J. 1974. *Eur. J. Pharmacol.* 26:285–87
132. Passo, S. S., Assaykeen, T. A., Goldfien, A., Ganong, W. F. 1971. *Neuroendocrinology* 7:97–104
133. Michelakis, A. M., McAllister, R. G. 1972. *J. Clin. Endocrinol.* 34:386–94
134. Stokes, G. S., Weber, M. A., Thornell, I. R., Stokes, L. M., Sebel, E. F. 1974. *Prog. Biochem. Pharmacol.* 9:29–44
134a. Leonetti, G. et al 1975. *Clin. Sci.* 48:491–99
135. Rojo-Ortega, J. M., Casado-Perez, S., Boucher, R., Genest, J. 1969. *Renal Renin Content Does Not Always Represent Renin Secretion.* Presented at 4th Int. Congr. Nephrol., Stockholm, June 22–27
136. Hansson, L. 1973. *Acta Med. Scand.,* Suppl. 550
137. Stokes, G. S., Weber, M. A., Thornell, I. R. 1974. *Br. Med. J.* 1:60–62
138. Gysling, E., De Wurstemberger, B. 1974. *Schweiz. Med. Wochenschr.* 104:1797–98
139. Otsuka, K., Assaykeen, T. A., Goldfien, A., Ganong, W. F. 1970. *Endocrinology* 87:1306–17
140. Ahlquist, R. P. 1948. *Am. J. Physiol.* 135:586–600
141. Tobert, J. A. et al 1973. *Clin. Sci.* 44:461–73
142. Lands, A. M., Arnold, A., McAuliff, J. P., Ludwena, F. L., Brown, T. G. 1967. *Nature London* 214:597–98
143. Lefkowitz, R. J. 1974. *Circulation* 49:783–86
144. Assaykeen, T. A. 1973. *Evidence for Beta-2-Adrenergic Receptor of Renin Release in Dogs.* Presented at 55th Ann. Meet. *Endocr. Soc.,* Chicago
145. Amery, A., Billiet, L., Fagard, R. 1974. *N. Engl. J. Med.* 290:284
146. Weber, M. A., Stokes, G. S., Gain, J. M. 1974. *J. Clin. Invest.* 54:1413–19
147. Aberg, H. 1974. *Int. J. Clin. Pharmacol.* 9:98–100
148. Barrett, A. M. 1971. *Postgrad. Med. J.* 45:7–12
149. Prichard, B. N., Boakes, A. J., Day, G. 1971. *Postgrad. Med. J.* 47:Suppl. 1, 84–92

150. Esler, M. D., Nestel, P. J. 1973. *Br. Heart J.* 35:469-74
151. Esler, M. D. 1974. *Clin. Pharmacol. Ther.* 15:484-89
152. Streeten, D. H. P., Anderson, G. H., Freiberg, J. M., Dalakos, J. G. 1975. *N. Engl. J. Med.* 292:657-62
153. Bravo, E. L., Tarazi, R. C., Dustan, H. P. 1973. *J. Lab. Clin. Med.* 83: 119-28
154. Bravo, E. L., Tarazi, R. C., Dustan, H. P. 1975. *N. Engl. J. Med.* 292: 66-70
154a. Guthrie, G. P. et al 1976. In *Effects of Antihypertensive Therapy,* ed. M. P. Sambhi. Miami: Symposium Specialists. In press
155. Pettinger, W. A., Keeton, K. 1975. *J. Clin. Invest.* 55:236-43
156. Pettinger, W. A., Mitchell, H. C. 1975. *N. Engl. J. Med.* 292:1214-17
157. Channick, B. J., Adlin, E. V., Marks, A. D. 1969. *Arch. Intern. Med.* 123: 131-40
158. Jose, A., Kaplan, N. M. 1969. *Arch. Intern. Med.* 123:141-46
159. Marshall, S. J., Grim, C. E. 1973. *Clin. Res.* 21:699
160. Drayer, J. I. M., Kloppenberg, P. W. C., Benraad, T. J. 1974. *Clin. Sci.* 48:91-96
161. Brunner, H. R., Sealy, J. E., Laragh, J. H. 1973. *Circ. Res.* 32-33:Suppl. I, 99-109
162. Crane, M. G., Harris, J. J., Johns, V. J. 1972. *Am. J. Med.* 52:457-66
163. Brunner, H. R. et al 1972. *N. Engl. J. Med.* 286:441-49
164. Dunn, M. J., Tannen, R. L. 1974. *Kidney Int.* 5:317-25
165. Genest, J., Boucher, R., Kuchel, O., Nowaczynski, W. 1973. *Can. Med. Assoc. J.* 109:475-78
166. Helmer, O. M., Judson, W. E. 1968. *Circulation* 38:965-76
167. Mroczek, W. J., Finnerty, F. A., Catt, K. J. 1973. *Lancet* 2:464-68
168. Gulati, S. C., Channick, B. J., Adlin, E. V., Biddle, C. M., Marks, A. D. 1975. *Arch. Intern. Med.* 135:260-63
169. Tuck, M. L., Williams, G. H., Cain, J. P., Sullivan, J. M., Dluhy, R. G. 1973. *Am. J. Cardiol.* 32:637-42
169a. Genest, J. et al 1975. *Can. Med. Assoc. J.* 113:421-31
170. Gunnells, J. C. Jr., McGuffin, W. L. 1975. *Ann. Rev. Med.* 26:259-75
171. Kem, D. C., Kramer, N. J., Gomez-Sanchez, C., White, M., Kaplan, N. M. 1973. *J. Clin. Invest.* 52:46a

172. Sambhi, M. P., Crane, M. G., Genest, J. *Ann. Intern. Med.* 79:411-24
172a. Laragh, J. H., Sealy, J., Brunner, H. R. 1972. *Am. J. Med.* 53:649-63
173. Schalekamp, M. A., Schalekamp-Kuyken, M. P., Burkenhager, W. H. 1970. *Clin. Sci.* 38:101-10
174. Kaplan, N. M. 1975. *J. Am. Med. Assoc.* 231:167-70
175. Finnerty, F. A. Jr. 1971. *J. Am. Med. Assoc.* 216:1634-35
176. Adlin, E. V., Marks, A. D., Channick, B. J. 1972. *Arch. Intern. Med.* 130: 855-58
177. Weinberger, M. H., Perkins, B. J., Yu, P. 1973. In *Mechanisms of Hypertension,* ed. M. P. Sambhi, 332-42. Amsterdam: Excerpta Med.
178. Stroobandt, R., Fagard, R., Amery, A. K. P. C. 1973. *Am. Heart J.* 86:781-87
179. Doyle, A. E., Jemms, G., Johnston, C. I., Lewis, W. J. 1973. *Br. Med. J.* 2:206-7
180. Christlieb, A. R., Gleason, R. E., Hickler, R. B., Lauler, D. P. 1974. *Ann. Intern. Med.* 81:7-10
181. Veterans' Admin. Coop. Study Group Antihypertensive Agents 1967. *J. Am. Med. Assoc.* 202:1028-34
182. Veterans' Admin. Coop. Study Group Antihypertensive Agents 1970. *J. Am. Med. Assoc.* 213:1143-52
183. Oxman, H. A. et al 1972. *Circulation* 46:Suppl. II, 104-10
184. Soc. Actuaries 1959. Build and Blood Pressure Study. Vol. 1. Chicago: Soc. Actuaries
185. Kannel, W. B., Schwartz, M. J., McNamara, P. M. 1969. *Dis. Chest* 56:43-52
186. Kannel, W. B., Wolf, P. A., Verter, J., McNamara, P. M. 1970. *J. Am. Med. Assoc.* 214:301-10
187. McKee, P. A., Costelli, W. P., McNamara, P. M., Kannel, W. B. 1971. *N. Engl. J. Med.* 285:1441-46
188. Melby, J. C. 1975. *J. Am. Med. Assoc.* 231:399-404
189. Gifford, R. W. Jr. 1969. *Milbank Mem. Fund. Q.* 47:170-86
190. Finnerty, F. A. 1975. *J. Am. Med. Assoc.* 231:402-3
191. Ferguson, R. K. 1975. *Ann. Intern. Med.* 82:761-65
192. Chobanian, A. V., Burrows, A. V., Hollander, W. 1961. *J. Clin. Invest.* 40: 416-22
193. Tarazi, R. C., Dustan, H. P., Frohlich, E. D., Gifford, R. W. Jr., Hoffman, G. C. 1970. *Arch. Intern. Med.* 125:835-42

194. Novak, L. P., Strong, C. G., Hunt, J. C. 1972. In *Hypertension '72*, ed. J. Genest, E. Koiw, 444–59. Heidelberg: Springer

195. Biglieri, E. G., Herron, M. A., Brust, N. 1966. *J. Clin. Invest.* 45:1946–54

196. Brown, J. J. et al 1972. See Ref. 194, pp. 313–19

197. Biglieri, E. G., Stockigt, J. R., Schambelan, M. 1972. *Am. J. Med.* 52:623–32

198. Filipecki, S. et al 1972. *J. Clin. Endocrinol. Metab.* 35:225–29

199. Melby, J. C., Dale, S. L., Grekin, R. J., Gaunt, R., Wilson, T. 1972. See Ref. 194, pp. 350–60

200. Genest, J., Nowaczynski, W., Kuchel, O., Sasaki, C. 1972. See Ref. 194, pp. 293–98

201. Sennett, J. A. et al 1975. *Circ. Res.* 36:Suppl. 1, 2–9

201a. Funder, J. W., Robinson, J. A., Feldman, D., Wynne, K. N. 1975. The Affinity of 16β-Hydroxy-dehydroepiandrosterone for Mineralocorticoid Receptors. Presented at 57th Ann. Meet. Endocr. Soc., New York, June 18–20

202. Woods, J. W., Liddle, G. W., Staut, E. G., Michelakis, A. M., Brust, A. B. 1969. *Arch. Intern. Med.* 123:366–79

203. Spark, R. F. 1972. *N. Engl. J. Med.* 787:348–49

204. Collins, R. D. et al 1970. *J. Clin. Invest.* 49:1415–26

205. Grim, C. E. 1973. *Clin. Res.* 21:493

206. Nowaczynski, W., Kuchel, O., Genest, J. 1973. See Ref. 52, pp. 244–55

207. Nowaczynski, W., Kuchel, O., Genest, J. 1971. *J. Clin. Invest.* 50:2184–90

208. Nowaczynski, W. et al 1975. *J. Steroid Biochem.* 6:767–78

209. Laragh, J. H. 1973. *Am. J. Med.* 55:261–74

210. Collins, R. D., Weinberger, M. H., Gonzales, C., Nokes, G. W., Luetscher, J. A. 1970. *Clin. Res.* 18:167

211. Esler, M. D., Westel, P. J. 1973. *Am. J. Cardiol.* 32:643–49

212. Padfield, P. L. et al 1974. *Lancet* 1:548–50

213. Hunyor, S. N. Zweifler, A. J. Hansson, L. 1973 *Circulation* 48:Suppl. 4, 83

214. Vaughn, E. D. et al 1973. *Am. J. Cardiol.* 32:522–32

215. Douglas, J. C., Hollifield, J. W., Liddle, G. W. 1974. *J. Am. Med. Assoc.* 227:518–21

216. Schalekamp, M. A. et al 1973. *Am. J. Med.* 55:379–90

217. Biglieri, E. G., Forsham, P. H. 1961. *Am. J. Med.* 30:564–76

218. Helmer, O. M., Judson, W. E. 1968. *Circulation* 38:965–76

219. Bikenhäger, W. H. et al 1972. *Eur. J. Clin. Invest.* 2:115–22

220. Meyer, P. et al 1967. *Circulation* 36:570–76

221. Cohen, E. L., Rovner, D. R., Conn, J. W. 1966. *J. Am. Med. Assoc.* 197:973–78

222. Hollenberg, N., Epstein, M., Bosch, R. I., Merrill, J. P., Hickler, R. B. 1969. *Circ. Res.* 24:Suppl. I, 113–22

223. Kurtzman, N. A., Pillay, V. K. G., Rogers, P. W., Nash, D. 1974. *Arch. Intern. Med.* 133:195–99

224. Hollifield, J. W. et al 1975. *Arch. Intern. Med.* 135:859–64

225. Koch-Weser, J. 1973. *Am. J. Med.* 32:499–510

RELATIONS BETWEEN STRUCTURE AND BIOLOGICAL ACTIVITY OF SULFONAMIDES

♦6652

Thomas H. Maren
Department of Pharmacology and Therapeutics, University of Florida
College of Medicine, Gainesville, Florida 32610

Five major and biologically diverse types of drugs have resulted from the discovery of sulfanilamide (*p*-aminobenzene sulfonamide). Each type has been the fulcrum for enormous intellectual and medical progress. It is not the prime purpose of this review to deal with these notable advances; such reviews are available in the separate fields, and will be cited. I wish rather to deal with the five related chemical types, primarily to show the specific structural features that yield activity in each of the cases. Nowhere in pharmacology can the theoretical organic chemist see more clearly the profound results of molecular change; nowhere can the biologist have more useful probes for physiological or biochemical mechanisms; nowhere can the physician have a group of drugs whose actions are more realistic and reliable.

Figures 1–5 show the basic structures. On the left for each category is shown the simplest stem structure; many molecules from such a stem are but weakly active. One of the main goals of this review is to show the progression from such stem compounds to those with much greater potency and medical utility, examples of which are shown at the right of the figures. The following classes of drugs are dealt with in this chapter: antibacterial sulfonamides and sulfones, carbonic anhydrase inhibitors, antidiabetic (insulin-releasing) sulfonamides, saluretics of the "thiazide" and high ceiling sulfonamide type, and certain antithyroid drugs.

ANTIBACTERIAL SULFONAMIDES AND SULFONES

An astonishingly complete and thoughtful monograph (1) covers the pioneering and most productive years (1935–1946) of sulfonamide chemistry, in which some 5000 compounds were made and tested. Newer drugs made in the next 20 years (2) showed variation in excretion, distribution, and metabolism, but contributed little to relations between antibacterial action and chemical structure. The principal

309

advances since 1946 are the knowledge that sulfonamides and sulfones interfere with the assembly of folic acid at the step that adds *p*-aminobenzoic acid (PABA) (3), and the development of cell-free enzyme systems to study the synthetic steps (4).

The stage was then set for a true evaluation of structure-activity relations. The Bell-Roblin theory of 1942 had been based on the activity of 50 sulfonamides against growth of *Escherichia coli* (5). This work emphasized the N'-substituted sulfanila-mides, exemplified by sulfadiazine (Figure 1). This paper had tremendous intellectual impact and is still widely used as an example of how molecular forces are significant for chemotherapy. The theory was based on the known competition between PABA and the sulfonamides and the fact that, at pH 7, PABA yields the negative COO⁻ ion. Then, "the more negative the SO_2 group of an N' substituted sulfanilamide derivative, the greater the bacteriostatic activity of the compound." Experimental data yielded maximum activity for drugs with pK_a of 6–7, and their theoretical treatment suggested that such drugs had maximum negativity of the SO_2 group.

Two major problems arose with the Bell-Roblin formulation. First, the data are obtained in whole cells, so drug activity is a composite of true antibacterial effect

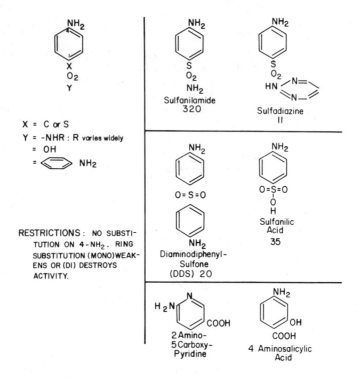

Figure 1   Antibacterial sulfonamides and sulfones. Concentration (μM) for 50% inhibition of synthesis of dihydropteroic acid in presence of 10 μM PABA (6).

and penetration. Highly ionized drugs are weakly active (5); but when sulfanilic acid (Figure 1) was tested in a cell-free system for folate synthesis, it proved almost equal to sulfadiazine (4). Second, there were numerous exceptions to the parabolic relation of activity vs pK_a; sulfaguanidine and diaminodiphenylsulfone (DDS) (Figure 1) have no acidic pK_a yet are highly active in either intact cells (5) or the cell-free system (6). Other exceptions included active compounds disubstituted on the $-SO_2N<$group, which have no acidic pK_a (7).

Early work in the field had shown that isosteres of benzene could also produce active compounds; the analog of PABA, $2-NH_2-5-COOH$ pyridine (Figure 1), was bacteriostatic for *E. coli* and reversed by PABA. Some activity was also found among thiophenes and pyrimidines with NH_2 and COOH arranged in homologous fashion to PABA (8).

Substituents in the ring of PABA yield active compounds, although on a weight basis they are relatively weak (8, 9). The most important member of this class is *p*-aminosalicylic acid (Figure 1), which appears somewhat specific for the tubercle bacillus, although active as a PABA antagonist for other organisms as well (10).

It is thus clear that the five different but related structures of Figure 1 are all active and may be regarded as subsets of an ideal molecular shape that interferes with the assimilation of PABA into folic acid. Before attempting to define this molecular shape, we may briefly set down the specific reactions involved.

The first organic step in the synthesis of folic acid is the condensation of $2-NH_2-$ 4-OH-6 hydroxymethylpteridine (Pt) pyrophosphate with PABA to form dihydropteroic acid. The reaction occurs between the $-CH_2O-PO_3H-$ group of Pt pyrophosphate and the $-NH_2$ group of PABA to form a $-CH_2-NH-$ link. It is here that the sulfonamides are thought primarily to act by competing in some fashion with the condensation of PABA. A secondary site is the conjugation between Pt pyrophosphate and *p*-aminobenzoylglutamate. The same chemical link is involved, yielding $-CH_2-NH-$. Evidence for both of these is reviewed and diagrammed in (11), largely from the work of (4). From consideration of these pathways, it is not surprising that all inhibitors of these reactions (or of bacterial growth, reversed by PABA) contain an aromatic NH_2 group or radicals that are readily converted to such a group. It seems likely, but is not finally proven, that sulfonamides (and sulfones) act as false substrates for PABA in these reactions, forming a dihydropteroic sulfonamide or a false folate–incorporating sulfonamide (4). Such compounds remain to be identified.

The basic molecular shape of the "sulfonamide" or "sulfone" inhibitors is shown on the left of Figure 1. As suggested in the brief review of active compounds just given, a wider range of substituents on C^1 is permitted than is suggested by inspection of available sulfonamide drugs, in which the substituent is always $-SO_2NHR$. This is evident from the structures on the right of Figure 1. In the cell-free system, $-SO_3H$ is highly active (4), and even $-COOH$ is inhibitory when modified by an adjacent OH group (10). Furthermore, ionization of the group on C^1 is not demanded, despite an enormous amount of work on this issue. DDS is virtually as active as sulfadiazine (6), and certain N'N' dialkyl compounds are as active as their monosubstituted analogs (12).

A recent paper attempts again to link activity with increased ionization of $-SO_2NHR$ (13) but neglects DDS and sulfaguanidine and the N'N' dialkyl compounds. It is likely that in a closely knit homologous series, or in studies of a single drug at different pH, ionization will increase activity, although not quantitatively.

There does not seem to be any measurable (as yet) property of the SO_2 group that confers activity, as had been postulated (5, 12). It is intuitively clear that reactivity of the N^4 amino group is essential for competition at the PABA steps, but that the properties of the group at C^1 directly bear on this. These properties remain elusive; however, I conclude this section by considering some papers that attempt to relate structure to activity, as a means of tentative identification of the requirements at C^1.

Structure-action relations cannot be obtained rigorously in bacterial growth studies because of the problem of drugs penetrating bacterial cells. Such studies might well yield highly effective drugs, as a composite of activity and access to cells, but will probably not give the key to synthetic or inhibitory mechanisms. In terms of sulfonamides inhibiting the condensation of Pt pyrophosphate + PABA, four papers using cell-free dihydropteroate synthetase from *E. coli* are relevant (4, 6, 12, 13). These data show, as indicated above, that ionization on substituents of C^1 is not a factor, and that drugs can be weak acids, weak bases, or carry no ionic charge. Indeed, the weak base, DDS, is virtually as potent as the weak acid sulfadiazine (6). A weakness of an interesting study purporting to show relation between pK_a and cell-free activity is the narrow range of pK_a and chemical type studied (13). The same criticism applies to correlations with NMR-measured shifts of primary (N^4) amine protons, with the additional caveat that these shifts are of the precursor amines used in the synthesis, not the sulfonamide itself (13).

Inspection of the 50-odd structures studied in these four papers conveys the general impression that any substituent that is electron-rich and attached to $-SO_2-$ at C^1 is associated with high activity; electron-poor substituents are weak. Thus the aromatic ring of DDS, the O atom of sulfanilic acid, and the heterocyclic rings of the drugs in common use (cf sulfadiazine) are potent, while sulfanilamide and its N' alkyl derivatives are weak. The potent compounds inhibit PABA incorporation into folate at concentrations about half that of PABA (inhibition index ranging from 0.3 to 0.8), while weak compounds have indices of 20–30 (4, 12). Figure 1 shows inhibitory concentrations for the several drugs, in the presence of a fixed concentration of PABA (6).

The effect of electron pressure on the N^4 amine is crucial, since this is the reactive part of the molecule. Nevertheless, no definitive property of N^4 has been shown to correlate with activity across the wide range of drug type shown on the right of Figure 1. Attempts to make such a correlation with either basic pK_a of the amine or chemical shift are unconvincing, since a very narrow range of pK_a or shift is covered, the precursor amine rather than the sulfonamide was studied, data are from a small homologous series of N^1 benzenesulfonamides, and activity was measured by cell growth (7).

The intimate nature of N^4 reactivity must also await more detailed knowledge of how sulfonamides and sulfones are interpolated in the folate pathway. Although there are several points at which the drugs may replace PABA, it is not yet clear what products are formed; neither the postulated Schiff base (7) from Pt aldehyde nor the presumed "false folate"–incorporating sulfonamide (4) has been isolated. This matter is discussed in reference 11.

CARBONIC ANHYDRASE INHIBITORS

The criteria for activity in this class are the simplest in pharmacology; all unsubstituted aromatic sulfonamides (aryl SO_2NH_2) inhibit carbonic anhydrase, and no other class of organic compounds approaches these in activity. Figure 2 shows representative compounds. Several hundred chemicals of this class have been tabulated according to activity (relative to sulfanilamide) and structural type. It was not possible to make any general rules, but interesting insights within certain series of compounds were made (14). The dissociation constants (K_I) of some 60 drugs against red cell carbonic anhydrase of various species have been tabulated. K_I was a function of inhibition of the catalytic hydration of CO_2. In addition, twelve representative drugs are discussed in terms of K_I, physical and chemical properties, and their effects in vivo. The history of their development is also given, stemming

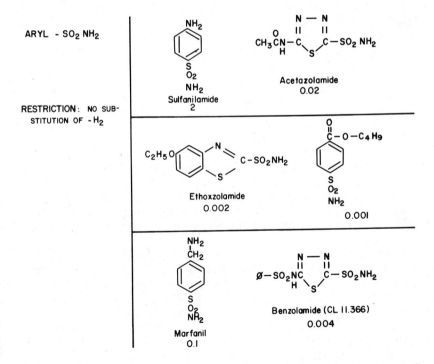

Figure 2   Carbonic anhydrase inhibitors. Concentration (μM) for K_I against human red cell carbonic anhydrase C (15).

from unexplained clinical and chemical findings with sulfanilamide when it was first used in 1935–1937 (15). As is evident from the structural requirements for carbonic hydrase inhibition, such findings never occurred when sulfanilamide gave way to the N^1-substituted compounds now used in antibacterial chemotherapy (Figure 1).

The nature of the reaction between sulfonamides and the active site of carbonic anhydrase has been reviewed (16, 17). An important element is the measurement of the overall association (k_a) and dissociation (k_d) rate constants (18) which are the bases for the net activity, by the relation $k_d/k_a = K_I$. As known for a long time, K_I varies greatly, some 10^5-fold, among all drugs studied (15). For the 24 compounds in which rate constants were measured, k_a varied 240-fold and k_d 80-fold. It then becomes relevant to discuss structure-activity relations in terms, largely, of k_a. Furthermore, the effect of the charge of the sulfonamide group (as judged by measuring k_a, k_d, or K_I at differing pH) is upon k_a (19).

The inquiry into structure-activity relations has naturally led into the question of the form in which the sulfonamides react, whether undissociated weak acid (SH) or anion (S⁻). This has been studied by relating pH to either their rates of inhibition of CO_2 hydration (20, 21) or the actual rates of association between sulfonamide and enzyme (18, 19, 22). Analysis of the data has been complicated by the fact that the enzyme (as weak base) ionizes in the same pH range (7–8) as many of the drugs. When k_a is plotted against pH, bell-shaped curves are generated with k_a maximal at pH 7–9, depending on the drug used. Data were consistent with either

(a)   E + SH

          or   complex RSO₂NH⁻CA = S⁻E + H⁺

(b)   EH⁺ + S⁻

Ancillary evidence supported b, particularly the ultraviolet difference spectroscopy of the sulfonamide in the complex showing the form S⁻, and the fact that the cyanate (pK_a 4) acts only as the anion. There are no sulfonamides in critical range (pK_a 6 or below) for an unequivocal test of activity of species S⁻ vs SH, but, if anions act by a mechanism similar to that of sulfonamides, the NCO⁻ experiment is important (16).

However, mechanism b fails when it is realized that several drugs of $pK_a = 10$, salicylazobenzenesulfonamide (17, 18), and esters of –OOC ⬡ SO₂NH₂ (23), are highly active when tested at pH 6.5. To act as the anion in the overall reaction (mechanism b), their k_a would have to be $> 10^{10}$ M⁻¹ sec⁻¹, essentially an impossibly great speed for collision between a drug and macromolecule (19).

It has therefore been suggested that "the initial formation of the complex is more or less independent of ionization state of the sulfonamide" (16, 17). If this is accepted, it means that a or b (or both) must apply in any given case, but we cannot have E + S⁻ or EH⁺ + S, since these would not generate the bell-shaped curves that all investigators have found for the sulfonamides and the weak anions (pK_a 7–10) HS⁻ and CN⁻.

The matter now has been freshly investigated, with results that clarify the situation and resolve these dilemmas (23). Association rates between enzyme and drug for six homologous series of sulfonamides were studied with emphasis on esters and amides of benzene sulfonamide. Figure 2 shows the butyl ester, one of the most active inhibitors known. As noted above, activity was largely a function of the association rate constant k_a. Substitution of ester or amide on the para position of the benzene ring gave far greater activity than ortho or meta substitution. A wide range of activity was studied, with K_I from 4×10^{-5} to 4×10^{-10} M. The principal advance lay in considering the reaction of drug and human red cell carbonic anhydrase C as a two-step reaction, first to the apoenzyme [equivalent to an intermediate complex (En D_1)], followed by isomerization to a final coordinating complex (En D_2). For the first time it was possible to measure affinity of drugs to the apoenzyme (K_{apo}) and to compare them with overall dissociation constants (K_I) or affinity constants (K_{holo}). Finally, estimations could be made of the rate constants, according to the following scheme

$$\text{En} + \text{D} \underset{k_{-1}}{\overset{k_1}{\rightleftharpoons}} [\text{En D}_1] \underset{k_{-2}}{\overset{k_2}{\rightleftharpoons}} [\text{En D}_2] \rightleftharpoons (\text{En D})_x.$$

In general, it was found that $k_1/k_{-1} = K_{apo}$ was about 10^3 M^{-1} while K_{holo} (reciprocal of K_I) was about 10^8M^{-1}. However, the initial "on" rate constant k_1, assumed from diffusion, is very fast (about 10^8 sec^{-1}) and is a significant factor in the overall activity.

We may now contrast the two reactions: the first, to form En D_1, is not dependent on the active Zn site, is not pH dependent, does not require an intact RSO$_2$NH$_2$ (binding is observed with RSO$_2$NH acetyl), and its affinity constant K_{apo} is proportional to lipid solubility. It is thus a typical hydrophobic reaction. The second or coordination step, to form En D_2, appears to involve the active site, is pH dependent, and probably involves the charged species of both enzyme and drug. As the authors point out (23), their earlier stricture (19) relative to rates that appeared faster than diffusion (discussed above) is irrelevant, since diffusion is not a factor in the second or isomerization step.

This study is a valuable contribution to molecular pharmacology. Specifically it enables us to understand, for the first time, how inhibition of carbonic anhydrase appearing similar in overall kinetics can be accomplished by either hydrophilic (i.e. anions and partially charged sulfonamides) or hydrophobic (uncharged organic sulfonamides) substances. Perhaps optimum activity occurs when important elements of both are present in the same molecule. The two-step system yields the latitude of interpretation demanded by the large body of data in the literature. It is evident that the hydrophobic (step 1) interaction ($K_{apo} = k_1/k_{-1}$) can vary at least 40-fold (almost certainly more if the chemical series were extended) and the second or isomerization stage ($k_2/k_{-2} = K_2$) some 2000-fold. Thus both the structurally nonspecific binding (step 1) and that concerned with active site, charge, and intact RSO$_2$NH$_2$ structure (step 2) are significant (23). Step 2 appears to link the activity of inorganic anions with that of the sulfonamides. Further work, hopefully, will include the heterocyclic sulfonamides represented by Figure 2, so that precise structural relations for K_2 (independent of hydrophobic binding) can be found.

Certain structural relations may be tentatively established as a result of the studies described (14–23). These pertain to overall activity, since not enough data exist to characterize fully K_2, the specific drug-enzyme step.

The first "rule" is that activity of $K_I < 10^{-4}$M requires an unsubstituted group R–SO$_2$NH$_2$. As Figure 2 shows, a wide variety of structures has been studied, whose K_I range is almost 10^5. Clearly there is no simple guide to structure-action relations, and this is now explicable in terms of the two-step sequence just described (23). High activity has generally been associated with resonating heterocyclic structures (e.g. ethoxzolamide, benzolamide, acetazolamide; see reference 15); these may be particularly effective in the second or coordination step. The esters of p-sulfonamide benzoic acid appear to owe their high activity to the first or hydrophobic step, with a moderate affinity in the second step. It appears, however, that affinity in the first step alone could not yield $K_I < 10^{-4}$M (23), which shows why the specific RSO$_2$-NH$_2$ structure, yielding k_{-2}/k_2 of 10^{-6} M and overall K_I to 10^{-9} M, is necessary for high activity.

Second, R should be aromatic; alkyl compounds (23a) are exceedingly weak ($K_I > 10^{-4}$M). Such activity may be due to contamination by aromatic sulfonamides during synthesis or, in terms of the above model, some affinity of the alkyl sulfonamide in the nonspecific first step.

Third, within homologous series of benzene sulfonamides, ester or amide substitution on the para position yields far more active compounds than ortho or meta substitution. This is due to superior affinity at both steps, but chiefly at the specific second (23).

Fourth, very large, or bulky, fused ring systems with multiple substituents seem to repress activity. Thus the "diuretic sulfonamides" or saluretics to be considered below are relatively weak inhibitors (15, 23a). Some of these compounds show unusual increments of activity during incubation with enzyme in absence of substrate; this merits further attention in terms of mechanism (23a). This phenomenon may be the basis for the curious pharmacology of 2-amino-4-phenylsulfonylbenzenesulfonamide (NSD 3004), which appears to bind carbonic anhydrase in red cells in vivo with much greater affinity than would be predicted from in vitro assays against the enzyme in high CO$_2$ (24 and papers cited). This type of dissociation (not evident in the drugs shown in Figure 2) (15) may be related to multiple ring systems or a sulfoxide group, and may indicate a degree of irreversible binding not generally seen in sulfonamide-carbonic anhydrase reactions.

Fifth, within a homologous series, activity increases with lipid solubility of the undissociated molecule (23). This appears to reflect increased affinity in the hydrophobic initial step.

Lastly, within a given group of drugs, introduction of an acidic group appears to increase activity, in degree relative to the strength of the acid group. Thus, in the series of thiadiazole-5-sulfonamides, there is increasing activity from 2-NH$_2$ to 2-acetylamino (acetazolamide) to 2-benzenesulfonamido (benzolamide). The same relation is found between sulfanilamide and 4-acetylsulfanilamide (15). This appears reasonable in terms of ionic interactions in the coordination step 2, just described.

Attempts have been made to predict structure-activity relations of carbonic anhydrase inhibitors in terms of Hammett's factor, pK_a, chemical shift of $-SO_2NH_2$ protons, valence force of $S = O$ bond, and hydrophobic factors. The correlations do not seem convincing, in part because very few of the highly active and diverse heterocyclic drugs were studied (25). Significantly, if the foregoing model is accepted, overall activity could never be related to a given set of forces, since at least four rate constants, which vary independently, are involved.

Thus there are reasonable guides to the strength of the highly specific group $aryl-SO_2NH_2$ as inhibitors of vertebrate carbonic anhydrase, but there are no single or set of molecular configuration(s) absolutely predicting degree of activity.

The nature of the inhibition of catalytic hydration (or dehydration) is outside the scope of this review. In brief, the sulfonamides appear to inhibit hydration (of CO_2) noncompetitively, and dehydration (of HCO_3^-) competitively (15). This agrees with the ionic nature of the dominant second step of sulfonamide enzyme binding in the above model.

Finally, it now appears that the dissociation constants for acetazolamide and human red cell enzymes may be 5- to 10-fold less when measured in the CO_2 hydration reaction, compared to HCO_3^- dehydration; further work is in progress on this critical point (25a).

INSULIN-RELEASING SULFONAMIDES

Unlike the two classes of sulfonamides that have just been discussed, the chemistry of interaction at the active site is unknown for the present class. The intriguing game of structural analogy cannot be played, and only empirical relations can be discussed. This class is defined physiologically by hypoglycemic action in animals and man whose pancreases contain cells capable of preparing and secreting insulin.

The discovery of these so-called sulfonylureas (26) was made accidentally when blood sugar was found to be low during treatment with the antibacterial sulfonamide, sulfathiadiazole (Figure 3). This compound has a thiourea skeleton, and later developments showed that most, if not all, aromatic sulfonylureas or thioureas reduced blood sugar in animals or humans with potential insulin stores. The standard drug for many years was tolbutamide (Figure 3), a sulfonylurea with no antibacterial activity (no free aryl NH_2) and no activity against carbonic anhydrase (no free aryl SO_2NH_2).

Further work, however, (27, 28) showed that the urea structure was not essential, and that $C = O$ or $C = S$ could give way to C–N, as in glycodiazine (Figure 3). The fundamental structure is simply R_1SO_2NH-, and there are few restrictions on R_1. Of course, not all compounds with this group are active, but it is worth noting that compounds in the classes of Figures 1, 2, and 4 have the possibility of lowering blood sugar.

During the past two decades, some 12,000 compounds, an extraordinary number, have been synthesized and tested, largely in the German pharmaceutical industry. Although the compounds have been duly recorded and divided into appropriate chemical classes (27, 28), this has not been accompanied by a quantitative measure of activity. For certain key compounds, we do have the parenteral dose needed to

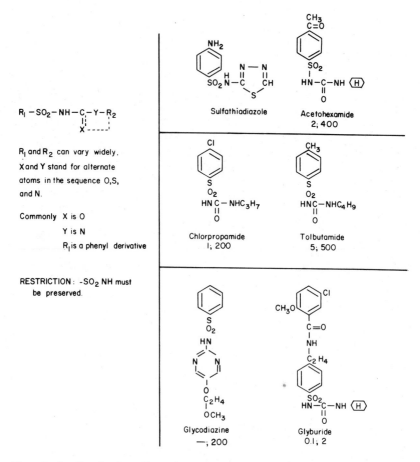

Figure 3 Insulin-releasing sulfonamides. Minimum oral dose mg/kg, for 10% reduction in blood glucose in rat; human single oral dose, mg (28).

lower blood sugar in standard tests in the rat, and these numbers, along with clinical doses, will be used as a measure of activity. It is important to note that in vivo activity has, in the few cases studied, been correlated successfully with the release of insulin in vitro from slices of pancreas (29). It is also important that quantitative potency of several drugs could be measured in dog and man by both fall in blood sugar and rise in insulin concentration after intravenous doses (30). Using these data, I attempt some generalizations about structure and degree of activity.

In the tolbutamide or chlorpropamide type (Figure 3), best activity results when R_2 is C_3H_7 to C_6H_{13}. If C = 2, activity declines; it is zero when C is 12. If R_2 is H (p-toluenesulfonylurea) the drug is inactive. The effect of p-Cl in chlorpropamide is to increase activity fourfold over tolbutamide. Other halogens or CF_3 in the para position do not enhance activity. If R is cycloaliphatic, activity is enhanced, as in acetohexamide (Figure 3), and in such compounds the cycloalkyl C can be 7 or 8. The changes so far described lead to a modest (about four to sixfold) increase in activity over tolbutamide, for instance, in the experimental drug V 14826, p-chlorbenzenesulfonyl-cycloheptyl urea. A further variation of this compound is the inclusion of N in the seven-membered cycloalkyl ring of R_2 to yield the semicarbazide link of azepinamide, which is stated to be about ten times as active as tolbutamide.

A truly striking change in activity is brought about by p-substitution with acylaminoalkyl groups; these findings resulted in glyburide (Figure 3), which is about 100 times as active as tolbutamide, either in vivo or in vitro (29). The basis for the increase in activity is p-C_2H_4NHCO–aryl–; the nature and substituents of the aryl ring may not be critical. This pragmatic finding has not resulted in any systematic or theoretical treatment. Again, as in the other classes of drugs under review, molecular changes relatively far from the core or basic structure essential to activity have a large influence on the potency.

Recent developments in the field show the subtlety of the problem. In glycodiazine (Figure 3) and congeners, there are no substituents on the benzene ring, and the sulfonyl urea link has given way to $-SO_2NH-C-N_2$, in which the nitrogens are incorporated into a pyrimidine ring, with alkoxy side chain. Despite elimination of two seemingly important elements, glycodiazine is about twice as active as tolbutamide. Yet when p-benzene substitution is made with the 5-chlor-2-methoxy-benzamidoethyl chain (as in glyburide, Figure 3), very large activation occurs. Clearly, this acylamino-alkyl group is an important clue in structure-action relations.

Many other relations, particularly within the many subclasses of antidiabetic sulfonamides, have been indicated (28). However, there has been little attempt to correlate activity with any chemical or physical property, such as we have seen for the antibacterial and carbonic anhydrase inhibitory drugs. Such work should lie in the future, along with studies of the reaction by which these drugs effect the release of insulin.

THIAZIDE AND HIGH CEILING SALURETICS

Figures 4 and 4A show the structures of the saluretics. All have 1,3-disulfamyl or 1-sulfamyl-3-carboxy groups attached to a benzene ring. Pharmacologically, they cause increased renal excretion of sodium and chloride in roughly equimolar amounts. Their mechanism of action is not known. Although all the useful drugs of this class have unsubstituted R–SO_2NH_2 groups and so are carbonic anhydrase inhibitors in vitro, they are usually weak inhibitors. All (except dichlorphenamide, see below) are used in doses that do not inhibit renal carbonic anhydrase physiologically, i.e. they do not alkalinize the urine. This saluretic class is complicated by the existence of a most important subclass (Figure 4A) of high ceiling compounds; these have certain chemical and pharmacological properties in common with those of Figure 4. But at their maximal dose, the high ceiling compounds elicit about three times as much NaCl excretion as from maximal doses of drugs of Figure 4. There

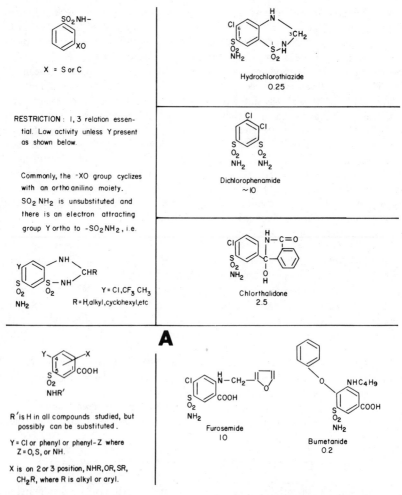

Figure 4 Thiazide saluretics and (*A*) High ceiling saluretics. Minimum i.v. dose for maximum Na$^+$ or Cl$^-$ effect in dog, mg/kg (31).

are also differences in the renal mechanisms and structure. This section lists the basic structure requirements of both classes 4 (thiazide and related types) and 4A (high ceiling sulfonamides), as well as some of the elements that determine potency in these classes.

Thiazide and Related Types

The first few years of research in this field culminated in an important review by its leaders (31). Two additional, excellent monographs are available, emphasizing the chemical (32) and pharmacological (33) sides of the structure-activity relation. The latter (33) includes an invaluable listing of the quantitative natriuretic potency of 50 of these drugs in animals and in man. Activity, based on dose, covers a 2000-fold range! From these papers, we may lay out the structure-activity relations in class 4.

The original research stemmed from attention to renal carbonic anhydrase inhibition, but the crucial finding was the difference between benzenesulfonamide or p-chlorbenzenesulfonamide, and 1,3-disulfonamide-6-chlorbenzene. The second sulfonamide group, meta to the first, yielded a chloruretic (saluretic) compound, while the monosulfonamide (Figure 2) showed only the renal effects of carbonic anhydrase inhibition, HCO_3^- and not Cl^- excretion. In the disulfonamide class, addition of a second Cl to the ring yielded dichlorophenamide (Figure 4); because this is sufficiently active against carbonic anhydrase, it is a drug of both classes, i.e. it may be used in glaucoma and as a saluretic.

Ring closure of another of these disulfonamides, chlorodisulfamylaniline, yielded the more active chlorothiazide. Further work yielded hydrochlorothiazide (Figure 4), still more (10 times) active as a chloruretic, but less so as a carbonic anhydrase inhibitor. In hydrochlorothiazide, we see again the fundamental features necessary for activity, the 1,3-disulfamyl relation and the adjacent Cl. Compounds without the halogen have activity, but are very weak (31; and work in the reviewer's laboratory).

Further activity was obtained by continuing in the 3–4 saturated series, and making alkyl substitutions in position 3. The 3-cyclopentylmethyl derivative (cyclopenthiazide, not shown) is about 100 times as active as hydrochlorothiazide. It is interesting, but unexplained, that, although the role of Cl in position 6 is presumably that of electron attraction, CF_3 in this position does not enhance activity. The increasing activity in the series chlorothiazide $\longrightarrow$ hydrochlorothiazide $\longrightarrow$ cyclopenthiazide corresponds with increasing ether/water partition coefficient, although it was recognized that additional (unknown) factors are also at work. There is no relation between pK_a and renal activity (31). The possible relations between lipid solubility, pK_a, drug disposition, and renal activity are well illustrated in a neglected paper, and show that no single or obvious pattern is at work (34).

The advent of chlorthalidone (Figure 4) made it clear that a carbamyl function can substitute effectively for the second (meta) sulfamyl group. The activity of this drug is equal to that of chlorothiazide; its distinction lies in long duration of action. Further departures from the original benzothiadiazine structure are discussed, including such esoterica as replacement of the benzene ring by pyridine and inclusion of boron in the thiadiazine ring (32). It is significant that, even in these types, activity follows only if the fundamental features just described are retained.

The precise nature of the sulfamyl group(s) in these compounds was debated for many years, along with the closely related issue of whether all or part of their pharmacological effect was due to carbonic anhydrase inhibition. Initially, many workers stated or implied that the renal effects were, in some way, due to inhibition of the enzyme (31, 35, 36), and the question is unfortunately still raised (32). It has now been shown clearly that the $R-SO_2NH_2$ group could be substituted, although in all the useful compounds it was free. The free sulfonamide in the 7 position of hydrochlorothiazide was altered to $-SO_2NHR$, where R was alkyl or acyl, or to $-SO_2-CH_3$. None of these compounds inhibit carbonic anhydrase, yet all were chloruretic (37). Data on 7-acetylhydrochlorothiazide were particularly convincing. This result was not unexpected, since some of the compounds most potent as chloruretics (i.e. cyclopenthiazide) were the weakest as carbonic anhydrase inhibitors and did not alkalinize the urine (31, 33). The minimal requirement for activity thus appears to be the structure shown on the left of Figure 4, although, for maximum activity, the free SO_2NH_2, group and adjacent halogens are necessary. The free SO_2NH_2, however, does not work here through carbonic anhydrase inhibition, since the renal effects of fully effective saluretic doses (of hydrochlorothiazide, for example) are qualitatively different from those of the monosubstituted sulfonamides (Figure 2), whose renal effects are solely due to carbonic anhydrase inhibition (15, 33).

A surprising and significant finding was that a compound of the general type of Figure 4, with both features that usually enhance activity (6-halogen and 3-alkyl), is not only virtually devoid of diuretic action, but blocks the renal effect of other thiazides (i.e. hydrochlorothiazide). This compound, 3,4-dihydro-2-methyl-3-(β-oxopropyl)-7-sulfamyl-6-trifluoromethyl-2H-1,2,4-benzothiadiazine-1,-1-dioxide-1-phthalazinylhydrazone (EX 4877), appears to occupy the renal thiazide receptor (37a). The special structural feature may be a ring-substituted hydralazine linked to the 3-alkyl group. It is surprising that these studies have not been pursued, since they could illuminate the nature of this important receptor, which is still entirely unknown. Comparison of the antagonist EX 4877 and the agonists of Figure 4 shows possibilities for making compounds substituted on the 3 position to reveal whether the hydrazine or the additional ring (or other features) are responsible for blockade.

The relation between structure and activity for the antidiuretic action of this type of thiazide drug has received special attention (38). It was found that the same structural criteria that elicit saluresis are responsible for free water retention; this is an interesting but not unexpected finding, in view of theories linking the site of distal sodium reabsorption with that of elaboration of osmotically unobligated water. These and other physiological mechanisms underlying the actions of diuretics have been reviewed (39).

High Ceiling Sulfonamide Saluretics

Figure 4A shows a new and separate class of compounds; although derived from thiazide research they have structural similarities with compounds of Figure 4. Chief of these is the meta relation between sulfamyl and carboxy groups on the benzene ring. However, when a series of 5-sulfamylanthranilic acids was synthesized (40), a much higher ceiling of activity was reached. This is clearly shown in the human pharmacology of furosemide (Figure 4A), the first and chief drug of the class (41). Dose and potency comparison was made with six of the "thiazides"; furosemide elicited two to three times the sodium excretion at plateau or peak doses of all those drugs. Details of the pharmacology and renal action of furosemide have been well reviewed (33), and physiological differences from the thiazide type have been discussed (39).

With regard to structure-activity relations, it is important to note that the sulfamyl group does appear in all compounds of this class, but that carbonic anhydrase inhibition is relatively low and furosemide does not alkalinize the urine (33). In some experimental compounds the $-SO_2NH_2$ group has one or two N substituents (40) but, since these may be subject to metabolic removal (35), it is not clear whether the sulfamyl group need be intact. Of paramount interest is the finding that furosemide and hydrochlorothiazide do not have a common mode of action (42). This was determined by blocking the renal action of hydrochlorothiazide with the specific antagonist EX 4877 (see above), in which case the effect of furosemide was retained.

Supporting this concept is further work in the structure-activity field. Two departures (at least) are possible from the furosemide type—whose structure does conform to the basic criterion of the thiazides. First, it was possible to move the –NHR groups from ortho (i.e. anthranilic acid type) to meta relative to COOH; second, and most significant, the activating halogen ortho to the sulfonamide group was found unnecessary and, in fact, yielded compounds in the metanilic acid series with low activity (43). This interesting research produced bumetanide (Figure 4A), which showed "high ceiling" diuretic activity in animals (43) and man (44) at about one fiftieth the dose of furosemide. The activating groups ortho to the sulfonamide group now appear to be –Y–phenyl where Y = NH, S, or O (43). Of further significance is the fact that these new activating groups yielded inert compounds when substituted for the halogen in the thiazide series (45).

The structure-action relations of the high ceiling types are currently being extended past furosemide and bumetanide to cover dozens of compounds with 2-, 3-, and 4- substituents of 5-sulfamylbenzoic acid. The most recent paper that summarizes work of this group is cited (46). It is now shown that the NH function is not necessary on positions 2 or 3. The most active compounds have a connecting link to the phenyl in the 4 position and a bulky substituent at 3. Figure 4A shows the various possibilities. Perhaps the most potent diuretic yet to be described (active in dog at 1 μg/kg) is 4-benzoyl-5-sulfamoyl-3-(3-thenyloxy)benzoic acid. The authors also explain the activity of a series of benzisothiazoles not containing a free $-SO_2-NH_2$, by ring cleavage, which yields the free sulfonamide, meta to –COOH.

A clear criterion for this high ceiling type is the –COOH group, which links it to ethacrynic acid, the other main high ceiling type of seemingly quite different structure. The basic structural criteria for class 4A have not been elucidated absolutely. It would be interesting if these did turn out to be similar to ethacrynic acid, since the two types do share, for the most part, a common renal pharmacology (33).

ANTITHYROID COMPOUNDS

The sulfonamides belong to one of three distinct classes of organic compounds that interfere with the synthesis of thyroid hormone (Figure 5). Activity is not actually related to the sulfonamide group, but to the R–NH₂ component, which occurs in all antibacterial sulfonamides (Figure 1). None of these sulfonamides or other aromatic amines are in clinical use as antithyroid drugs. However, there are several reasons for inclusion here: historical development, recognition of possible anti-

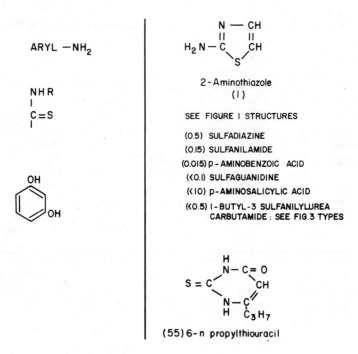

ARYL —NH₂

NHR
|
C = S
|

2-Aminothiazole
(I)

SEE FIGURE I STRUCTURES

(0.5) SULFADIAZINE
(0.15) SULFANILAMIDE
(0.015) p - AMINOBENZOIC ACID
(<0.1) SULFAGUANIDINE
(<10) p-AMINOSALICYLIC ACID
(<0.5) I-BUTYL-3 SULFANILYLUREA
  CARBUTAMIDE : SEE FIG.3 TYPES

(55) 6-n propylthiouracil

Figure 5 Antithyroid drugs. Relative (to 2-aminothiazole) antithyroid activity based on reduction of I content of rat thyroid. Compiled from (50) and (55).

thyroid activity as an unwanted side effect of drugs of other classes, and the theoretical and possible practical importance of the fact that the sulfonamides (or amines) may work at a site in thyroxine biosynthesis different from that of the thioureas.

The discovery of the antithyroid drugs, like that of the carbonic anhydrase inhibitors and the antidiabetic sulfonylureas, was an accident during a study of the antibacterial sulfonamides. Goiter was observed in rats during work on the effect of sulfaguanidine on intestinal flora (47). This, together with similar chance observations on phenylthiourea during the same year, set off an explosive round of research on physiological mechanisms, chemical syntheses, and structure-action relations of antithyroid drugs. Work of the first few years was summarized by its leading figure (48) and has been brought forward to the present (49). At the end of ten years, almost 1000 compounds had been carefully evaluated (50) but relatively little work of this type has been done since.

It was soon found that goiter was a compensatory change resulting from drug-induced hypothyroidism (48). The possibility of developing drugs for the treatment of hyperthyroidism was immediately conceived, and screening was set up in many pharmaceutical houses. As in all the other classes of drugs discussed, these procedures were rewarded by the discovery of new compounds, hundreds of times as active as those that furnished the lead. However, these were all in the thiourea, rather than in the arylamine series (Figure 5). Nevertheless, enough work was done to delineate clearly the structural features necessary for activity in the arylamine group.

Drugs were evaluated quantitatively largely by their effect in lowering the iodine content of rat thyroid in vivo (51; reviewed in 50). The activity and structural specificity of sulfanilamide-like compounds were also studied in the synthesis of diiodotyrosine and thyroxine from labeled iodine, in thyroid slices in vitro (52). Extension of quantitative structure-activity relations to man was made possible by external counting of injected ^{131}I in the region of the thyroid, following intravenous injection (53). Syntheses of these varied data make it possible to arrive at intrinsic structural relations unmarred by species peculiarities or factors of metabolic alteration of the drugs.

The simple fact emerges that all aromatic primary amines, $R-NH_2$, are probably active. In many cases such activity is either not observed (as aniline itself) or is weak (as p-aminobenzoic acid) in the rat test (50), but at $10^{-3}M$ in vitro all such compounds inhibit organic synthesis of iodide (52, 54). Although in vivo data suggest that the free amino group is necessary (50), several substituted amines (cf acetanilide) were active in vitro (52). Similarly, acetazolamide (Figure 2), which failed to alter thyroid morphology or function in several species studied (15), did lower uptake of radioiodine in thyroid slices (54). The in vitro test also uncovered the activity of certain aromatic hydroxy compounds; however, these studies are marred by lack of dose-response curves (52).

The most active compound of the amine class is 2-aminothiazole (Figure 5), which has about one fiftieth the potency of 6-n-propylthiouracil in the rat. However, the startling fact emerges that, in man, 2-aminothiazole is three times as active as 6-n-propylthiouracil in the inhibition of iodine uptake to the thyroid (53).

The only compound of this class that has caused hypothyroidism and goiter in man is p-aminosalicylic acid (Figure 1). This occurs as a toxic side effect of the chemotherapy of tuberculosis, in which the unusually large dose of 5-10 g per day is given (49, 55). It is clear that, in the structural specificity of amine antithyroid drugs (Figure 5) and antibacterial sulfonamides (Figure 1), the $R-NH_2$ group is shared. Thus all the latter drugs will have the potential for inhibiting thyroid hormone synthesis. As noted, this has not generally been observed in man, although clearly demonstrable in rat (50) and in tissue slices (52, 54). Other primary amines in clinical use include the sulfonylurea, carbutamide, and the inhibitor of adrenal steroid synthesis, amphenone. They are goitrogenic in rat, and inhibit thyroidal ^{131}I uptake in man, but have not caused hypothyroidism or goiter in man (reviewed in 55).

The arylamine class of antithyroid drugs thus fundamentally has nothing to do with the sulfonamide group itself. The association arose out of the chance observation with sulfaguanidine (47) and the fact that many antibacterial sulfonamides, all bearing the arylamine group, were available for investigation. However, it is worth noting that the sulfonamides may have an antithyroid mechanism different from the thioureas or possibly from the anilines themselves. This difference is revealed by the fact that iodide greatly potentiates the inhibitory action of the sulfonamides (i.e. sulfadiazine) but not of the thioureas (55). The sulfonamides may therefore be useful probes in thyroid physiology, as they have been in all the systems reviewed.

Literature Cited

1. Northey, E. H. 1948. *The Sulfonamides and Allied Compounds.* New York: Reinhold
2. Zbinden, G. 1964. *Adv. Chem. Ser.* 45:25–38
3. Woods, D. D. 1954. *Ciba Symposium on Chemistry and Biology of Pteridines.* Boston: Little, Brown
4. Brown, G. M. 1961. *J. Biol. Chem.* 237:536–40
5. Bell, P.H., Roblin, R. O. 1942. *J. Am. Chem. Soc.* 64:2905–17
6. McCullough, J. L., Maren, T. H. 1973. *Antimicrob. Agents Chemother.* 3: 665–69
7. Seydel, J. K. 1968. *J. Pharm. Sci.* 57:1455–78
8. Johnson, O. H., Green, D. E., Pauli, R. 1944. *J. Biol. Chem.* 153:37–47
9. Wyss, O., Rubin, M., Strandskov, F. B. 1943. *Proc. Soc. Exp. Biol. Med.* 52: 155–58
10. Wacker, A., Kolm, H., Ebert, M. 1958. *Z. Naturforsch.* 13B:147–49
11. Gale, E. F., Cundliffe, E., Reynolds, P. E., Richmond, M. H., Waring, M. J. 1972. *The Molecular Basis of Antibiotic Action.* London: Wiley
12. Thijssen, H. H. W. 1974. *J. Pharm. Pharmacol.* 26:228–34
13. Miller, G. H., Doukas, P. H., Seydel, J. K. 1972. *J. Med. Chem.* 15:700–706
14. Bar, D. 1963. *Actual. Pharmacol.* 15:1–44
15. Maren, T. H. 1967. *Physiol. Rev.* 47:595–781
16. Coleman, J. D. 1975. *Ann. Rev. Pharmacol.* 15:221–42
17. Lindskog, S. et al 1971. *The Enzymes,* ed. P. D. Boyer, 5:587–665. New York: Academic
18. Taylor, P. W., King, R. W., Burgen, A. S. V. 1970. *Biochem. J.* 9:2638–45
19. Taylor, P. W., King, R. W., Burgen, A. S. V. 1970. *Biochem. J.* 9:3894–3902
20. Kernohan, J. D. 1966. *Biochim. Biophys. Acta* 118:405–12
21. Lindskog, S., Thorslund, A. 1969. *Eur. J. Biochem.* 3:453–60
22. King, R. W., Maren, T. H. 1974. *Mol. Pharmacol.* 10:344–48
23. King, R. W., Burgen, A. S. V. 1976. *Proc. R. Soc. London.* In press
23a. Maren, T. H., Wiley, C. E. 1968. *J. Med. Chem.* 11:228–32
24. Lung, J., Pedersen, H. E., Olsen, P. Z., Hvidberg, E. F. 1971. *Clin. Pharmacol. Ther.* 12:902–12
25. Kakeza, N., Yata, N., Kamada, A., Aoki, M. 1969. *Chem. Pharm. Bull.* 17:2558–64
25a. Maren, T. H., Rayburn, C. S., Liddell, N. E. 1976. *Science,* Vol. 191
26. Loubatieres, A. 1969. *Oral Hypoglycaemic Agents,* ed. G. D. Campbell, 1–22. New York: Academic
27. Bänder, A. See Ref. 26, pp. 23–37
28. Aumüller, W., Heerdt, R. 1971. *Oral Wirksame Antidiabetika. Handbook of Experimental Pharmacology,* ed. H. Maske, 29:1–249. Heidelberg: Springer
29. Schwarz, H., Ammon, J., Yeboah, J. E., Hildebrandt, H. E., Pfeiffer, E. F. 1969. *Diabetologica* 4:10–15
30. Beyer, J., Haupt, E., Cordes, V., Sell, G., Schöffling, K. 1973. *Arzeim. Forsch.* 23:1668–73
31. Beyer, K. H., Baer, J. E. 1961. *Pharmacol. Rev.* 13:517–62
32. Sprague, J. M. 1968. *Topics in Medicinal Chemistry,* ed. J. L. Rabinowitz, R. M. Myerson, 2:1–63. New York: Wiley
33. Peters, G., Roch-Ramel, F. 1969. *Handbook of Experimental Pharmacology, Diuretics,* ed. H. Herken, 24:257–405. Heidelberg: Springer
34. Yu, Y.-W., Shao, C.-Y., Sung, C.-Y. 1964. *Sci. Sin.* 13:775–88
35. Kobinger, W., Katic, U., Lund, F. J. 1961. *Arch. Pharmakol. Exp. Pathol.* 240:469–82
36. Pulver, R., Stenger, E. G., Exer, B. 1962. *Arch. Pharmakol. Exp. Pathol.* 244:195–210
37. Maren, T. H., Wiley, C. E. 1964. *J. Pharmacol. Exp. Ther.* 143:230–42
37a. Ross, C. R., Cafruny, E. J. 1963. *J. Pharmacol. Exp. Ther.* 140:125–32
38. Crawford, J. D., Frost, L., Welsh, M., Terry, M. L. 1962. *J. Pharmacol. Exp. Ther.* 135:382–93
39. Suki, W. N., Eknoyan, G., Martinez-Maldonado, M. 1973. *Ann. Rev. Pharmacol.* 13:91–106
40. Sturm, K., Siedel, W., Weyer, R., Ruschig, H. 1966. *Chem. Ber.* 99:328–44
41. Timmerman, R. J., Springman, F. R., Thomas, R. K. 1964. *Curr. Ther. Res. Clin. Exp.* 6:88–94
42. Small, A., Cafruny, E. J. 1967. *J. Pharmacol. Exp. Ther.* 156:616–21
43. Feit, P. W. 1971. *J. Med. Chem.* 14:432–39
44. Davies, D. L. et al 1974. *Clin. Pharmacol. Ther.* 15:141–55
45. Feit, P. W., Nielsen, O. B. T., Bruun, H. 1972. *J. Med. Chem.* 15:437–44

46. Nielsen, O. B. T., Bruun, H., Bretting, C., Feit, P. W. 1975. *J. Med. Chem.* 18:41–50
47. Mackenzie, J. B., Mackenzie, C. G., McCollum, E. V. 1941. *Science* 94:518–19
48. Astwood, E. B. 1945. *Harvey Lect.* 40:195–235
49. Astwood, E. B. 1970. *The Pharmacological Basis of Therapeutics,* ed. L. S. Goodman, A. Gilman, 1466–1500. New York: Macmillan. 4th ed.
50. Anderson, G. W. 1951. *Medicinal Chemistry,* ed. C. M. Suter, 1–150. New York: Wiley
51. Astwood, E. B., Bissell, A., Hughes, A. M. 1945. *Endocrinology* 37:456–81
52. Taurog, A., Chaikoff, I. L., Franklin, A. L. 1945. *J. Biol. Chem.* 161:537–43
53. Stanley, M. M., Astwood, E. B. 1947. *Endocrinology* 41:66–84
54. Krieger, D. T., Moses, A., Ziffer, H., Gabrilove, J. L., Soffer, L. J. 1959. *Am. J. Physiol.* 196:291–94
55. Greer, M. A., Kendall, J. W., Smith, M. 1964. *The Thyroid Gland,* ed. R. Pitt-Rivers, W. R. Trotler, 1:357–89. London: Butterworth

BEHAVIORAL PHARMACOLOGY AND TOXICOLOGY[1]

❖6653

G. Bignami

Laboratori di Chimica Terapeutica, Istituto Superiore di Sanità, 00161 Roma, Italy

If a survey of behavioral pharmacology and toxicology in the seventies must be a review, rather than an extensive treatise, it must be limited to a fraction of the relevant topics. The reader who is skeptical of conventional caveats and apologies can peruse the six volumes that make up just one third of the new *Handbook of Psychopharmacology* (1) or count the references in papers on drugs, CNS functions, and behavior that have appeared in this and related serials since the general reviews by Weiss & Laties (2), Himwich & Alpers (3), and Kumar, Stolerman & Steinberg (4). In fact, the original plan of this paper included a fairly broad range of topics, and also a review of reviews on various aspects of psychopharmacology and behavioral toxicology. However, the sheer size of the materials collected,[2] hundreds of references to reviews and books in various areas of neuropsychopharmacology, only for the period from 1970–1975, required the elimination of the general reference section. Furthermore, the psychopharmacology section had to be limited to drug-behavior interactions obtained in recent years with barbiturates, benzodiazepines, and 5-hydroxytryptamine (5-HT) system agents that have an antipunishment action. Finally, the behavioral toxicology section has been devoted mainly to two lines of work that have considerable interest from both a methodological and a theoretical viewpoint: to some aspects of the stimulus functions of drugs and to some of the effects of drugs and other chemicals on behavioral development.

[1]Generic names of drugs were used whenever possible. US adopted names have been used where several generic names are extant. When no generic names were available, well-known (abridged) chemical names were adopted. When used more than once these were replaced by common abbreviations indicated in the text.

[2]The literature survey pertaining to this review was concluded at the end of May 1975. The survey was greatly facilitated by the material received from several colleagues in different countries, who were asked to send reprints, preprints, and information on work being prepared for publication.

This introduction must be extended by a brief discussion of the philosophies underlying various approaches in neuropsychopharmacology, which are not obvious to the nonspecialist. On the one hand, it is not difficult to understand the rationale of increasingly sophisticated screening programs, which attempt to assess the properties of new agents, or that of studies concerned with correlations between behavioral and physiological-biochemical events. On the other hand, it is sometimes difficult to accept the hard fact that most of the interactions between treatments and several organismic and test variables are not presently amenable to explanations in physiological-biochemical terms. As a consequence, considerable efforts are required to establish provisional models of drug action in behavioral terms.

The analysis that follows considers in some detail two approaches leading to data of considerable interest. The first can be broadly categorized as a functional analysis of behavior changes induced by treatments. In fact, this approach uses a wide variety of response outputs generated mainly by schedules of intermittent reinforcement in order to identify the variables that can influence either size or direction of drug-induced changes. The second makes use of provisional models of behavior organization in terms that are neither strictly functional nor strictly physiological, but intermediate between the two; in other words, it makes recourse to so-called assumed processes or mechanisms in the analysis of input-output relationships (and of drug effects thereon). Of course, both the above distinction and that between physiological-biochemical and behavioral models are far from rigid. Nevertheless, there still remains a substantial difference between a functional analysis saying, "These effects of amphetamine are amenable (or not amenable) to a rate dependence model" (see below) and an analysis saying, "These same effects of amphetamine are suggestive of an attentional (or a motor, or a motivational, or an associative) bias." On the other hand, both behavioral approaches make use of a wide variety of effects in different, or even opposite, directions. When these are obtained with the same drug and different experimental contingencies (or by measuring different outputs given a particular contingency) the inevitable result is a complex (interactionist) model of drug action. This is not easily reconciled with a brain-behavior (correlational) approach, because even simple drug-behavior interactions have not yet been accounted for in physiological-biochemical terms (e.g. the opposite effects of amphetamine on locomotor and on some "exploratory" activities).

BARBITURATES, BENZODIAZEPINES, AND 5-HT SYSTEM AGENTS

Any discussion of psychotropic drug effects should start with a summary of studies concerning "unlearned" behaviors—spontaneous activities of various kinds, feeding and drinking responses, sexual and social responses—and then go on with data on stimulus reactivity, habituation, and operant behaviors maintained by sensory reinforcement (e.g. illumination changes) and by intracranial reinforcement (self-stimulation). This approach, however, would make it impossible to deal in any detail with studies that can best illustrate the complexity of drug-behavior interactions. Therefore, the following sections deal with drug effects on responses controlled by schedules of positive reinforcement, on differential response (discriminations), on behavior suppressed by punishment, on response maintained by negative reinforcement (escape-avoidance), and on changes in response caused by nonreinforcement (extinction, frustrative nonreward). Finally, an attempt is made to analyze some of the evidence on drugs that share one of the important properties of barbiturates and benzodiazepines (the antipunishment action), namely, 5-HT depletors and antagonists.

Operant Schedules with Positive Reinforcement

A well-known review published by Kelleher & Morse in 1968 (5) pointed out the uselessness of labels such as *stimulant* and *depressant drugs*. In fact, the results obtained with operant schedules[3] showed a series of remarkable analogies between amphetamine, on the one side, and barbiturates and benzodiazepines (or even neuroleptics), on the other, consisting mainly of similar rate-dependent changes in various situations. A well-known example can be drawn from fixed-interval (FI) schedules, in which several agents can increase the low rates observed in the early portions of the intervals (i.e. when a considerable delay separates the experimental subject from the next available reward), and reduce the high rates observed later in the same intervals. Of course, Kelleher & Morse (5) also pointed out that rate dependence cannot be put on a par with the laws of physics and chemistry, as exemplified by critical differences between barbiturates and benzodiazepines—enhancing low rates in the presence of a punishment contingency—and amphetamine, having either slight or no antipunishment effects.

In recent years the study of barbiturate and benzodiazepine effects on behaviors controlled by schedules of positive reinforcement has been extended in several directions. In the first place, previous reports of a relative insensitivity to drug of high and regular rates generated by small- and medium-sized fixed ratios (FRs) have been ascribed to the insufficiency of the measurements made before computers became available (7). In fact, a fine-grain analysis of pentobarbital effects in pigeons showed a consistent reduction of postreinforcement pauses and an increased cohesion of response patterns, two changes in good agreement with each other, with enhancements of low rates reported previously, and with the antisatiety effects of several barbiturates. The use of FRs of increasing size indicated a greater persistence of response in spite of less and less favorable reinforcement contingencies after administration of phenobarbital or chlordiazepoxide to pigeons (8). Furthermore, rats performing in extended FR sessions were employed to assess interactions between drug treatments and behavior changes induced by satiation. Interestingly enough, out of several agents that were able to increase response controlled by other schedules, phenobarbital, meprobamate, and chlordiazepoxide showed an antisatiety action, while diazepam did not, and oxazepam worked in the opposite direction (9, 10). On the other hand, unexplained differences between the effects of various

---

[3]No attempt can be made here to describe the schedules mentioned. While the standard reference must remain the textbook by Ferster & Skinner (6), much essential information can be found in condensed form in the review by Kelleher & Morse (5).

benzodiazepines on variable-interval (VI) response in rats appeared also in a study comparing several compounds. Only oxazepam gave a conventional profile—rate increases at low doses and rate decreases at higher doses—while only rate decreases reached statistical significance after chlordiazepoxide and diazepam, and no changes were observed over a wide dosage range with temazepam (11). One could speculate here that the use of schedules generating borderline rates (lower than those that are easily increased and higher than those that can be only decreased) could be exploited to analyze further subtle differences within a given drug category. In fact, another study showed few, if any, enhancing effects on FI response after chlordiazepoxide, inconsistent enhancements after diazepam, and marked enhancements after phenobarbital (12). As concerns benzodiazepines, these data obtained with pigeons, in contrast with those obtained in similar schedules either in the same or in different species (5, 13), indicate that the analysis of treatment and test factors interacting to produce widely differing changes in response is far from complete.

The rate dependence of pentobarbital effects in pigeons was further confirmed by the use of conjunctive FR-FI schedules. However, given the same baseline rate, drug-induced enhancements of FR response were less marked than those of FI response when the two components were scheduled on separate keys (14). Furthermore, reductions of high FR rates in pigeons, also after pentobarbital, were found to be about the same in multiple and in mixed FR-FI schedules, while high (terminal) FI rates appeared more resistant to reduction in mixed, than in multiple schedules (15). These interactions led to a discussion of treatment effects as a function of stimulus control of behavior, especially because a well-known study had shown an attenuation of the typical effects of pentobarbital on FI response in pigeons when the behavior was under the control of a succession of exteroceptive stimuli (so-called FI with superimposed clock) (16). In a recent study, also using pigeons, indentical VI periods were associated to different key colors, leading to substantial differences in response rates in spite of identical contingencies in various portions of the schedule. These differences were markedly reduced by diazepam, due mainly to rate enhancements during the presentation of the less preferred colors (green, yellow, and red) after 0.62 and 2.5 mg/kg, and to a rate reduction during the presentation of the favorite color (blue) after a higher dose (5 mg/kg) (16a). In another investigation, again with pigeons, even-numbered minutes in a long FI went with a stimulus identical with that presented when food was delivered (S^D), while odd-numbered minutes went with one or the other of several stimulus conditions never associated with food delivery (S^Δ). Enhancements of low rates were obtained with amobarbital in the presence of both types of stimuli, but they were less marked in some of the S^Δ conditions apparently exerting a strong inhibitory control (17).

Complex manipulations of the relationships between stimuli, responses, and reinforcements were also performed in a study on pigeons, in which one component of a multiple VI-VI schedule was substituted either by VI with a prereinforcement signal (which led to marked response reduction in the VI + signal component, and to a marked response enhancement in the regular VI component), or by administration of gratis food at irregular intervals, variable time (VT), which led to a marked rate reduction in VT itself, and to a moderate reduction in the regular VI component. This study allowed a striking separation between the effects of amphetamine, which lost its ability to enhance low rates, and those of phenobarbital, which maintained such ability both in VI + signal and in VT (18).

Equally interesting results were obtained by measuring not only schedule-controlled responses, but also schedule-induced (adjunctive) responses, that is, behaviors such as drinking an excess amount of water that can develop upon exposure to schedules of intermittent reinforcement. For example, a study showed that adjunctive licking could remain basically unaffected after doses of pentobarbital and amphetamine, which increased response in second-order schedules (19). An experiment showed that the development of adjunctive drinking can take place at a normal, or even at a higher rate during the chronic administration of chlordiazepoxide (19a). Another study measured both schedule-controlled and adjunctive components of the same output—licking on a FI schedule by rats—and showed a remarkable insensitivity of the latter to chlordiazepoxide at doses that induced substantial increases of the former (20). The same study also revealed differences between chlordiazepoxide and amphetamine, since both schedule-controlled and adjunctive responses were insensitive to the latter agent until depressant effects appeared at higher doses. Somewhat different results were obtained in a study with squirrel monkeys, which used the same FI contingency and showed chlordiazepoxide enhancements of both schedule-controlled lever pressing and schedule-induced water or ethanol consumption (21).

Additional differences in drug profiles were obtained by extending operant studies to mouse responses in a multiple FR-FI schedule. A preliminary report of this work suggests that amphetamine has conventional effects (enhancement of low FI rates and reduction of high FR rates), while both FI and FR response enhancements are indicated for pentobarbital (22). Regarding schedules with differential reinforcement of low rates (DRL), previous studies showing enhanced response frequencies and reduced reinforcement frequencies after barbiturates and benzodiazepines were replicated with similar results in the same and in other spaced-responding schedules (23–25). However, response-enhancing effects of chlordiazepoxide (and also, of amphetamine) were negligible or absent in a study with pigeons, while higher doses of both agents were able to reduce response rates (26). Another remarkable exception to drug enhancement of responses emitted at low rates was obtained by superimposing a classical alimentary stimulus (i.e. a signal paired with gratis food) during VI sessions, leading to a suppression similar to that induced by classically conditioned aversive stimuli. No attenuation of such suppression was obtained with chlordiazepoxide and with diazepam in rats and monkeys, while additional tests limited to chlordiazepoxide and to rats showed a drug disinhibition of responses suppressed by a fear signal (see below). Symmetrically opposite results were obtained with amphetamine, which enhanced low rates during the presentation of classical alimentary CS, but not during the presentation of classical aversive CS (27).

In summary, recent work with operant schedules has shown (a) several important differences both within and between drug groups, (b) several differences in rate-dependence functions obtained with given drugs, due to differences in test variables including those that affect stimulus control of behavior, and (c) some remarkable exceptions to the rate-dependence phenomenon, to be discussed again in a later section.

Experiments on Discriminations

Several experiments with either discrete-trial or operant discriminations were carried out in an attempt to answer particular questions, that is, should the disruption of differential response by barbiturates and benzodiazepines be ascribed to (a) a general psychomotor depression (overall response reduction, leading to a relative increase of incorrect responses), or to (b) attentional, associative, or motivational changes (parallel decreases of correct responses and increases of incorrect responses), to be further separated from each other by appropriate control experiments, or (c) an impairment of response control (selective reappearance of previously suppressed responses)? Although most data on aversively motivated behaviors are not examined until later, the following discussion must consider several results obtained with alimentary and defensive discrimination tasks. A fairly large portion of the available data on discriminations (28–33)—to be considered in conjunction with (a) the enhancements of low rates in operant schedules (see above) and (b) the enhancements of avoidance and extinction rates (see later sections)—apparently supports a response disinhibition model of benzodiazepine and barbiturate effects. A closer analysis of the data, however, shows a wide variety of interactions between treatment factors and species, stimulus, response, and other experimental factors. In some instances the results were only superficially in contrast with a disinhibition hypothesis since, for example, one can easily understand why an impairment of response control should lead to more marked changes in a successive, than in a simultaneous discrimination (28).

In other instances treatment factors seem to dominate the picture, as in a series of experiments on delayed matching in which both the presence or absence of an influence of the delay factor, and the balance between "go" (omission) and "no go" (commission) errors, depended on the agent used. Disinhibitory phenomena seemed to be absent in the case of several barbiturates, while mixed profiles of remarkable complexity were obtained with various benzodiazepines (34, 35). Furthermore, several studies using vigilance (signal detection) tasks with either positive or negative reinforcement gave variable ratios of "go" and "no go" errors after secobarbital in monkeys, as shown by the data reported in (36, 37) and in several previous papers quoted therein. Because omission errors accounted for most, if not all, of the disruption observed with chlorpromazine, it can be shown that the variability of the barbiturate profile should be considered as a genuine drug-task interaction, rather than as a consequence of differences between tasks per se.

The present discussion cannot be extended to include all available experiments, for example those concerning repeated acquisition of response chains (38, 39, 39a), those on discrimination behaviors requiring a joint use of exteroceptive and response-produced cues (40, 40a), those on discrimination of the pressure exerted on an operandum (41), and those on alternation behaviors (42, 43, 43a). However, the above and several other results indicate that drug-induced changes of differential response are not amenable to simple models such as disinhibition or rate dependence. This is also shown by studies finding improved differential response after amobarbital (44) and after chlordiazepoxide (45), due to a selective reduction of lever presses during nonreinforced signals. Finally, it must be emphasized that the above inconsistencies cannot be explained by using higher or lower cost of incorrect response as a criterion of classification. In fact, a closer analysis of the above and of several previous studies would reveal that presence or absence of given changes, for example response disinhibition, cannot be related systematically to the consequences, at the reinforcement level, of inappropriate response.

An analysis of discriminative functions of barbiturates and benzodiazepines (state-dependent learning) is outside the scope of this discussion, especially since the reader can be referred to several recent papers and reviews in (46, 47). It can only be mentioned here that dissociation phenomena caused by transitions from the drug to the no-drug state, or vice versa, have been repeatedly exploited in experiments on habit reversal. Interestingly enough, state changes facilitated the acquisition of behavior incompatible with that established previously not only in several experiments using presession treatments (48–54), but also in a study using one-trial discrimination learning and treatments administered immediately after the first exposure (55). Another line of work to which considerable efforts were devoted in the sixties [see (56, 57) and the papers quoted therein] regards the tranquilizer prevention of "fixations," that is, those stereotypes that are caused by exposure to insoluble problems and that interfere with discrimination learning when the problem is made soluble. Benzodiazepine effects in situations causing "neurosis" have also been investigated by tests in which monkeys become inactive (58), or in which rats make an increasing use of an escape ("time out") platform (59), when discrimination is made more and more difficult. Treatment with diazepam (58) or with chlordiazepoxide (59) was found to facilitate discrimination by reducing the above phenomena. Both fixation induced by exposure to insoluble problems in the Lashley jumping stand (56, 57) and neurosis triggered by increasingly difficult discriminations between signals corresponding to reward and punishment (58, 59) are generally ascribed to the high aversiveness of the situation. Therefore, the above effects appear to be directly related to the antipunishment properties discussed in the following section. Drug studies exploiting lack of adaptation to experimental contingencies are not limited to paradigms that mimic those originally used in the famous experiments by the Pavlovian school. For example, dogs of a "genetically nervous" strain with low performances in a simple bar-press task with food reinforcement showed operant rates similar to those of a "stable" strain after treatment with chlordiazepoxide (60). The authors of this study, however, have emphasized "the superficial nature of the improved behavior," based on the fact that most of the animals stopped bar pressing and assumed rigid ("frozen") postures within two days after medication withdrawal (60a).

In summary, from the considerable amount of work on discrimination some firm conclusions can be drawn concerning facilitation of habit reversal by state changes, and facilitation of discrimination behavior disrupted by events that can be classified as aversive. On the other hand, little progress has been made in the understanding of mechanisms responsible for drug effects on several types of discrimination—an uncomfortable conclusion indeed, if one considers that these compounds are used not only as sedative-hypnotics, but also at times when people must engage in their regular activities.

Behavior Suppressed by Punishment

When considering the most popular types of barbiturate and benzodiazepine effects —those on behaviors modified by punishment (present section) and those on behaviors maintained by negative reinforcement (next section)—one quickly discovers that the simplified "antiemotional" explanations that prevailed until about the midsixties have been seriously questioned over the past few years. However, at least one category of effects has withstood experimental testing in a wide variety of different situations, namely, the drug attenuation of the suppression of ongoing behaviors by response-contingent punishment (5, 61, 62). It is well known that this antipunishment effect, which is best shown by approach-avoidance (Geller type) schedules, cannot be ascribed to an antinociceptive action of barbiturates and benzodiazepines. This is shown by the negative results obtained with potent analgesic agents (5), and also by recent results indicating that the size of the analgesic action of chlordiazepoxide in spatial preference and titration tests is much less than that of its antipunishment action (63, 64).

Barbiturate and benzodiazepine effects on behavior suppressed by response-contingent punishment have been confirmed by a great number of studies published over the past few years, most of which cannot even be listed with the literature cited. Some of these studies must be mentioned because they made accurate comparisons of rate-dependent effects on punished and unpunished behavior (13, 65–67), or analyzed interactions between treatment and other factors such as punishment intensity (68), or took into account nonmonotonic (Kamin type) response changes in the first 24 hr after punishment of an approach response (69). Other studies provided indications on central sites of action by showing that oxazepam given systemically could alleviate the intensified suppression caused by localized cholinergic treatment of the hypothalamus (70) and of the dorsal raphe (71). Several experiments obtained changes in the expected direction by a variety of methods, such as a simplified test measuring punishment effects on licking responses (66a, 72), discrete-trial approach-avoidance tasks with either shocks (73) or air blasts (74) as the punishing events, and maze tasks in which performance tends to deteriorate with heating of the floor (75).

Antipunishment effects usually measured in rats, pigeons, and monkeys have also been observed in goldfish treated with phenobarbital (76) and in pigs treated with diazepam or with phenobarbital (77, 77a), while the effects of chlordiazepoxide were surprisingly small in the latter species (78). A study pointed out that antipunishment effects obtained with amobarbital, normally disappearing upon abrupt discontinuation of treatment, can be carried over to the no-drug state if the drug is withdrawn gradually (79). By the use of repeated treatments it could be shown that no tolerance to oxazepam develops with respect to antipunishment properties, while depression of unpunished behavior can be rapidly attenuated (80). A similar result was obtained by using flurazepam at doses sufficient to depress unpunished response, and exerting little effect on punished low rates. Repeated treatments led to an attenuation of the response suppression, and to an appearance of a marked antipunishment action (81). Analogies and differences between drugs were repeatedly investigated. For example, a study using rats showed chlordiazepoxide enhancements of both unpunished and punished responses over a fairly wide dosage range, while a strong tendency toward reduction of unpunished VI rates by pentobarbital was paralleled by a slight antipunishment action (82). On the other hand, no substantial differences between the antipunishment effects of the two drugs were observed in a study using pigeons, in which the treatments also exerted similar effects on unpunished behavior (66).

As illustrated in the above-mentioned review by Kelleher & Morse (5), behavior suppression by stimuli paired with noncontingent shock is not alleviated by barbiturates and benzodiazepines as consistently as suppression by contingent shock. Furthermore, the same reviewers hypothesized that the former type of suppression might be substantially insensitive to drugs, while disinhibition, when observed, could perhaps be ascribed to adventitious punishment phenomena. In fact, positive results had been obtained by the use of short intervals between the conditioned stimulus (CS) and the unconditioned stimulus (UCS), that is, in situations in which noncontingent shock can be easily "perceived" as if it were response-contingent. This type of explanation has been rejected by Millenson & Leslie in a paper that provides several of the more recent references (83). These investigators have attempted to show that the apparently inconsistent results obtained in tests with noncontingent shock were due either to the treatment schedules (acute treatments more effective than chronic treatments) or to the procedures used for the measurement of classically conditioned emotional responses (CERs) (operant and instrumental outputs more sensitive to drug than consummatory outputs). Assuming for a moment that these criteria of classification have general validity, several problems would still remain without solution. In fact, it would be difficult to understand why the use of chronic treatment schedules, or of consummatory behaviors, should allow the drugs to exert disinhibiting effects in the case of response-contingent shock (see several of the papers quoted above), while leading to inconsistent, or even to opposite (paradoxical) effects (84) in the case of CER situations, not to speak of the inconsistencies between studies comparing drug effects on CER acquisition and performance (85, 86).

Some recent experiments have shown a benzodiazepine attenuation of suppression in CER tests using both short (27) and long (87) CS-UCS intervals. The latter study used overtrained animals with well-developed "inhibition of delay"—or "temporal discrimination"—i.e. with normal or near normal response rates at the beginning of the CS presentation period and an increasing suppression in successive portions of the 5-min CS-UCS interval. A breakdown of the data revealed a rate dependence of oxazepam effects, because high rates in the initial portions of the intervals were reduced while low rates in later portions were increased. An effort was also made to compare more directly the effects of drugs as a function of presence or absence of a response-shock contingency, which was achieved by using pigeons performing in a FI schedule (88). Some of the animals received response-contingent shocks, while others were "yoked" to the former ones so as to receive noncontingent shocks. Both pentobarbital and chlordiazepoxide produced the expected attenuation of suppression with the punishment procedure, while only pentobarbital was effective in yoked animals. A similar experiment used rats performing in a VI schedule, and showed much larger disinhibiting effects of chlordiazepoxide in the animals punished with response-contingent shock, than in those receiving noncontingent shock (88a); (this study must also be recommended for a concise analysis of the mechanisms that may be responsible for different consequences of contingent vs noncontingent shock). Finally, one can mention here a study that made use of an insufficiently exploited sensitization phenomenon, namely, the enhancement by prior exposure to strong noncontingent shock of the suppressant effects of mild contingent shock. By treating animals during the initial shock exposure it was shown that the dose of pentobarbital required to prevent sensitization was quite high, at least when compared to those that are sufficient to disinhibit punished response (89).

The above picture is further complicated by passive avoidance and classical conditioning studies other than those measuring the suppression of ongoing alimentary responses. As concerns the former, disinhibiting effects were obtained with several benzodiazepines and barbiturates (90–92). One of the studies, however, showed by appropriate controls that the chlordiazepoxide impairment of passive avoidance should be largely ascribed to state-dependence phenomena (92). Two studies measured activity in a Y maze and passive avoidance of the arm in which rats had previously been shocked (note, however, that this initial shock exposure had not been made contingent upon entry into the arm itself). Passive avoidance was attenuated both by amobarbital (93) and by chlordiazepoxide (94), but its extinction was either unaffected or retarded. Passive avoidance of "naturally" fearful situations was attenuated by benzodiazepines and barbiturates in the case of an elevated (open-side) arm test in a Y maze, but not in the case of a brightly illuminated arm test (95, 96). A marked disruption of rat passive avoidance was also found with posttrial pentobarbital treatment. The appropriate controls, however, showed that this effect was due to a retrograde state-dependent learning similar to what has been mentioned when speaking of facilitation of habit reversal by changes of state (55, 97, 98). Finally, an experiment exploited the disturbances of rat passive avoidance that are caused by changes in the illumination cycle. The effects of chlordiazepoxide administered in the drinking water were mainly in the direction of an accelerated recovery of passive avoidance abilities after phase shifts (99).

As concerns responses to classically conditioned fear stimuli the sole purpose of comparing drug effects on a wide variety of different outputs can be that of showing the slight heuristic value of terms such as "antiemotional (antifear) action." Overt responses of rats to buzzers previously paired with shock were markedly reduced by chlordiazepoxide and by phenobarbital (100). Several motor and autonomic responses elicited in cats by clicks paired with aversive midbrain stimulation were attenuated by chlordiazepoxide and by nitrazepam (101). A study showed a chlordiazepoxide reduction of classically conditioned (nictitating membrane) responses in rabbits (102). On the other hand, the same group showed that treatment prior to tone-shock pairings did not prevent the CS from acquiring avoidance-enhancing properties (103). A similar result was obtained in rats with exposure to CS-UCS pairings in the no-drug state, followed by treatment sessions in the amobarbital state in which the effects of the classical CS on avoidance response were measured in an extinction paradigm (104). Such maintenance of the response-enhancing properties of classical CS both in a drug-no-drug (103) and in a no-drug-drug (104) paradigm excludes both an antifear effect of the drugs used, and a state-dependence explanation of the failure to obtain significant deviations from the controls. Interestingly enough, the latter experiment was paralleled by another study in which a stimulus previously paired to amobarbital treatment was able to exert a depressant effect on active avoidance response (105).

In summary, several data show that barbiturate and benzodiazepine effects in situations with either contingent or noncontingent exposure to aversive events cannot be explained on the basis of one-factor models of drug action. Many of these data open the door to a more systematic analysis of interactions between treatment factors (different drugs, acute versus chronic schedules), organismic factors (species and strains), and test factors such as operant (instrumental) versus consummatory ongoing behaviors, CS modality and intensity, UCS duration and intensity, temporal relationships between CS and UCS, and of course presence versus absence of a response-shock contingency. Several factors that can favor, or prevent, the transfer of drug-induced changes from the treatment to the no-treatment state should also be investigated by acquisition and performance experiments and by different schedules of treatment withdrawal, given the interest of these phenomena in human psychopharmacology.

Behavior Maintained by Negative Reinforcement

The experiments on behaviors maintained by negative reinforcement have provided much evidence that is again incompatible with unqualified antifear models of barbiturate and benzodiazepine action. Most of the earlier studies, which cannot be reviewed here, had shown that active avoidance depression by these agents, even when not entirely ascribable to sedation or to motor incapacitation, was far from being as selective as the one obtained with phenothiazines and butyrophenones. Some of these earlier studies using operant escape-avoidance techniques had already pointed out a complex profile of rate increases and decreases after drug treatments, mostly in agreement with a rate-dependence model (106). A more recent study used monkeys performing in a multiple VI escape schedule with response termination of noise paired to irregularly pulsed shock in one component, and response termination of continuous shock of low intensity in the other component. In agreement with previous results denying a specific antiavoidance action of benzodiazepines, chlordiazepoxide was found to be more effective in reducing response rates in the latter, than in the former component of the schedule (107).

On the other hand, many experiments carried out over the past decade have shown that several barbiturates and benzodiazepines, when given at doses lower than those endowed with an antiavoidance action, can facilitate the acquisition and/or the performance of two-way (shuttle box) and lever-press avoidance responses (81, 108–121). Furthermore, some experiments carried out in parallel with one of the two-way studies mentioned above showed no effects of chlordiazepoxide on the acquisition of one-way avoidance and a depressant action of the same drug on the acquisition of pole-climbing avoidance (119, 122). The attempts to explain the avoidance facilitation obtained in particular situations have generally made recourse to models emphasizing drug effects on suppression phenomena that interfere with active response. (These are ascribed to the general aversiveness of the tasks, to the confounding of safe and unsafe parts of the apparatus in bidirectional tests, and to adventitious punishment of outputs that are just about to fulfill a response criterion when a scheduled shock is turned on.) In other words, facilitation is explained by a greater drug influence on response suppression, than on response activation, in agreement with the fact that antipunishment effects have repeatedly been shown to be more specific than antiavoidance effects.

Given the variable balance between activation and suppression phenomena in apparently similar avoidance tasks, leading to different acquisition rates and performance asymptotes, one could disregard several failures to show a facilitation, which have been reported in references 103, 123, and 124. Surprisingly enough, however, some experiments showed an absence of two-way avoidance facilitation with a drug effective in other experiments mentioned above (amobarbital), and in conditions allowing the appearance of response enhancements after treatment with a nonbarbiturate sedative (methylpentinol) (125, 126).

Several data should be analyzed in detail in order to account for at least part of the variability in avoidance changes, such as the interactions between treatment and strain factors in a mouse study using both active and passive avoidance (91); the drug modification of repertoires elicited by shock (127); the drug depression of pseudoconditioned response with unpaired presentations of noise and shocks (128); and the interactions between treatment and stimulus factors, allowing a drug facilitation in the presence, but not in the absence, of stimulus events providing a response feedback (109). Furthermore, state-dependence phenomena have been shown to vary from one situation to the other (109, 111, 112, 117, 119, 122, 129–131). When present, they consisted sometimes of symmetrical decrements with changes of state in either direction, and sometimes of an asymmetrical dissociation with decrements after drug-no-drug transitions, but not after no-drug-drug transitions. Complex interactions between treatments (drugs and doses), test factors (responses, use of special procedures such as forced extinction by flooding), and state-dependence phenomena should also be analyzed to understand a wide variety of drug effects on extinction of avoidance, for which the reader must be referred to the original studies (104, 119, 122, 132–136).

Finally, several experiments conducted in recent years have dealt with drug effects on heart rate, respiratory rate, blood pressure, temperature, and urine excretion in animals performing escape-avoidance tasks or exposed to classical contingencies (137–141). In agreement with the data showing a drug-induced reduction of plasma corticosterone changes upon exposure to nonspecific stress (142) or to escapable shock (143), these studies have pointed out an attenuation of the above responses by barbiturates and benzodiazepines. By consulting the original papers, however, the reader will quickly discover that the authors disagree with respect to relative effectiveness of drugs on specified motor outputs, such as avoidance and classically conditioned responses, and on other outputs.

In summary, the results concerning behaviors maintained by negative reinforcement support the conclusions outlined in the previous section. Many data suggest that avoidance facilitation can result from the attenuation of punishment suppression. Other data confirm that the relations between antipunishment and other drug effects are still poorly understood, while the evidence on interactions between treatment factors, response and other test factors, and state-dependence phenomena provides the basis for testing multifactorial models of drug action.

Changes in Positively Reinforcing Events: Extinction, Frustrative Nonreward, and Incentive Shifts

Experimental manipulations of positively reinforcing events have been shown to cause a wide variety of response changes, as shown by the extensive literature on extinction, frustrative nonreward, and incentive shifts. In particular, several theorists support the view that nonobtention of anticipated ("expected") rewards leads in the first place to emotional changes (frustration reaction), and in the second place to conditioning phenomena by which nonreward-related stimuli acquire control over instrumental or operant responses (144, 145). In order to simplify the discussion of drug-induced changes one can add here that several phenomena have been ascribed to the above processes, namely, (a) the higher running speeds observed during acquisition (particularly in the second part of it) with partial reinforcement (PRF) than with consistent reinforcement (CRF) (the partial reinforcement acquisition effect, PRAE); (b) the greater resistance to extinction after PRF than after CRF (the partial reinforcement extinction effect, PREE); (c) the greater running speed in the second alley of an apparatus with two goal boxes when an anticipated reward is missed in the first box (the double alley frustration effect, DAFE); and (d) the tendency to escape from a situation in which an anticipated reward is missed (escape from frustration, EFR). Given the above theoretical framework, and the resulting "fear = frustration hypothesis," it is not surprising that runway tests, or their operant equivalents, have often been used to confirm the antiemotional effects of benzodiazepines and barbiturates and also, after such effects are considered proved, to achieve a separation between emotional and nonemotional phenomena in PRF and other experiments with manipulation of reinforcing events.

Since two well-known studies published in the early sixties, showing respectively an antiextinction (146) and an anti-PRAE (147) effect of amobarbital in rats, several experiments with barbiturates and benzodiazepines, also using rats, have yielded results supporting the above assumptions. This applies to the drug retardation of extinction (148–154), to the attenuation or disappearance of the PRAE (155, 156), and to the attenuation of EFR (155). Furthermore, the drugs were found to prevent the response attenuation caused by a reduction of reward magnitude (157–159), while the response depression caused by reinforcement withdrawal in a discrete-trial lever-press task was antagonized by chlordiazepoxide, but not by phenobarbital and pentobarbital (160). A control study showed no drug influence on response enhancements caused by an increase of reward magnitude, thereby excluding the possibility that the above results might be ascribed to an impaired perception of changes in reinforcement size (161). A more complex experiment exploited response enhancements and reductions caused by signals paired to incentive shifts in opposite directions, and showed differential drug effects essentially similar to those outlined above (162).

From a certain point on, however, the results of both nonpharmacological and pharmacological experiments created a situation of an amazing complexity. Frustration models were substantially modified by theorists who emphasized the variable balance between emotional (aversive) and nonemotional (perceptual-cognitive) consequences of PRF, based mainly on experiments with different sequences of reward and nonreward (163). Alternative explanations of PRF consequences were also provided, based mainly on the finding that nonobtention of anticipated reinforcements can lead to opposite changes in consummatory outputs (depressed) and instrumental outputs (enhanced) (164).

On the pharmacologist's side, some experiments with barbiturates found either a minimal effect on extinction (44) or a decreased resistance to extinction (165), with complex interactions depending on schedules of treatment and of drug withdrawal (abrupt versus gradual) (166). A control experiment showed that this paradoxical acceleration of extinction was to a large extent independent of state changes (165). Another study using chlordiazepoxide showed the expected increase of response in extinction, but the drug was unable to affect the changes in response force (167). Furthermore, benzodiazepine effects on extinguished behavior have been far from consistent (65, 66a, 67). Repeated attempts to interfere with the DAFE by amobarbital treatment resulted in clear-cut failures (155, 168–171), while one success was scored by using rats made dependent on barbital (172). A drug attenuation of the PREE was demonstrated in animals trained without drug and extinguished with drug, but not in animals trained and extinguished in the drug state, while variable results were obtained with animals trained with drug and extinguished without drug (150, 151, 154, 155, 169). Therefore, few conclusions could be drawn concerning the relative role of drug effects on PRF consequences and of state-dependence phenomena. Finally, the complexity of the results obtained prevents a detailed analysis of a remarkable series of amobarbital studies concerning PRF and CRF with different spacing of trials (173), the PREE following a limited acquisition experience (174), different magnitudes of consistent reinforcement (175), and treatment schedules based on sequential hypotheses (differential effects of drug given either before nonrewarded trials followed by rewarded trials, or before rewarded trials followed by nonrewarded trials) (176). At this point the reader must be referred to a recent review that attempts to reconcile several of the above inconsistencies with the notion of an antiemotional mechanism of action of barbiturates and benzodiazepines (176a).

Speculations on the Nature of Drug-Behavior Interactions

A discussion of some of the factors that may influence the size, or even the direction, of barbiturate and benzodiazepine effects can exploit selected data obtained with agents that are known both for their rate-dependent effects and for their different profiles with respect to feeding and drinking responses. In fact, these consummatory behaviors are uniformly depressed by amphetamine, while they remain unaffected, or are enhanced, after barbiturate and benzodiazepine treatments (except, of course, at doses that cause heavy sedation and motor impairment). Given these differences, one can consider enhancements of low response rates as a function of response consequences at the reinforcement level. A hypothesis that response cost per se discriminates between drug profiles is quickly disproven by several data showing amphetamine, barbiturate, and benzodiazepine enhancements both in the absence, and in the presence of a reduction of reinforcement frequency (e.g. FI versus DRL schedules) (5). On the other hand, a striking attenuation of amphetamine changes has been observed sometimes when measuring "operants" drawn from the consummatory repertoire, such as FI-licking by rats (20), or when measuring responses with mixed consummatory and preparatory (instrumental) properties controlled by schedules with adverse consequences of hyperresponse, such as DRL key-pecking by pigeons (26). Furthermore, enhancements of low rates by chlordiazepoxide have been found when measuring FI-licking (20), that is, when the operant was drawn from the consummatory repertoire and the schedule was without adverse consequences of hyperresponding. In contrast, the usual effect of the same drug on DRL was at least markedly attenuated when key-pecking responses of pigeons were studied (26). Finally, the contrasting profiles of amphetamine and of barbiturates and benzodiazepines on punishment suppression were reversed in experiments on suppression by stimuli paired with gratis food, which are known to elicit classically conditioned consummatory responses at the expense of ongoing instrumental behavior (177). In such a situation, amphetamine-treated animals resumed operant response, while benzodiazepine-treated animals did not (27).

A more detailed analysis should consider several other data showing exceptions to the absence of antipunishment effects in amphetamine-treated animals, exceptions to the antipunishment properties of barbiturates and benzodiazepines, and also, exceptions to the exceptions (e.g. instances in which amphetamine enhanced responses drawn from the consummatory repertoire). Nevertheless the above data, when considered with the complex effects of barbiturates and benzodiazepines on extinction and frustrative nonreward, suggest that several types of interactions have not been sufficiently explored. Some of the critical factors, taken one by one, have indeed received much attention; for example, the differences between drugs belonging to the same class in particular situations; the different "reversal points" in nonmonotonic dose-response functions, depending on the test used; and quantitative differences in rate-dependence functions, depending on the schedule. Others seem to offer much space to future investigations, as suggested by the above interactions between (*a*) treatments that enhance, or depress, consummatory outputs; (*b*) responses drawn from different components of a species-specific repertoire (mainly preparatory, or mainly consummatory, or with mixed properties as in the case of bird pecks); and (c) schedules generating low rates either with, or without, adverse consequences of hyperresponse at the reinforcement level. Drug effects as a function of stimulus control of behavior are also amenable to a similar analysis.[4] In fact, nonpharmacological studies designed to maximize the separation between "consummatory" and "instrumental" properties of stimuli have shown that the two types of signals can elicit entirely different types of response changes in the dog (177). (Of course, this divergence is facilitated by the fact that instrumental and consummatory activities are more easily separated from each other in the dog than in other laboratory animals.) Finally, the finding (also in dogs) of opposite effects of partial reinforcement on consummatory activities (depressed) and on instrumental activities (enhanced) shows that alternative models of nonreward consequences (164) and of drug effects thereon must be explored by parallel measurements of several types of responses.

If the above or other similar phenomena can be shown to account for at least part of the observed variance, then the relations between behavioral and physiological-biochemical models of drug action can cease to be antagonistic. In fact, the problem would not be any more than of knowing all that happens in the CNS when a particular drug, given various contingencies, leads to different types of response changes; in Oppenheimer's terms, this is a useless attempt to explain "everything." A more rational solution might be to employ consistent physiological-biochemical data accounting for a series of basic events (e.g. drug-induced changes at the level of different sensory, response, and reinforcement systems) as building blocks in behavioral models—a combination of reductionist and nonreductionist philosophies for the purpose of explaining "anything."

Some Behavioral Data Pertaining to the 5-HT Hypothesis of Tranquilizer Effects

It may appear surprising that some of the effects of 5-HT system drugs are analyzed in an appendix to the above discussion on barbiturates and benzodiazepines, at the expense of other more conventional topics such as the analogies and differences between antianxiety agents and neuroleptics. The fact is that two types of effects of benzodiazepines at the biochemical level have been emphasized in relation to their antipunishment effects, namely, (a) the inhibition of cyclic adenosine monophosphate phosphodiesterase (cAMPD) (178, 179), and (b) the interference with 5-HT

---

[4]Several provisional inferences with potential heuristic value might be drawn by reexamining the interactions between treatment and stimulus factors as a joint function of drug type, response type, and relations between stimuli, responses, and reinforcements (e.g. cues signaling gratis food vs cues signaling the availability of response-produced food in an intermittently reinforced schedule vs cues signaling nonreinforcement, etc; see, for example, 16–18, 27, 65, 67). No use has been made in psychopharmacology of some techniques and tentative models in the literature on autoshaping, which emphasize the variable balance between consequences of stimulus-reinforcement relations and consequences of response-reinforcement relations, as a joint function of cue, reinforcement, and response categories.

turnover (71). As concerns the former, the reader must be referred to a study of correlations between antipunishment and anti-cAMPD effects of various agents (178) and to the data showing an enhanced suppression and an antagonism of chlordiazepoxide effects in a CER test by a cAMPD stimulator (imidazol-4-acetic acid) (179). Regarding the latter, it has been reported that effects of benzodiazepines on punished behavior and on 5-HT turnover are maintained with repeated treatments, while tolerance develops to depressant effects and to drug-induced changes of noradrenaline turnover (71). Furthermore, several experiments have shown an attenuated suppression in conflict and in CER situations after treatment with a 5-HT–depleting agent (parachlorophenylalanine, PCPA) or with 5-HT antagonists (cyproheptadine, cinanserin, methysergide, 2-bromlysergic acid diethylamide) (71, 180–189), while the administration of 5-hydroxytryptophan (5-HTP) counteracted the antipunishment action of PCPA and of cinanserin (180, 181, 184, 189).[5]

Two types of arguments have been used against the hypothesis that central 5-HT systems have a major role in punishment suppression, and more or less directly, against the hypothesis that antianxiety agents act mainly by interfering with 5-HT turnover. First, one study failed to show an antipunishment effect of cinanserin in a situation in which chlordiazepoxide was quite active, while both agents antagonized the reduction of response rate caused by N,N-dimethyltryptamine (193). In this regard, several effects of 5-HT system agents on operant and instrumental responses maintained by positive reinforcement are far from being amenable to any simple explanation. In fact, a response depression has been obtained with a variety of drugs that cause different or even opposite biochemical effects, such as 5-HTP, several substituted tryptamines, PCPA, and 5-HT antagonists (194–199), while subthreshold doses of 5-HTP acquired depressant properties after pretreatment with PCPA (200). The same group responsible for the latter study showed a similar phenomenon with subthreshold doses of LSD-25 in animals with 5-HT depletion induced either by PCPA or by midbrain raphe lesions (201, 202).

A second line of criticism has denied both (a) that the available data show a parallelism between 5-HT depletion and alleviation of punishment suppression by PCPA, and (b) that the measurements and statistical procedures used in previous studies could demonstrate a reliable antipunishment action of the drug (203). Additional experiments with the same agent yielded apparently negative results (203).

While the above controversy cannot be solved in the present context, it can be underlined that several effects of 5-HT–depleting drugs or lesions are quite different from those observed after benzodiazepines. It is true that some of these changes, such as the facilitation of avoidance response in several shuttle box and lever-press studies (204–210), are amenable to an explanation based on a reduction of punish-

---

[5]In one of these studies (188) an attenuation of punishment suppression was also observed with lysergic acid diethylamide (LSD-25), while other studies using either concurrent positive reinforcement and punishment (190), or previous or concurrent punishment of an active avoidance response (191, 192) seem to deny the generality of the antipunishment action of this drug. In any event, most of the complex effects of LSD-25 must be left outside of the present discussion.

ment suppression (see the section on behavior maintained by negative reinforcement.[6] However, several components of the 5-HT depletion syndrome (e.g. hyperreactivity) (215–218) create a wide area of nonoverlap with the tranquilizer syndrome.

The above situation suggests that simpler models of drug action, which were originally endowed with considerable heuristic value, should now be replaced by multifactorial working hypotheses. These need not reject the provisional assumption that some apparently similar effects of tranquilizers and of 5-HT system agents can be induced by similar mechanisms, while other explanations should be sought for several effects taking place in different directions. Attention can be focused here on some methodological problems, even though they belong to areas not included in the present review. In the first place, there is an obvious disproportion between studies of complex behaviors using intracerebral treatments or lesioned animals that have been carried out respectively with noradrenergic, dopaminergic, and cholinergic stimulants and blockers and with tranquilizers and 5-HT depletors and antagonists (219–223). In the case of the former agents, several qualitative and quantitative differences in the behavioral effects, depending on treatment or lesion site, have indicated that the complex syndromes obtained by systemic treatments can be separated into increasingly well-defined components. Another methodological problem is pointed out by the considerable time lags that usually separate the obtention of "expected" effects of one or the other drug and that of "paradoxical" effects of the same agent. This situation applies to several data discussed in previous sections, inasmuch as the enhancements of low rates of schedule-controlled behavior, of punished behavior, and of avoidance behavior have generally been obtained at a later time, and with lower doses, than depressant effects. As concerns other areas, the joint study of floor and ceiling phenomena and of nonmonotonic dose-response relationships has been recently extended to aggressive responses and to "predatory" behaviors such as mouse and frog killing by rats. Several important differences have been pointed out between the enhanced intraspecies aggression obtained with relatively low doses of tranquilizers, on the one side, and the indirect facilitation of aggression (mainly via interactions with other agents) and the enhanced interspecific killing obtained with 5-HT depletors, on the other side (224, 225). The fact remains that the use of situations that eliminate floor and ceiling effects and of nonmonotonic dose-response functions can still have a considerable potential in an analysis of the mechanisms of action of agents with partially overlapping profiles.

[6]As with most avoidance-enhancing drugs, negative data (presumably due to ceiling effects), or even opposite (depressant) effects were obtained when using pretrained animals with high response base lines (211, 212). Furthermore, the fact that the enhancing effects of raphe lesions on two-way avoidance are paralleled by a depression of one-way avoidance (205) is in line with the above interpretation—at least according to much literature on CNS lesions such as that reviewed by McCleary (213). On the other hand, the available evidence does not allow direct comparisons between the effects of 5-HT system drugs (204, 214) and those of barbiturates and benzodiazepines in passive-avoidance tests other than those that measure the suppression of operant or consummatory behaviors.

BEHAVIORAL TOXICOLOGY

Although behavioral toxicology has only recently gained status as a semiautonomous discipline (226–232), several lines of research in this area have been firmly established for fairly long periods of time. In fact, with more space available one could refer (a) to much work carried out in animal and human subjects in order to assess the adverse behavioral effects of alcohol, tobacco smoke, and several drugs of abuse; (b) to a great deal of data on behavioral effects of nutritional or hormonal deficits and imbalances; (c) to several investigations attempting to establish animal models of human diseases marked by disturbances of mental development (e.g. phenylketonuria); and (d) to an increasing number of studies dealing with behavioral changes induced by ionizing and nonionizing radiation, hypoxia, carbon monoxide, several compounds used in the manufacturing industry, pesticides, air and water pollutants, food additives, and so forth. The present section, however, must leave out most of the studies using behavioral measurements largely as convenient dependent variables, which can be easily located via computerized indexing and abstracting services, and can be handled without trouble also by investigators who do not specialize in behavioral research. Considered here are mainly those data that have remarkable methodological interest, and at the same time require an understanding of behavior organization beyond the general information level of the nonspecialist.

Some Consequences of Stimulus Functions of Drugs and Chemicals

In recent years an increasing number of behavioral investigations on stimulus functions of various agents have been carried out by pharmacologists and psychologists, sometimes without any direct reference to the toxicological implications of the results obtained. Stimulus functions of physical and chemical agents are usually subdivided into discriminative (CS), unconditioned (UCS), and reinforcing functions (46). The term *CS function* implies that changes in the "internal state" caused by a treatment can become a signal controlling one or the other behavioral output, by taking up a role in response modulation similar to that of conventional stimuli of one or the other modality. While the reader must be referred to the available reviews for more systematic information (46, 47), a limited discussion is in order here to show both the difficulties encountered when interpreting the results in this area, and the relevance of state-dependence phenomena for drug abuse and for the understanding of dissociative side effects of drugs.

The studies so far carried out have indicated that any agent can acquire CS functions in experiments in which different response outputs must be emitted to meet reinforcement requirements, if the only available cue is a treatment administered before a particular session, for example, food obtained or shock avoided by turning to the left, or by pressing the left lever, after the administration of a given drug, and by going to the right, or by pressing the right lever, after administration of saline. However, when turning to comparisons between different drugs, or between different doses of the same drug, considerable attention must be given to the particular paradigm in which an apparent similarity, or an apparent difference, has been observed. For example, several experiments by the same group of investigators showed that (a) rats trained in two-lever tasks with alcohol versus placebo gave the "alcohol" response when tested with pentobarbital; (b) rats trained in similar tasks to discriminate pentobarbital from placebo gave either the "placebo," or the "pentobarbital" response when tested with alcohol, depending on the reinforcer; and (c) rats could be taught to use one of the levers when treated with pentobarbital, and to use the other lever when treated with alcohol (233). The overall conclusion is obviously that the stimulus properties of the two agents have some element in common (the a and part of the b results). At the same time, however, one can be confident that the two states are discriminable from each other (the c result). Finally, the presence or absence of generalization from one to the other set of internal stimuli generated by the two agents must depend on which component of a given set has gained control of behavior during the original discrimination training —the a and the b results; for additional examples of these asymmetrical transfer phenomena see also (234). It goes without saying that any attempt to draw a conclusion from any one of the three types of data summarized above would have led to a considerably distorted picture of the analogies and differences between the pentobarbital and the alcohol states.

This and much other evidence shows that the results of experiments on state dependence are best understood by making reference to the basic facts of conventional experiments on discrimination and stimulus generalization, up to and including those concerned with psychophysical measurements. In fact, the variable data in a and b are similar to those that can be obtained when subjects are taught to discriminate between stimuli A and B (corresponding to different response-reinforcement contingencies), and then tested to see whether a third stimulus (X) will elicit an A- or a B-type response, or a mixture of the two. Assume now that this experiment has shown that X elicits an A-type response in one or more paradigms. It cannot be concluded from this that A and X are not discriminable from each other; such a conclusion can be had only by training with different response-reinforcement contingencies in the presence of A and X. Furthermore, if a first attempt fails, it cannot be inferred that A and X have a substantial identity (psychophysically speaking). In fact, the literature abounds with data showing that stimuli known to be discriminable from each other cannot be used, or are used only with considerable difficulty, as differential signals in particular discrimination tasks. Therefore, only a gradual accumulation of negative findings in different tests in which two states are pitched against each other can eventually demonstrate that the states themselves are indistinguishable.

Other data on state dependence have been obtained by imposing shifts from a treatment to a no-treatment state and vice versa (or from one treatment to another and vice versa) in conventional tasks that can be learned without relying on drug-induced stimuli. These data show that transfer, or no transfer (dissociation), of behavior acquired in a given state to a different one depends on complex interactions between treatment and test factors. For example, T-maze avoidance studies showed several years ago that transitions from the phenobarbital to the no-drug state, or vice versa, had an adverse effect on response initiation (start time), but not on response execution (running time), nor on response choice (proportion of correct turns) (235). Other experiments with the same drug pointed out a successful transfer in either direction of an immobility (freezing) response, but not of an active escape response (236). Finally, it was shown that in particular conditions a state change can facilitate discrimination reversal as discussed previously (evidence for state dependence), even in the absence of a retention deficit with respect to the original discrimination (evidence against state dependence) (48).

In theory, several types of phenomena could account for the contrasting consequences of state changes as a function of test factors, but unfortunately, no single set of interactions obtained with a particular agent has so far been fully explained. Some possibilities have little to do with stimulus functions per se; that is, it is conceivable that general behavioral changes due either to treatment initiation, or to withdrawal of an agent to which the organism has been accustomed, can have widely differing consequences on the transfer of various types of responses from one state to another. On the other hand, by taking recourse to conventional discrimination data one could show that response control can come more under one, or more under the other type of stimulus, depending on the characteristics of the task. In other words, when the experimenter provides a set of relevant (conventional) stimuli, and also superimposes another set of stimuli (those derived from the drug-induced changes of the *milieu intérieur*), he cannot foresee whether or not elements from the two sets will be used as compound signals, and if they are, which particular aspects of the behavior will show dissociative phenomena. Conversely, state dependence in tasks learned on the basis of relevant treatment cues (chlordiazepoxide versus placebo) has been shown to vary as a function of the exteroceptive stimuli superimposed on the internal cues (237, 238).

No great efforts are required to explain the toxicological implications of the various types of findings. The greater or lesser discriminability of a drug state, as well as the greater or lesser analogies between two or more drug states (including different doses of the same drug), have obvious relevance in the analysis of abuse phenomena, and should be given increasing attention when assessing the effects and side effects of psychotropic drug treatments (or treatment changes). Furthermore, with some remarkable exceptions (concerning, e.g. alcohol), little is known about the factors that determine whether or not behaviors acquired in particular states are transferred to other states in human subjects. Finally, no attention has been so far given to possible dissociative effects of a variety of chemicals to which individuals can be exposed for variable periods of time, for example at work, but not elsewhere; or at home, but not elsewhere.

UCS and reinforcing functions of various agents have no smaller interest than CS functions, although some of them are so well known (and well reviewed) that they need not be discussed in detail. This applies to positively reinforcing properties of various agents, which have been extensively investigated by preference and self-administration tests in several species, in the framework of research on abuse phenomena (239–244). Furthermore, several studies on conditioning of drug treatment and of drug withdrawal effects have been carried out in an attempt to separate "physical" and "psychic" aspects of drug dependence (46, 241, 243, 244a). While a few of these experiments, not pertaining directly to the abuse problem, will have to be mentioned later, some attention must be given here to several recent results concerning either behavior suppression by treatments with aversive properties, or escape-avoidance behaviors established and maintained with treatments used as the UCS.

In addition to conventional tests carried out with preference-rejection paradigms, recent research has increasingly exploited the so-called Garcia paradigm, which allows the study of conditioned aversion phenomena ("bait shyness") (245, 246). In fact, when particular cues (mainly gustatory ones in nonvisual animals, such as rodents, and visual ones in species that select food mainly on the basis of visual cues, such as diurnal birds) are associated with an experience of "malaise" or "illness" caused by a physical or chemical agent, they can acquire suppressant properties similar to those of a conventional CS in a classical (CER) paradigm. Furthermore, conditioned suppression can develop in spite of CS-UCS delays much longer than those that allow classical fear conditioning with conventional exteroceptive signals (e.g. tones or lights) and conventional UCS (e.g. painful shock). Few problems arise with the fact that conditioned aversions are easily established (a) with ionizing radiations, and with substances such as cyclophosphamide and lithium, at doses sufficient to cause overt signs of physical illness (245), and (b) with subtoxic doses of agents that are well known for the "unpleasant" quality of the experience they produce, such as apomorphine (245) and antimuscarinics (247, 247a). Equally, one can easily understand why positively reinforcing and punishing properties of the alcohol (247a, 248–250) and of the morphine (247a, 248, 251) experiences should be related to each other in a complex fashion. Other recent results however, were quite unexpected. This applies, to conditioned aversions obtained with doses of lithium (252), chlorpromazine (247), and benzodiazepine derivatives (247, 247a, 248) either within or not much above the therapeutic range, and with doses of amphetamine within the self-administration range (247a, 253–258). On the other hand, the conditioned aversions recently obtained with several barbiturates and with the nonbarbiturate hypnotic methaqualone (247a, 258a) are in contrast with previous negative results concerning one of the compounds [phenobarbital (247)]. Furthermore, negative results have been obtained with the tricyclic antidepressant imipramine (247), while the data so far available on cannabis derivatives (247a, 259–262) appear to be insufficient to conclude for a specificity, or a nonspecificity —with respect to doses endowed with conventional psychotropic effects (263, 264) —of the aversions obtained.

Although with the present state of knowledge any classification must be provisional, and perhaps arbitrary, it can have at least heuristic value to separate aversive properties of therapeutic agents that are seldom, if ever, self-administered (such as chlorpromazine and lithium) from those of agents that are often self-administered and lead to abuse phenomena (ethanol, morphine, amphetamines, hypnotic-sedatives, and tranquilizers). The former appear to have considerable relevance in a rational risk-benefit analysis, if the goal of a therapy must be that of maximizing returns, while minimizing both conventional side effects and subjective disturbances. The latter have relevance both from the above viewpoint, for example, when considering the extensive therapeutical applications of tranquilizers, and from the view-point of abuse phenomena. Within this category are most of the results that are hotly debated, since similar phenomena are ascribed to widely differing mechanisms by various authorities. For example, a more detailed analysis of the literature on behavior suppression by amphetamine (253–258) could show that these phenomena are ascribed to the development of genuine conditioned aversions by some experi-menters, and to a conditioning of the anorexigenic effects of the drug by others. Furthermore, the data showing a suppressant action on ongoing operant behavior of stimuli previously associated with chlorpromazine or LSD-25 have also been interpreted as the consequence of a conditioning of drug-induced changes, rather than of punishment suppression (265, 266). Finally, some drug profiles can be quite complex with respect not only to induction of both self-administration and condi-tioned aversions at similar doses, but also to their influences on negatively reinforc-ing properties of other agents. For example, chlordiazepoxide was found to attenuate conditioned aversions induced either by amphetamine or by lithium (254, 267), which is obviously in agreement with the antipunishment properties measured in conventional tests.

The provisional conclusion must be that the relations between positively reinforc-ing, punishing, and other properties of any given agent can be clarified only by a further extension of the available tests. Traditional preference-rejection tests, self-administration tests, and conditioned aversion (Garcia-type) tests have recently been joined by choice procedures using conditioned reinforcers, that is, exterocep-tive stimuli previously paired to different drugs, or to different doses of the same drug (267a), and by escape-avoidance techniques allowing one to assess whether an animal tolerates, or escapes and avoids, scheduled infusions. The combined use of these and of self-administration techniques has already yielded a series of interesting results. For example, monkeys made dependent on morphine by treatments imposed by the experimenters escaped and avoided nalorphine and naloxone infusions, while monkeys made dependent in a self-administration paradigm went on self-adminis-tering nalorphine in substitution tests, even though this precipitated a severe absti-nence syndrome (268). When the studies were extended to animals without prior addiction, the results clearly separated several treatments that were accepted (nalox-one, cocaine, codeine, pentazocine, and propiramfumarate infusions) from others that were escaped and avoided (nalorphine and cyclazocine infusions) (269); for additional evidence on the mixed positively reinforcing and punishing properties of narcotic antagonists see (270, 271). Furthermore, a recent study showed a contrast between the acceptance of pentobarbital up to a fairly high dosage level (0.1 mg/kg per infusion) and escape-avoidance of both chlorpromazine (down to 0.005 mg/kg per infusion) and LSD-25 (down to 0.001 mg/kg per infusion) (272). Finally, an indirect confirmation of the results on chlorpromazine aversiveness obtained in Garcia-type and escape-avoidance tests was provided by self-administration studies, using monkeys that performed in an operant (FR) schedule with cocaine as the reinforcer. In fact, substitution tests yielded amphetamine and morphine rates higher than saline rates, imipramine rates comparable to saline rates, and chlor-promazine rates significantly lower than saline rates (273).

Selected (Mainly Developmental) Data on Psychotropic Drugs, Pesticides, Food Additives, Mercury, and Lead

This section deals with some of the effects of prenatal or early postnatal treatments with psychotropic drugs, and comments upon some results showing that exposure of immature organisms to various chemicals can lead to behavioral changes that are not usually obtained by treating adult animals. Several studies conducted in the sixties, which have been reviewed in (274–278), showed various types of deviations from normal behavior development after pre- or postnatal administration of psychotropic agents. More recently, several suggestions have been made concerning biochemical changes underlying altered behavior maturation, especially regarding the effects on catecholamine and indole amine metabolism of early exposure to amphetamines (279–281), chlorpromazine (280, 281), haloperidol (282, 283), LSD-25 (284), ethanol (285), and PCPA (286). Other studies have either attempted a better definition of treatment variables or investigated interactions of considerable interest between treatment and other factors. For example, the data on the effects of pre- and postnatal morphine in the rat were extended by results showing opposite effects of different dosage levels on avoidance acquisition at a later time—facilitation after smaller doses, and depression after higher doses (287). Several experiments using prenatal amphetamine treatments showed correlations between enhanced activity, enhanced active avoidance, and impaired passive avoidance (279, 288, 289), while postnatal treatments with an enhancing effect on neonatal locomotor activity did not modify adult two-way avoidance learning (289a). Previous work on adverse effects of prolonged postnatal treatments with phenothiazines on later avoidance in the rat were also extended in several directions. First, the use of shorter (6-day) trifluoperazine treatments showed that the avoidance deficits were the consequence of cumulative damage, rather than of a selective effect during particular critical periods (290). Second, depressed avoidance was observed in the first and second generation obtained from females that had received phenothiazines postnatally (291–294). One of these studies using a cross-fostering control showed that nursing of the young by dams that had previously received postnatal phenothiazine treatments was not necessary to obtain depression of avoidance (294). Finally, one experiment with 0.16–0.33 mg/kg of trifluoperazine administered daily for 25 days yielded nonmonotonic dose-response relationships with respect to avoidance performance of the offspring of females that had received postnatal treatment (293). These data are highly suggestive of multiple mechanisms of action at least in part in opposition to each other, because cross-generational effects on avoidance were larger after lower doses, than after higher doses. On the other hand, impairments of behavioral development including avoidance deficits have also been obtained in recent years by treating neonate rabbits with other types of neuroleptics [butyrophenones, pimozide; see (294a) and other papers by the same group quoted therein].

Another group of investigators used prenatal chlorpromazine treatments inducing a greater susceptibility to seizures at 30 days of age, and higher avoidance abilities at 90 days. In this instance the cross-fostering procedure showed that at least part of the changes occurred in animals not exposed in utero, but nursed by previously treated mothers (295). On the other hand, cross-fostering controls indicated that the effects on the offspring of Δ^9-tetrahydrocannabinol administered at a fairly high dose to pregnant rats (10 mg/kg daily for three days) (retarded growth, reduced rearing and grooming, retarded development of cliff avoidance and of visual placing reflexes) were due entirely to prenatally suffered damage (296). Similar procedures, however, do not seem to have been employed when dealing with more subtle changes induced by prenatal cannabis exposure, for example, the retardation of learning in a Lashley III maze (297). Finally, several studies using postnatal strychnine (298–301), methamphetamine (302) and PCPA (286), and prenatal imipramine (303) indicated that the effects of drugs on behavior development can depend on the characteristics of the environment in which the animals are raised.

In summary, the results so far obtained suggest that pre- or early postnatal treatments by psychotropic agents can influence behavior development in widely differing ways, ranging from direct effects on brain mechanisms at the time of exposure to altered mother-offspring interactions at a time when the drug is no longer present. This evidence places a considerable burden on future experimentation, because it shows that it is not enough to consider the interactions between the most obvious factors such as species, type of drug, doses, time and duration of exposure, behavioral tests, and so forth. As a consequence, there arises the need for a standardization of procedures allowing the assessment of indirect mechanisms of action (e.g. prenatal and postnatal maternal effects) in order to ensure that the data obtained in different laboratories are amenable to direct comparisons.

The literature on the behavioral effects of pesticides shows that organophosphate and carbamate compounds have been used very extensively both in toxicological investigations, and in studies of biochemistry-behavior correlations exploiting the well-known effects of the compounds on central cholinergic systems. For an overview of this subject see (304), and for more recent data and references on tolerance mechanisms see one of the latest papers by the most active group in this area (305). Comparatively speaking, behavioral data on organochlorine compounds are much less extensive than those on anticholinesterase agents. However, the concern created by the persistence in the environment of agents such as DDT has led to a number of studies of the behavioral effects of organochlorine insecticides in fish [see recent data and references in (306)] and to a multi-year research project using behavioral (mainly discrimination) and electrophysiological measurements in sheep (307). Furthermore, ready access to the literature on behavioral and electrophysiological changes induced by organochlorine compounds in several laboratory species is provided by a recent review (307a) and by several recent papers reporting changes in activity, avoidance, discrimination, operant and maze behavior, maternal and aggressive behavior, and electrical activity (308–315).

A survey of the studies concerned with early treatments by pesticides shows that few cues are presently available to understand the mechanisms by which these compounds affect behavioral development. In fact, a series of experiments carried out in mice by one investigator (although with different co-workers and in different laboratories) showed changes in maturation of seizure sensitivity after prenatal DDT, aldrin, chlordane, and parathion, while prenatal chlordane, but not DDT or parathion, led to later enhancements of open-field activity, and prenatal chlordane or DDT, but not parathion nor aldrin, retarded avoidance behavior (316–321). T-maze performance of mice has also been found to be altered by pre- and neonatal exposure to DDT (322). On the other hand, postnatal exposure to an anticholinesterase fungicide (maneb) had correlated effects on activity (depressed) and passive avoidance (facilitated). Response changes per se, however, were not sufficient to account for all the effects observed, since active avoidance was also facilitated (323).

Some recent findings—including alteration of reproductive functions in rats and mice after prenatal or neonatal exposure to DDT, or to some of its analogs, or to polychlorinated biphenyls (PCBs) (324, 324a); the altered development of ambulation and rearing in rats after prenatal administration of the herbicide 2,4,5-trichlorophenoxyacetic acid (2,4,5-T, with less than 1-ppm of 2,3,7,8-tetrachlorodibenzo-p-dioxin) (325, 325a)—confirm the suspicion that the weak estrogenic action of several organochlorine compounds might have a role in behavior modification by early treatments. In fact, all reproductive and nonreproductive behaviors so far mentioned are known to be influenced by hormonal treatments during critical periods.[7] On the other hand, biochemical studies on DDT and chlordane have shown complex changes in the metabolism of acetylcholine, noradrenaline, 5-HT, and amino acids in the brain (307a, 326–330), which provides a basis for a more thorough comparison of the mechanisms of action of organochlorine compounds with those of better-known agents.

Although this discussion cannot be extended to a wide range of substances that can enter the organism via foods and beverages, recent studies using nitrites (331), butylated hydroxyanisole and butylated hydroxytoluene (332), cyclamates (333, 334), and monosodium glutamate (MSG) (335–337) can be mentioned to point out the growing concern for developmental changes induced by various types of agents. These studies have sometimes provided interesting cues concerning possible mechanisms of action, as shown by some of the data on MSG. For example, the obesity-hyperactivity syndrome observed after neonatal exposure of mice (335) should be confronted with the irreversible inhibition of pituitary prolactin and growth hormone secretion induced by similar treatments in the same species (338), again leading to speculations about possible interferences with "organization" of CNS systems by hormonal influences during critical periods of development. Also in this instance the available data suggest a large difference in sensitivity between developing and mature organisms, as exemplified by the transient and apparently nonspecific depression by large doses of MSG of fixed ratio and of avoidance response in adult rats (339, 340).

In a discussion of mercury compounds, the behavioral and electrophysiological studies dealing with exposure in adulthood, or during relatively late postnatal periods, for example, those reported or discussed in (341–356) should again be

---

[7]Note, however, that the results have been often contradictory ones, even in the hands of the same investigators (325, 325a), and also that 2,4,5-T treatments were given during the first half of pregnancy (325, 325a), that is, too early for those "organizational" effects on reproductive functions and behavior that are usually described in the literature on hormones.

contrasted with those using pre- and early postnatal treatments (231, 357–362). The results obtained by the former approach have shown a variable sensitivity to mercury treatments of the tests used, as indicated by the comparisons carried out in the Rochester research project (354–356). Furthermore, some experiments have pointed out that the intake of diets contaminated by mercury can be reduced by aversion phenomena (342, 344). These, however, do not seem to afford an efficient protection, as indicated by the well-known data on humans and animals that pertain to the Minamata, to the Iraq, and to other accidents. On the other hand, the developmental studies mentioned above, which used both rodents and birds, revealed a uniformly high sensitivity of immature organisms. Furthermore, these results include an impressive series of different phenomena, ranging from deficits observed relatively early in life [e.g. the changes in the neonatal sequence of development in rats, involving eye opening and neuromotor coordination (360)] to the effects appearing only at a much later time, such as the general debilitation and the gross neurological changes observed in mice about the end of the first year of life (361, 361a).

Finally, similar research trends have made their appearance in the analysis of behavioral effects of lead. Most of these studies have used postnatal exposure of rat and mouse offspring via the milk of treated dams, sometimes combined with later treatment of weanlings by different dietary levels of lead compounds (363–369). Although no in-depth discussion of the results is possible here, several points deserve to be emphasized. First, the available data have convincingly shown a much higher sensitivity of immature, than of adult animals; for consequences of treatments given later in life see (368, 370–372). Second, a recent dose-response study has revealed a separation of gross neurological disorders caused by higher doses from more subtle behavioral changes following exposure to lower doses (mainly hyperactivity) (364). Third, the lead intake via contaminated food, which normally leads to aversion phenomena, was found to be increased by the reduction of dietary calcium (373), a finding with obvious implications with respect to lead pica in humans. Fourth, the offspring from female rats receiving lead acetate during lactation showed both an enhanced fluid consumption and a greater aversion for lead acetate solutions than did the control offspring (364a). Fifth, rats made hyperactive by early exposure to lead showed paradoxical changes after drug treatments, namely, a further enhancement of activity levels after phenobarbital, and a reduction of activity after d- or l-amphetamine and other stimulants (367, 367a, 369). Amphetamine, however, maintained its well-known ability to enhance low rates of avoidance responses (369). Finally, a series of studies was carried out in sheep by the Iowa behavioral toxicology program (374–377). Not only did these experiments confirm the greater liability to damage in the pre- and early postnatal stages, than in adulthood; but also, they pointed out that impairments of behavioral development can take place with lead blood levels below those considered acceptable by EPA for pregnant women (up to 30 μg/100 ml) and for children (up to 40 μg/100 ml).

Since a fairly optimistic attitude has been maintained throughout the present discussion, concerning the progress made by behavioral toxicology in recent years, a final caveat is in order here. In fact, most of the studies mentioned above have followed, rather than preceded, the demonstration of adverse effects in humans, while satisfactory criteria for extrapolation from animals to man in previsional experiments have not been established. Given the complexity of developmental studies, it is understandable that dose-response experiments should have been the exception, rather than the rule. Furthermore, if one considers the thresholds that have been measured (or if one even optimistically assumes that thresholds will be found to be immediately below the effective dosage levels in experiments with a single treatment schedule), one can expect considerable trouble at the moment of deciding on safety factors. In fact, nonbehavioral previsional toxicology uses safety factors for the extrapolation from animals to man that are generally about one hundred. One could easily show at this point that maximum allowable levels of exposure for most agents mentioned here would have to be brought down to a near zero level in the case of expectant or nursing mothers and of young children, if the conventional procedure were extended to the results of studies of behavioral development.

GENERAL DISCUSSION AND CONCLUSIONS

A more general evaluation of the state of the art of behavioral pharmacology in the midseventies can emphasize both the risks and the benefits of an increasing complexity of working hypotheses that are used when dealing with drug-behavior interactions, with both explanatory and heuristic purposes. In fact, the diminishing returns obtained by the use of simpler models inevitably leads to serious problems of communication not only among behavior specialists and neurophysiologists, biochemists and clinicians, but also among behavioral pharmacologists with different orientations. This review tries to compensate at least in part for the minimal cross-referencing between studies using a functional approach and studies centered on assumed processes and mechanisms. At the opposite end, several developments deserve to be classified as potential, if not yet actual, benefits. In fact, it is increasingly realized that in this, as in other areas of the biological sciences (378), reductionist ("molecular") and nonreductionist ("molar") approaches need not to be pitched against each other, since they can be shown to be complementary (see the section on the nature of drug-behavior interactions).

Thus the philosophies underlying the extrapolations from the animal laboratory to the clinic are being gradually revised, and the relative roles of the two types of research are defined more clearly.

Animal psychopharmacology and behavioral toxicology, although necessarily subdivided into several specialized areas, appear to be at their best when not hampered by arbitrary distinctions between effects and side effects of the agents studied, nor by chicken-and-egg questions about which level of explanation is most appropriate. In recent years they have attempted to provide sophisticated interaction models that take into account several phenomena of increasing complexity, including differential changes in various portions of species-specific repertoires, changes in stimulus reactivity, changes depending on various response-reinforcement relationships, rate-dependence phenomena, and stimulus functions of drugs. Even though the latter have been given only a minimum of attention in the section on behavioral toxicology, they can be used to show how the extremes of a continuum are, in reality, quite close to each other. In fact, the study of discriminative functions of drugs fulfills both the need to know more about critical stimulus factors in conditioning and learning (or, if preferred, in behavior control), and the need to understand dissociative side effects of psychotropic agents as well as the "substitution potentials" of various drugs of abuse. Correspondingly, the study of positively and negatively reinforcing functions fulfills both the need to clarify the physiological-biochemical substrates of reinforcement processes (or, in a functional analysis, equivalence and nonequivalence phenomena with different reinforcers), and that of understanding abuse phenomena as well as aversive side effects of therapeutic agents. As pointed out in the behavioral toxicology section, positively reinforcing and aversive properties are often found to coexist in animal experiments; therefore, one cannot expect to obtain simple answers when complex biological factors and even more complex social-cultural factors interact with each other in humans.

Several other examples could be drawn from the literature of behavioral pharmacology and toxicology to show the increasing need for strict relations between the basic and the mission-oriented aspects of any given problem. In the fifties the uneven development of appropriate interactions and feedbacks between research in reproductive and developmental biology and research on desired and undesired effects of drugs and chemicals led both to remarkable successes (e.g. the development of oral contraceptives) and to dramatic failures (e.g. thalidomide). In the seventies, it appears that the effort to understand the basic facts of behavioral development, as well as their physiological and biochemical substrates, goes in hand with remarkable efforts to assess the risks of the exposure to potentially noxious drugs and chemicals during critical maturation periods. The coming years will undoubtedly be marked by much uneasiness. In fact, the right questions have come to the surface, while appropriate answers to these questions are far from available. This is tantamount to affirming that both type I and type II errors can be made in large numbers at the operational level.

In any event, a few examples and general comments cannot suffice to clarify the complex relations between animal research and human applications in the realm of psychotropic drugs and other chemicals that affect behavior. Some may regret the pioneer age when terms such as *antiavoidance* and *antipsychotic*, or *anticonflict* and *antianxiety*, were almost synonyms; or when limited data on the general toxicity of a new agent were deemed to suffice for the completion of a risk-benefit analysis. A more realistic and responsible approach cannot be based solely on an increasingly broad range of previsional studies in animals. In fact, the value and the limits of extrapolations from animals to man can be thoroughly assessed only with the help of a much more extensive knowledge of basic analogies and differences between mechanisms than what is presently available. Animal psychopharmacologists and behavioral toxicologists have shown that, on the average, different species can vary with respect to behavioral changes induced by various agents more than they vary with respect to other types of changes—a logical consequence of the fact that behavioral specialization is both a "final common path" in adaptation to different environments, and an essential mechanism in the evolution and isolation of species.

However, the problems encountered when drawing comparisons between animal species are dwarfed by the inordinate proliferation of interacting factors in the human species, as shown by the apparently irreconcilable opinions on the reliability and meaning of one or the other type of data (379), and even more by the conflicts between judgments of value (380-383).

ACKNOWLEDGMENTS

This review is part of a program in experimental psychology and behavioral pharmacology sponsored jointly by Istituto Superiore di Sanità (ISS) and by Istituto di Psicologia, Consiglio Nazionale delle Ricerche (IP-CNR), Roma, Italy (1969 to date). The author wishes to acknowledge the help and advice received from Dr. G. L. Gatti (ISS) and from Dr. Marina Frontali (IP-CNR).

Literature Cited

1. Iversen, L. L., Iversen, S. D., Snyder, S. H., eds. 1975. *Handbook of Psychopharmacology. Sect. 1. Basic Neuropharmacology.* New York: Plenum. 6 vols. 2155 pp.
2. Weiss, B., Laties, V. G. 1969. *Ann. Rev. Pharmacol.* 9:297-326
3. Himwich, H. E., Alpers, H. S. 1970. *Ann. Rev. Pharmacol.* 10:313-34
4. Kumar, R., Stolerman, I. P., Steinberg, H. 1970. *Ann. Rev. Psychol.* 21:595-628
5. Kelleher, R. T., Morse, W. H. 1968. *Ergeb. Physiol. Biol. Chem. Exp. Pharmakol.* 60:1-56
6. Ferster, C. B., Skinner, B. F. 1957. *Schedules of Reinforcement.* New York: Appleton. 741 pp.
7. Weiss, B., Gott, C. T. 1972. *J. Pharmacol. Exp. Ther.* 180:189-202
8. Thompson, D. M. 1972. *J. Exp. Anal. Behav.* 17:287-92
9. Wedeking, P. W. 1973. *Physiol. Behav.* 10:707-10
10. Wedeking, P. W. 1974. *Pharmacol. Biochem. Behav.* 2:465-72
11. Longoni, A., Mandelli, V., Pessotti, I. 1971. *Pharmacol. Res. Commun.* 3:165-73
12. Bignami, G., Gatti, G. L. 1969. *Psychopharmacologia* 15:310-32
13. Wuttke, W., Kelleher, R. T. 1970. *J. Pharmacol. Exp. Ther.* 172:397-405
14. Barrett, J. E. 1974. *J. Exp. Anal. Behav.* 22:561-73
15. Leander, J. D., McMillan, D. E. 1974. *J. Pharmacol. Exp. Ther.* 188:726-39
16. Laties, V. G., Weiss, B. 1966. *J. Pharmacol. Exp. Ther.* 152:388-96
16a. Sahgal, A., Iversen, S. D. 1975. *Psychopharmacologia* 43:175-79

17. McKearney, J. W. 1970. *J. Exp. Anal. Behav.* 14:167-75
18. Thompson, D. M., Corr, P. B. 1974. *J. Exp. Anal. Behav.* 21:151-58
19. Wuttke, W., Innis, N. K. 1972. *Schedule Effects: Drugs, Drinking, and Aggression,* ed. R. M. Gilbert, J. D. Keehn, 129-47. Toronto: Univ. Toronto Press. 261 pp.
19a. Sanger, D. J., Blackman, D. E. 1975. *Q. J. Exp. Psychol.* 27:499-505
20. McKearney, J. W. 1973. *Psychopharmacologia* 30:375-84
21. Barrett, J. E., Weinberg, E. S. 1975. *Psychopharmacologia* 40:319-28
22. Wenger, G. R., Dews, P. B. 1975. *Fed. Proc.* 34:766 (Abstr.)
23. Sanger, D. J., Key, M., Blackman, D. E. 1974. *Psychopharmacologia* 38:159-71
23a. Sanger, D. J., Blackman, D. E. 1975. *J. Pharmacol. Exp. Ther.* 194:343-50
24. Stretch, R., Dalrymple, D. 1968. *Psychopharmacologia* 13:49-64
24a. Smith, J. B., Clark, F. C. 1975. *J. Exp. Anal. Behav.* 24:241-48
25. Thomas, J. R. 1973. *Pharmacol. Biochem. Behav.* 1:421-26
26. McMillan, D. E., Campbell, R. J. 1970. *J. Exp. Anal. Behav.* 14:177-84
27. Miczek, K. A. 1973. *Pharmacol. Biochem. Behav.* 1:401-11
28. Hasegawa, Y., Ibuka, N., Iwahara, S. 1973. *Psychopharmacologia* 30:89-94
28a. Frontali, M., Amorico, L., De Acetis, L., Bignami, G. 1976. *Behav. Biol.* In press
29. Ison, J. R., Rosen, A. J. 1967. *Psychopharmacologia* 10:417-25
30. Iwahara, S., Matsushita, K. 1971. *Psychopharmacologia* 19:347-58

31. Schallek, W., Kuehn, A., Kovacs, J. 1972. *Neuropharmacology* 11:69–79
32. Wedeking, P. W. 1969. *Psychon. Sci.* 15:232–33
33. Yamaguchi, K., Iwahara, S. 1974. *Psychopharmacologia* 39:71–79
34. Nicholson, A. N., Wright, C. M., Ferres, H. M. 1973. *Neuropharmacology* 12:311–17
35. Nicholson, A. N., Wright, C. M. 1974. *Neuropharmacology* 13:919–26
36. Pragay, E. B., Mirsky, A. F. 1973. *Psychopharmacologia* 28:73–85
37. Mirsky, A. F., Tecce, J. J., Harman, N., Oshima, H. 1975. *Psychopharmacologia* 41:35–41
38. Thompson, D. M. 1973. *J. Pharmacol. Exp. Ther.* 184:506–14
39. Thompson, D. M. 1974. *J. Pharmacol. Exp. Ther.* 188:701–13
39a. Thompson, D. M. 1975. *J. Exp. Anal. Behav.* 23:429–36
40. Branch, M. N. 1974. *J. Pharmacol. Exp. Ther.* 189:33–41
40a. Rosenberg, J., Woods, J. H. 1975. *Bull. Psychon. Soc.* 5:33–35
41. Falk, J. L. 1969. *Physiol. Behav.* 4:421–27
42. Douglas, R. J., Scott, D. W. 1972. *Psychon. Sci.* 26:164–65
43. Iwahara, S., Oishi, H., Yamazaki, S., Sakai, K. 1972. *Psychopharmacologia* 24:496–507
43a. Hughes, R. N., Greig, A. M. 1975. *Physiol. Psychol.* 3:155–56
44. Rosen, A. J. 1970. *Arch. Int. Pharmacodyn. Ther.* 188:112–18
45. Geller, I., Hartmann, R., Blum, K. 1971. *Psychopharmacologia* 20:355–65
46. Thompson, T., Pickens, R., eds. 1971. *Stimulus Properties of Drugs.* New York: Appleton. 221 pp.
47. Overton, D. A., Winter, J. C., eds. 1974. *Fed. Proc.* 33:1785–1835
48. Bindra, D., Reichert, H. 1967. *Psychopharmacologia* 10:330–44
49. Bliss, D. K. 1973. *J. Comp. Physiol. Psychol.* 84:149–61
50. Bliss, D. K., Sledjeski, M., Leiman, A. L. 1971. *Neuropsychologia* 9:51–59
51. Caul, W. F. 1967. *Psychopharmacologia* 11:414–21
52. Iwahara, S., Sugimura, T. 1970. *Jpn. J. Psychol.* 41:142–50
53. Meltzer, D., Merkler, N. L., Maxey, G. C. 1966. *Psychon. Sci.* 5:413–14
54. Porsolt, R. D., Joyce, D., Summerfield, A. 1971. *Act. Nerv. Super.* 13:75–77
55. Wright, D. C., Chute, D. L., McCollum, G. C. 1974. *Pharmacol. Biochem. Behav.* 2:603–6
56. Feldman, R. S. 1968. *Psychopharmacologia* 12:384–99
57. Feldman, R. S., Kaada, B. R., Langfeldt, T. 1973. *Pharmacol. Biochem. Behav.* 1:379–87
58. Jarosch, E., Nitsch, F. M. 1968. *Int. Pharmacopsychiatry* 1:168–83
59. Bremner, F. J., Cobb, H. W., Hahn, W. C. 1970. *Psychopharmacologia* 17:275–82
60. Angel, C., Murphree, O. D., DeLuca, D. C. 1974. *Dis. Nerv. Syst.* 35:220–23
60a. Murphree, O. D., Angel, C., DeLuca, D. C. 1974. *Biol. Psychiatry* 9:99–101
61. Garattini, S., Mussini, E., Randall, L. O., eds. 1973. *The Benzodiazepines.* New York: Raven. 685 pp.
62. Randall, L. O., Schallek, W., Sternbach, L. H., Ning, R. Y. 1974. *Psychopharmacological Agents,* ed. M. Gordon, 3:175–281. New York: Academic. 403 pp.
63. Houser, V. P., Paré, W. P. 1973. *Psychopharmacologia* 32:121–31
64. Houser, V. P. 1975. *Behav. Biol.* 12:383–92
65. Hanson, H. M., Witoslawski, J. J., Campbell, E. A. 1967. *J. Exp. Anal. Behav.* 10:565–69
66. McMillan, D. E. 1973. *J. Exp. Anal. Behav.* 19:133–45
66a. Miczek, K. A., Lau, P. 1975. *Psychopharmacologia* 42:263–69
67. Miczek, K. A. 1973. *Psychopharmacologia* 28:373–89
68. McMillan D. E. 1973. *Psychopharmacologia* 30:61–74
69. Hablitz, J. J., Braud, W. G. 1972. *Learn. Motiv.* 3:51–58
70. Margules, D. L., Stein, L. 1967. *Neuro-Psycho-Pharmacol. Proc. Int. Congr. Coll. Int. Neuro-Psycho-Pharmacol., 5th,* 108–120
71. Stein, L., Wise, C. D., Berger, B. D. 1973. See Ref. 61, 299–326
72. Vogel, J. R., Beer, B., Clody, D. E. 1971. *Psychopharmacologia* 21:1–7
73. Sepinwall, J., Grodsky, F. S., Sullivan, J. W., Cook, L. 1973. *Psychopharmacologia* 31:375–82
74. Yen, H. C. Y., Krop, S., Mendez, H. C., Katz, M. H. 1970. *Pharmacology* 3:32–40
75. Soubrié, P., Schoonhoed, L., Simon, P., Boissier, J. R. 1972. *Psychopharmacologia* 26:317–20
76. Geller, I., Croy, D. J., Ryback, R. S. 1974. *Pharmacol. Biochem. Behav.* 2:545–48
77. Dantzer, R., Roca, M. 1974. *Psychopharmacologia* 40:235–40

360   BIGNAMI

77a. Dantzer, R. 1975. *J. Pharmacol.* 6:323–40
78. Dantzer, R., Baldwin, B. A. 1974. *Psychopharmacologia* 37:169–77
79. Sherman, A. R. 1967. *Behav. Res. Ther.* 5:121–29
80. Margules, D. L., Stein, L. 1968. *Psychopharmacologia* 13:74–80
81. Cannizzaro, G., Nigito, S., Provenzano, P. M., Vitikova, T. 1972. *Psychopharmacologia* 26:173–84
82. Blum, K. 1970. *Psychopharmacologia* 17:391–98
83. Millenson, J. R., Leslie, J. 1974. *Neuropharmacology* 13:1–9
84. Stein, L., Berger, B. D. 1969. *Science* 166:253–56
85. Cicala, G. A., Hartley, D. L. 1967. *J. Comp. Physiol. Psychol.* 64:175–78
86. Scobie, S. R., Garske, G. 1970. *Psychopharmacologia* 16:272–80
87. Maser, J. D., Hammond, L. J. 1972. *Psychopharmacologia* 25:69–76
88. McMillan, D. E., Leander, J. D. 1975. *Arch. Int. Pharmacodyn. Ther.* 213:22–27
88a. Huppert, F. A., Iversen, S. D. 1975. *Psychopharmacologia* 44:67–75
89. Wiley, R. G., Dilts, S. L., Berry, C. A. *Arch. Int. Pharmacodyn. Ther.* 192:231–37
90. Aron, C., Simon, P., Larousse, C., Boissier, J. R. 1971. *Neuropharmacology* 10:459–69
91. Fuller, J. L. 1970. *Psychopharmacologia* 16:261–71
92. Oishi, H., Iwahara, S., Yang, K.-M., Yogi, A. 1972. *Psychopharmacologia* 23:373–85
93. Kumar, R. 1971. *Psychopharmacologia* 19:163–87
94. Kumar, R. 1971. *Psychopharmacologia* 19:297–312
95. Morrison, C. F., Stephenson, J. A. 1970. *Psychopharmacologia* 18:133–43
96. Morrison, C. F., Stephenson, J. A. 1972. *Psychopharmacologia* 24:456–61
97. Chute, D. L., Wright, D. C. 1973. *Science* 180:878–80
98. Wright, D. C., Chute, D. L. 1973. *Psychopharmacologia* 31:91–94
99. Davies, J. A., Navaratnam, V., Redfern, P. H. 1974. *Br. J. Pharmacol.* 51:447–51
100. Bainbridge, J. G., Greenwood, D. T. 1971. *Neuropharmacology* 10:453–58
101. Ross, N., Monti, J. M. 1971. *Psychopharmacologia* 22:31–44
102. Chisholm, D. C., Couch, J. V., Moore, J. W. 1971. *Psychon. Sci.* 23:203–4

103. Chisholm, D. C., Moore, J. W. 1970. *Psychopharmacologia* 18:162–71
104. Kamano, D. K. 1973. *Psychopharmacologia* 28:45–50
105. Kamano, D. K. 1973. *Physiol. Psychol.* 1:321–23
106. Cook, L., Catania, A. C. 1964. *Fed. Proc.* 23:818–35
107. Dinsmoor, J. A., Bonbright, J. C. Jr., Lilie, D. R. 1971. *Psychopharmacologia* 22:323–32
108. Bignami, G., De Acetis, L. Gatti, G. L. 1971. *J. Pharmacol. Exp. Ther.* 176:725–32
109. Bignami, G., De Acetis, L. 1973. *Pharmacol. Biochem. Behav.* 1:277–83
110. Cannizzaro, G., Nigito, S., Provenzano, P. M., Vitikova, T. 1972. *Arzneim. Forsch.* 22:772–76
111. Goldberg, M. E., Hefner, M. A., Robichaud, R. C., Dubinsky, B. 1973. *Psychopharmacologia* 30:173–84
112. Iwahara, S. 1971. *Jpn. Psychol. Res.* 13:207–18
113. Leathwood, P. D., Bush, M. S., Mauron, J. 1975. *Psychopharmacologia* 41:105–9
114. Martin, L. K., Powell, B. J. 1970. *Psychon. Sci.* 18:44–45
115. Pirch, J. H., Osterholm, K. C. 1974. *Res. Commun. Chem. Pathol. Pharmacol.* 8:203–11
116. Robichaud, R. C., Sledge, K. L., Hefner, M. A., Goldberg, M. E. 1973. *Psychopharmacologia* 32:157–60
117. Sachs, E., Weingarten, M., Klein, N. W. Jr. 1966. *Psychopharmacologia* 9:17–30
118. Sansone, M., Renzi, P., Amposta, B. 1972. *Psychopharmacologia* 27:313–18
119. Taber, R. I., Latranyi, M. B., Steiner, S. S. 1967. *Pharmacologist* 9:200 (Abstr.)
120. Davidson, A. B. 1970. *Proc. 78th Ann. Conv. Am. Psychol. Assoc.* 5:807–8
121. Takaori, S., Yada, N., Mori, G. 1969. *Jpn. J. Pharmacol.* 19:587–96
122. Steiner, S. S., Fitzgerald, H. L., Taber, R. I. 1967. *Pharmacologist* 9:200 (Abstr.)
123. Chisholm, D. C., Moore, J. W. 1970. *Psychon. Sci.* 19:21–22
124. Kamano, D. K., Arp, D. J. 1964. *Psychopharmacologia* 6:112–19
125. Gupta, B. D., Holland, H. C. 1969. *Psychopharmacologia* 14:95–105
126. Gupta, B. D., Holland, H. C. 1969. *Int. J. Neuropharmacol.* 8:227–34
127. Emley, G. S., Hutchinson, R. R. 1971. *Proc. 79th Ann. Conv. Am. Psychol. Assoc.* 6:759–60

128. Izquierdo, I. 1974. *Psychopharmacologia* 38:259–66
129. Henriksson, B. G., Järbe, T. 1971. *Psychopharmacologia* 20:186–90
130. Iwahara, S., Noguchi, S. 1972. *Jpn. Psychol. Res.* 14:141–44
131. Pusakulich, R. L., Nielson, H. C. 1972. *Exp. Neurol.* 34:33–44
132. Christy, D., Reid, L. 1975. *Bull. Psychon. Soc.* 5:175–77
133. Cooper, S., Coon, K., Mejta, C., Reid, L. 1974. *Physiol. Psychol.* 2:519–22
134. Kamano, D. K. 1972. *Behav. Res. Ther.* 10:367–70
135. Kamano, D. K., Powell, B. J., Martin, L. K., Ogle, M. E. 1967. *Psychol. Rec.* 17:97–102
136. Ziskind, D., Amit, Z., Baum, M. 1974. *Psychopharmacologia* 38:231–38
137. Benson, H. J., Herd, J. A., Morse, W. H., Kelleher, R. T. 1970. *J. Pharmacol. Exp. Ther.* 173:399–406
138. Bloch, S., Pragay, E. B., Mirsky, A. F. 1973. *Pharmacol. Biochem. Behav.* 1:29–34
139. Corson, S. A., O'Leary Corson, E. 1967. *Neuro-Psycho-Pharmacol. Proc. Int. Congr. Coll. Int. Neuro-Psycho-Pharmacol., 5th,* 857–78
140. Delini-Stula, A., Morpurgo, C. 1970. *Int. J. Psychobiol.* 1:71–75
141. Delini-Stula, A. 1971. *Psychopharmacologia* 20:153–59
142. Bassett, J. R., Cairncross, K. D. 1974. *Arch. Int. Pharmacodyn. Ther.* 212:221–29
143. Lahti, R. A., Barsuhn, C. 1974. *Psychopharmacologia* 35:215–20
144. Amsel, A. 1967. *Psychol. Learn. Motiv.* 1:1–65
145. Gray, J. A. 1970. *Psychol. Rev.* 77:465–80
146. Barry, H. III, Wagner, A. R., Miller, N. E. 1962. *J. Comp. Physiol. Psychol.* 55:464–68
147. Wagner, A. R., 1963. *J. Exp. Psychol.* 65:474–77
148. Gray, J. A., Araujo-Silva, M. T. 1971. *Psychopharmacologia* 22:8–22
149. Dudderidge, H. J., Gray, J. A. 1974. *Psychopharmacologia* 35:365–70
150. Ison, J. R., Pennes, E. S. 1969. *J. Comp. Physiol. Psychol.* 68:215–19
151. Iwahara, S., Nagamura, N., Iwasaki, T. 1967. *Jpn. Psychol. Res.* 9:128–34
152. Molinengo, L., Ricci-Gamalero, S. 1969. *Arch. Int. Pharmacodyn. Ther.* 180:217–31
153. Tessel, R. E., Lash, S. 1968. *Proc. 76th Ann. Conv. Am. Psychol. Assoc.* 3:149–50
154. Tessel, R. E. 1969. *The effects of chlordiazepoxide and sodium amobarbital on the partial reinforcement effects in the runway.* MA thesis. Univ. Illinois, Chicago. 30 pp.
155. Gray, J. A. 1969. *J. Comp. Physiol. Psychol.* 69:55–64
156. Iwahara, S., Iwasaki, T., Nagamura, N., Masuyama, E. 1966. *Jpn. Psychol. Res.* 8:131–35
157. Rosen, A. J., Glass, D. H., Ison, J. R. 1967. *Psychon. Sci.* 9:129–30
158. Rosen, A. J., Tessel, R. E. 1970. *J. Comp. Physiol. Psychol.* 72:257–62
159. Vogel, J. R., Principi, K. 1971. *Psychopharmacologia* 21:8–12
160. Heise, G. A., Laughlin, N., Keller, C. 1970. *Psychopharmacologia* 16:345–68
161. Ison, J. R., Northman, J. 1968. *Psychon. Sci.* 12:185–86
162. Ridgers, A., Gray, J. A. 1973. *Psychopharmacologia* 32:265–70
163. Capaldi, E. J. 1967. *Psychol. Learn. Motiv.* 1:67–156
164. Søltysik, S., Gasanova, R. 1969. *Acta Biol. Exp. Warsaw* 29:29–49
165. Griffiths, R. R., Thompson, T. 1973. *Psychol. Rep.* 33:323–34
166. Griffiths, R. R., Thompson, T. 1974. *Pharmacol. Biochem. Behav.* 2:331–38
167. Fowler, S. C. 1974. *Pharmacol. Biochem. Behav.* 2:155–60
168. Freedman, P. E., Rosen, A. J. 1969. *Psychopharmacologia* 15:39–47
169. Gray, J. A., Dudderidge, H. 1971. *Neuropharmacology* 10:217–22
170. Ison, J. R., Daly, H. B., Glass, D. H. 1967. *Psychol. Rep.* 20:491–96
171. Ludvigson, H. W. 1967. *Psychon. Sci.* 8:115–16
172. Norton, P. R. E. 1971. *Br. J. Pharmacol.* 41:317–30
173. Capaldi, E. J., Berg, R. F., Sparling, D. L. 1971. *J. Comp. Physiol. Psychol.* 76:290–99
174. Ziff, D. R., Capaldi, E. J. 1971. *J. Exp. Psychol.* 87:263–69
175. Capaldi, E. J., Sparling, D. L. 1971. *Psychon. Sci.* 23:215–17
176. Capaldi, E. J., Sparling, D. L. 1971. *J. Comp. Physiol. Psychol.* 74:467–77
176a. Gray, J. A. 1976. *Handbook of Psychopharmacology, Sect. 2, Behavioral Pharmacology in Animals,* ed. L. L. Iversen, S. D. Iversen, S. H. Snyder. New York: Plenum. In press
177. Konorski, J. 1967. *The Integrative Activity of the Brain.* Chicago: Univ. Chicago Press. 531 pp.
178. Beer, B., Chasin, M., Clody, D. E., Vo-

gel, J. R., Horovitz, Z. P. 1972. *Science* 176:428–30
179. Clody, D. E., Beer, B., Lenard, L. G. 1972. *Proc. 80th Ann. Conv. Am. Psychol. Assoc.* 7:825–26
180. Geller, I., Blum, K. 1970. *Eur. J. Pharmacol.* 9:319–24
181. Geller, I., Hartmann, R. J., Croy, D. J. 1974. *Res. Commun. Chem. Pathol. Pharmacol.* 7:165–74
182. Graeff, F. G. 1974. *J. Pharmacol. Exp. Ther.* 189:344–50
183. Graeff, F. G., Schoenfeld, R. I. 1970. *J. Pharmacol. Exp. Ther.* 173:277–83
184. Hartmann, R. J., Geller, I. 1971. *Life Sci.* 10: Part I, 927–33
185. Robichaud, R. C., Sledge, K. L. 1969. *Life Sci.* 8: Part I, 965–69
186. Stein, L., Wise, C. D. 1974. *Adv. Biochem. Psychopharmacol.* 11:281–91
187. Stevens, D. A., Fechter, L. D. 1969. *Life Sci.* 8: Part II, 379–85
188. Wise, C. D., Berger, B. D., Stein, L. 1970. *Proc. 78th Ann. Conv. Am. Psychol. Assoc.* 5:821–22
189. Wise, C. D., Berger, B. D., Stein, L. 1973. *Biol. Psychiatry* 6:3–21
190. Appel, J. B. 1971. *Psychopharmacologia* 21:174–86
191. Key, B. J. 1961. *Psychopharmacologia* 2:352–63
192. Bovet, D., Robustelli, F., Bignami, G. 1965. *C. R. Hebd. Seances Acad. Sci.* 260:4641–45
193. Winter, J. C. 1972. *Arch. Int. Pharmacodyn. Ther.* 197:147–59
194. Campbell, A. B., Brown, R. M., Seiden, L. S. 1971. *Physiol. Behav.* 7:853–57
195. Cole, J. M., Pieper, W. A. 1973. *Psychopharmacologia* 29:107–12
196. Ho, B. T., McIsaac, W. M., An, R., Harris, R. T., Walker, K. E., Kralik, P. M., Airaksinen, M. M. 1970. *Psychopharmacologia* 16:385–94
197. Rosen, A. J., Buga, J. 1969. *Arch. Int. Pharmacodyn. Ther.* 180:299–308
198. Rosen, A. J., Cohen, M. E. 1973. *Neuropharmacology* 12:501–8
199. Winter, J. C. 1969. *J. Pharmacol. Exp. Ther.* 169:7–16
200. Boggan, W. O., Freedman, D. X., Appel, J. B. 1973. *Psychopharmacologia* 33:293–98
201. Appel, J. B., Lovell, R. A., Freedman, D. X. 1970. *Psychopharmacologia* 18:387–406
202. Appel, J. B., Sheard, M. H., Freedman, D. X. 1970. *Commun. Behav. Biol.* 5:237–41
203. Blakely, T. A., Parker, L. F. 1973. *Pharmacol. Biochem. Behav.* 1:609–13

204. Brody, J. F. Jr. 1970. *Psychopharmacologia* 17:14–33
205. Srebro, B., Lorens, S. A. 1975. *Brain Res.* 89:303–25
206. Lorens, S. A. 1973. *Pharmacol. Biochem. Behav.* 1:487–90
207. Schlesinger, K., Schreiber, R. A., Pryor, G. T. 1968. *Psychon. Sci.* 11:225–26
207a. Steranka, L. R., Barrett, R. J. 1974. *Behav. Biol.* 11:205–13
208. Takaori, S., Tanaka, C. 1970. *Jpn. J. Pharmacol.* 20:607–9
208a. Vorhees, C. V., Schaefer, G. J., Barrett, R. J. 1975. *Pharmacol. Biochem. Behav.* 3:279–84
209. Tanaka, C., Yoh, Y.-J., Takaori, S. 1972. *Brain Res.* 45:153–64
210. Tenen, S. S. 1967. *Psychopharmacologia* 10:204–19
211. Cuomo, V., Marino, A. 1974. *Pharmacol. Res. Commun.* 6:531–37
212. Yen, H. C. Y., Katz, M. H., Krop, S. 1971. *Arch. Int. Pharmacodyn. Ther.* 190:103–9
213. McCleary, R. A. 1966. *Progr. Physiol. Psychol.* 1:209–72
214. Rake, A. V. 1973. *Psychopharmacologia* 29:91–100
215. Barchas, J., Usdin, E., eds. 1973. *Serotonin and Behavior.* New York: Academic. 642 pp.
216. Costa, E., Gessa, G. L., Sandler, M., eds. 1974. *Adv. Biochem. Psychopharmacol.* 10:1–329, 11:1–428
217. Sandler, M., Gessa, G. L., eds. 1975. *Sexual Behavior—Pharmacology and Biochemistry.* New York: Raven. 354 pp.
218. Chase, T. N., Murphy, D. L. 1973. *Ann. Rev. Pharmacol.* 13:181–97
219. Bignami, G. 1976. *Acta Neurobiol. Exp.* 36: In press
220. Glick, S. D. 1976. *Behavioral Pharmacology,* ed. S. D. Glick, J. Goldfarb. St. Louis: Mosby. In press
221. Grossman, S. P., Sclafani, A. 1971. *Pharmacological and Biophysical Agents and Behavior,* ed. E. Furchtgott, 269–344. New York: Academic. 402 pp.
222. Harvey, J. A., Schlosberg, A. J., Yunger, L. M. 1975. *Fed. Proc.* 34:1796–1801
223. Margules, D. L., Margules, A. S. 1973. *Efferent Organization and the Integration of Behavior,* ed. J. Maser, 203–28. New York: Academic. 375 pp.
224. Krsiak, M. 1974. *Res. Commun. Chem. Pathol. Pharmacol.* 7:237–57
225. Miczek, K. A., Barry, H. III. 1976. See Ref. 220

226. Brimblecombe, R. W. 1968. *Mod. Trends Toxicol.* 1:149–74
227. Porter, R., Birch, J., eds. 1970. *Chemical Influences on Behaviour.* London: Churchill. 221 pp.
228. Van Gelder, G. A., Carson, T. L., Smith, R. M., Buck, W. B., Karas, G. G. 1973. *J. Am. Vet. Med. Assoc.* 163:1033–35
229. Weiss, B., ed. 1975. *Fed. Proc.* 34:1754–1903
230. Weiss, B., Laties, V. G., eds. 1975. *Behavioral Toxicology.* New York: Plenum. 469 pp.
231. Weiss, B., Spyker, J. M. 1974. *Pediatrics* 53:851–56
232. Xintaras, C., Johnson, B. L., De Groot, I., eds. 1974. *Behavioral Toxicology. Early Detection of Occupational Hazards.* Washington DC: US Dep. of Health Educ. Welfare. 508 pp.
233. Barry, H. III 1974. *Fed. Proc.* 33:1814–24
234. Järbe, T.U.C., Henriksson, B. G. 1974. *Psychopharmacologia* 40:1–16
235. Bindra, D., Reichert, H. 1966. *Psychon. Sci.* 4:95–96
236. Bindra, D., Nyman, K., Wise, J. 1965. *J. Comp. Physiol. Psychol.* 60:223–28
237. Connelly, J. F., Connelly, J. M., Epps, J. O. 1973. *Psychopharmacologia* 30:275–82
238. Connelly, J. F., Connelly, J. M., Phifer, R. 1975. *Psychopharmacologia* 41:139–43
239. Braude, M. C., Harris, L. S., May, E. L., Smith, J. P., Villarreal, J. E., eds. 1973. *Adv. Biochem. Psychopharmacol.* 8:1–592
240. Clouet, D. H., Iwatsubo, K. 1975. *Ann. Rev. Pharmacol.* 15:49–71
241. Goldberg, L., Hoffmeister, F., eds. 1973. *Psychic Dependence.* Berlin: Springer. 244 pp.
242. Schuster, C. R., Thompson, T. 1969. *Ann. Rev. Pharmacol.* 9:483–502
243. Schuster, C. R., Johanson, C. E. 1974. *Res. Adv. Alcohol Drug Probl.* 1:1–31
244. Singh, J. M., Miller, L. H., Lal, H., eds. 1972. *Drug Addiction. I. Experimental Pharmacology.* Mount Kisco, NY: Futura. 288 pp.
244a. Lynch, J. J., Fertziger, A. P., Teitelbaum, H. A., Cullen, J. W., Gantt, W. H. 1973. *Cond. Reflex* 8:211–23
245. Revusky, S., Garcia, J. 1970. *Psychol. Learn. Motiv.* 4:1–84
246. Garcia, J., Hankins, W. G., Rusiniak, K. W. 1974. *Science* 185:824–31
247. Berger, B. D. 1972. *J. Comp. Physiol. Psychol.* 81:21–26

247a. Vogel, J. R., 1976. *Neurobiology of Drug Dependence. I. Behavioral Analysis of Drug Dependence,* ed. H. Lal, J. Singh. New York: Futura. In press
248. Cappell, H., LeBlanc, A. E., Endrenyi, L. 1973. *Psychopharmacologia* 29:239–46
249. Eckardt, M. J., Skurdal, A. J., Brown, J. S. 1974. *Physiol. Psychol.* 2:89–92
250. Lester, D., Nachman, M., Le Magnen, J. 1970. *Q. J. Stud. Alcohol* 31:578–86
251. Coussens, W. R., Crowder, W. F., Davis, W. M. 1973. *Psychopharmacologia* 29:151–57
252. Bignami, G., Pinto-Scognamiglio, W., Gatti, G. L. 1973. *Proc. Eur. Soc. Study Drug Toxic.* 15:33–42
253. Cappell, H., LeBlanc, A. E. 1971. *Psychopharmacologia* 22:352–56
254. Cappell, H., LeBlanc, A. E. 1973. *J. Comp. Physiol. Psychol.* 85:97–104
255. Carey, R. J. 1973. *Pharmacol. Biochem. Behav.* 1:227–29
256. Carey, R. J. 1973. *Pharmacol. Biochem. Behav.* 1:265–69
257. Martin, J. C., Ellinwood, E. H. Jr. 1973. *Psychopharmacologia* 29:253–61
258. Martin, J. C., Ellinwood, E. H. Jr. 1974. *Psychopharmacologia* 36:323–35
258a. Vogel, J. R., Nathan, B. A. 1975. *Pharmacol. Biochem. Behav.* 3:189–94
259. Corcoran, M. E., 1973. *Life Sci.* 12: Part I, 63–72
260. Corcoran, M. E., Bolotow, I., Amit, Z., McCaughran, J. A. Jr. 1974. *Pharmacol. Biochem. Behav.* 2:725–28
261. Elsmore, T. F. 1972. *Proc. 80th Ann. Conv. Am. Psychol. Assoc.* 7:817–18
262. Elsmore, T. F., Fletcher, G. 1972. *Science* 175:911–12
263. Miller, L. L., Drew, W. G. 1974. *Psychol. Bull.* 81:401–17
264. Paton, W. D. M. 1975. *Ann. Rev. Pharmacol.* 15:191–220
265. Cameron, O. G., Appel, J. B. 1972. *Psychon. Sci.* 27:302–4
266. Cameron, O. G., Appel, J. B. 1972. *J. Exp. Anal. Behav.* 17:127–37
267. Cappell, H., LeBlanc, A. E., Endrenyi, L. 1972. *Physiol. Behav.* 9:167–69
267a. Johanson, C. E., Schuster, C. R. 1975. *J. Pharmacol. Exp. Ther.* 193:676–88
268. Goldberg, S. R., Hoffmeister, F., Schlichting, U., Wuttke, W. 1971. *J. Pharmacol. Exp. Ther.* 179:268–76
269. Hoffmeister, F., Wuttke, W. 1973. *Psychopharmacologia* 33:247–58
270. Goldberg, S. R., Hoffmeister, F., Schlichting, U. U. 1972. See Ref. 244, pp. 31–48

271. Hoffmeister, F., Wuttke, W. 1973. See Ref. 239, pp. 361–69
272. Hoffmeister, F. 1975. *J. Pharmacol. Exp. Ther.* 192:468–77
273. Hoffmeister, F., Goldberg, S. R. 1973. *J. Pharmacol. Exp. Ther.* 187:8–14
274. Joffe, J. M. 1969. *Prenatal Determinants of Behaviour.* Oxford: Pergamon. 366 pp.
275. Kornetsky, C. 1970. *Psychopharmacologia* 17:105–36
276. Vernadakis, A., Weiner, N., eds. 1974. *Adv. Behav. Biol.* 8:1–537
277. Werboff, J. *Principles of Psychopharmacology,* ed. W. G. Clark, J. Del Giudice, 343–53. New York: Academic. 814 pp.
278. Young, R. D. 1967. *Psychol. Bull.* 67:73–86
279. Middaugh, L. D., Blackwell, L. A., Santos, C. A. III, Zemp, J. W. 1974. *Dev. Psychobiol.* 7:429–38
280. Tonge, S. R. 1973. *Br. J. Pharmacol.* 47:425–27
281. Tonge, S. R. 1973. *J. Neurochem.* 20:625–27
282. Kellogg, C., Lundborg, P., Roos, B. E. 1972. *Brain Res.* 40:469–75
283. Lundborg, P., Roos, B. E. 1974. *J. Pharm. Pharmacol.* 26:816–18
284. Baker, P. C., Hoff, K. M. 1975. *Gen. Pharmacol.* 6:19–22
285. Branchey, L., Friedhoff, A. J. 1973. *Psychopharmacologia* 32:151–56
286. Schaefer, G. J., Buchanan, D. C., Ray, O. S. 1973. *Life Sci.* 12: Part I, 401–411
287. Banerjee, U. 1975. *Psychopharmacologia* 41:113–16
288. Nasello, A. G., Astrada, C. A., Ramirez, O. A. 1974. *Psychopharmacologia* 40:25–31
289. Seliger, D. L. 1973. *Physiol. Psychol.* 1:273–80
289a. Sobrian, S. K., Weltman, M., Pappas, B. A. 1975. *Dev. Psychobiol.* 8:241–50
290. Gauron, E. F., Rowley, V. N. 1972. *Psychopharmacologia* 26:73–78
291. Gauron, E. F., Rowley, V. N. 1969. *Psychopharmacologia* 16:5–15
292. Gauron, E. F., Rowley, V. N. 1971. *Eur. J. Pharmacol.* 15:171–75
293. Gauron, E. F., Rowley, V. N. 1971. *Psychol. Rep.* 29:497–98
294. Gauron, E. F., Rowley, V. N. 1973. *Psychopharmacologia* 30:269–74
294a. Ahlenius, S., Engel, J., Lundborg, P. 1975. *Arch. Pharmacol.* 288:185–93
295. Golub, M., Kornetsky, C. 1974. *Dev. Psychobiol.* 7:79–88
296. Borgen, L. A., Davis, W. M., Pace, H. B. 1973. *Pharmacol. Biochem. Behav.* 1:203–6
297. Gianutsos, G., Abbatiello, E. R. 1972. *Psychopharmacologia* 27:117–22
298. Le Boeuf, B. J., Peeke, H. V. S. 1969. *Psychopharmacologia* 16:49–53
299. Peeke, H. V. S., Le Boeuf, B. J., Herz, M. J. 1971. *Psychopharmacologia* 19: 262–65
300. Schaefer, G. J., Buchanan, D. C., Ray, O. S. 1974. *Behav. Biol.* 10:253–58
301. Stein, D. G. 1971. *Commun. Behav. Biol.* 6:335–40
302. Rosenzweig, M. R., Bennett, E. L. 1972. *J. Comp. Physiol. Psychol.* 80:304–13
303. Coyle, I. R., Singer, G. 1975. *Psychopharmacologia* 41:237–44
304. Bignami, G., Rosić, N., Michalek, H., Milošević, M., Gatti, G. L. 1975. See Ref. 230, 155–210
305. Russell, R. W., Overstreet, D. H., Cotman, C. W., Carson, V. G., Churchill, L., Dalglish, F. W., Vasquez, B. J. 1975. *J. Pharmacol. Exp. Ther.* 192:73–85
306. Weis, P., Weis, J. S. 1974. *Environ. Res.* 7:68–74
307. Van Gelder, G. A. 1975. See Ref. 230, 217–37
307a. Hrdina, P. D., Singhal, R. L., Ling, G. M. 1975. *Adv. Pharmacol. Chemother.* 12:31–88
308. Bourgeois, A. E., Casey, A. 1974. *Psychol. Rep.* 35:997–98
309. Burt, G. S. 1975. See Ref. 230, 241–62
310. Joy, R. M. 1974. *Neuropharmacology* 13:93–110
311. Paulsen, K., Adesso, V. J., Porter, J. J. 1975. *Bull. Psychon. Soc.* 5:117–19
312. Peterle, A. F., Peterle, T. J. 1971. *Bull. Environ. Contam. Toxicol.* 6:401–5
313. Smith, R. M., Cunningham, W. L. Jr., Van Gelder, G. A., Karas, G. G. 1975. *J. Toxicol. Environ. Health.* In press
314. Sobotka, T. J. 1971. *Proc. Soc. Exp. Biol. Med.* 137:952–55
315. Sós, J., Dési, I. 1972. *Recent Dev. Neurobiol. Hung.* 3:133–65
316. Al-Hachim, G. M. 1971. *Psychopharmacologia* 21:370–73
317. Al-Hachim, G. M., Al-Baker, A. 1973. *Br. J. Pharmacol.* 49:311–15
318. Al-Hachim, G. M., Fink, G. B. 1967. *Psychol. Rep.* 20:1183–87
319. Al-Hachim, G. M., Fink, G. B. 1968. *Psychol. Rep.* 22:1193–96
320. Al-Hachim, G. M., Fink, G. B. 1968. *Psychopharmacologia* 13:408–12
321. Al-Hachim, G. M., Fink, G. B. 1968. *Psychopharmacologia* 12:424–27

322. Craig, G. R., Ogilvie, D. M. 1974. *Environ. Biochem. Physiol.* 4:189–99
323. Sobotka, T. J., Brodie, R. E., Cook, M. P. 1972. *Dev. Psychobiol.* 5:137–48
324. Kihlström, J. E., Lundberg, C., Örberg, J., Danielsson, P. O., Sydhoff, J. 1975. *Environ. Biochem. Physiol.* 5:54–57
324a. Gellert, R. J., Heinrichs, W. L. 1975. *Biol. Neonate* 26:283–90
325. Sjödén, P.-O., Söderberg, U. 1972. *Physiol. Behav.* 9:357–60
325a. Sjödén, P.-O., Söderberg, U. 1975. *Physiol. Psychol.* 3:175–78
326. Hrdina, P. D., Singhal, R. L., Peters, D.A.V., Ling, G. M. 1971. *Eur. J. Pharmacol.* 15:379–82
327. Hrdina, P. D., Singhal, R. L., Peters, D.A.V., Ling, G. M. 1972. *Eur. J. Pharmacol.* 20:114–17
328. Hrdina, P. D., Peters, D.A.V., Singhal, R. L. 1974. *Eur. J. Pharmacol.* 26:306–12
329. Kar, P. P., Matin, M. A. 1974. *Eur. J. Pharmacol.* 25:36–39
330. Matin, M. A., Kar, P. P. 1974. *Pharmacol. Res. Commun.* 6:357–62
331. Gruener, N. 1974. *Pharmacol. Biochem. Behav.* 2:267–69
332. Stokes, J. D., Scudder, C. L. 1974. *Dev. Psychobiol.* 7:343–50
333. Stone, D., Matalka, E., Riordan, J. 1969. *Nature London* 224:1326–28
334. Stone, D., Matalka, E. 1970. *Fed. Proc.* 29:657 (Abstr.)
335. Araujo, P. E., Mayer, J. 1973. *Am. J. Physiol.* 225:764–65
336. Berry, H. K., Butcher, R. E., Elliot, L. A., Brunner, R. L. 1974. *Dev. Psychobiol.* 7:165–73
337. Pradhan, S. N., Lynch, J. F. Jr. 1972. *Arch. Int. Pharmacodyn. Ther.* 197:301–4
338. Nagasawa, H. Yanai, R., Kikuyama, S. 1974. *Acta Endocrinol. Copenhagen* 75:249–59
339. Tadokoro, S., Higuchi, Y., Kuribara, H., Okuzumi, K. 1974. *Pharmacol. Biochem. Behav.* 2:619–25
340. Pinto-Scognamiglio, W., Amorico, L., Gatti, G. L. 1972. *Farmaco Ed. Prat.* 27:19–27
341. Beliles, R. P., Clark, R. S., Yuile, C. L. 1968. *Toxicol. Appl. Pharmacol.* 12:15–21
342. Braun, J. J., Snyder, D. R. 1973. *Bull. Psychon. Soc.* 1:419–20
343. Klein, S. B., Atkinson, D. J. 1973. *Bull. Psychon. Soc.* 1:437–38
344. Klein, S. B., Barter, M. J., Murphy, A. L., Richardson, J. H. 1974. *Physiol. Psychol.* 2:397–400
345. Lahue, R. 1973. *Bull. Environ. Contam. Toxicol.* 10:166–69
346. Lehotzky, K., Mészáros, I. 1974. *Acta Pharmacol. Toxicol.* 35:180–84
347. Morganti, J. B., Lown, B. A., Stineman, C., Massaro, E. J. 1974. *Psychol. Rep.* 35:901–2
348. Post, E. M., Yang, M. G., King, J. A., Sanger, V. L. 1973. *Proc. Soc. Exp. Biol. Med.* 143:1113–16
349. Richardson, R. J., Murphy, S. D. 1974. *Toxicol. Appl. Pharmacol.* 29:289–300
350. Salvaterra, P., Lown, B., Morganti, J., Massaro, E. J. 1973. *Acta Pharmacol. Toxicol.* 33:177–90
351. Thaxton, J. P., Parkhurst, C. R. 1973. *Proc. Soc. Exp. Biol. Med.* 144:252–55
352. Vitulli, W. F. 1974. *Psychol. Rep.* 35:3–9
353. Weir, P. A., Hine, C. H. 1970. *Arch. Environ. Health* 20:45–51
354. Weiss, B. 1974. *Behavioral Methods for Investigating Environmental Health Effects.* Presented at CEC - EPA - WHO Int. Symp. Environ. Health, Paris
354a. Evans, H. L., Laties, V. G., Weiss, B. 1975. *Fed. Proc.* 34:1858–67
355. Weiss, B. 1973. *Behav. Res. Methods Instrum.* 5:67–79
355a. Laties, V. G. 1975. *Fed. Proc.* 34:1880–88
356. Weiss, B., Simon, W. 1975. See Ref. 230, 429–35
357. Hughes, J., Annau, Z., Goldberg, A. M. 1972. *Fed. Proc.* 31:552 (Abstr.)
357a. Heinz, G. 1975. *Bull. Environ. Contam. Toxicol.* 13:554–64
358. Olson, K., Boush, G. M. 1975. *Bull. Environ. Contam. Toxicol.* 13:73–79
359. Rosenthal, E., Sparber, S. B. 1972. *Life Sci.* 11: Part I, 883–92
360. Sobotka, T. J., Cook, M. P., Brodie, R. E. 1974. *Biol. Psychiatry* 8:307–20
361. Spyker, J. M. 1975. See Ref. 230, 311–44
361a. Spyker, J. 1975. *Fed. Proc.* 34:1835–44
362. Spyker, J. M., Sparber, S. B., Goldberg, A. M. 1972. *Science* 177:621–23
363. Brown, D. R. 1975. *Toxicol. Appl. Pharmacol.* 32:628–37
364. Michaelson, I. A., Sauerhoff, M. W. 1974. *Toxicol. Appl. Pharmacol.* 28:88–96
364a. Morrison, J. H., Olton, D. S., Goldberg, A. M., Silbergeld, E. K. 1975. *Dev. Psychobiol.* 8:389–96
365. Sauerhoff, M. W., Michaelson, I. A. 1973. *Science* 182:1022–24
366. Silbergeld, E. K., Goldberg, A. M. 1973. *Life Sci.* 13:1275–83

367. Silbergeld, E. K., Goldberg, A. M. 1974. *Exp. Neurol.* 42:146–57
367a. Silbergeld, E. K., Goldberg, A. M. 1975. *Neuropharmacology* 14:431–44
368. Snowdon, C. T. 1973. *Pharmacol. Biochem. Behav.* 1:599–603
369. Sobotka, T. J., Cook, M. P. 1974. *Am. J. Ment. Defic.* 79:5–9
370. Avery, D. D., Cross, H. A., Schroeder, T. 1974. *Pharmacol. Biochem. Behav.* 2:473–79
371. Bullock, J. D., Wey, R. J., Zaia, J. A., Zarembok, I., Schroeder, H. A. 1966. *Arch. Environ. Health* 13:21–22
372. Brown, S., Dragann, N., Vogel, W. H. 1971. *Arch. Environ. Health* 22:370–72
373. Snowdon, C. T., Sanderson, B. A. 1974. *Science* 183:92–94
374. Carson, T. L., Van Gelder, G. A., Buck, W. B., Hoffman, L. J., Mick, D. L., Long, K. R. 1973. *Clin. Toxicol.* 6:389–403
375. Carson, T. L., Van Gelder, G. A., Karas, G. G., Buck, W. B. 1974. *Environ. Health Perspect.* May, Issue 7:233–37
376. Carson, T. L., Van Gelder, G. A., Karas, G. G., Buck, W. B. 1974. *Arch. Environ. Health* 29:154–56
377. Van Gelder, G. A., Carson, T. L., Smith, R. M., Buck, W. B., 1973. *Clin. Toxicol.* 6:405–17
378. Simpson, G. G. 1964. *This View of Life.* New York: Harcourt Brace. 308 pp.
379. Tobias, L. L., MacDonald, M. L. 1974. *Psychol. Bull.* 81:107–25
380. Berger, F. M. 1972. *Adv. Pharmacol. Chemother.* 10:105–18
381. Crane, G. E. 1973. *Science* 181:124–28
382. Crane, G. E. 1974. *Trans. NY Acad. Sci.* 36:644–57
383. Cole, J. O. 1974. *Trans. NY Acad. Sci.* 36:658–62

SELECTIVE SUPPRESSION OF HUMORAL IMMUNITY BY ANTINEOPLASTIC DRUGS

❖6654

G. H. Heppner and P. Calabresi[1]

Department of Medicine, Roger Williams General Hospital and Division of Biological and Medical Sciences, Brown University, Providence, Rhode Island 02912

Within the last few years there has been a tremendous increase in knowledge of clinical and experimental immunology. We are becoming aware of the complexity of immune responses as they really occur, as opposed to the relatively simple responses described in textbooks and studied in model systems. Not only are there humoral (antibody-mediated) and cell-mediated immunities, with their cellular counterparts, the B- and T-cell systems (1), but also there are further subpopulations of lymphoid cells, with differing functions and responses to antigens, and with interaction between them a continuing process. In an immune response to a single antigenic stimulus, there may be, in addition to cells producing antibody, helper T cells that cooperate with B cells in the triggering of antibody production (1), suppressor T cells that somehow limit the extent of the immune response (2), and effector T cells that are involved in the manifestations (such as cytotoxicity, delayed hypersensitivity, contact sensitivity, or skin allograft rejection) of specific cell-mediated immunity (3), presumably through the release of lymphokine(s) (4). It is not known whether all these functions are carried out by the same or different T-cell populations. A similar level of functional complexity has not yet been described for B cells, although the different classes of immunoglobulins and the sensitivity of antibody production to feedback regulation (5) indicate that complexity and interaction are operative here also. Thus, it is apparent that the concept *immunosuppression* is far too naive. However, if ways could be found to affect selectively the different parts of the immune response, the possibility for "fine-tuning" the system would lead to much more subtle immunoregulatory capabilities than now exist.

[1]Our experimental work described in this review was supported by US Public Health Service Grants GM-16538 and CA-13943.

The purpose of this paper is to review the relatively limited literature that suggests that selective immunosuppression may be possible. Because the goal of our own work has been to use immunosuppressives in such a way as to maximize host resistance to neoplasia, this review, except for a brief discussion, is limited to observations with antineoplastic agents. Very little work has been published on the suppression of cell-mediated immunity without concomitant antibody suppression (but see 6–8), so we have restricted our review to selective suppression of humoral immunity. As will be seen, selective immunosuppression is barely out of the descriptive stage, and regulation beyond the antibody versus cell-mediated level is just beginning.

SELECTIVE SUPPRESSION OF HUMORAL IMMUNITY: GENERAL DISCUSSION

Before reviewing studies on selective suppression with antineoplastic drugs, we mention a number of other procedures that have been reported to have similar selective effects. Indeed, even the classical methods of immunosuppression may show selectivity. For example, Nossal & Pike (9) have shown that B cells of adult strain CBA mice are more sensitive than T cells to high dose irradiation (800 r). In their study the number of splenic B cells fell by a factor of 200 during the first day after irradiation, whereas the total spleen cell number fell by a factor of 10. Kuening & Bos (10) found that sublethal total body irradiation (450 r) in rabbits selectively destroyed splenic lymphoid follicles and germinal centers (B-dependent areas) without affecting periarteriolar sheath lymphocytes. In our own experience (unpublished observations), 600 r total body irradiation suppressed the ability of strain C_3HeB/FeJ adult male mice to produce 19S antibody to sheep red blood cells (SRBC), as measured by Jerne plaque assay, as long as 30 days after irradiation, whereas the ability to develop contact sensitivity to oxazolone was not significantly affected even when sensitization was assessed 24 hr after irradiation. [Sensitivity to oxazolone was assessed five days after immunization, a time when T cells are principally responsible for the hypersensitivity reaction (11)].

Other immunosuppressive treatments that have been shown to be more effective for both the number and function of B cells than for T cells include prostaglandin E in rats (12, 13) and cytoplasmic components of group A streptococci in mice (14). The immunosuppression induced by graft-vs-host disease has been reported to be longer lasting for humoral immunity than for rejection of skin allografts in mice (15), although cellular immunity seems to be more markedly depressed than humoral immunity in human allogeneic bone marrow chimeras (16). In the latter case, however, the graft recipients were patients with acute lymphocytic leukemia (17).

A most interesting example of selective immunosuppression comes from the work of Jose & Good (18) on the effect of amino acid deficiencies on immunity. Diets moderately deficient in phenylalanine-tyrosine, valine, threonine, methionine-cystine, isoleucine, or tryptophan resulted in depressed production of both hemagglutinating antibodies and serum blocking factors (see below) in strain C_3H mice, although cell-mediated immunity, as measured by an in vitro cytotoxicity test, to allogeneic tumor cells remained intact. Limitation of arginine, histidine, or lysine had only a slight effect, but limitation of leucine depressed cell-mediated immunity without suppressing antibody production.

Passive administration of specific antibody can be an effective method of inhibiting both antibody production (19) as well as sensitization to allogeneic tissue grafts (19) and development of delayed hypersensitivity to antigens, such as SRBC (20). However, administration of high concentrations of antibody has been found to inhibit antibody production but to enhance delayed hypersensitivity to flagellin, polymerized flagellin, and SRBC in rats, with lower concentrations having the inverse effect (21). This suggests that control of the amount of antibody given could result in regimens selectively suppressive for B- or T-cell immunity. The stage in immunization at which the suppressing serum is taken is also a factor (20).

Another approach to shifting the effective balance between humoral and cell-mediated immunity is preferential stimulation of the T-cell system. This has been accomplished by either acetoacetylation of the antigen (22, 23) or, in the case of red blood cell antigens, by fixation with formaldehyde or glutaraldehyde (24). Thus, acetoacetylation of flagellin turned that antigen from a strong antibody inducer into one that exclusively induced delayed hypersensitivity reactions in rats (22). Likewise, guinea pigs sensitized to acetoacetylated carcinoembryonic antigen (CEA) developed delayed skin reactivity with only low levels of antibody (23). Immunization of mice to fixed chicken red blood cells gave poor primary antibody responses, but subsequent injection of the fixed antigen resulted in normal or better secondary responses, with T-cell specificity, demonstrating that the initial immunization had resulted in effective helper T-cell priming without concomitant B-cell sensitization (24).

This brief survey of selective immunosuppression is not meant to be all-inclusive, but simply to illustrate other approaches to the problem beyond the use of antineoplastic, immunosuppressive drugs. On a practical level, however, it demonstrates that selective effects may be more common than are realized and that analysis of the immune status in experimental animals or patients requires the use of several different types of assays, even in the case of such standard immunosuppressive treatments as X irradiation.

SELECTIVE SUPPRESSION OF HUMORAL IMMUNITY BY ANTINEOPLASTIC DRUGS

6-Mercaptopurine (6-MP)

One of the first reports of selective suppression of humoral immunity was with 6-MP. Kimball, Herriot & Allison (7) found that a dose of 75 mg/kg per day, given on days 0 to 3, only had a minimal effect on retention of strain C_3H skin allografts by AKR mice but markedly suppressed the production of hemagglutinating antibody to SRBC. Stewart (25) likewise found that 6-MP had no significant effect on allograft survival, even when donor and recipient differed only at weak histocompatibility loci and when drug treatment was extended for longer periods of time (15 mg/kg per day; days −1 to 14). On the other hand Schwartz (26) found in guinea pigs that administration of 10 mg/kg per day on days 0 to 4 suppressed delayed hypersensitivity to a protein antigen (in Freund's adjuvant) without affecting anti-body production. Clearly species differences may play a role in these divergent observations.

Cyclophosphamide (CY)

Cyclophosphamide was first used to suppress the B-cell immune system in chickens (27). Birds treated with doses ranging from 4 to 8 mg/day, for the first three days after hatching, showed depressed levels of serum IgM and IgG immunoglobulin levels and also failed to produce normal levels of antibodies to antigens (bovine serum albumin, SRBC, and *S. typhimurium*) at 7 and 11 weeks of age. Their ability to make a cell-mediated immune response (graft vs host reaction) was only slightly affected.

Subsequently, Turk & Poulter (28) showed in adult mice and guinea pigs that either a single i.p. dose of 300 mg/kg, or three such doses given on alternate days, destroyed lymphocytes in B-dependent areas of spleen and lymph nodes, but had much less effect on T-dependent areas. In mice it could also be shown that the proportion of θ antigen (T-cell marker) carrying lymphocytes in peripheral lymphoid organs was over 90% after three injections of CY, as opposed to approximately 24%, 50%, and 57% in control spleens, mesenteric lymph nodes, and peripheral lymph nodes, respectively (29). Dumont (30) essentially confirmed these results, and also identified two T-cell subpopulations, differing in electrophoretic mobility, which also differed in sensitivity to CY. Restoration of T cells began by day 8 after CY (300 mg/kg), but B-cell regeneration was only evident after day 16. Normal levels of both systems were reached by day 30.

In addition to the effect on cell number and lymphoid organ morphology, treatment with 300 mg/kg CY was shown to affect immunological function. Dumont (30) found that responsiveness of spleen cells from treated animals to *E. coli* lipopolysaccharide (LPS), a B-cell mitogen in mice, was initially abolished and then showed the same recovery curve as the B-cell number. Responsiveness to Concanavalin A (Con A), a T-cell mitogen, was also diminished but not to as great an extent as responsiveness to LPS. Recovery of normal Con A responsiveness likewise occurred more quickly than did that of LPS.

Turk and associates (31) showed in guinea pigs that 300 mg/kg of CY greatly enhanced development of contact sensitivity to 2,4-dinitrofluorobenzene or to oxazolone when the antigen was administered three days after the drug. The extent of the reaction following challenge with the antigen seven days after sensitization was greater both in intensity and duration than in control animals. Antibody production to the dinitrophenyl (DNP) hapten, however, was suppressed in the treated animals, compared to antibody production in controls. Lymph node fragments (rich in T cells) from sensitized, nontreated guinea pigs further enhanced the sensitivity of the sensitized, CY-treated animals when placed in their peritoneal cavities; transfer of spleens (rich in B cells) from two such donors, however, partially reversed the effects of CY. One spleen had no effect. Removal of the spleen from guinea pigs four days after sensitization to dinitrofluorobenzene (DNFB) or oxazolone had an effect similar to that of the CY treatment in prolonging the reaction to challenge antigen.

These, and further similar data (32), were interpreted as evidence that B cells normally exercise a suppressor function in the development of T-cell-mediated hypersensitivity. Elimination of the B cells by CY also eliminates this suppression. Efforts to substitute immune serum for spleen cells in the transfer experiment met with no success, although the amount of serum (10 ml from guinea pigs sensitized seven days previously to administration of the antigen) may have been too small. However, it was stated (32) that living B cells are necessary for inhibition of the CY effect.

Further work on selective suppression of antibody formation by CY has been reported by Lagrange, Mackaness & Miller (33). They found that 200 mg/kg CY, given i.v., would permit the use of greater doses of SRBC than normally effective to elicit delayed hypersensitivity to that antigen in strain CD-1 mice. Induction of delayed hypersensitivity to SRBC in mice is strongly dose-dependent, with high doses resulting in failure of sensitization, apparently due to production of an antigen-antibody-complex blocking factor. Mice in whom sensitization has been blocked by high doses of antigen remain refractory to subsequent administration of SRBC. Even in such blocked mice, however, CY treatment can at least partially restore reactivity to further sensitization, as well as inhibit a secondary antibody response to the antigen (34).

It should be emphasized that CY given prior to sensitization does not always enhance the development of delayed hypersensitivity. In studies made along with those using DNFB and oxazolone as antigens (see above), Turk, Parker & Poulter (31) found that 300 mg/kg CY, given three days prior to sensitization with BCG, resulted in depressed reactivity to tuberculin-PPD at challenge seven days later. Jokipii & Jokipii (35) also found suppression of reactivity to azobenzenearsonate-N-acetyl-1-tyrosine (Ars-Tyr) in similarly treated guinea pigs. This latter finding is especially interesting in that the reactivity to Ars-Tyr appears to be a pure T-cell response. Furthermore, Dennert, Hatlen & Tucker (36) have recently examined the time dependence of selective immune suppression by CY. They confirmed the ability of CY to increase selectively the proportion of splenic T cells in unimmunized mice and also showed that pretreatment with the drug before the antigen resulted in spleens with higher T helper cell activity for red cell antigens and greater T cytotoxic cell activity for allogeneic tumor cell antigens. Simultaneous administration of drug and tumor cells also resulted in greater cytotoxicity by spleen cells than in untreated controls. When CY was given after antigen, however, the degree of selectivity was much less. A three-day course (30 mg/kg) resulted in suppression of T helper cell, as well as B cell, response to SRBC, although it only partially inhibited T cytotoxicity to tumor cell antigen. Prolonged drug administration (six days) totally inhibited the cytotoxicity reaction.

Cytosine Arabinoside (ara-C, 1-D-Arabinofuranosylcytosine)

The possibility that ara-C could be used as a selective immunosuppressive was originally seen in studies on development of immune responses to allogeneic tumor cells in mice. Administration of ara-C to strain $C_{57}B1$ mice early (days 1–5) after injection of strain DBA/2-derived tumor cells resulted in suppression of anti-tumor cell antibody, but did not alter development of cell-mediated immunity (37). Administration of the drug on days 6 to 10, however, suppressed both responses. Ara-C was also shown to suppress antibody production to SRBC in dogs, without affecting kidney allograft rejection (38).

Extension of these observations resulted in a more complete elucidation of the circumstances under which ara-C can selectively suppress humoral immunity in mice. Similar to the findings in (37), Griswold, Heppner & Calabresi (39) demonstrated that although administration of drug i.p. on days 1–5 or 6–10 after immunization, in doses of 20 or 40 mg/kg per day, suppressed 19S and 7S antibody production in strain C_3H mice, rejection of skin from $C_{57}Bl$ donors was only suppressed with the latter treatment period. Thus, time of administration is an important parameter. Another factor is drug dosage. Induction of contact sensitivity to oxazolone in strain A/J mice was not inhibited by 20 mg/kg per day on days 1 to 5, but was somewhat suppressed by the higher dose of 40 mg/kg per day (40). The third factor contributing to selective suppression by ara-C is the nature of the antigen; the 40 mg/kg per day dose given early suppressed hypersensitivity to oxazolone, but not to methylated bovine serum albumen (MBSA), nor did it affect skin allograft rejection.

As with similar experiments with CY, ara-C, given at times that would selectively suppress antibody production, was found to enhance development of a cell-mediated reaction. For example, mice sensitized to MBSA, and given ara-C early in the sensitization period, showed much greater reactivity than untreated, sensitized mice to antigenic challenge 14 days later (41).

Recently, treatment of unsensitized mice with ara-C has also been found to have a greater effect on levels of B cells in the spleen than on T cells, although the difference is not as great as with CY (see above). Data of A. Anaclerio, G. Heppner, and P. Calabresi (to be published) show that the percentage of splenic B cells in unsensitized C_3H mice treated with the 20 mg/kg per day, days 1 to 5 regimen, has dropped from about 45% to 32% and 35% on days 4 and 5 respectively, with only a slight, insignificant drop in numbers of T cells. No ara-C-induced differences were found in the number of T and B cells in peripheral lymph nodes.

Methotrexate (MTX), Leucovorin (LCV), and 5-Fluorouracil (5-FU)

The discussion above summarizes results from our laboratory on selective humoral suppression by ara-C. It is apparent that there are several difficulties with using ara-C for this purpose. The time, dose, and antigen parameters are quite stringent and make control of the suppression uncertain. In hopes of overcoming these difficulties, we first turned to 5-FU because conflicting reports on its immunosuppressive capacities in the literature suggested that it might be a selective agent. Also, there is a report that 5-FU, and 5-fluoro-2'-deoxyuridine, could potentiate secondary delayed hypersensitivity reactions in cancer patients (42).

At 13 mg/kg per day for the first five days after sensitization, 5-FU suppressed 19S and 7S antibody production to SRBC in C_3H mice, but even higher doses (up to 40 mg/kg per day) did not suppress various cell-mediated immune responses (40, 41). As with ara-C, 5-FU (10 to 30 mg/kg per day, days 1 to 5) enhanced the development of hypersensitivity to MBSA (40), and to oxazolone in some cases (43).

Two problems with 5-FU in mice, however, also interfere with its use as a selective immunosuppressant: (a) the degree of suppression of antibody production is variable and oftentimes inadequate, and (b) toxicity becomes significant in long-term studies. The combination of MTX, LCV, and 5-FU has been developed to overcome these problems. The combination is administered on day 2 after exposure to antigens [with replicating antigens, such as tumor cells (see below), it is given at weekly intervals]. The doses are 1 mg/kg MTX, 1 mg/kg LCV, and 50 mg/kg 5-FU. MTX and LCV are given simultaneously or separated by a short time interval (15–30 min). 5-FU is given 1 to 6 hr after MTX. The order and timing of the combination are important. If MTX and 5-FU are given simultaneously, only additive suppression of humoral immunity is seen, whereas potentiated inhibition is found when there is an interval between them (43, 44). If 5-FU is given before MTX, the selectivity of the combination becomes equivocal. LCV was added to the combination to counteract potential toxicity problems due to MTX (45). It does not substantially change the immunosuppressive properties (44), although in some cases it seems to enhance the selectivity for humoral immunity (43). This latter is not a consistent finding, however.

In experiments similar to those described above for ara-C, MTX, LCV, and 5-FU have been found to suppress 19S (43) and 7S (44) antibody production to SRBC, but to have no significant effect on skin allograft rejection or contact sensitivity to oxazolone (43, 44). Hypersensitivity to MBSA is markedly stimulated. For example, in an experiment in which sensitized, saline-treated C_3HeB/FeJ mice developed 19 ± 6 μliters of edema upon footpad challenge with MBSA, mice given MTX, LCV, and 5-FU developed 90 ± 8 μliters. Studies on the effect of the combination on lymphoid organ morphology or on numbers of T and B cells have not yet been made.

Bisdioxopiperazines

Two other agents with demonstrated selective immunosuppressive activity are 1,2-bis(3,5-dioxopiperazin-1-y1) ethane (ICRF 154) and (±)-1,2-bis(3,5-dioxopiperazin-1-y1) propane (ICRF 159) (36, 42, 43). These agents are comparable to CY in increasing the proportion of splenic T cells in unsensitized mice, and also, if given prior to immunization with red blood cells, in increasing T helper cell activity (36). Dennert, Hatlen & Tucker (36) found increased T cytotoxic cell activity to allogeneic tumor cell antigen in mice pretreated with ICRF 154, but not with ICRF 159. Turk & Parker (47), however, found that ICRF 159 enhanced development of contact sensitivity in guinea pigs. As with CY, enhanced T-cell function is only clearly demonstrated when these drugs are given prior to, or simultaneously with, antigen, although administration after antigen seems to have a somewhat greater suppressive effect on B than on T cells (36, 46).

Other Drugs

The above drugs are those that, to our knowledge, have been investigated for selective immune effects in some detail. It may be that many agents will be shown to have similar activity, especially when advantage is taken of dose and timing parameters. For example, Turk & Parker (47) have reported that melphalan and azathioprine can enhance induction of contact sensitivity in guinea pigs.

Mechanisms of Selective Immunosuppression of Humoral Immunity by Antineoplastic Drugs

A full understanding of the mechanisms involved in selective immunosuppression will not be possible until more complete information is available as to which drugs are, or are not able, to produce the effect, and under what circumstances (timing, dose, antigen, etc). It is already apparent, however, that no single class of anti-tumor drugs is involved (48); some selective activity has been found in all groups, including alkylating agents and antimetabolites; folic acid antagonists, antipurines, and antipyrimidines; phase-specific and nonspecific agents. All the agents so-far identified, however, have greater activity on cells undergoing proliferation than on resting cells. The influence of cell proliferation on sensitivity to immunosuppressive agents has long been appreciated (49). Indeed, the rationale cited by Turk & Poulter (28) for looking for selective effects by CY was that it was more likely to be active on short-lived than on long-lived lymphocytes. Since B cells, and some T cells, are shorter lived than the majority of T cells, agents that discriminate on the basis of frequency of division should be selective. In this regard, the fact that CY and ICRF 154, when given at appropriate times, eliminate B cells and an electrophoretically (30) and functionally (36) distinct class of T cells, seems to confirm this hypothesis. Likewise, the sensitivity of selective suppression to the time of drug administration in relation to antigen exposure also suggests that differential proliferation is involved in the effect. However, different drugs are selectively active at different times in the immune response: CY and the bisdioxopiperazines when given before antigen; ara-C, 5-FU, and MTX, LCV, and 5-FU when given after. It may also be that different subpopulations of lymphocytes differ in certain metabolic pathways that render them more or less sensitive to different drugs.

From the immunological point of view one of the most interesting features of selective suppression of humoral immunity is that it is frequently accompanied by an actual increase in cell-mediated immunity. This has been noted in studies with antibody-induced suppression of humoral immunity and acetoacetylated antigen induction of cell-mediated immunity (22) as well as with selectively suppressive drug treatments (31, 36, 41). The opposite effect, depressed cell-mediated immunity accompanied by enhanced antibody synthesis, has also been seen (50). This seesaw relationship, which has been discussed by Bretscher (50), could have quite complicated mechanisms, including feedback interrelationships, perhaps involving antigen-antibody complexes, and the sharing of common nutrients, informational molecules, or cells that can be diverted from one immune system to another. The preferential stimulation of suppressor cells could also be involved (32). These mechanisms would work at the levels of induction or production of immune factors. Heightened cell-mediated reactivity, under conditions of antibody suppression, could also be due to removal of an efferent block, in particular antigen-antibody complexes (serum blocking factors) which in many in vitro circumstances have been shown to be capable of inhibiting expression of cell-mediated immune reactions (41).

USES OF SELECTIVE IMMUNOSUPPRESSION OF HUMORAL IMMUNITY BY ANTINEOPLASTIC DRUGS

As stated above, the ability to suppress selectively one or another type of immune reactivity would allow "fine-tuning" of the immune response. So far our abilities in this regard are quite primitive. Nevertheless selective suppression is becoming increasingly used in three types of experimental work: (*a*) analysis of the nature of complex immune reactions, (*b*) investigation of the site of action of other immunological modifiers, and (*c*) development of ways to strengthen cell-mediated immune reactivity to solid tumors.

The Nature of Complex Immune Reactions

Although delayed hypersensitivity and contact sensitivity are classified as cell-mediated immune responses, many such reactions are in actuality mixed, with B-cell, T-cell, and also macrophage participation. In mixed reactions the B-cell response may act to augment the T-cell immunity, as in the case of macrophage-cytophilic antibodies (51), or counteract it, as in the case of serum blocking factors (antigen-antibody complexes). Clearly, selective suppression of humoral immunity could be used, in the analysis of mixed reactions, first, for identifying them, and then for assessing which type of humoral response is involved. This approach has been reported in at least two studies. Turk & Parker (47), using CY, melphalan, and ICRF 159, demonstrated that the "Jones-Mote" type of hypersensitivity in guinea pigs was in all likelihood a mixed reaction in which B-cell reactivity acted to suppress the T-cell component. Guinea pigs were treated with either drug, and then three days later immunized with 1 μg ovalbumin (OA) in Freund's incomplete adjuvant. Seven days after sensitization they were challenged by intradermal injection of 100 μg OA. The degree of skin reactivity in the drug-treated animals was greater than that in controls at 24, 48, 72, and 96 hr after challenge, although the extent and time course of the difference varied among the three drugs.

Griswold, DiLorenzo & Calabresi (11) used selective suppression with ara-C and 5-FU to show that oxazolone-induced contact sensitivity in mice does not involve a humoral blocking reaction, in addition to the already described cytophilic antibodies (51, 52) and T lymphocytes. Early (days 1–5) administration of low doses of ara-C or 5-FU had no effect on the development of sensitivity to oxazolone, in contrast to a great stimulation of reactivity to MBSA.

The Site of Action of Immunological Modifiers

So far the major use of selective humoral suppression to aid in investigation of the site of action of other immunological modifiers has been the work of Mackaness, Lagrange and co-workers. They showed that the effects of infection with BCG (the relatively nonvirulent bacillus Calmette-Guérin strain of tubercle bacilli) and administration of CY were synergistic in augmenting the induction of delayed hypersensitivity to SRBC in mice (53). Previously (see above), they had shown that CY alone could enhance hypersensitivity to that antigen, apparently by inhibiting the development of anti-SRBC antibodies. BCG infection was likewise shown to enhance hypersensitivity, but also to enhance antibody production. However, the delayed hypersensitivity was less subject to suppression by humoral blocking factors (antigen-antibody complexes) in BCG-infected animals, than in uninfected controls, possibly as a result of enhanced clearing of these factors by a stimulated reticuloendothelial system. Thus, the synergistic effects of the combination BCG and CY in producing heightened hypersensitivity were explained by an absolute increase in cell-mediated immunity (BCG), a reduction in susceptibility of the cell-mediated immunity to antibody modulation (BCG), and an inhibition of antibody production (CY).

More recently this same group has used selective suppression by CY in their studies on the ability of LPS to either stimulate or depress immunity in mice. LPS, given three days prior to antigen, diminished the development of delayed hypersensitivity to SRBC (54). LPS is a B-cell mitogen in mice, and indeed it could be shown that antibody production was increased in the treated animals. To show that the increase in antibody was causally related to the depressed cell-mediated reaction, CY was administered simultaneously with LPS. Under these circumstances the delayed hypersensitivity reaction was enhanced.

Strengthening of Cell-Mediated Immunity to Solid Tumors

Our major interest in selective inhibition of humoral immune responses relates to work on the nature of immunity to solid cancers. It has been shown that factors, probably antigen-antibody complexes (55), exist in sera of tumor-bearing animals and cancer patients that can block in vitro the expression of cell-mediated cytotoxic or cytostatic immunity (56, 57). Since these serum blocking factors seem to be associated with progressing disease (58, 59), prevention of their development might strengthen host defense reactions against cancer. We have tested this hypothesis by selective immunosuppression with ara-C (60), 5-FU (40), and MTX, LCV, and 5-FU (to be published).

Strain C_3H mice were implanted with syngeneic, early transplants of spontaneously arising mammary tumors and treated for the first five days with low (10 or 20 mg/kg per day) or high (40 mg/kg per day) doses of ara-C. In a typical experiment the tumors grew to palpable size after about four weeks in control mice. In mice given high doses of drug, the tumors appeared after about two weeks. In mice treated with low doses tumor appearance took about six weeks. The exact times for tumor outgrowths to appear differed from experiment to experiment. Also, with some tumors a dose of 20 mg/kg per day was a high dose, resulting in early tumor appearance. In these cases, however, 10 mg/kg per day delayed tumor growth.

Ara-C only influenced tumor growth when tumors capable of inducing cell-mediated immunity were used. With a tumor that was shown by in vitro techniques to be incapable of inducing cell-mediated cytotoxicity (although serum blocking factors were produced) neither 20 or 40 mg/kg per day of ara-C had any effect.

Using in vitro assays we were able to demonstrate directly the selective inhibition of serum blocking factors. Sera from mice given low doses of ara-C, which demonstrated retardation of tumor growth, failed to block cell-mediated immunity until about two weeks prior to tumor appearance. Sera from mice given high doses of drug also failed to block cell-mediated immunity; however, lymph node cells from these mice failed to kill tumor cells in vitro, whereas lymph node cells from mice given low doses of ara-C not only killed tumor cells but also continued to do so when reactivity of lymph node cells from untreated mice could no longer be demonstrated.

Selectively suppressive treatments with 5-FU and MTX, LCV, and 5-FU have shown effects similar to those of ara-C on the outgrowth of syngeneic mammary tumor cells. In the latter case, treatment, given at weekly intervals, has been effective in slowing, and even preventing, tumor growth, not only when begun soon after tumor implantation, but also after tumors have been allowed to grow unchecked for several weeks before treatment. In fact, MTX, LCV, and 5-FU is moderately effective in delaying reappearance of the tumor following incomplete surgical removal of large tumors. Earlier, low doses of ara-C were also found to be effective in preventing regrowth after surgery (60).

In experiments analogous to these, CY has been found, under appropriate circumstances, to interfere with growth of established polyoma virus–induced sarcomas in rats (61). Sequential in vitro assays have demonstrated serum blocking factors prior to treatment, and in untreated rats with progressively growing tumors, but not after treatment, when the tumors have regressed to about 50% of their pretreatment size (62).

That ara-C, MTX, 5-FU, or CY should interfere with tumor growth is not surprising, for they have all been originally developed as antineoplastic agents. What is surprising is that they inhibit tumor growth under circumstances in which they selectively inhibit antibody production, but may actually increase it if both humoral and cell-mediated immunity are suppressed. Clinically these drugs are often used under conditions thought to be advantageous for killing of tumor cells. These conditions, however, may not be optimal for the selectivity of the drugs for humoral immunity, and thus the host's ability to withstand tumor growth may be weakened. Perhaps in the future, chemotherapeutic regimens will be designed to maximize host reactivity to cancer, as well as to kill tumor cells directly (63).

CONCLUSION

Immune responses are complex, consisting of humoral and cell-mediated immunity, with both augmenting and suppressing interactions between them. The ability to suppress selectively one type of immune response, without directly affecting others, would allow more sensitive and precise immunoregulation than is now possible. Selective suppression of humoral immunity has been reported under a number of circumstances, but, in particular, with several antineoplastic drugs, including 6-mercaptopurine, cyclophosphamide, cytosine arabinoside, 5-fluorouracil, a combination of methotrexate, leucovorin, and 5-fluorouracil, and the bisdioxopiperazines, ICRF 154 and 159. Exploitation of the selective effects of these drugs is leading to new ways of analyzing complex immune responses, investigating the action of other immunological modifiers, and using antineoplastic drugs to strengthen host defense reactions against cancer.

Literature Cited

1. Good, R. A. 1972. *Clin. Immunobiol.* 1:1–28
2. Kirkwood, J. M., Gershon, R. K. 1974. *Prog. Exp. Tumor Res.* 19:157–64
3. Tucker, D. F., Dennert, G., Lennox, E. S. 1974. *J. Immunol.* 113:1302–12
4. David, J. R. 1973. *N. Engl. J. Med.* 288:143–49
5. Weigle, W. O. 1975. *Adv. Immunol.* 21:87–111
6. Freedman, H. H., Fox, A. E., Morrison, G., Shavel, J. 1972. *Proc. Soc. Exp. Biol. Med.* 139:909–12
7. Kimball, A. P., Herriot, S. J., Allison, P. S. 1967. *Proc. Soc. Exp. Biol. Med.* 126:181–84
8. Quagliata, F., Phillips-Quagliata, J. M., Floersheim, G. L. 1972. *Cell. Immunol.* 3:198–212
9. Nossal, F. J. V., Pike, B. L. 1973. *Immunology* 25:33–45
10. Kuening, F. J., Bos, W. H. 1966. *Germinal Centers in Immune Responses*, pp. 250–51. New York: Springer
11. Griswold, D. E., DiLorenzo, J., Calabresi, P. 1974. *Cell. Immunol.* 11:198–204
12. Zurier, R. B., Quagliata, F. 1971. *Nature London* 234:304–5
13. Quagliata, F., Lawrence, V. J. W., Phillips-Quagliata, J. M. 1973. *Cell. Immunol.* 6:457–65
14. Gaumer, H. R., Schwab, J. H. 1972. *Cell. Immunol.* 4:394–406
15. Trieber, W., Lapp, W. S. 1973 *Transplantation* 16:211–16
16. Halterman, R. H., Graw, R. G., Fuccillo, D. A., Leventhal, B. G., 1972. *Transplantation* 14:689–97
17. Sen, L., Bordella, L. 1974. *Br. J. Haematol.* 27:477–87
18. Jose, D. G., Good, R. A. 1973. *J. Exp. Med.* 137:1–9
19. Uhr, J. W., Möller, G. 1968. *Adv. Immunol.* 8:81–127
20. Rowley, D. A., Fitch, F. W., Stuart, F. P., Köhler, H., Cosenza, H. 1973. *Science* 181:1133–41
21. Liew, F. Y., Parish, C. R. 1972. *Cell. Immunol.* 5:499–519
22. Parish, C. R. 1973. *Cell. Immunol.* 6:66–79
23. Chao, H. F., Peiper, S. C., Aach, R. D., Parker, C. W. 1973. *J. Immunol.* 111:1800–1803
24. Dennert, G., Tucker, D. F. 1972. *J. Exp. Med.* 136:656–61
25. Stewart, P. B. 1969. *Transplantation* 7:498–505
26. Schwartz, R. S. 1966. *Fed. Proc.* 125:165–68
27. Lerman, S. P., Weidanz, W. P. 1970. *J. Immunol.* 105:614–19
28. Turk, J. L., Poulter, L. W. 1972. *Clin. Exp. Immunol.* 10:285–96
29. Poulter, L. W., Turk, J. L. 1972. *Nature London* 238:17–18
30. Dumont, F. 1974. *Int. Arch. Allergy Appl. Immunol.* 47:110–23
31. Turk, J. L., Parker, D., Poulter, L. W. 1972. *Immunology* 23:493–501
32. Katz, S. I., Parker, D., Turk, J. L. 1974. *Mayo Clin. Proc.* 49:537–40
33. Lagrange, P. H., Mackaness, G. B., Miller, T. E. 1974. *J. Exp. Med.* 139:1529–39
34. Mackaness, G. B., Lagrange, P. H. 1974. *J. Exp. Med.* 140:865–70
35. Jokipii, A. M. M., Jokipii, L. 1973. *Cell. Immunol.* 9:477–81
36. Dennert, G., Hatlen, L. E., Tucker, D. F. 1975. *J. Natl. Cancer Inst.* 54:621–29
37. Calabresi, P. 1967. *Proc. 5th Int. Cong. Chemother.*, pp. 409–21
38. Gray, G. D., Perper, R. J., Mickelson, M. M., Crim, J. A., Zukowski, C. F. 1969. *Transplantation* 7:183–87
39. Griswold, D. E., Heppner, G. H., Calabresi, P. 1972. *Cancer Res.* 32:298–301
40. Calabresi, P., Griswold, D. E., Poplin, E. A., Heppner, G. H. 1973. *Proc. 5th Int. Congr. Pharmacol.* 5:421–30
41. Heppner, G. H., Griswold, D. E., DiLorenzo, J., Poplin, E. A., Calabresi, P. 1974. *Fed. Proc.* 33:1882–85
42. Blomgren, S. E., Wolberg, W. H., Kisken, W. A. 1968. *Cancer Res.* 25:977–79
43. DiLorenzo, J. A., Griswold, D. E., Bareham, C. R., Calabresi, P. 1974. *Cancer Res.* 34:124–28
44. DiLorenzo, J. A., Griswold, D. E., Heppner, G. H., Calabresi, P. 1975. *Proc. Am. Assoc. Cancer Res.* 16:691
45. Calabresi, P., Parks, R. E. Jr. 1971. *The Pharmacological Basis of Therapeutics*, ed. L. S. Goodman, A. Gilman, pp. 1360–64. New York: Macmillan
46. Hellman, K. 1972. *Proc. R. Soc. Med.* 65:264
47. Turk, J. L., Parker, D. 1973. *Immunology* 24:751–58
48. Johnson, R. K., Goldin, A. 1975. *Cancer Treatment Rev.* 2:1–31
49. Berenbaum, M. C. 1969. *Antibiot. Chemother.* 15:155–76

50. Bretscher, P. A. 1974. *Cell. Immunol.* 13:171–95
51. Askenase, P. W. Hayden, B. J. 1974. *Immunology* 27:563–76
52. Zembala, M., Asherson, G. L. 1970. *Cell. Immunol.* 1:276–89
53. Mackaness, G. B., Lagrange, P. H., Ishibashi, T. 1974. *J. Exp. Med.* 139:1540–52
54. Lagrange, P. H., Mackaness, G. B., Miller, T. E., Pardon, P. 1975. *J. Immunol.* 114:442–46
55. Sjögren, H. O., Hellström, I., Bansal, S. C., Hellström, K. E. 1971. *Proc. Natl. Acad. Sci. USA* 68:1372–75
56. Hellström, K. E., Hellström, I. 1970. *Ann. Rev. Microbiol.* 24:373–98
57. Hellström, I., Hellström, K. E., Sjögren, H. O., Warner, G. A. 1971. *Int. J. Cancer* 7:1–16
58. Hellström, I., Warner, G. A., Hellström, K. E., Sjögren, H. O. 1973. *Int. J. Cancer* 11:280–92
59. Heppner, G. H., Stolbach, L., Byrne, M., Cummings, F. J., McDonough, E., Calabresi, P. 1973. *Int. J. Cancer* 11:245–60
60. Heppner, G. H., Calabresi, P. 1972. *J. Natl. Cancer Inst.* 48:1161–67
61. Steele, G., Pierce, G. E. 1974. *Int. J. Cancer* 13:572–78
62. Steele, G., Sjögren, H. O., Ankerst, J. 1974. *Int. J. Cancer* 14:743–52
63. Mott, M. G. 1973. *Lancet* 1:1092–94

MORPHOLOGICAL METHODS FOR EVALUATION OF PULMONARY TOXICITY IN ANIMALS

♦6655

D. L. Dungworth, L. W. Schwartz, W. S. Tyler
California Primate Research Center and School of Veterinary Medicine, University of
California, Davis, California 95616

R. F. Phalen
Department of Community and Environmental Medicine, California College of Medicine,
University of California, Irvine, California 92664

INTRODUCTION

The mammalian respiratory system has a variety of important functions in addition to the primary one of gaseous exchange (1, 2). The corresponding diversity of structural components of the respiratory tract, compounded by the inhomogeneity of morphologic responses of the lung to damaging agents, necessitates extremely careful selection and implementation of the several morphological methods required for its examination. Methods must be sensitive enough to reveal the presence and nature of subtle effects, and also to provide information on which useful hypotheses of pathogenesis can be based.

This review is designed to present the important considerations in the choice of methods and is a guide to references describing them in more detail. It is not intended to be a detailed critique of methods or a complete laboratory protocol. Much of the review deals with the routine necessary for the satisfactory search for and documentation of toxic effects. Emphasis is on the sine qua non for detecting subtle effects, which provide the most discriminating information relevant to pulmonary toxicity. The remainder of the review briefly addresses special methods for investigating various aspects of the pathogenesis of pulmonary lesions likely to be encountered and which are necessary for furthering the understanding of pulmonary pathobiology.

ROUTINE EVALUATION

Gross Examination

The methods to be described in this and subsequent sections are postmortem procedures, although most are applicable to surgical specimens. Radiographic studies, therefore, are not discussed. They can provide indications of gross and subgross morphologic changes in vivo, however, and are particularly pertinent to chronic studies involving the larger experimental animals.

TRACHEOBRONCHIAL TREE AND PARENCHYMA   The animal is deeply anesthetized by sodium pentobarbital and killed by exsanguination. The trachea and lungs are carefully exposed after the diaphragm is punctured, and search is made for abnormalities of the pleural cavity and its parietal and visceral surfaces (e.g. excessive fluid, adhesions). The trachea is transected 3–5 rings distal to the larynx, and the distal portion with attached lungs and other thoracic viscera removed. The surfaces of the trachea and lungs are examined for signs of abnormalities (e.g. indications of edema, hemorrhage, consolidation, emphysema, scarring, possible tumor nodules). These can be documented photographically or schematically in outline drawings. The partially collapsed state of the normal regions of the excised lung results in exaggerated appearance of the abnormalities and enables detection of small lesions that sometimes cannot be discerned in the inflated state. The extent to which the major airways and pulmonary parenchyma need be opened depends on the amount of gross damage. If there is no sign of edema or an exudative lesion, the examination of airways and parenchyma is left until after fixation. Even where major airways are opened, samples of lungs should be retained for perfusion fixation by the airways. The weight and fluid-displacement volume of the lungs can be obtained after tying off the major vessels and dissecting away the heart and mediastinum, if the degree and nature of the abnormalities observed indicate these would be useful quantitative parameters. The volume of fresh unfixed lungs is better measured from radiographs, however, as recommended by Dunnill et al (3).

NASOPHARYNX AND LARYNX   These structures should be surveyed for damage and the need for more extensive examination determined. In laboratory rodents, the nasal sinuses and turbinates can be examined by removing the overlying nasal bone with forceps or by sagittal section. In larger animals such as the dog, a sagittal section is made. Except in cases of tumors or severe upper respiratory irritation by inhaled materials, microscopic methods are usually necessary for detection of changes in these regions.

Fixation

CHOICE OF FIXATIVE AND METHOD OF FIXATION   Criteria for suitable fixation are production of least artifact, reproducibility, and simplicity and cost. The major aim with respect to production of least artifact is to retain as close as possible the in vivo appearance of the lung immediately preceding death. With pulmonary tissue, in addition to the usual fixation artifacts that have to be considered (e.g. shrinkage, mechanical distortion, changes in cellular organelles), there is the need to prepare pulmonary parenchyma for microscopic examination such that the correct configurations and relationships of airspaces are retained. Fixation by immersing small pieces of lung in various fluids is a common routine procedure. With the exception of severe exudative processes or where there are solid lesions such as tumors, however, immersion-fixed lungs do not provide proper definition of either normal or abnormal components. The preferred method of distending the lungs by perfusion of fixative through the airways eliminates these disadvantages by returning the lung to a state similar to that in vivo.

The work of Heard and colleagues (4, 5) is the basis for most of the methods of perfusion via the airways used today. After the lungs have been examined grossly, they are inflated with fixative via the trachea at 30 cm of fluid pressure measured from the surface of the fixative bath in which the lungs are immersed. We have used pumps to provide the necessary height of fixative in the reservoir for large animals (e.g. horses) but have found the marriott bottle to be the most suitable device for lungs from animals the size of dogs or monkeys down to mice. We routinely use 30 cm of water pressure, since this is clearly on the plateau of the pressure-volume curve for all of these species and should not result in tearing or rupture of tissues. Fixation of dog lungs at 25 cm of water pressure has resulted in incompletely filled or distended alveoli. This is characterized by folds in the interalveolar septum, which at total lung capacity should be straight. Specimens prepared at pressures that result in incomplete distension of the alveoli and airways are not suitable for morphometric analysis using stereological procedures, and are less suitable for scanning electron microscopy because of local variations in the degree of distension and therefore interrelationships of the component parts. The airway perfusion method can be applied equally well to one lung or, as is sometimes necessary in large animals, to one lobe or bronchopulmonary segment. A more extensive discussion of general methods of fixation can be found in the report by Dunnill et al (3).

Fixation by perfusion through the airways not only maintains the dimensions and configurations of the tissues at approximately total lung capacity, but also provides a large volume of fixative in intimate contact with the various surfaces, which is essential to rapid fixation. The distance the fixative must diffuse for complete penetration is minimal. This method has for general studies the additional advantage of providing a relatively unobstructed view of cell surfaces for scanning electron microscopy by flushing off mucous coat and alveolar lining material. It has the disadvantage of causing some translocation of exudates and particles and of providing a specific artifact of increased tissue spaces around pulmonary vessels, the so-called edema artifact.

The choice of fixative is also a major consideration in view of the large numbers of fixatives that have been used for the respiratory system. The main components of these fixatives are usually one or more aldehydes, buffer, and various salts with high purity water so that the fixative has a constant pH and osomolality. Many investigators today use a mixture of glutaraldehyde and formaldehyde made from paraformaldehyde, which results in rapid penetration and thorough fixation. Cacodylic acid is generally preferred as the buffer because it results in resilient lungs; that is, blocks of lung compressed by cutting rapidly resume their original fixed volume when placed in fresh fixative. A small amount of calcium is commonly added to the fixative to preserve phospholipids associated with pulmonary surfactant as well as those that are components of the various cell membranes. Although iso-osmotic fixatives are used, we prefer a hypertonic fixative (approximately 550 milliosmoles). All of the above desirable characteristics are achieved using a modification of Karnovsky's formaldehyde/glutaraldehyde fixative with added calcium chloride (paraformaldehyde, 40 g/liter; glutaraldehyde, 100 ml of 50% solution/liter; calcium chloride, 0.5 g/liter; cacodylic acid, 12.8 g/liter) which is diluted 1 to 4.5 before use with cacodylic acid (32 g/liter) and the pH adjusted to 7.2 with 1.0 N HCl (6). The fixative is relatively simple to prepare and can be stored in the refrigerator for several months. It has the advantage of being a good storage fluid for keeping fixed tissues at room temperature. Using this fixative at 30 cm of pressure, fixation is rapid and complete. Fixation times of 2 and 4 hr are acceptable, but we prefer to maintain the 30 cm of pressure overnight or for 18 hr. Samples cut from these lungs are placed in fresh room temperature fixative where they may be stored without damage or deterioration for more than one year.

Fixation of lungs at a standard pressure of 30 cm of the fluid provides the most reproducible appearance for general purposes. Considerations of reproducibility and least artifact become more critical relative to morphometry. Here again, for purposes of pathology we find perfusion of the excised lung to be the method of choice. The alternative approach such as used for morphometry of normal lungs is perfusion via the trachea with the lungs in situ within the thoracic cavity (7).

Perfusion of excised lungs by trachea or major bronchus is a relatively simple procedure for rodents, once a series of delivery tubes leading from marriott bottle reservoirs is provided. Larger reservoirs are needed for lungs of larger species. Although the perfusion method cannot be performed as rapidly as immersion of samples in fixative, the greater effectiveness in enabling detection and evaluation of subtle or mild lesions more than outweighs the greater cost in time taken. Where large numbers of animals per treatment group are involved, at least a significant proportion of lungs should be fixed by airway perfusion.

FIXATION OF LUNG BY PERFUSION THROUGH AIRWAYS   As will be evident from the foregoing discussion, our preferred routine method of fixation is perfusion by the airways with modified Karnovsky's fixative at 30 cm of fluid pressure (6). We find that after partial collapse of the lungs has occurred on excision, no degassing is necessary to obtain complete distribution of the perfusate. Degassing is in fact contraindicated for most purposes because it increases the cumbersomeness of the technique, lessens the degree of reproducibility of reinflation, and makes redistribution of components of any lesion more likely.

FIXATION OF LUNG BY IMMERSION   Massively consolidated or edematous parenchyma, or large solid lesions such as tumors, have to be fixed by immersion in fixative fluid. For subsequent study by light microscopy, formol-Zenker is preferable to formalin because it heightens the contrast of hematoxylin and eosin staining, especially the eosinophilia of proteinaceous transudates or exudates. The shrinkage caused by immersion in fixative is used to advantage in enumeration of tumor nodules in lungs of strain A mice, which is the basis of a carcinogenesis bioassay system (8). Tissue to be examined by electron microscopy is immersed in the modified Karnovsky's fixative described previously.

Immersion fixation is also used when the redistribution of intraluminal particles, cells, or exudates might interfere with the objectives of the study, as in determining the fate of inhaled particles (9, 10).

FIXATION OF NASOPHARYNX AND LARYNX   After gross examination, these structures in small animals (i.e. rodents) can be fixed in toto in the modified Karnovsky's fixative after flushing surfaces with fixative to remove trapped air bubbles and mucous coat. Samples of tissues from recognized lesions and representative portions of the nasoturbinate region, pharynx, and larynx need to be dissected out in large animals.

Sampling for Microscopic Examination

The size and diversity of components of the respiratory tract pose a considerable sampling problem in the thorough search for lesions. This is compounded by the inhomogeneity of morphologic responses of the tract to irritants, as was mentioned in the introduction. These two features together require that sampling be both wide in distribution and specific in anatomic localization. The number of large blocks taken for examination by light microscopy and scanning electron microscopy will be determined by the compromise between thoroughness and the practical limit in terms of cost of preparation and examination. But there is a minimum below which the risk of spurious conclusions due to serious sampling errors becomes unacceptable. Any sampling of parenchyma must take into account vertical (gravitational) gradients affecting the distribution patterns of certain lesions and the difference between hilar and peripheral regions of lobes.

TRACHEOBRONCHIAL TREE AND PARENCHYMA   The sampling procedure varies according to the size of the lung. In the case of rodents such as rats and hamsters, sampling of the trachea presents few problems other than the need to be aware of possible differences in the mucosa over the cartilaginous and intercartilaginous portions of the trachea as has been found in the rat (11). A block containing a longitudinal section of distal trachea and the bifurcation into bronchi suffices for nonparenchymal regions. The preferred planes of section for rodents' lungs are illustrated in Figure 1. These are vertical sections in the sagittal plane for the left lung and from the hilus along the axis of major airways for the cranial, middle, and caudal lobes of the right lung. All of these blocks can be sectioned whole for histologic examination. Although the sagittal section of the left lung is a common section for major attention, we prefer the sections from the right middle and caudal lobes. One reason is that unless the section of the left lung is cut very close to the midline, most of the airways are cut transversely. The longitudinal sections of airways present in blocks from the right middle and caudal lobes reveal bronchial and acinar orientations of lesions much more readily, especially by scanning electron microscopy (SEM). A second reason is that the blocks from the right lung are of a more convenient size to mount whole for light microscopy.

More care in sampling is required for lungs of larger animals such as dogs and monkeys because of the bulk of tissue to be surveyed and the increased likelihood of regional variations in response being manifested. To minimize sampling errors, standard parenchymal sampling sites covering both dorsoventral and hilarperipheral axes should be chosen. The nine sampling sites we take from parenchyma of the four lobes of the right lung of the dog are illustrated in Figure 2. Because we frequently use one lung of dogs and monkeys for biochemical studies or those

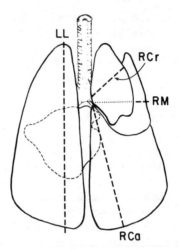

Figure 1   Schematic outline of the dorsal view of a rat's lungs illustrating the vertical planes of section for sampling tissue. The contour of the accessory lobe is indicated by the narrow broken line. LL, left lung; RCr, right cranial lobe; RM, right middle lobe; RCa, right caudal lobe.

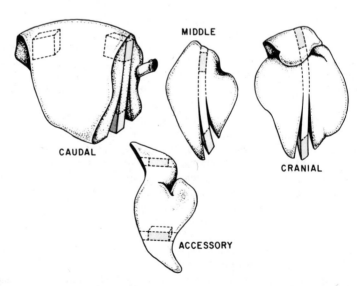

Figure 2   Schematic outline of the lateral view of the four lobes of a dog's right lung illustrating nine sampling sites.

requiring special fixation, such as freezing, we derive most morphologic information on the basis of one lung. If the two lungs are available, samples can be taken from both. Samples of major airways typically consist of proximal trachea, bifurcation of trachea, and lobar bronchus.

Evaluation of pulmonary toxicity invariably involves the comparison of lungs from two or more groups of animals. For this specific comparison, by qualitative or quantitative (morphometric) means, we use the same sampling sites for tissue blocks in all animals (12) rather than the method of stratified random sampling using a random number table together with a numbered sampling grid (13). The latter method relates more to statistical confidence with which the sample represents the lung from which the sample is taken, rather than to precise comparison among different lungs where the lesion can be affected by specific anatomic location.

When detailed comparisons are required within or among groups of animals, a useful approach is to select a specific bronchopulmonary segment of the lung for more specific study. Sections of segmental bronchus, terminal bronchiole, and more distal lobular tissue can be sliced out of the desired bronchopulmonary segment under a dissecting microscope. These sections, as well as those of trachea and lobar bronchus, can then be closely compared.

NASOPHARYNX AND LARYNX   Blocks are taken representing proximal and distal regions of nasal sinuses and turbinates, and the pharynx and larynx. Again, more are required for larger animals. For some studies it is desirable to dissect mucosa from the nasal septum or turbinates and prepare it as a whole mount for morphological examination. Further details of the use of whole mounts and sections of nasal regions can be found elsewhere (14, 15).

Microscopic Examination

The need for examination of a wide sampling of pulmonary tissue has already been stressed. Requirements for cost effectiveness in the evaluation of lungs from large numbers of animals in toxicity trials means that the microscopic methods most useful are those that provide for examination of large samples, that is, light microscopy (LM) and SEM. For initial detection and analysis of lesions we use correlated LM and SEM. The best way to do this generally is to take complementary blocks of tissue from the same sampling site, embed one in plastic suitable for large 1 μ sections and process the other for SEM. The surface and sectioned views can then be compared for interpretation. The advantage of the large 1 μ section is that it not only provides the best resolution for LM, but also enables precise selection of anatomic locations for thin sections to be examined by transmission electron microscopy (TEM).

This is a discussion of routine microscopic methods and we recognize that the word can take on shades of difference in meaning according to the objectives of the investigations. Often, most microscopic screening has to be by LM of paraffin-embedded tissue because of the bulk of specimens. Equally so, it must be realized that in the search for subtle effects or in the description of damage once it is found, at least a significant number of lungs from animals in the critical experimental groups should be examined by correlated LM, SEM, and TEM.

LIGHT MICROSCOPY   Survey by LM of sections carefully prepared from vacuum-embedded paraffin blocks and stained by hematoxylin and eosin provides the basis for other modes of microscopic investigation (Figure 3). More definitive study of cellular components of lesions is made on the 1 μ sections cut from large plastic-embedded blocks and these provide the essential link between LM and TEM (see segment on TEM below). The paraffin sections also provide the basis for a large variety of special staining methods (16).

SCANNING ELECTRON MICROSCOPY The large, approximately 12 X 10 X 4 mm samples of tissue selected for SEM are the complementary halves of blocks used for LM and are cut so as to include longitudinal sections of airways in the surface to be examined (Figures 4–6). The tissue blocks are dehydrated in graded ethanol and then dried by the critical point procedure using CO_2 (6, 17). The dried tissue is attached to standard SEM stubs put in a high vacuum coating device on a tilting and rotating stage and coated first with carbon then with gold-palladium (18). Such tissues can be stored in a desiccator for prolonged periods and still be useful for SEM.

Although not a routine procedure, to enable precise correlation between surface features seen by SEM and cross-sectional features of selected areas, blocks can be removed from the SEM stub after evaluation and prepared for LM and TEM. They are placed in 100% ethanol, which is next substituted by propylene oxide, and are then embedded in an Epon-Araldite mixture. The tissue is examined by LM of 1 μ sections, and specific regions can be selected for TEM (18). Information on

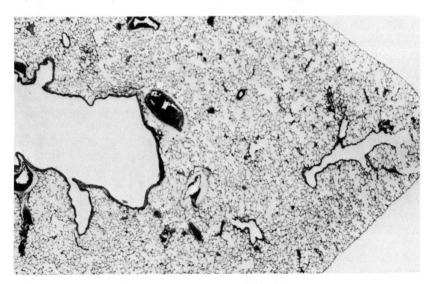

Figure 3   Light microscopy of properly prepared paraffin sections provides a relatively simple and rapid means of screening all levels of the tracheobronchial tree and parenchyma. Normal rat lung, H & E stain, 12 X.

interior aspects of tissues and cells can be obtained by SEM after the tissue has been fractured either before (19) or after (20) drying. It can also be obtained from plastic-embedded tissue after iodine and acetone surface etching (21).

TRANSMISSION ELECTRON MICROSCOPY   Because lesions in the lung are frequently focal and have a specific orientation relative to the acinar structure of the pulmonary parenchyma, it is essential to know precisely the anatomic location in the small airways or acinus from which the TEM blocks are taken. This precise location can be learned by several routes. The oldest is a modification of the procedure used by Grimley (22) wherein large, 2 X 2 cm blocks of tissue are embedded as for TEM, and alternate 30 μ and 10 μ sections cut on a large microtome commonly used for metal or bone. The 10 μ sections are evaluated using light microscopy, and the precise lesion area is dissected from the adjacent 30 μ section, cemented on a block from a beem capsule, and ultrathin sections cut (23). It has the disadvantage of relatively low resolution for LM due to the thickness of the section. This can be avoided by embedding slightly smaller blocks (i.e. 12 X 10 mm) and cutting 1 μ sections on a Sorval JB-4 microtome using glass knives. These thin sections can be stained using various dyes and provide high resolution for evaluation of the tissue by LM (Figures 7A, B). The areas of interest are selected in the one-micron section, identified in the block, and the surrounding tissue removed leaving a plastic mesa containing the required region (24). This mesa is sectioned in the usual manner and examined by TEM (Figure 7C).

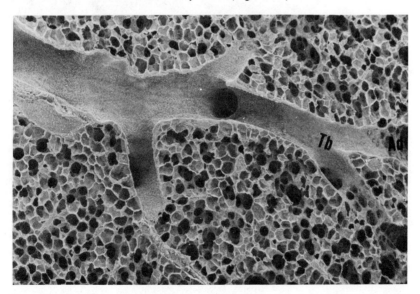

Figure 4   SEM enables evaluation of surfaces and is intermediate in resolution between LM and TEM. It allows the examination of relatively large areas and provides a great depth of field as illustrated in this micrograph of normal rat lung. Tb, terminal bronchiole; Ad, alveolar duct; 30 X.

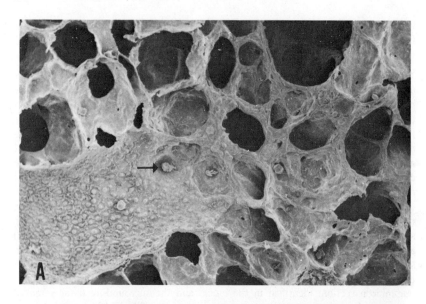

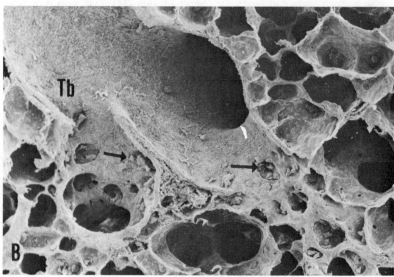

Figure 5 *A*. The transition region from terminal bronchiole to alveolar duct is an area frequently damaged by inhaled irritants. Occasional macrophages (*arrow*) can be observed within proximal alveoli of this alveolar duct from a normal rat, 170 X. *B*. Compared to the normal, in the rat following exposure to ozone (0.8 ppm for 7 days) the terminal bronchiole has a flattened surface appearance (Tb) and proximal alveoli contain clusters of infiltrating inflammatory cells and debris (*arrows*), 160 X.

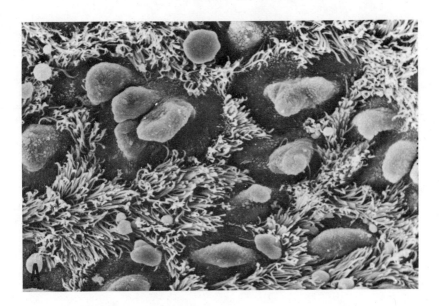

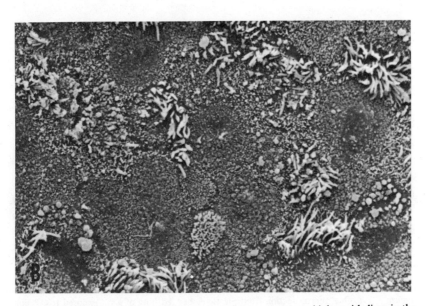

Figure 6 *A.* Highly magnified SEM view of normal terminal bronchiolar epithelium in the rat, 2800 X. *B.* In contrast, note the loss of surface projections of nonciliated bronchiolar (Clara) cells and the shortening and reduced density of cilia in a rat exposed to 0.8 ppm ozone for 7 days, 2300 X.

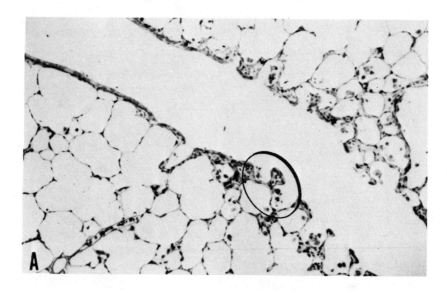

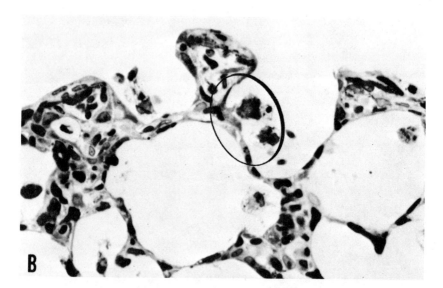

Figure 7   A. One micron section from plastic-embedded lung of a rat exposed to 0.8 ppm ozone for 2 days provides good resolution of cellular detail by LM and localization of specific region of interest (*circled*). Richardson trichrome, 111 X. *B.* Higher magnification of area circled in *A,* 500 X.

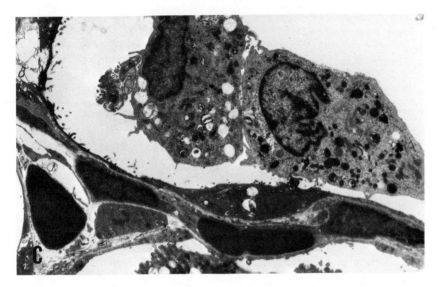

Figure 7   C. Using the mesa technique, a portion of the lesion, such as circled in *B,* can be selected and thin sections from the same region of the block examined by TEM. Uranyl acetate and lead citrate, 3750 X.

SPECIAL METHODS FOR GROSS AND SUBGROSS EVALUATION

Whole Lung Sections

The technique of preparing whole sections from human lungs was first described by Gough & Wentworth (25) and was used in their studies of emphysema in man. The sections can be useful as permanent records or illustrations of whole lung involvement in certain types of disease processes. Subsequent developments of the technique and their use in the measurement or grading of emphysema in human lungs is briefly discussed in a report by Dunnill et al (3). Preparation of lung macrosections and their permanent mounting by their lamination between sheets of transparent plastic film has also been described (26, 27).

Vascular Injection Technique

A technique using thin slices of lungs in which the vessels have been injected with multicolored latex has been used in studies of the comparative subgross pulmonary anatomy of a variety of mammals (28, 29). A major focus of attention in these studies was the comparative anatomy of the vascular tree. Vascular injection and casting have been used in investigations of the vascular changes accompanying emphysema in man (30).

Airway Casting

This is useful for development of mathematical models for behavior of inspired gases and particles (31) and for the study of airway disease (32) and the pathogenesis of emphysema (33).

Replica casts of airways down to and including alveoli can be prepared in situ for large and small animals (31). The method involves replacement of air by cyclic ventilation with CO_2, filling of the lungs with degassed saline, and slowly injecting silicone rubber through the trachea while allowing saline to drain from the thorax via slits between ribs. After curing (2–20 hr) the organ is removed from the thorax and the tissue digested away. Morphometric measurements that may be made on such casts include branching angles and dimensions of airways and alveoli. In some cases alveolar pores can be seen and their relative sizes determined via the scanning electron microscope.

The major limitation in using airway casts is that all but the simplest measurements made on them may require considerable time, effort, and skill. On the other hand, a replica cast captures and preserves the entire airway structure, allowing precise determination of the spatial and structural distribution of lesions.

SPECIAL METHODS OF MICROSCOPIC EVALUATION

A variety of investigative methods is needed in the search for pathogenetic mechanisms underlying disease processes in the lung, as it is for any organ. These methods are relevant to studies of both cellular biology and pathobiology, and unavoidably investigations into the one have considerable impact on the other. The techniques in question have for the most part either been in use for a relatively short time, or are in the process of being explored. Only an introduction to these topics is therefore provided.

Histochemistry

Histochemistry and cytochemistry are essential for the full elucidation of the pathogenesis of toxic changes in inhomogeneous organs such as the lung, because it is necessary to localize biochemical changes to the specific cells or cell populations involved.

Many specialized methods of tissue preparation and incubation are required for the broad spectrum of histochemistry. Enzyme histochemistry and histochemistry for certain other cellular components are best done on cryostat sections. As with all sections of pulmonary parenchyma, distended cryostat sections are much easier to evaluate and provide more useful information. Usually the tissue is distended with a cryostat embedding material, commonly 4% gelatin, as originally described by Tyler & Pearse (34). This embedment has the double advantage of distending the lung and also providing a medium that permits much more complete sections than can be obtained if the lung is handled like other organs or tissues. Without such embedding, only fragments of sections are obtainable. These are extremely difficult to evaluate in terms of total distal airway and parenchymal morphology. Freezing of the gelatin-infiltrated section is generally accomplished using Freon 22® cooled to near its freezing point of −160°C. Freezing directly in liquid nitrogen is considerably slower and frequently distorts the tissue blocks. While most cryostat sections tend to be thicker and therefore provide less resolution than paraffin sections, with appropriate equipment it is possible to cut serial frozen sections at 5 or 6 μm. Such sections are suitable for a wide variety of histochemical procedures, which are commonly applied to the serial section in order to obtain correlated biochemical and morphological information at the cellular level.

Histochemical procedures have been diversified significantly in recent years (35) and include methods for many enzymes as well as cell inclusions and intercellular material. Many of these procedures can be applied at both the light and electron microscopic levels of observation of the lung (36–40) and some are suitable for automated image analysis (41). The studies of Spicer et al (42) and Lamb & Reid (43, 44) concerning toxic effects of inhaled gases on respiratory mucopolysaccharides are especially noteworthy. Another example is the fluorescent amine technique of Falck that has been used in studies of serotonin-producing cells of neuroepithelial bodies present in respiratory mucosa (45).

A promising new area of chemical analysis that can be applied to the respiratory system is that of analyzing X rays, cathodoluminescence, or back-scattered electrons generated by the interaction of the electron beam of an SEM or TEM with the atoms of cellular components, inclusions, or histochemical final reaction products in situ, thus providing elemental analysis of endogenous or foreign materials in cells and tissues (46–49).

Autoradiography

Autoradiography has been used to determine the cytokinetics of pulmonary cells responding to damage caused by toxic environments, such as in the demonstrations that alveolar type 2 epithelial cells are the precursors of type 1 epithelial cells (50, 51). The second major use of autoradiographic techniques is for tracing the intracellular pathways traversed by radiolabeled precursors of known or hypothesized cell products (52–54). A third use is in studying the deposition and fate of inhaled particles (55).

Morphometry

Morphometry is necessary for precise correlation of structure and function in both normal and diseased organs. It can provide accurate measurement of the severity of damage in diseased organs, and it is the only means of confirming, by statistical methods, the existence of significant subtle lesions in a particular treatment group of experimental animals.

A systematic approach to a quantitative morphologic analysis of the architecture of the pulmonary system using manual methods has been provided by Dunnill (56), Weibel (57), and Thurlbeck (58). Those authors established the formulae and methods necessary to obtain statistically reliable quantitative values for the pulmonary system. Recently quantitation of the pulmonary system has been automated by use of computed pattern recognition techniques (59) and automated measuring microscopes (60). The greatest application of automation has been with automated measuring microscopes. They have been used to quantitate selected features of conducting airways in normal and experimental bronchitis (61) and of distal airspaces in normal (62), emphysematous (63), and experimental, pollutant-damaged lung (12, 64). Pattern recognition techniques have also recently been used to classify and measure the distal airways on an automated measuring microscope (65).

Freeze-Fracture

Freeze-fracture is a method of looking at replicas of fractured surfaces at very high resolution using TEM. Like the SEM, it provides a view of surfaces rather than cross sections. Thus for low magnification and low resolution of natural or fractured surfaces, the SEM is the most appropriate instrument, whereas for high magnification, high resolution freeze-fracture or freeze-etch is the most appropriate technique.

Freeze-fracture procedures avoid the necessity for including chemical interactions, which may cause artifacts in the preparation of tissue, and reveal an en face view of membranous surfaces. In the pulmonary system, the method has been used for study of cell organelles, particularly during secretion and phagocytosis (66), for visualization of the alveolar lining layer (67), and in the examination of endothelial cells relative to their capability for metabolizing circulating vasoactive agents (68). The method is also necessary for the study of normal and abnormal cell junctions (69).

Tracer Techniques

These have been used in studies of the permeability of the pulmonary vasculature in both normal and edematous lungs. Horseradish peroxidase, hemoglobin, microperoxidase, ferritin, and colloidal particles have been used (70–74). The investigations on pathways of clearance of inhaled iron oxide aerosols (10) or intratracheally instilled ferritin or colloidal carbon (9) referred to earlier also involved the use of tracers.

Thick Histologic Sections

These were principally used in the study of human emphysema (75). To some extent they have been superseded by SEM, but they still have an important role in documenting the pattern of collagenous and elastic fibers in interalveolar septa and determining their abnormalities during the pathogenesis of diseases such as emphysema.

ADDITIONAL SPECIAL METHODS OF FIXATION

No one fixation procedure is appropriate for all investigative purposes. To the extent that considerations of methods of fixation are intimately related to the techniques of evaluation for which they are to be employed, common fixation techniques have already been discussed. There remain several, however, that have special indications to be matched with the specific aims of the investigator.

Vapor Fixation

Methods have been developed for the use of formalin vapor (76, 77) or formalin steam (78) but have little to offer in the way of advantages and nothing at all in convenience. Air fixation likewise has no usefulness other than to provide a convenient gross anatomical reference. A recent method of vapor fixation using osmium tetroxide suspended in cooled fluorocarbon has been briefly reported by Kilburn & McKenzie (79). The mixture was injected intratracheally into breathing hamsters to fix the lungs while inflated and to lessen the chance of translocation of cells and particles on luminal surfaces of airways.

Vascular Perfusion

The primary use of this method has been in the demonstration of extracellular lining layers of alveoli and bronchioles by electron microscopy (80, 81). Translocation of cells and particles should be less than by intratracheal perfusion, which may make this method useful for localization of these components.

Rapid-Freeze Method

This method was developed by Staub & Storey (82). It provides an accurate representation of the morphologic state of the lung "frozen" at a point in time in its cycle of dynamic events. The animal's lungs are frozen while it is alive, at the desired phase of the respiratory cycle. The procedure does require thoracotomy with good exposure of the lungs. Carefully controlled ventilation is required to maintain physiological state with the ability to momentarily hold the lung at the desired degree of inflation or vascular perfusion. Freon 22 cooled to near its freezing point of $-160°C$ or propane cooled to $-175°C$ is used as the cryogenic agent for rapid freezing as each of them absorbs significantly more heat per unit volume of weight than liquid nitrogen, which rapidly absorbs heat, then boils, forming an air interface which effectively reduces the transmission of additional heat from the specimen to the cryogenic agent. Only the first few millimeters of tissue under the pleura are extremely rapidly frozen; deeper tissue is frozen considerably more slowly. Tissues frozen in this manner may be freeze-dried or freeze-substituted for subsequent critical point drying followed by evaluation in the SEM (6) or followed by embedding in paraffin or plastic for light microscopy (23) or TEM. In the SEM, the general architecture of the pulmonary tissues is well preserved and available for evaluation, but the surface detail of the cells is obscured by the mucous coat or alveolar lining layer in the airways or alveoli respectively.

ACKNOWLEDGMENTS

We are grateful for the assistance that we have received from our associates, M. E. G. Brummer, W. L. Castleman, D. M. Hyde and P. M. Lowrie. The work cited from our group is supported in part by NIH grants ES00628 and RR00169. Preparation of this review was aided by USAF contract F33615-76-C-5005 and by California Air Resources Board contract 4–611 with the Department of Community and Environmental Medicine, California College of Medicine, University of California, Irvine, California.

Literature Cited

1. Heinemann, H. O., Fishman, A. P. 1969. *Physiol. Rev.* 49:1–47
2. Fishman, A. P., Pietra, G. G. 1974. *New Engl. J. Med.* 291:953–59
3. Dunnill, M. S., Fletcher, C. M., Cumming, G., Heath, D. A., Heppleston, A. G., Lamb, D., Leopold, J. G., Wagner, J. C. 1975. *Thorax* 30:241–51
4. Heard, B. E. 1958. *Thorax* 13:136–49
5. Heard, B. E., Esterly, J. R., Wootliff, J. S. 1967. *Am. Rev. Respir. Dis.* 95:311–12
6. Nowell, J. A., Pangborn, J., Tyler, W. S. 1972. *Scanning Electron Microsc./1972*, pp. 305–12
7. Forrest, J. B., Weibel, E. R. 1975. *Respir. Physiol.* 24:191–202
8. Shimkin, M. B., Stoner, G. D. 1975. *Adv. Cancer Res.* 21:1–58
9. Lauweryns, J. M., Baert, J. H. 1974. *Ann. NY Acad. Sci.* 221:244–75
10. Sorokin, S. P., Brain, J. D. 1975. *Anat. Rec.* 181:581–626
11. Schwartz, L. W., Dungworth, D. L., Mustafa, M. G., Tarkington, B. K., Tyler, W. S. 1976. *Lab. Invest.* In press
12. Hyde, D. M., Wiggins, A., Dungworth, D. L., Tyler, W. S., Orthœfer, J. 1976. *J. Microsc. Oxford.* In press
13. Dunnill, M. S. 1964. *Thorax* 19:443–48
14. Bang, B. G., Bang, F. B. 1961. *Proc. Soc. Exp. Biol. Med.* 106:516–21
15. Adams, D. R. 1972. *Am. J. Anat.* 133:37–49
16. Luna, L. G. 1968. *Manual of Histologic Staining Methods of the Armed Forces Institute of Pathology.* New York: McGraw-Hill. 258 pp.
17. Anderson, T. F. 1951. *Trans. NY Acad. Sci. Ser. II* 13:130–34
18. Brummer, M. E. G., Lowrie, P. M., Tyler, W. S. 1975. *Scanning Electron Microsc./1975*, pp. 333–40
19. Humphreys, W. J., Spurlock, B. O., Johnson, J. S. 1974. *Scanning Electron Microsc./1974*, pp. 275–82
20. Watson, J. H. L., Page, R. H., Swedo, J. L. 1975. *Scanning Electron Microsc./1975*, pp. 417–24
21. Pachter, B. R., Penha, D., Davidowitz, J. 1974. *Scanning Electron Microsc./1974*, pp. 746–52
22. Grimley, P. M. 1965. *Stain Technol.* 40:259–63
23. Plopper, C. G., Dungworth, D. L., Tyler, W. S. 1973. *Am. J. Pathol.* 71:375–94
24. Lowrie, P. M., Tyler, W. S. 1973. *Proc. 31st Ann. Meet. Electron Microsc. Soc. Am.*, 324–25. Baton Rouge: Claitors
25. Gough, J., Wentworth, J. D. 1960. *Recent Advances in Pathology*, p. 80. London: Churchill. 7th ed.
26. Côté, R. A., Korthy, A. L., Kory, R. C. 1963. *Dis. Chest* 43:1–7
27. Kory, R. C., Rauterkus, L. T., Korthy, A. L., Côté, R. A. 1966. *Am. Rev. Respir. Dis.* 93:758–68
28. McLaughlin, R. F., Tyler, W. S., Canada, R. O. 1961. *Am. J. Anat.* 108:149–65
29. McLaughlin, R. F., Tyler, W. S., Canada, R. O. 1966. *Am. Rev. Respir. Dis.* 94:380–87
30. Wyatt, J. P., Fischer, V. W., Sweet, H. C. 1964. *Am. Rev. Respir. Dis.* 89: Part 1, 533–60; Part 2, 721–35
31. Phalen, R. F., Yeh, H.-C., Raabe, O. G., Velasquez, D. J. 1973. *Anat. Rec.* 177:255–63
32. Horsfield, K., Cumming, G., Hicken, P. 1966. *Am. Rev. Respir. Dis.* 93:900–906
33. Pump, K. K. 1973. *Am. Rev. Respir. Dis.* 108:610–20
34. Tyler, W. S., Pearse, A. G. E. 1965. *Thorax* 20:149–52
35. Pearse, A. G. E. 1968–1972. *Histochemistry, Theoretical and Applied*, Vol. 1, Boston: Little, Brown; Vol. 2, Baltimore: Williams & Wilkins. 2 vols. 3rd ed.
36. Castleman, W. L., Dungworth, D. L., Tyler, W. S. 1973. *Lab. Invest.* 29:310–19
37. Goldfischer, S., Kikkawa, Y., Hoffman, L. 1968. *J. Histochem. Cytochem.* 16:102–9
38. Sorokin, S. P. 1967. *J. Histochem. Cytochem.* 14:884–97
39. Cutz, E., Conen, P. E. 1971. *Am. J. Pathol.* 62:127–42
40. Schneeberger, E. E. 1972. *J. Histochem. Cytochem.* 20:180–91
41. Sherwin, R. P., Margolick, J. B., Azen, S. P. 1973. *Am. Rev. Respir. Dis.* 108:1015–18
42. Spicer, S. S., Chakrin, L. W., Wardell, J. R. Jr. 1974. *Am. Rev. Respir. Dis.* 110:13–24
43. Lamb, D., Reid, L. 1968. *J. Pathol. Bacteriol.* 96:97–111
44. Lamb, D., Reid, L. 1969. *Br. Med. J.* 1:33–35
45. Lauweryns, J. M., Cokelaere, M., Theunynck, P. 1973. *Science* 180:410–13
46. Johari, O. 1972. *Scanning Electron Microsc./1973*, pp. 364–74

47. Määttä, K., Arstila, A. U. 1975. *Lab. Invest.* 33:342–46
48. Funahashi, A., Pintar, K., Siegesmund, K. A. 1975. *Arch. Environ. Health* 30:285–89
49. Yakowitz, H. 1975. *Scanning Electron Microsc./1975,* pp. 1–10
50. Evans, M. J., Cabral, L. J., Stephens, R. J., Freeman, G. 1973. *Am. J. Pathol.* 70:175–98
51. Adamson, I. Y. R., Bowden, D. H. 1974. *Lab. Invest.* 30:35–42
52. Chevalier, G., Collet, A. J. 1972. *Anat. Rec.* 174:289–310
53. Petrik, P., Collet, A. J. 1974. *Am. J. Anat.* 139:519–34
54. Kikkawa, Y., Yoneda, K., Smith, F., Packard, B., Suzuki, K. 1975. *Lab. Invest.* 32:295–302
55. Felicetti, S. A., Silbaugh, S. A., Muggenburg, B. A., Hahn, F. F. 1975. *Health Phys.* 29:89–96
56. Dunnill, M. S. 1962. *Thorax* 17:320–28
57. Weibel, E. R. 1963. *Morphometry of the Human Lung.* New York: Academic. 151 pp.
58. Thurlbeck, W. M. 1967. *Am. Rev. Respir. Dis.* 95:765–73
59. Levine, M. D., Reisch, M. L., Thurlbeck, W. M. 1970. *IEEE Trans. Biomed. Eng.* BME-17, pp. 254–62
60. Cole, M. 1966. *Microscope* 15:148–60
61. Mawdesley-Thomas, L. E., Healey, P. 1973. *Arch. Environ. Health* 27:248–50
62. deBignon, J., André-Bougaran, J. 1969. *C. R. Acad. Sci. Ser. D* 269:409–12
63. Anderson, A. E. Jr., Foraker, A. G. 1971. *Am. J. Clin. Pathol.* 56:239–43
64. Sherwin, R. P., Margolick, J. B., Azen, S. P. 1973. *Arch. Environ. Health* 26:297–99

65. Hyde, D. M., Hallberg, D., Wiggins, A., Tyler, W. S., Dungworth, D. L., Orthoefer, J. 1976. *Proc. 6th Conf. Environ. Toxicol.,* Dayton, Ohio, 1975. In press
66. Lauweryns, J. M., Gombeer-Desmecht, M. 1973. *Pathobiol. Ann.* 8:257–82
67. Untersee, P., Gil, J., Weibel, E. R. 1971. *Respir. Physiol.* 13:171–85
68. Smith, U., Ryan, J. W., Smith, D. S. 1973. *J. Cell Biol.* 56:492–99
69. Hyde, D. M., Tyler, W. S., Dungworth, D. L. 1976. *Zentralbl. Veterinaermed. Reihe C.* In press (Abstr.)
70. Pietra, G. G., Szidon, J. P., Leventhal, M. M., Fishman, A. P. 1969. *Science* 166:1643–46
71. Szidon, J. P., Pietra, G. G., Fishman, A. P. 1972. *New Engl. J. Med.* 286:1200–1204
72. Schneeberger, E. E., Karnovsky, M. J. 1971. *J. Cell Biol.* 49:319–34
73. Williams, M. C., Wissig, S. L. 1975. *J. Cell Biol.* 66:531–55
74. Reese, T. S., Karnovsky, M. J. 1967. *J. Cell Biol.* 34:207–17
75. Pump, K. K. 1974. *Chest* 65:431–36
76. Blumenthal, B. J., Boren, H. G. 1959. *Am. Rev. Respir. Dis.* 79:764–72
77. Wright, B. M., Slavin, G., Kreel, L., Callan, K., Sandin, B. 1974. *Thorax* 29:189–94
78. Weibel, E. R., Vidone, R. A. 1961. *Am. Rev. Respir. Dis.* 84:856–61
79. Kilburn, K. H., McKenzie, W. 1975. *Science* 189:634–37
80. Gil, J., Weibel, E. R. 1969/1970. *Respir. Physiol.* 8:13–36
81. Gil, J., Weibel, E. R. 1971. *Anat. Rec.* 169:185–200
82. Staub, N. C., Storey, W. F. 1962. *J. Appl. Physiol.* 17:381–90

CUTANEOUS PHARMACOLOGY AND TOXICOLOGY

♦6656

Howard Maibach

Department of Dermatology, University of California Medical School, San Francisco, California 94143

This is the first review of cutaneous pharmacology and toxicology in this series. The choice of topics is highly personal—based on my experience and interests. This has been a period of greatly increased activity in this field; space limitations make this approach mandatory.

IRRITATION

Irritation is defined as nonimmunologically mediated dermatitis resulting from contact with a chemical. Some older texts imply that irritant dermatitis occurs in all subjects on first exposure. Actually, this holds only for the severest of irritants sometimes found in industry and laboratories but not for most drugs and consumer products. Some but not all irritants are also contact sensitizers.

Recent advances in the understanding of irritant dermatitis are conceptual rather than mechanistic or technical. By custom, standard toxicology texts classify chemicals as irritant or nonirritant; perusal of the Merck Index gives numerous examples (1). This nomenclature remains useful for industrial chemicals. For cutaneous drugs and consumer products it is realistic to accept that under appropriately exaggerated circumstances all chemicals—even water—are irritating. Current bioassays utilize this principle; a new chemical or product is compared to a similar agent for which there has been extensive human use. Rather than list a numerical score with somewhat arbitrary limits for acceptability, the new agent may be judged more, less, or equally as irritating as the standard.

Another conceptual advance considers chemicals as having a cumulative irritancy potential rather than an irritancy potential from single exposure. When dermatitis develops after repeated exposures of weeks to years, contact sensitization is generally assumed. While sensitization *may* occur in this situation, cumulative irritancy is even more likely with numerous chemical classes.

The Draize, Woodard & Calvery assay enjoys general acceptance (2). Finkelstein, Laden & Miechowski noted the limitations of the Draize method and started the trend to repetitive applications (3). Kligman & Wooding adapted repetitive irritancy testing (10 applications) to man (4).

Lanman, Elvers & Howard extended this to 21 application days in man, employing an all-or-none reading of dermatitis as their criterion to determine whether irritation has occurred (5). This was modified by Phillips, Steinberg, Maibach & Akers to utilize a five-point grading scale each day (6). This latter study and a sequel by Steinberg et al provide the most complete documentation of the relationship of animal and human irritancy assays (7).

In general the rabbit assay yields good correlation for man with chemicals and concentrations at either extreme—a great deal of irritation or almost no irritation (6). The rabbit can be employed for further definition of the middle ground by repetitive applications. Comparative human and repetitive rabbit data are summarized in the recent studies of Steinberg et al, Marzulli & Maibach (6, 8).

The rabbit is the animal commonly used for these assays; undoubtedly many others would be adequate. The advantages are cost and ease of handling; most important, the rabbit skin develops erythema and induration that is easily quantitated and is similar to that of man. The guinea pig could be utilized for similar reasons (9).

If methods based on these principles were generally used, the frequency and severity of irritant dermatitis would decrease. It is commonly held that most nonindustrial dermatitis is on an immunologic rather than an irritant basis in nature. Our experience in diagnostic patch testing in a university-based contact dermatitis clinic and in predictive testing for irritation and allergy convinces us that the opposite is the case: cumulative irritation is much more frequent than contact sensitization, that is, with most consumer, skin-care, and cosmetic products.

PHOTOTOXICITY

Phototoxicity is a nonimmunologic, light-induced skin response (dermatitis) to a photoactive chemical likened to an exaggerated sunburn. The photoactive chemical may reach the skin by direct application or via the blood stream, following ingestion or parenteral administration. Whether systemically or topically administered, the chemical may require metabolic transformation to become photoactive. It is a form of irritation that requires light.

Biophysical aspects of the phototoxic reaction were reviewed by Harber & Baer (10). Pathak & Fitzpatrick characterize phototoxic substances (11). Epstein has reviewed the general aspects of photosensitization (12).

Until recently there was considerable confusion as to the mechanism of phototoxicity in man and the method of diagnostic proof. Reproduction of the disease was sporadic, suggesting the possibility of an allergic mechanism rather than irritation.

Clarification of the issues rests on two technical and conceptual phenomena: appreciation of percutaneous penetration of the chemical and an appropriate light source. With adequate penetration and sufficient light energy, phototoxicity is ubiquitous with some phototoxic agents. Penetration can be obtained with intrader-mal injection, or by removal of much of the stratum corneum with repeated applica-tions of a sticky tape (cellophane tape). The appropriate light source can either be natural sunlight with its erythema rays (below 3100 Å) removed by an appropriate filter (window glass or appropriate plastic film) or artificial light from which the erythema rays have been removed. The high intensity black light is a convenient source (13, 14).

With this information phototoxicity can readily be demonstrated in man in a predictive assay (13). In less permeable skin sites such as the forearm, it is necessary to remove the stratum corneum; in more permeable anatomic areas including the neck and scrotum, higher concentrations of the phototoxic agent may obviate the need for stripping.

Presumably almost all animals could be used as a model for predictive toxicity. With bergamot the hairless mouse and the rabbit appeared somewhat more sensitive than the guinea pig. The pig (swine) was less responsive. The squirrel monkey appeared resistant; the hamster showed changes requiring histologic examination as dermatitis was not noted on gross examination. In practical terms this allows for a more than reasonable selection of test animals for laboratories to choose from. Until additional experience with test animals is obtained, new chemicals likely to be used widely in man might also be examined in human skin.

Similar techniques are suitable for the identification of systemic phototoxic chemi-cals (15, 16).

What is not clear is whether clinical examples of phototoxicity that have escaped recognition will be found; for example, Hjorth & Moeller identified a peculiar eruption which they termed bikini dermatitis (17). They demonstrated the patho-physiology as phototoxicity secondary to a dye in a bathing suit. We suspect that other syndromes may have the same mechanism. A likely syndrome requiring such investigation is the cholasma or melasma appearing with greater frequency in men.

If industrial and government laboratories employed the current predictive meth-odology, photoxicity would become an antique relegated to ancient textbooks.

DIAGNOSTIC TECHNIQUES IN ALLERGIC CONTACT DERMATITIS

During the last decade dermatologists realized that standardization of the methods of patch testing was inevitable if the results obtained in various clinics are to be comparable. The initial effort of preparing a standardized technique was performed by Magnusson & Hersle (18).

Anatomical Site of Testing

The region used for testing may determine the number of weak reactions to a substance; thus, testing on the anterior thighs yields only 50% of the reactions obtained in the region of maximum reactivity on the upper back. Areas less suitable for testing are the medial surface of the upper arm and the whole surface of the calves.

Adhesive Tape

The concentrations used for patch testing are usually established on the results obtained by occlusive testing. If nonocclusive systems are used, fewer patients will develop irritation, but less of the test materials are absorbed, and false negative reactions may occur.

Some vehicles may impart an added occlusive effect to the tests performed under a nonocclusive tape. Liquids are particularly prone to give false negatives with porous tapes.

The concentrations used for testing are all-important. Usually the concentration required extensively exaggerates the exposure during conditions of use. Thus, a concentration of 5% nickel sulfate may be needed to reproduce a dermatitis caused by the few molecules of nickel released from nickel-plated bra clips.

The concentration selected for patch testing always represents a compromise intended to eliminate false negative reactions but also to avoid false positive reactions and sensitization.

Test Units

Many different test units have been devised by industry and by individual dermatologists. Few have been subjected to systematic comparative study. One study (Magnusson) revealed a striking incidence of false negative reactions with several test units used to the present day. In Magnusson's and Hersle's study AL-TEST (IMECO) was by far superior to the other units evaluated (18). This system ensures adequate contact between test substance and skin, adequate occlusion, and facilitates the reading by leaving an area of skin around the test material free of contact with the adhesive tape. A recent test unit devised by Pirilä is promising, by occupying a smaller area of skin. So far, this test unit has not been compared with those hitherto used.

Epidemiology

The incidence of sensitivity to lanolin, paraben esters, and other substances which are by themselves rarely sensitizing is determined by the number of cases of stasis dermatitis and leg ulcers referred for testing. Thus few cases are seen and tested, while testing is routine in Copenhagen and Munich. Several other sensitivities are particularly frequent in patients with leg eczema, such as reaction to balsam and to local anesthetics.

A study comparing the sensitivities found at six Scandinavian clinics showed that the 20 most frequent allergens were the same in all clinics, although their relative rank could vary. In a later study comparing the sensitivities demonstrated at a number of European clinics with those obtained in Scandinavia, benzocaine was found to be particularly frequent in Germany and Sweden, while sulfonamides were frequent sensitizers in Germany and in Italy where sulfonamides are commonly used for first aid treatment.

Education of the public has failed to reduce the incidence of contact dermatitis. Nickel garter clasps were abandoned, but not because of the risk of sensitization. Primula obconica dermatitis has become rare not because of a shortage of customers for this plant but because of the reluctance on the part of the florists to stock a plant that carries a well-known risk to the shop employees. If a strong sensitizer is inadvertently marketed by a manufacturer, extensive damage may be avoided by alerting the public through radio or TV. To my knowledge this has only happened once, namely in Norway when a dishwashing agent containing a sensitizing impurity had given rise to a series of cases of dermatitis shortly after it had been released for general sale. Obviously most products of this character have been carefully screened before being put on the market. It is debatable whether a general alert should be given when medium or weak sensitizers are detected on the market. The phrasing of the warning would need to be unnecessarily frightening in order to persuade a housewife to discard a soap powder, toilet soap, etc.

In two epidemics in Denmark caused by an antiseptic toilet soap and an optic whitener in several soap powders it proved possible to withdraw the products within a few months after the cause of dermatitis had been detected.

The reader is referred to a series of collaborative research efforts documenting these points (18–27). These studies provide our first insights into the relative frequency of allergic contact dermatitis to a given agent; these are more satisfactory epidemiologic data than available from single investigator case reports. Much remains to be done before totally satisfactory epidemiologic data based on actual usage are available.   –

ALLERGIC CONTACT DERMATITIS: PREDICTIVE ASSAYS

Allergic contact dermatitis receives its share of enthusiastic effort in skin research. This serves at least two purposes: (*a*) aiding in the management of human allergic contact dermatitis and (*b*) serving as a convenient animal or human model of delayed hypersensitivity itself. The latter aspect receives more emphasis than the former. This review summarizes but one aspect of this broad area—the ability to predict the proclivity of a chemical to produce this syndrome in man. Although many animals including the mouse can be sensitized, the guinea pig remains the animal of choice for this purpose. The correct performance of the assay is fraught with conceptual and technical difficulty. Fortunately, in appropriately experienced laboratories the assay will correctly identify most moderate-grade human sensitizers (28). Numerous techniques have been reported, but few investigators have validated their model. The original methodologic studies of Landsteiner and Chase led to the officially accepted FDA test (29, 30). Subsequent modifications led to defined methods for applying the allergen topically (31); others have combined topical exposure with intradermal injection with Freund's adjuvant (31a–32). The most complete validation with man exists for the latter. It is likely that no single technique will be applicable to all classes of potential sensitizers; a more reasonable approach will be the identification of those factors requisite for a relevant assay for a given class.

All human sensitization assays are adapted from the guinea pig assay. A voluminous literature extols a dozen or so modifications; a current summary stresses that —as with the guinea pig assay—validation with standard sensitizers is essential (33). The test must be tested.

Most modifications stress either the number of patch test exposures, timing, or the addition of a use-test phase. The critical factor in avoiding false negative responses is the concentration tested (34, 35). By increasing the concentration to some multiple of the planned usage, the Draize test correlates well with the clinical sensitization experience. Kligman has employed this factor and added detergent-related enhancement in a maximization test. He currently has modified the operational steps attempting to avoid several previous pitfalls (36).

CUTANEOUS METABOLISM

Recent studies have shown that skin is indeed a metabolically vigorous tissue. Some aspects of its biochemical activities have been reviewed and discussed by Hsia (37), who pointed out that biochemistry of the skin is a potentially fertile field for new investigation. The ability of the skin to utilize glucose has been well documented (38–40) and the enzymes necessary for glycolysis and for pentose shunt have been demonstrated (41–43). It has been reported that glucose 6-phosphate dehydrogenase of rat skin can be effectively inhibited by the steroid, dehydroepiandrosterone (44). The study indicated that about half of the NADPH necessary for lipid synthesis in the skin might be supplied from the pentose shunt. It is interesting that the uptake of glucose by the skin is enhanced in vitro by insulin (45, 46), and by prostaglandin E_2 (47) although the mechanisms involved are not clear. It has also been shown that the skin is an active site for the synthesis of sterols (48, 49), prostaglandin E_2 (47), and a variety of other lipids (50–52). Of interest is the finding that lipid synthesis in the skin can be inhibited by clofibrate in vitro (53), suggesting that the skin may be a useful model tissue for evaluation of potential hypolipemic drugs.

There have been many studies on steroid metabolism in the skin in recent years. These studies are interesting because many biological activities of the skin and its appendages are regulated by steroid hormones, such as the enlargement of sebaceous glands in response to androgens (54), the relationship between the development of male pattern baldness and androgens (55), the swelling of sexual skin in female chimpanzees caused by estrogens, and detumescence by progesterone (56). In clinical dermatology, preparations containing corticosteroids are among the most frequently prescribed topical medications. It is now well established that the skin not only responds to steroid hormones, but also transforms them into various metabolites. Indeed, cutaneous metabolism of steroids has become an active field of investigation in the past decade. The hormones so far studied include the estrogens (57, 58), the androgens (59–64), the corticoids (65–67), and the progestins (68, 69). In each case, active metabolism has been observed. The subject of steroid metabolism in human skin has been reviewed (70, 71). It is significant that some of the metabolites formed in the skin have greater hormonal potency than the parent steroid; for example, dehydroepiandrosterone, a weakly androgenic steroid secreted by the adrenal cortex, is transformed by skin into the potent androgen, testosterone (61, 71), which is further transformed into 5α-dihydrotestosterone (59, 60). The last-mentioned steroid is currently regarded as the target tissue–active androgen that affects genetic expression in the target cells (72, 73). These findings suggest that skin does not simply receive messages from steroid hormones that are supplied by the endocrine glands, but that it actively alters the hormone molecules, so that the hormonal activities are modified to suit the need of the tissue. This view is supported by the finding of variations of steroid metabolism during the hair cycle (74, 75); the formation of 5α-dihydrotestosterone from testosterone is most active during the resting phase (telogen), whereas the metabolism of estradiol to form estrone is most active during the growing phase (anagen).

Progress has been made in the understanding of steroid enzymes of the skin. The studies of 17β-hydroxysteroid dehydrogenase (76) and testosterone 5α-reductase (77, 78) revealed specific structural requirements for steroid inhibitors of these enzymes. Using these findings, Voigt & Hsia (79, 80) tested the antiandrogenic effects of 4-androsten-3-one-17β-carboxylic acid and its methyl ester and found that these compounds, when applied topically, prevented the action of testosterone propionate from enlarging the flank organ of female hamsters. In a similar line of research, Mauvis-Jarvis et al (81) showed inhibition of the 5α reduction of testosterone in men treated topically with progesterone. It is hopeful that the enzymic studies may provide a rational basis for the development of therapeutic agents for controlling endocrine abnormalities.

Relevant to drug metabolism in the skin is a recent report by Levin & Conney (82), who demonstrated the enzyme system that hydroxylates benzopyrene in neonatal foreskin. When the skin specimen was cultured in a medium containing the carcinogen, an increase in the hydroxylation activity was induced.

Ziboh & Hsia (83) reported that topical application of prostaglandin E_2 cleared the scaly lesions in the skin of rats fed a diet deficient in essential fatty acids. The importance of essential fatty acids in maintaining healthy skin had been demonstrated long ago (84). It appears possible that the action of these acids may be via the synthesis of prostaglandins which are required for normal keratinization of the epidermis. The therapeutic usefulness of prostaglandins in dermatology is yet to be explored.

IN VIVO PERFUSION TECHNIQUE

The skin perfusion technique was first used by Fox & Hilton to investigate mediators of eccrine sweating in man (85). Greaves and Sondergaard modified the method to make it suitable for prolonged periods of perfusion (86). Two needles (length, 36 mm; internal diameter, 1 mm) are inserted in parallel in the deep dermis 10 mm apart, pointing in opposite directions lengthwise in the flexor surface of the forearm. Both needles have 4 holes 0.635 mm diameter equally spaced along opposite sides of the shaft. Sterile Tyrode solution, warmed to 32–34°C, is infused through one needle and recovered through the other into siliconized glass tubes in an ice bath. Continuous and uniform withdrawal of the perfusate was obtained by applying suction (0.5 atm pressure) with a peristaltic pump. To increase recovery the area of perfusion was confined by applying elastic bands round the forearm proximal and distal to the needles.

The Tyrode is infused at a rate of 2 ml per min and 40–80% of the infused solution is recovered in the perfusate. Plethysmographic studies showed that the volume of the forearm remained constant after the first 15 min of perfusion.

The perfusate issuing from the inflamed skin is then assayed using the cascade superfusion technique of Vane in which the perfusate trickles over a series of different isolated organ preparations mounted inside a heated, humidified cabinet (87). The perfusate is also stored for further pharmacological and biochemical analysis.

Using this technique Greaves and his colleagues have obtained much new information on the nature of pharmacological events in cutaneous inflammation. The special value of this method compared with earlier methods lies in its directness and as well as in its supplying human data on inflammation.

In early experiments Greaves carried out skin perfusions of three types of urticaria: whealing of cutaneous mastocytosis, factitious urticaria, and cutaneous anaphylaxis. In all three urticarial reactions histamine was recovered from involved skin (86, 88) although other, so far unidentified, activity was found in perfusates of urticaris pigmentosa. In these reactions there was a close correlation between histamine release and whealing.

A more unexpected situation was found in allergic contact eczema (89). Patch tests were applied to the flexor surface of the forearm in sensitized subjects. Perfusion of inflamed skin at these sites was carried out 48 hr later. Pharmacological analysis of the perfusates with solvent partition, thin-layer chromatography, and parallel quantitative bioassay revealed that a mixture of prostaglandins E_1, E_2, F_{1a}, and F_{2a} were present in the perfusates. These findings are of great potential significance since prostaglandin E is highly vasoactive (90).

Findings in cutaneous inflammation due to exposure to UVR varied according to the time interval between irradiation and perfusion. During the first 8 hr there was no detectable pharmacological activity. At 8–20 hr most perfusate contained histamine. At 20–48 hr prostaglandin-like acidic lipid material was found in addition to histamine (91). These results illustrate how skin perfusion can be used to obtain a "pharmacological profile" of an inflammatory reaction.

However, there are some limitations in interpretation of results using this method. These have been fully reviewed by Greaves & Søndergaard (92). Recovery experiments indicate that only a small percentage of released or locally synthesized activity is recovered in the perfusate, because of factors that include dilution by the subcutaneous "pool" of Tyrode solution, local enzymic degradation, and diffusion. Furthermore the variation in concentration of an agent in successive perfusate samples does not necessarily reflect changes in rate of formation or release. These changes could, for example, be due at least in part to variation in rates of diffusion through tissues, variation in permeability of lymphatics on blood vessels, or variation in chemical or enzymic degradation. Released pharmacological agents may themselves modify the pharmacological situation in inflamed skin; for instance, prostaglandin E has histamine-liberating properties (90).

Although skin perfusion has undoubtedly produced unique evidence on the pharmacology of inflammation, much work is required to improve the methodology and in particular the quantitativeness of the technique. Achievement of this aim would have the additional advantage of enabling the method to be used in the analysis of mode of action of anti-inflammatory drugs.

RETINOIC ACID

Vitamin A (retinol) was one of the first vitamins to be characterized chemically and physiologically. Still little is known about its metabolism and actual mechanisms of action accounting for the variety of biochemical events controlled by this drug. Many of its supposed attributes have been deduced from studies of vitamin A–deficient animals and humans, but this may lead to false conclusions because of the difficulty in limiting the deficiency to only vitamin A.

Studies indicate that Tretinoin (all *trans* retinoic acid) may be the active form of the vitamin in most of the body tissues since it can replace vitamin A except for the functions of vision and reproduction. The clinical effects of tretinoin have been best studied in the skin where it seems to have the unique potential to induce as well as control epithelial growth.

Metabolic studies have demonstrated that retinoic acid is metabolized rapidly and is present in low levels in tissues and plasma. Only recently have methods become available for the separation and detection of metabolites of vitamin A that are sensitive and relatively free of artifacts. Retinyl palmitate, an ester of retinoic acid, retinal, retinol, retinoic acid, and a polar metabolite appear in various tissues of the rat 12 hr after a dose of 2 μ of 11-^{14}C-retinyl acetate. There is also evidence that retinal is oxidized in intestinal epithelium and skin to retinoic acid. Retinoic acid not only can mimic many of the biologic functions of retinol but also has a sparing action on the vitamin A reservoir in the liver. This conversion of retinol to retinoic acid is apparently irreversible.

The main products of retinoic acid metabolism may be β-glucuronide which is found in the bile (93) and products of decarboxylation found in urine (94). Homogenates of kidney and liver also appear to have the ability to decarboxylate retinoic acid (95).

SUMMARY

The fields of cutaneous pharmacology and toxicology existed as long as man used topical therapy; some medicaments were helpful and others harmful. This review documents recent progress in these fields in terms of the experimental method. Emphasis has been given to conceptual and methodologic progress rather than a list of new molecules. As signs of the advent of the maturity of these fields, a graduate school course has recently been completed, one text has been published (7), and at least two are in preparation. It is likely that the next review of this topic in this series will reflect this considerable progress in terms of relevance to man.

ACKNOWLEDGMENT

I acknowledge with many thanks the assistance of Drs. R. Berger, M. Greaves, S. L. Hsia, N. Hjorth, and F. Marzulli.

Literature Cited

1. Merck Index, Merck Co.
2. Draize, J. H., Woodard, G., Calvery, H. P. 1944. *J. Pharmacol. Exp. Ther.* 82:377–90
3. Finkelstein, P., Laden, K., Miechowski, W. 1965. *Toxicol. Appl. Pharmacol.* 7:74–78
4. Kligman, A., Wooding, W. 1967. *J. Invest. Dermatol.* 49:78
5. Lanman, B. M., Elvers, W. B., Howard, C. S. 1968. In *Proc. Joint Conf. Cosmet. Sci.*, Toilet Goods Assoc., Washington DC, pp. 135–45
6. Phillips, L., Steinberg, M., Maibach, H., Akers, W. 1972. *Toxicol. Appl. Pharmacol.* 21:369–82
7. Steinberg, M., McCreesh, A., Akers, W., Maibach, H. 1975. In *Animal Models in Dermatology*, ed. H. Maibach, pp. 1–11. Edinburgh: Livingstone
8. Marzulli, F., Maibach, H. 1975. *Food Cosmet. Toxicol.* 15:533–40
9. Roudabush, R., Terhaar, C., Fassett, D., Dziuba, S. 1965. *Toxicol. Appl. Pharmacol.* 7:559–65
10. Harber, L., Baer, R. 1972. *J. Invest. Dermatol.* 58:324–42
11. Pathak, M., Fitzpatrick, T. 1972. *Radiat. Drug Ther.* 6:1–6
12. Epstein, J. 1972. *Arch. Dermatol.* 106:741–48
13. Marzulli, F., Maibach, H. 1970. *J. Soc. Cosmet. Chem.* 21:685–715
14. Burdick, K. 1966. *Arch. Dermatol.* 93:424–25
15. Maibach, H., Sams, W., Epstein, J. 1967. *Arch. Dermatol.* 95:12–15
16. Kligman, A., Goldstein, F. 1973. *Arch. Dermatol.* 107:548–50
17. Hjorth, N., Moeller, H. 1975. In press
18. Magnusson, B., Hersle, K. 1965. *Acta Derm. Venereol.* 45:123–27
19. Fregert, S. et al 1969. *Trans. St. John's Hosp. Dermatol. Soc.* 55:17
20. Magnusson, B. et al 1969. *Acta Derm. Venereol.* 46:396
21. Wilkinson, D. S. et al 1970. *Acta Derm. Venereol.* 50:287
22. Magnusson, B. et al. 1966. *Acta Derm. Venereol.* 49:396
23. Wilkinson, D. S. et al 1970. *Trans St. John's Hosp. Dermatol. Soc.* 56:19
24. Fregert, S. et al 1968. *Arch. Dermatol.* 98:144
25. Malten, K. et al 1968. *Berufsdermatosen* 16:135
26. North Am. Contact Dermatitis Res. Group 1973. *Arch. Dermatol.* 108:537–40

27. North Am. Contact Dermatitis Res. Group 1976. *Contact Dermatitis.* In press
28. Bueller, E. 1975. See Ref. 7, pp. 56–66
29. Landsteiner, K., Jacobs, J. 1936. *J. Exp. Med.* 64:625
30. Draize, J. 1959. In *Appraisal of the Safety of Chemicals in Foods, Drugs and Cosmetics.* Austin: Assoc. Food Drug Officials US
31. Buehler, E. 1965. *Arch. Dermatol.* 91:171
31a. Maguire, H. C. Jr. 1973. *J. Soc. Cosmet. Chem.* 24:151
31b. Magnusson, B., Kligman, A. 1969. *J. Invest. Dermatol.* 52:268
32. Kligman, A. 1966. *J. Invest. Dermatol.* 47:393
33. Marzulli, F., Maibach, H. 1976. *Contact Dermatitis.* 2:In press
34. Marzulli, F., Maibach, H. 1974. *Food Cosmet. Toxicol.* 12:219–27
35. Marzulli, F., Carson, T., Maibach, H. 1968. In *Proc. Joint Conf. Cosmet. Sci.* Sponsored by TGA and Soc. Cosmet. Chem. in cooperation with FDA, Washington DC
36. Kligman, A., Epstein, W. 1975. *Contact Dermatitis* 1:231
37. Hsia, S. L. 1971. *Essays Biochem.* 7:1–38
38. Fusaro, R. M., Johnson, J. A. 1970. *The Dermal Glucose Compartment in the Dermis,* ed. W. Montagna, J. P. Bentley, R. L. Dobson. New York: Meredith
39. Freinkel, R. K. 1960. *J. Invest. Dermatol.* 34:37–42
40. Pomerantz, S. H., Asbornsen, M. T. 1961. *Arch. Biochem. Biophys.* 93:147–52
41. Yardley, H. J., Godfrey, G. 1963. *Biochem. J.* 86:101–3
42. Halprin, K. M., Ohkawara, M. D. 1966. *J. Invest. Dermatol.* 46:43–50
43. Adachi, K., Uno, H. 1968. *Am. J. Physiol.* 215:1234–39
44. Ziboh, V. A., Dreize, M. A., Hsia, S. L. 1970. *J. Lipid Res.* 11:346–54
45. Kahlenberg, A., Kalant, N. 1966. *Can. J. Biochem.* 44:801–8
46. Ziboh, V. A., Wright, R., Hsia, S. L. 1971. *Arch. Biochem. Biophys.* 146:93–99
47. Ziboh, V. A., Hsia, S. L. 1971. *Arch. Biochem. Biophys.* 146:100–109
48. Gaylor, J. L. 1963. *J. Biol. Chem.* 238:1643–48
49. Kandutsch, A. A., Russell, A. E. 1960. *J. Biol. Chem.* 235:2256–61

50. Wilkinson, D. I. 1970. *J. Invest. Dermatol.* 54:132–38
51. Hsia, S. L., Fulton, J. E. Jr., Fulghum, D., Buch, M. M. 1970. *Proc. Soc. Exp. Biol. Med.* 135:285–91
52. Vroman, H. E., Nemecek, R. A., Hsia, S. L. 1969. *J. Lipid Res.* 10:507–14
53. Fulton, J. E. Jr., Hsia, S. L. 1972. *J. Lipid Res.* 13:78–85
54. Strauss, J. S., Pochi, P. E. 1969. *Arch. Dermatol.* 100:621–36
55. Ludwig, E. 1968. In *The Role of Sexual Hormones in Pattern Alopecia in Biopathology of Pattern Alopecia,* ed. A. Baccaredda-Boy, G. Moretti, J. R. Frey, pp. 50–60. Basle: Karger
56. Graham, C. E., Collins, D. C., Robinson, H., Preedy, J. R. K. 1972. *Endocrinology* 91:13–24
57. Frost, P., Weinstein, G. D., Hsia, S. L. 1966. *J. Invest. Dermatol.* 46:584–85
58. Weinstein, G. D., Frost, P., Hsia, S. L. 1968. *J. Invest. Dermatol.* 51:4–10
59. Gomez, E. C., Hsia, S. L. 1968. *Biochemistry* 7:24–32
60. Wilson, J. D., Walker, J. D. 1969. *J. Clin. Invest.* 48:371–79
61. Cameron, E. H. D., Baillie, A. H., Grant, J. K., Milne, J. A., Thomson, J. 1966. *J. Endocrinol.* 35:xix–xx
62. Sansone, G., Reisner, R. M. 1971. *J. Invest. Dermatol.* 56:366–72
63. Faredin, I., Fazekas, A. G., Toth, I., Kokai, K., Julesz, M. 1969. *J. Invest. Dermatol.* 52:357–61
64. Takayasu, S., Adachi, K. 1972. *Endocrinology* 90:73–80
65. Hsia, S. L., Hao, Y. L. 1966. *Biochemistry* 5:1469–74
66. Hsia, S. L., Hao, Y. L. 1967. *Steroids* 10:489–500
67. Malkinson, F. D., Lee, M. W., Cutukovic, I. 1959. *J. Invest. Dermatol.* 32:101–7
68. Frost, P., Gomez, E. C., Weinstein, G. D., Lamas, J., Hsia, S. L. 1969. *Biochemistry* 8:948–52
69. Rongone, E. L. 1969. *Proc. Soc. Exp. Biol. Med.* 130:253–56
70. Hsia, S. L. 1971. In *Steroid Metabolism in Human Skin in Modern Trends in Dermatology,* ed. P. Borrie, 4:69–88. London: Butterworth
71. Julesz, M., Faredin, I., Toth, L. 1971. *Steroids in Human Skin.* Budapest: Akad. Kiado
72. Liao, S., Fang, S. 1969. In *Receptor-Proteins for Androgens and the Mode of Action of Androgens on Gene Transcription in Ventral Prostate in Vitamins and Hormones,* ed. R. S. Harris, I. G. Wool, J. A. Loraine, P. L. Munson, pp. 17–90. New York & London: Academic
73. Bruchovsky, N., Wilson, J. D. 1968. *Biol. Chem.* 243:2012–21
74. Rampini, E., Voigt, W., Davis, B. P., Moretti, G., Hsia, S. L. 1971. *Endocrinology* 89:1506–14
75. Rampini, E., Davis, B. P., Moretti, G., Hsia, S. L. 1971. *J. Invest. Dermatol.* 57:75–80
76. Davis, B. P., Rampini, E., Hsia, S. L. 1972. *J. Biol. Chem.* 247:1407–13
77. Voigt, W., Fernandez, E. P., Hsia, S. L. 1970. *J. Biol. Chem.* 245:5594–99
78. Voigt, W., Hsia, S. L. 1973. *J. Biol. Chem.* 248:4280–85
79. Voigt, W., Hsia, S. L. 1973. *Endocrinology* 92:1216–22
80. Hsia, S. L., Voigt, W. 1974. *J. Invest. Dermatol.* 62:224–27
81. Mauvais-Jarvis, P., Kuttenn, F., Bandot, N. 1974. *J. Clin. Endocrinol. Metab.* 38:142–47
82. Levin, W., Conney, A. H., Alvares, A. P., Merkatz, I., Kappas, A. 1972. *Science* 176:419–20
83. Ziboh, V. A., Hsia, S. L. 1972. *J. Lipid Res.* 13:458–67
84. Burr, G. O., Burr, M. M. 1929. *J. Biol. Chem.* 82:345–55
85. Fox, R. H., Hilton, S. M. 1958. *J. Physiol.* 142:219
86. Greaves, M. W., Søndergaard, J. 1970. *Arch. Dermatol.* 101:418
87. Vane, J. R. 1964. *Br. J. Pharmacol.* 23:360
88. Søndergaard, J., Greaves, M. W. 1971a. *Acta Derm. Venereol.* 51:98
89. Greaves, M. W., Søndergaard, J., McDonald-Gibson, W. 1971. *Br. Med. J.* 2:258
90. Søndergaard, J., Greaves, M. W. 1971b. *Br. J. Dermatol.* 84:424
91. Søndergaard, J., Greaves, M. W. 1971c. *J. Pathol.* 101:93
92. Greaves, M. W., Søndergaard, J. 1971. *Acta Derm. Venereol.* 51:50
93. Dunagin, P. E., Zachman, R., Olson, J. 1965. *Science* 148:65
94. Sundaresan, P. R., Sundaresan, G. M. 1973. *Int. J. Vitam. Nutr. Res.* 43:61
95. Kleiner-Bossaler, A., Reluca, H. 1971. *Arch. Biochem. Biophys.* 142:371

EFFECTS OF DRUGS ON THE ELECTRICAL ACTIVITY OF THE BRAIN: ANESTHETICS

❖6657

Wallace D. Winters

School of Medicine, Department of Pharmacology, University of California, Davis, California 95616

The emergence of the newer anesthetics such as ketamine and enflurane tested the concept that all anesthetics are depressants. It was with this in mind that the editors requested this chapter, which reviews neurophysiological studies mainly in cats that collate the various states induced by the anesthetics into an organized schema. I apologize to those readers who expected a broader review of the anesthetic state and/or a less biased approach. On the other hand, I hope that this review serves as a focus for the reorganization of our concept of anesthesia and its relation to other drug-induced states.

INTRODUCTION

Both basic scientists and clinicians tend to consider a subject asleep or anesthetized when lying down and hyperexcited when moving around. This view is only partially correct. In the hyperexcited, cataleptic, and preconvulsant states, subjects are immobile but their CNS is highly activated. We often cannot determine either the behavioral or functional brain state of subjects by mere observation. The loss of righting reflex, as the classic pharmacological test for determining CNS depression, sleeping time, or anesthesia time, is misleading since this tests only for immobility and not for the functional activity of the CNS. To determine the state of consciousness of a subject, it is necessary to examine the level of excitability of the brain. By placing electrodes in various parts of the brain and examining the brain wave activity during various states of normal behavior, such as wakefulness and sleep, and during drug-induced states, the effects induced by these states on CNS activity can be interpreted (1–3).

This presentation attempts to correlate some of the acquired data into a meaningful interpretation of the action of the CNS anesthetics.

413

Agents used as anesthetics form a diffuse group which are generally classified as CNS depressants (4, 5). Pharmacologists often view anesthesia as a progression of decreasing CNS irritability leading to depression and finally death (Figure 1). In contrast, increasing states of irritability represent an opposite continuum leading to hyperexcitation, convulsions, and finally death (6). The progressive depression induced by the anesthetic agent diethyl ether was fitted into a schema by Guedel (7). The schema implies a progressive decrease in CNS excitability (Figure 1) as follows: stage I, analgesia; stage II, delirium; stage III, surgical anesthesia; and stage IV, medullary paralysis.

The first two stages of anesthesia, however, are characterized by motor excitation and ataxia in stage I, and hallucinatory and cataleptoid behavior in stage II. These two stages constitute a stage of excitation or increased stimulation rather than CNS depression (4, 8–10). Ataxia is considered, by some, to imply CNS depression; however, it actually indicates an inability to coordinate motor activity. The ataxia

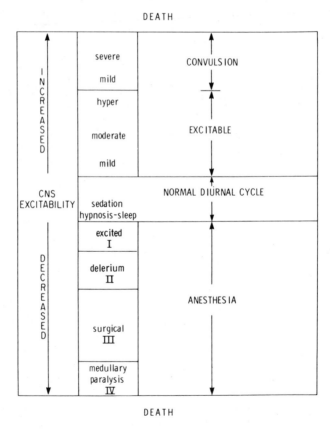

Figure 1 Classical unidimensional schema of CNS excitation and depression (29).

that appears during stage 1 anesthesia is correlated with elevated levels of neuronal activity, not depression (4, 5).

In addition, prior to clinical trial, both diethyl ether and nitrous oxide were well-known nonmedically as stimulants, euphoriants, and hallucinogens (11). Likewise, other anesthetics have confusing histories. α-Chloralose has been described as a convulsant-anesthetic agent (12), is often used in animals as an anesthetic for neurophysiological studies (13), and was used clinically to activate the electroencephalogram (EEG) of suspected epileptic patients (14). γ-Hydroxybutyrate (GHB) was reported to be a possible neurotransmitter in sleep (15) and also was utilized as an anesthetic in several thousand neurosurgical patients (16). Several investigators reported (16–18) a similarity in EEG activity between anesthetic doses of GHB and pentobarbital. However, subsequent studies demonstrated that GHB (2, 19, 20) has behavioral and neurophysiological properties distinctly different from those of pentobarbital and, in fact, in high doses is a convulsant.

Phencyclidine (Sernyl®) was introduced as an anesthetic in clinical trials in 1957 (21, 22). This drug induced amnesia, analgesia, catalepsy, anesthesia, and convulsions as well as profound postoperative delirium and acute psychotic reactions which prevented it from being accepted as an anesthetic in man. It is presently used widely in veterinary medicine as an immobilizing agent for short surgical procedures. In addition, this agent is used widely as a street drug (23), called PCP, Peace, Angel's Dust, Horse Tranquillizer, or Hog. A less potent derivative of phencyclidine, ketamine, with similar properties is used as an anesthetic mainly in the young or elderly and less frequently in young adults for limited surgical procedures. Domino et al (24) performed a controlled study of ketamine in twenty adult volunteer prisoners. He found ketamine to be less potent than phencyclidine; it did not induce convulsions, but did induce analgesia and anesthesia. The principal disadvantage of ketamine was its adverse psychic effects during emergence, such as hallucinations and changes in mood, body image, and affect, some of which were so frightening to some of the subjects that they preferred not to repeat the drug. Domino et al noted that in some subjects, ketamine induced an alarming rise in systolic and diastolic blood pressure and heart rate, along with sweating, lacrimation, hyperactive tendon reflexes, and a rise in blood glucose levels. In addition, during the catalepsia many of the protective reflexes, such as laryngeal, pharyngeal, eyelid, and corneal, were maintained. EEG studies in these volunteers demonstrated a hypersynchronous slow-wave pattern during catalepsia. To date there are no reports of significant street abuse of this drug.

Enflurane (Ethrane®) is a gaseous anesthetic with properties similar to those of ketamine (25) but is more efficacious in terms of CNS excitation in that it readily induces seizures at doses slightly higher than those that induce anesthesia (26). The close association of some anesthetic agents with states not usually considered to represent anesthesia, such as seizures and street abuse to induce hallucinations, suggests that we must alter our pharmacological concept that there is a stereotypical anesthetic state characterized by CNS depression. For a review of the neurophysiology of anesthesia see references 27–29. We later look further into the characterization of the anesthetic state but first look at some concepts of the functional organization of the CNS. In 1951, Himwich (30) developed the concept of horizontal levels within the brain that were reversibly affected sequentially by increasing depths of anesthesia. As the subject progresses through the various depths, the cerebral cortex is depressed before the subcortical diencephalon, then the mesencephalon and pons are gradually depressed, and finally deepest anesthesia occurs when the vital centers in the medulla are depressed.

More recent developments in neurophysiology have given strong support for an alternate concept of CNS function and drug action. Rather than horizontal stratification of the brain, Livingston (31) visualized the CNS as composed of three highly interrelated but vertical systems: the specific sensory, the nonspecific sensory, and the motor system. The nonspecific sensory system is seen as responsible for interrelating and modulating all sensory-motor interrelationships. This nonspecific system is located essentially within the midline structures, running from the medulla up to the diencephalon, and contains the ascending reticular activating system described by Moruzzi & Magoun (32). Since the reticular formation was demonstrated to be a vital system for the control of wakefulness, several investigators have attempted to relate both sleep and anesthesia to altered functioning of this reticular system. The reticular formation is very sensitive to changes in the spontaneous wake-sleep cycle (3) and is likewise sensitive to states induced by various anesthetics (33–36).

CONTINUUM OF STATES

Based on the results of neurophysiological studies of anesthetics, excitatory, hallucinogenic, and convulsant agents in cats, Winters et al (4, 5) proposed a multidirectional schema of the progression of states of CNS excitation and depression to replace what was implied in the unidirectional schema of Guedel (7). The schema (Figure 2) states (5) that anesthetics and CNS excitants induce an initial excitation (stage I) characterized by increased motor activity including ataxia. Some anesthetics then bypass stage II and directly induce surgical anesthesia (stage III) characterized by a loss of responsiveness to stimuli, slow regular respiration, and CNS depression. Other anesthetics induce stage II prior to stage III. Stage II is characterized by bizarre postures and inappropriate behavior—hallucinatory (A, B) and cataleptoid (C). During stage II-C, as in stage III, the subject is relatively unresponsive to stimuli. Many anesthetics do not induce stage III following II but either induce only stage II or progress to heightened levels of CNS excitation, i.e. myoclonic jerking followed by generalized seizures. Further CNS depression during stage III will progress to stage IV (medullary paralysis) with depressed respiration and/or cardiovascular function terminating in death. During stage II and myoclonus, the respiratory and cardiovascular systems are not depressed and may be markedly stimulated. Both progressions are reversible, providing the subject does not die from respiratory and cardiovascular collapse either during the convulsions or stage IV.

Both the arousal response to stimuli and the righting reflex are absent during stage II-C and stage III. Thus, behaviorally it is difficult to differentiate between these two divergent states.

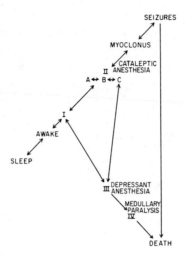

Figure 2 Schematic representation of the stages of anesthesia. Stage I, II, III, and IV, myoclonus, seizures, and death are shown. CNS excitation is implied above the awake level and CNS depression below.

In a recent review, Winters (37) discussed in detail the induced behavior and neurophysiology of the states of CNS excitation including stage I, II-A, II-B, II-C, myoclonus, and seizures; the induction of these states by various drug types, i.e. anesthetics, hallucinogens, and convulsants; and the progression of loss of awareness and recall during stages II-A, -B, and -C. Briefly stage II-A is characterized as a hallucinatory state identical with the state induced by hallucinogens or subconvulsant doses of pentylenetetrazol. Stage II-B and II-C are further progressions of this behavior with increased immobility and fixed postures characteristic of catalepsy. Stage II-A is related to a level of consciousness in which the subject is aware of and can recall the bizarre experience; while in stage II-B the subject is not aware but has recall; and while in stage II-C the subject is not aware and does not have recall. Descriptions of bizarre experiences following anesthesia are likely related to experiences recalled during emergence back to consciousness from II-C through II-B, II-A to stage I.

EEG

The characteristic electrical patterns of the EEG during the various drug-induced stages of CNS activity help to distinguish the divergent states of CNS activity. In cats (5, 8, 38) these patterns (Figure 3) are as follows: during stage I the mesodiencephalic and cortical EEG consists of an activated pattern with high frequency, low voltage wave-form activity (desynchronization). During stage II, the initial phase, A, is characterized by intermittent bursts of high amplitude 2.5 Hz waves (hypersynchrony) associated with hallucinatory behavior. During II-B the hypersynchronous waves are continuous and the bizarre actions of the cats are more intense. During

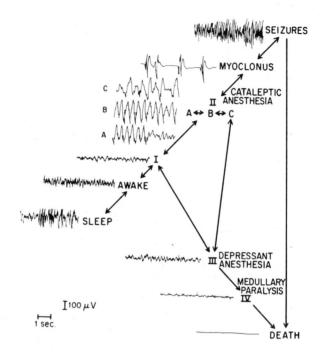

Figure 3 The cortical EEG (cat) representative of each stage is depicted. (See Figure 2.)

II-C the animals lose the righting reflex and maintain abnormal, bizarre postures that are cataleptoid and their EEG pattern changes to 1.5 Hz slow waves with occasional spiking. More profound CNS excitation is characterized by spontaneous and stimuli-induced myoclonic jerking and concomitant 400–500 μV large amplitude spike bursts followed by increasingly prolonged periods of relative electrical silence. This phase can continue or culminate in a generalized tonic-clonic seizure with high frequency, high voltage EEG discharge in all leads lasting as long as one minute. On the other hand, during stage III the general pattern is not as stereotyped as it is for the continuum of CNS excitation; there is a mixture of 10–12 Hz spindle-like bursts and irregular high amplitude slow waves. As anesthesia deepens the amplitude of the spindle bursts and slow-wave activity between bursts become progressively smaller until the burst suppression phase is reached. At this time the animal is unresponsive to all stimuli and has marked muscle relaxation. During burst suppression the spike bursts do not usually exceed 50 μV in amplitude, there are no after bursts, and the low amplitude spikes do not change in response to tactile or sensory stimuli. The intervals of isoelectric activity are progressively prolonged as the amplitude of spike bursts is reduced until the EEG is totally flat in deepest anesthesia. During emergence, each of the preceding EEG patterns reappear but are not as clear-cut as during induction.

GROUPING OF ANESTHETICS

Four general groups of anesthetic agents can be described according to the schema of the continuum of anesthetic states (Table 1). The first group of compounds is characterized by diethyl ether, which induces stage I and II and then progresses to stage III and IV. The second group includes nitrous oxide, trichlorethylene, and ketamine. These agents induce stage I and then stage II anesthesia but do not progress to stage III. While they do not usually induce seizures these agents may manifest generalized seizures if large doses are administrated. The third group is composed of phencyclidine, γ-hydroxybutyrate, α-chloralose, and enflurane. These agents induce stage I and II, then myoclonus and/or generalized seizures. The fourth group includes the barbiturates, halothane and methoxyflurane. These agents induce an initial stage I, followed by stage III, but do not manifest stage II activity. Higher doses induce stage IV medullary depression.

RETICULAR FORMATION MULTIPLE UNIT ACTIVITY

Reticular formation neuronal activity is an important control mechanism for the various states of wakefulness, sleep, and anesthesia. Studies were performed (3, 8, 38) utilizing the technique of continuous reticular multiple unit recording in intact freely moving animals. The multiple neuronal activity of the reticular formation during these various stages correlates with the EEG and behavior (Figure 4). During stage I the tonic activity of the reticular units is slightly increased over the awake control. During stage II, the excitability is equal or slightly greater than stage I. During myoclonus (spiking) and generalized seizures the intermittent neuronal activity is more profound and neuronal excitability is markedly increased. In contrast, during stage III the neuronal activity is markedly reduced and the neurons are relatively nonexcitable. The significance of these findings is discussed after a review of the actions of anesthetics on auditory evoked responses.

Table 1 Grouping of anesthetics according to induced stages

Drug	Anesthesia stage
Diethyl ether	I ⟷ II ⟷ III ⟷ IV
Nitrous oxide	I ⟷ II
Trilene®	
Ketamine	
Phencyclidine	I ⟷ II ⟷ seizures
γ-Hydroxybutyrate	
α-Chloralose	
Enflurane	
Barbiturates	I ⟷ III ⟷ IV
Halothane	
Methoxyflurane	

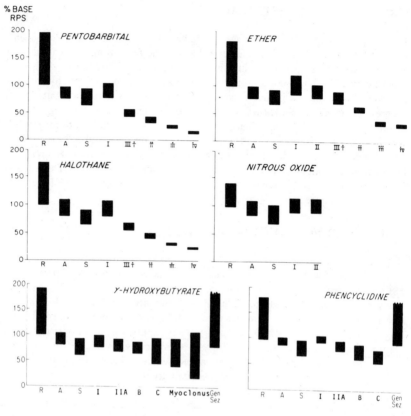

Figure 4   Bar graphs representing reticular neuronal activity during dream sleep (R), wakefulness (A), and spindle or slow wave sleep (S), and the various stages of CNS excitation (I, II, myoclonus, and generalized seizures) and depression (III, i, ii, iii, and iv). The height of the bar indicates neuronal excitability. [For details see method section (3).] [Modified from (8).]

AUDITORY EVOKED RESPONSE (AER)

A further evaluation of the excitability of the CNS is demonstrated by the studies on the averaged evoked response to auditory stimuli. The basis of these studies was to determine the manner in which auditory stimuli are received at the first relay nucleus (dorsal cochlear nucleus), the modulatory area (midbrain reticular formation), and the association cortex (suprasylvian gyrus). The assumption is that the amplitude of an evoked response indicates a degree of information significance, i.e. a large response contains more information regarding the stimulus than a small response (39).

During the control state, the auditory response is smallest during dream [rapid eye movement (REM)] sleep, larger during the awake state, and largest during spindle sleep (Figure 5). This correlation between the AER amplitude and configuration and the spontaneous behavioral state is also noted during the anesthetic states (1, 3, 8). The reticular response was absent during all stages of anesthesia. During stages I and II, the AER in the cochleus is equal and the cortical slightly smaller than the awake control. During stage III the AER in the cochleus is initially larger than during stages I and II and is slightly reduced during plane 4. The AER in the cortex was progressively reduced during stage III.

These data led to the conclusion that the reticular formation modulates the auditory signal peripheral to the cochlear nucleus (Figure 6). This would explain the reduced size of the evoked response during stages I and II when reticular activation is marked and modulation is likewise active. During the later phase of

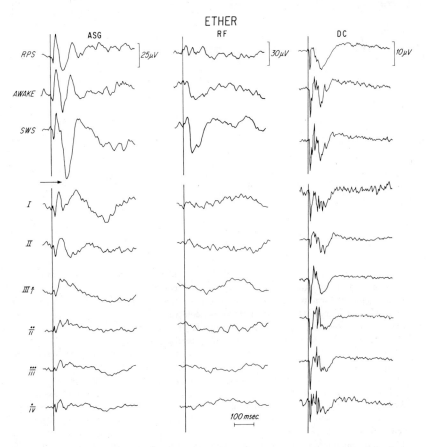

Figure 5 Comparison of the computed averaged auditory evoked response to 40 clicks during control [wakefulness, slow wave sleep, and rhombencephalic phase of sleep (RPS), REM or dream sleep] and ether (10–40%) anesthesia recordings from cat brain: anterior suprasylvian gyrus (ASG), midbrain reticular formation (RF), and dorsal cochlear nucleus (DC) (8).

stage II activity, the animal shows neither electrical nor behavioral arousal, the evoked potentials are slightly larger than controls, and the units appear to fire in synchronous bursts. Since the arousal response disappears concurrently with this intermittent bursting of units, it appears that the reticular unit activity has undergone a partial functional disorganization (40, 41) and while highly excitable, it exerts a reduced control over the level of arousal and sensory modulation (Figure 6). As

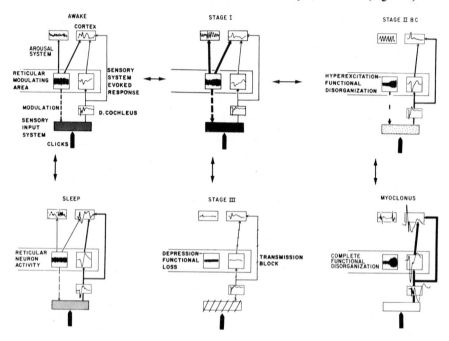

Figure 6 Diagrammatic representation of the control mechanism for sensory input and arousal. Each frame contains the depiction of characteristic evoked potentials at the dorsal cochleus, reticular formation and association cortex, reticular unit activity, and cortical EEG (*upper left box*). The six states shown are awake control to slow wave sleep or stage I, stage I passing to either stage II or stage III, and stage II passing to myoclonus. The sensory input system is depicted by the varying shades indicating degree of filtering as influenced by reticular modulation (*broken lines*). The thickness of the lines denotes qualitative degree of effectiveness; absence of the line denotes complete loss of action.

During control states the reticular unit activity and modulation of sensory input are greatest during wakefulness and least during sleep; therefore the evoked responses are least during wakefulness and greatest during sleep. Stage I results in slightly greater modulation than during wakefulness; thus auditory-evoked responses are slightly smaller. During stage III, reticular unit activity is markedly depressed, there is no sensory modulation, and there is a reduced transmission of sensory signal through CNS. Therefore, the AERs are reduced beyond the cochleus. In contrast, during myoclonus reticular units are hyperexcited but functionally disorganized, there is no sensory modulation and no transmission block; thus the AERs are large throughout the CNS. (Modified from 39.)

this functional disorganization becomes more profound, the EEG pattern changes to the spiking phase, and the bursting pattern of unit activity becomes more pronounced. At this time there is a more profound loss of reticular modulation, the sensory input becomes markedly elevated, and the evoked responses in all brain areas are enlarged (Figures 6, 7).

During stage III, plane i (Figures 5, 6), the reticular unit activity falls rapidly; thus the increase in size of the AER during plane i is indicative of the loss of reticular modulation function along with the loss of the arousal response. The reduction in the amplitude of the AER in the reticular formation and cortex during stages

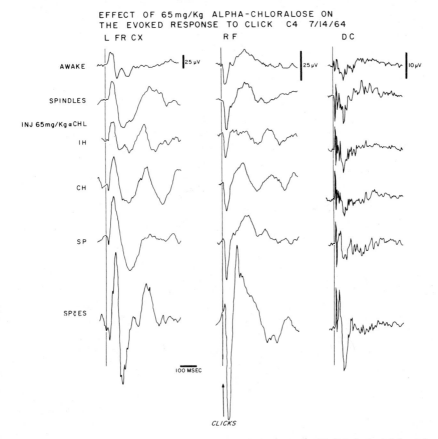

Figure 7 Comparison of the computed average evoked response to 40 clicks in the left frontal cortex (L FR CX), midbrain reticular formation (RF), and dorsal cochlear nucleus (DC) following injection of 65 mg/kg α-chloralose (α-CHL). Stage II-A, intermittent hypersynchrony (IH); stage II-B, continuous hypersynchrony (CH); stage II-C, spikes (SP); myoclonus, spikes with electrical silence (SP with ES) (39).

III–ii–iv while the cochlear response remains large suggests a further direct depressant action of the anesthetic on the transmission of the sensory signal from the cochlear nucleus to the reticular formation and cortex. Alternately this could be due to a direct reduction in responsiveness of the reticular and cortical neurons to the transmitted signal. Schlag & Brand (10) presented evidence that no such depressant action occurs on cortical neurons, since they were unable to demonstrate significant changes in the electrical activity of the isolated cortex prior to deepest anesthesia. The persistent AER in the cochlear nucleus even during deep anesthesia implies that anesthetics during stage III have little direct action on the auditory system peripheral to, and at, the cochlear nucleus. Rather the anesthetics exert a profound inhibition on neuronal transmission, thus preventing the propagation of the auditory response from the cochlear nucleus to the more central areas of the CNS (Figure 6).

DISCUSSION

The elevated reticular formation multiple unit activity during wakefulness and during drug-induced stages I and II is of interest in view of the reports by Rossi & Zirondoli (9) and Schlag & Brand (10) that connections between the midbrain reticular formation and cortex are necessary for the induction of cortical desynchronization during early stages of anesthesia. During stage III anesthesia there is a progressive fall in the level of reticular unit activity. Thus, since two of the four stages of anesthesia manifest properties of CNS excitation the anesthetic state should not be characterized solely as a progressive CNS depression (6). Nitrous oxide is not sufficiently potent to induce depths greater than stage II, and since its actions appear to be solely excitatory it should not be regarded as a CNS depressant. Studies of nitrous oxide action on dogs at greater than 1 atm indicate that anesthesia does occur followed by seizures at the higher atmospheres. Thus, at these higher atmospheres nitrous oxide functions as a cataleptic anesthetic similar to phencyclidine, α-chloralose, or γ-hydroxybutyrate (E. L. Frederickson, personal communication). While diethyl ether induces all four stages of anesthesia, pentobarbital and halothane have less of an initial excitant action than does ether in that they do not induce stage II hallucinatory action following the stage I excitation.

The interpretation of the mode of action of the various anesthetic agents as presented in the continuum of anesthetic stages suggests that the concept of a single anesthetic state is not valid. Because drugs induced both CNS catalepsy or depression (Figure 8), both of which are regarded as states of anesthesia, it seems that it is vital when using these agents that the user be keenly aware of the specific type of agent being used. In addition, a search for a unifying single neurochemical or neurophysiological mechanism to explain the basis of anesthetic action is frivolous. A functional definition of the anesthetic state (5) could be a drug-induced stage that makes the subject relatively unresponsive to painful stimuli and amnestic. This state can be achieved by CNS stimulation or depression (Figure 8). The ultimate neurological basis is the functional control of the reticular activating system. This system can be inhibited (stage III) resulting in functional depression or hyperexcitation (stage II-C) resulting in a functional disorganization, either of which will result in

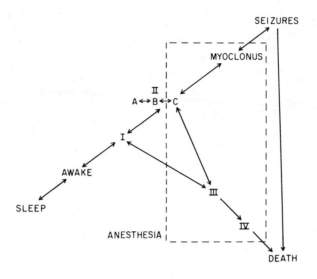

Figure 8 Schema indicating anesthetic states of cataleptic anesthesia (stage II-C and myo-clonus) or depressant anesthesia (stage III, IV). Cataleptic representing CNS excitation and depressant representing CNS depression.

a loss of reticular arousal action resulting in unresponsiveness (Figure 6). The amnestic effect of these agents can likewise be presumed to result from a functional disorganization of the CNS networks involved in the process of memory, by either depression or hyperexcitation (28).

SUMMARY

The major concepts presented in this review can be summarized as follows: 1. There is a multidirectional continuum of anesthetic states—some represented by CNS excitation and others by depression. 2. The reticular activating system is influenced by all anesthetics; some inhibit its action (stage III) and some hyperexcite the system resulting in a function disorganization (stage II-C). 3. Some agents traverse both excitation and depression, diethyl ether (I, II, III). 4. Others induce only stage II —catalepsia, e.g. nitrous oxide, ketamine, γ-hydroxybutyrate, α-chloralose, phen-cyclidine, trichlorethylene, and enflurane. 5. Others induce no stage II but progress directly from stage I to stage III, e.g. halothane and barbiturates. 6. Cataleptic agents may induce further CNS excitation manifested by seizures, e.g. γ-hydroxybu-tyrate, phencyclidine, ketamine, α-chloralose, trichlorethylene, and enflurane. 7. The functional definition of surgical anesthesia is: a stage induced by a drug that makes the subject relatively unresponsive to painful stimuli and amnestic. Thus, the subject does not respond during surgery and cannot recall what happened after-wards. This state can be achieved by functional disruption of CNS systems by marked stimulation or depression.

426   WINERS

Literature Cited

1. Winters, W. D. 1964. *Electroenceph-alogr. Clin. Neurophysiol.* 17:234–45
2. Winters, W. D., Spooner, C. E. 1965. *Electroencephalogr. Clin. Neurophysiol.* 18:287–96
3. Winters, W. D., Mori, K., Spooner, C. E., Kado, R. T. 1967. *Electroencephalogr. Clin. Neurophysiol.* 23:539–45
4. Winters, W. D., Mori, K., Bauer, R. O., Spooner, C. E. 1967. *Anesthesiology* 28:65–80
5. Winters, W. D., Ferrar-Allado, T., Guzman-Flores, C., Alcaraz, M. 1972. *Neuropharmacology* 11:303–16
6. Franz, D. N. 1975. *The Pharmacological Basis of Therapeutics,* ed. L. S. Goodman and A. Gilman, pp. 49–52. New York: Macmillan. 5th ed.
7. Guedel, A. E. 1937. *Inhalation Anesthesia: A Fundamental Guide.* New York: Macmillan. 172 pp.
8. Mori, K., Winters, W. D., Spooner, C. E. 1968. *EEG J.* 24:242–48
9. Rossi, G. F., Zirondoli, A. 1955. *EEG J.* 7:383–90
10. Schlag, J., Brand, H. 1958. *EEG J.* 10:305–24
11. Keys, T. E. 1963. *The History of Surgical Anesthesia.* New York: Dover. 21 pp.
12. Hanriot, M., Richet, C. 1897. *Arch. Int. Pharmacodyn.* 3:191–211
13. Monroe, R. R., Balis, G. U., Ebersberger, E. 1963. *Curr. Ther. Res. Clin. Exp.* 5:141–53
14. Monroe, R. R. 1959. *Arch. Gen. Psychiatry* 1:205–14
15. Jounay, M. M. et al 1960. *Agressologie* 1:417–27
16. Laborit, H. 1964. *Int. J. Neuropharmacol.* 3:433–52
17. Drakontides, A. B., Schneider, J. A., Funderburk, W. H. 1962. *J. Pharmacol. Exp. Ther.* 135:275–84
18. Hosko, M. J. Jr., Gluckman, M. I. 1963. *Pharmacologist* 5:254
19. Winters, W. D., Spooner, C. E. 1965. *Int. J. Neuropharmacol.* 4:197–200
20. Winters, W. D., Spooner, C. E. 1966. *Electroencephalogr. Clin. Neurophysiol.* 20:83–90
21. Luby, E. D., Cohen, B. D., Rosenbaum, G., Gottlieb, J. S., Kelley, R. 1959. *AMA Arch. Neurol. Psychiatry* 81:363

22. Domino, E. F. 1964. *Int. Rev. Neurobiol.* 6:303–47
23. Reed, A. Jr., Kane, A. W. 1972. *J. Psychedelic Drugs* 5(1):8–12
24. Domino, E. F., Chodoff, P., Corssen, G. 1965. *Clin. Pharmacol. Ther.* 6:279–91
25. Julien, R. M., Kavan, E. M. 1972. *J. Pharmacol. Exp. Ther.* 183(2):393–403
26. Lebowitz, M. H., Blitt, C. D., Dillon, J. B. 1972. *J. Int. Anesth. Res. Soc.* 51(3):355–63
27. Mori, K. 1975. *Neurophysiological Basis of Anesthesia,* Vol. 13, No. 1. Boston: Little, Brown
28. Brazier, M. A. 1972. *The Neurophysiological Background for Anesthesia.* Springfield, Ill.: Thomas
29. Brechner, V. L. 1973. *Pathological and Pharmacological Considerations in Anesthesiology.* Springfield, Ill.: Thomas
30. Himwich, H. E. 1951. *Brain Metabolism and Cerebral Disorders.* Baltimore: Williams & Wilkins
31. Livingston, W. K., Haugen, F. P., Brookhardt, J. M. 1954. *Neurology* 4:485–96
32. Moruzzi, G., Magoun, H. W. 1949. *Electroencephalogr. Clin. Neurophysiol.* 1:455–73
33. French, J. D., Verzeano, M., Magoun, H. W. 1953. *Arch. Neurol. Psychiatry* 69:519–29
34. French, J. D., King, E. E. 1955. *Surgery* 38:228–38
35. King, E. E. 1956. *J. Pharmacol. Exp. Ther.* 116:404–17
36. Killam, E. K. 1962. *Pharmacol. Rev.* 14:175
37. Winters, W. D. 1975. *Hallucinations: Behavior, Experience & Theory,* ed. R. K. Siegel, L. J. West, pp. 53–70. New York: Wiley
38. Winters, W. D., Mori, K., Wallach, M. B., Marcus, R. J., Spooner, C. E. 1969. *Electroencephalogr. Clin. Neurophysiol.* 27:514–22
39. Winters, W. D. 1968. *Psychopharmacology: A Review of Progress, 1957–1967,* ed. D. H. Efron, pp. 453–77. Washington DC: PHS Publ.
40. Schlag, J., Balvin, R. 1963. *Exp. Neurol.* 8:203–19
41. Winters, W. D., Spooner, C. E. 1966. *Electroencephalogr. Clin. Neurophysiol.* 20:83–90

DEVELOPMENTAL ASPECTS   ❖6658
OF THE HEPATIC CYTOCHROME
P450 MONOOXYGENASE SYSTEM

Allen H. Neims, Margaret Warner, Peter M. Loughnan, and
Jacob V. Aranda
Roche Developmental Pharmacology Unit, Departments of Pharmacology and
Therapeutics, and Pediatrics, McGill University, and the Montreal Children's Hospital
Research Institute, Montreal, Quebec

In addition to their intrinsic value as probes in the study of differentiation, the interactions between xenobiotics and the developing organism are of immediate therapeutic and toxicologic consequence (1). The magnitude of inadvertent exposure of the fetus and newborn to drugs is well documented. Surveys have revealed that the gravid woman is exposed to an average of three to ten drugs per pregnancy (2–5). In addition to transplacental acquisition of drugs and metabolites (6, 7), exposure of the perinate continues postnatally through suckling (8, 9). Recent advances in perinatal care continue to redefine the dimensions of exposure. The regionalization of high-risk obstetrical and neonatal care has been associated with evolution of an attitude of aggressive diagnostic and therapeutic intervention. Attention must now be devoted to the influence of drugs on the cardiorespiratory measurements involved in diagnostic fetal monitoring (10, 11). Indeed, the practice of fetal therapeutics has materialized with approaches designed to modify the maturational process (12), including glucocorticoids to prevent respiratory distress syndrome (13, 14) and phenobarbital to lessen the degree of hyperbilirubinemia (15, 16). Recent survey in a neonatal intensive care unit has revealed an average exposure of 3.4 drugs per infant excluding nursery routines (17); exposure was inversely related to birth weight, and 71 different drugs were utilized in the 320 consecutive infants surveyed.

    The adverse actions of drugs upon the human fetus and newborn have been tabulated recently (18–20). Delayed effects, such as vaginal adenocarcinoma after in utero exposure to diethylstilbesterol (21) and hyperkinetic behavioral anomalies in rats after neonatal exposure to lead (22), dramatize the scope of the problem (23). Nonetheless, the need for further information has been tempered by the moral dilemmas inherent to fetal and neonatal research (24). The recent appearance of

427

numerous books, clinics and symposia (25–32), and comprehensive reviews (33, 34) has allowed us to restrict the subject of this review to fetal and neonatal aspects of the mammalian hepatic cytochrome P450 monooxygenase complex in relation to developmental biology (35–37).

DEVELOPMENT OF HEPATIC MONOOXYGENASE ACTIVITY IN NONPRIMATE MAMMALS

Developmental aspects of the hepatic cytochrome P450 monooxygenase system in nonprimate mammals have been studied for almost two decades (38, 39), and comprehensive reviews are available (34, 40). The capacity of hepatic tissue to catalyze the xenobiotic monooxygenase reaction is presented schematically as a function of the age of the animal from which liver was obtained in Figure 1. The various developmental sequences depicted in Figure 1 apply to different species, including rat (41–48), mouse (49, 50), rabbit (39, 51–53), hamster (54), guinea pig (38, 55, 56), opossum (57), swine (34, 58–60), and ferret (61). The figure was compiled to emphasize the similarities, rather than the differences, in separate studies.

The specific developmental pattern(s) exhibited by each animal may vary with substrate (e.g. 47, 61), strain (62), sex (e.g. 41, 46), and details of tissue preparation (homogenate, postmitochondrial supernatant, or microsomal pellet) including the techniques of cell disruption and differential centrifugation (63). An important consideration involves the standard selected for expression of results since the liver undergoes appreciable anatomical and biochemical modification perinatally (64,

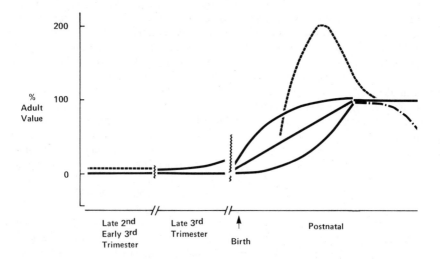

Figure 1 Patterns of development of hepatic monooxygenase activity for different nonprimate mammalian species. See text.

65). The standard employed (body weight or surface area; liver weight, DNA, or protein; microsomal protein or phospholipid; etc) has remained a function of the purpose of each investigation.

Aspects of each phase of development of hepatic monooxygenase activity merit discussion. In contrast to the substantial xenobiotic monooxygenase activity exhibited by midgestational human fetal liver preparations, studies of nonprimate fetal liver have not revealed comparable activity (34, 53, 55, 66), even in animals that achieve considerable maturity in utero (55) or experience a long gestational period (34). Although miniscule, catalytic activity and/or components of the monooxygenase system are measurable in liver from second or third trimester fetal swine (34, 58–60), guinea pig (55), rat (67), and mouse (50).

Many (e.g. 55, 67), but not all, investigations of nonprimate mammals have revealed a definite, albeit small, increase in monooxygenase activity near term. After birth, all animals studied to date have exhibited marked increases in hepatic monooxygenase activity, the time course of which can be measured in days, weeks, or even months. It seems likely that the rapidity with which this sequence occurs is determined at least in part by the relative state of maturity of each animal at birth. During postnatal maturation it has not been unusual to observe levels of hepatic monooxygenase activity that exceed subsequent adult values by two to three fold (45, 47, 55). After puberty, monooxygenase activity toward a few substrates decreases (43, 44, 48).

The influence of fetal and neonatal events upon expression of the sex differences has received recent attention. "Imprinting" by androgens of certain behavioral characteristics and the release of gonadotropins have been recognized for some time in rodents and primates (cf 68). De Moor & Denef (69, 70) observed that the masculine pattern of adult rat hepatic cortisol metabolism could be altered by neonatal castration. A male pattern was expressed after puberty in such animals only in association with the administration of testosterone in the neonatal period; similar androgen exposure in female pups elicited postpubertal masculine hydroxylation patterns. Gonadectomy and/or treatment with androgen after weaning were without relevant effect. The imprinting of hepatic steroid metabolism has been studied in detail by Einarsson and colleagues (71, 72). Chung et al (73) have demonstrated applicability of imprinting to the hepatic xenobiotic monooxygenase reaction, and some evidence has been presented for involvement of pituitary factor(s) (74). Levin et al (75) have evaluated the effects of imprinting on the relative proportions of fast and slow turning-over forms of cytochrome P450 in rat liver microsomal preparations. The significance of these findings deserves emphasis.

CORRELATES OF MONOOXYGENASE ACTIVITY

Various components and catalytic activities that have been associated with the hepatic monooxygenase complex (cytochrome P450, NADPH-cytochrome P450 reductase, NADPH-cytochrome c reductase, NADPH-oxidase, cytochrome b_5, and cytochrome b_5 reductase) have been studied singly or in combination in livers of developing rat (41, 42, 47, 48), rabbit (52, 53), swine (34, 60), guinea pig (55), and ferret (61). In general, the developmental sequences for cytochrome P450 and NADPH-cytochrome P450 reductase resemble closely the developmental patterns for monooxygenase activity depicted in Figure 1. In rabbit (53) and swine (34), the postnatal increments in the content of cytochrome P450 and the activity of NADPH-cytochrome P450 reductase occur synchronously. In rat (41, 76) and ferret (61), however, maturation of NADPH-cytochrome P450 reductase activity lags relative to the increase in cytochrome P450 content despite the presence of substantial NADPH-cytochrome c reductase activity at, or shortly after, birth (41, 61, 76, 77). Certain phenomena reviewed below could be involved in retarding the reducibility of cytochrome P450; these include developmental alterations in (a) the species of cytochrome P450, (b) endogenous ligands affixed to cytochrome P450, and (c) membrane composition and structure (see also reference 76).

In adult rats, the activity of NADPH-cytochrome P450 reductase is considered to be rate limiting with respect to microsomal hydroxylations (78). Although much effort has been devoted to detailed correlations of component data with monooxygenase activity for the purpose of identifying the rate-limiting component during development, we agree with the analysis by Short et al (34) who state, "It seems most likely that after birth the monooxygenase system develops largely as a unit, with some species and substrate variation in the postnatal increase in reducibility of cytochrome P450 by NADPH-cytochrome c reductase." In different developmental studies, the component (or catalytic activity) that correlates best with the development of overall monooxygenase activity has been found to vary with substrate (e.g. 51), species, and sex (41). Other possible rate determinants, such as a deficiency in NADPH or NADH, an age-dependent variation in the ratio of low/high spin iron in cytochrome P450, or an age-dependent change in the stimulatory effects of type I substrates, are not thought to be of quantitative significance (79). An important, unresolved problem relates to possible age-related variation in the relative proportions of different forms (80) of cytochrome P450 (including cytochrome P448), or even the existence of a distinct fetal or perinatal cytochrome (81).

Substrates that generate type I difference spectra with adult hepatic microsomes, elicit reverse type I (modified type II) spectra with preparations from neonatal animals (e.g. 34) and human fetuses (82–84). Although interpretation of the reverse type I difference spectrum is incompletely resolved (85), its occurrence in perinatal hepatic preparations raises the possibility that inhibitory, endogenous ligands are affixed to the monooxygenase complex. Ligand candidates include phospholipids present in immature endoplasmic reticulum (81) and a variety of steroids, the composition and proportions of which are known to fluctuate considerably during maturation (e.g. 86). More specifically, certain metabolites of progesterone inhibit the monooxygenase reaction (87–89). The potential affinity of steroidal ligands for the monooxygenase complex is emphasized by the findings of Juchau and co-workers (90) that relate to human placental preparations and the ability of androstenedione to prevent binding of carbon monoxide to cytochrome P450.

It is generally held that the monooxygenase complex is associated with the smooth endoplasmic reticulum (SER) (91). Electron microscopic investigations (34, 55, 76) of nonprimate mammalian liver have revealed little or no SER before birth;

its appearance postnatally mimics the development of monooxygenase activity (cf 34, 55, 76). The proliferation of SER requires net synthesis of membrane lipid as well as protein. Certain enzymes involved in phospholipid biosynthesis exhibit sharp increases in activity perinatally (92).

Studies with solubilized components of the monooxygenase complex have revealed an absolute requirement for phospholipids (93). The chain length and degree of unsaturation of the fatty acid moieties of phosphatidylcholine determine the extent of monooxygenase activity exhibited by the reconstituted system. In vivo, changes in the fatty acid composition of microsomal phosphatidylcholine have been observed during both postnatal development (94) and xenobiotic induction (95). The linoleic acid content of microsomal phosphatidylcholine parallels monooxygenase activity during phenobarbital induction and withdrawal; changes in oleic acid content correlate best with monooxygenase activity after 3-methylcholanthrene induction. Interestingly, one of the developmental changes in microsomal lipid composition of rabbit liver is an increase in the linoleic acid content of phosphatidylcholine after the tenth postnatal day (94). Finally, current concepts of the mechanism of action of membrane-bound multienzyme complexes have been summarized eloquently by Strittmatter and colleagues (96) for the case of cytochrome b_5 and its reductase; the potential influence of composition and physical state of the membrane upon monooxygenase activity during maturation clearly merits further investigation.

The inverse relationship between monooxygenase activity and microsomal lipid peroxidation is a subject of current investigative interest (97, 98), but quantitative comparisons are complex in part because of the deficiencies inherent in the use of malonic dialdehyde production as a measure of lipid peroxidation. The rate of microsomal lipid peroxidation has been found to increase after the neonatal period in rats and swine (99, 100). A chemically unidentified hepatic cytosol factor of ca 10,000 daltons by gel filtration is capable of inhibiting lipid peroxidation and enhancing monooxygenase activity (101, cf 102); this factor is present at birth and does not seem to fluctuate significantly during subsequent maturation (103).

DEVELOPMENT OF THE MONOOXYGENASE SYSTEM IN PRIMATE LIVER

Certain aspects of the development of hepatic monooxygenase activity in man differ significantly from the sequence depicted in Figure 1. Although little is known about perinatal events, the presence of substantial monooxygenase activity in the hepatic microsomes from the midgestational human fetus has been established. Reference is made to the excellent reviews on this subject in the past few years by Yaffe & Juchau (33), Pelkonen & Kärki (104), Rane et al (105), Short et al (34), and Netter (106). In 1969 and 1970, in vitro demonstration of hepatic xenobiotic monooxygenase activity in livers from late first and second trimester human fetuses was provided independently by various research groups. Pelkonen et al (107) found that the human fetal liver metabolized chlorpromazine, p-nitrobenzoic acid, and hexobarbital, and Arvela et al (108) observed 3,4-benzpyrene hydroxylase activity (cf 49).

Yaffe et al (109) demonstrated that hepatic microsomes obtained from 14 to 25 week abortuses catalyzed the hydroxylation of endogenous substrates such as laurate and testosterone, and significantly, that cytochrome P450, as well as the electron transport enzymes, were measurable. Gustafsson & Lisboa (110) had earlier demonstrated catalysis of the oxidation of testosterone by microsomal preparations from human fetal liver. Similarly, Juchau observed the reduction of p-nitrobenzoic acid (111).

Both hepatic monooxygenase activity (111–114) and SER (115, 116) are demonstrable as early as the sixth week of gestation. Current data suggest that an increase in monooxygenase activity occurs during the first trimester of gestation with subsequent plateau during the second trimester. Pelkonen (112, 113) observed a positive correlation between fetal weight and levels of hepatic monooxygenase activity for fetuses from 8 to 13, but not 13 to 21, weeks of gestation. Yaffe et al (109) also found no significant age-related increase in cytochrome P450, NADPH-cytochrome c reductase, or laurate hydroxylase during midgestation.

A bibliographic summary of data pertaining to monooxygenase activity and components in hepatic preparations from the midgestational human fetus is presented in Table 1. Many of the parameters that influence monooxygenase activity and its variability in animal studies discussed above apply also to study of human fetal tissue. Specifically, characteristics of cell disruption and differential centrifugation are different in fetal and adult liver (119, 124). Although striking interindividual variability exists, hepatic monooxygenase activity toward most substrates is lower than comparative human adult values. Levels of fetal hepatic monooxygenase activity relative to adult tissue vary as a function of substrate, ranging from a few percent [oxidation of 3,4-benzpyrene expressed per gram of liver (117)] to more than 100%

Table 1 Cytochrome P450 monooxygenase activity in early and midgestational human fetal liver

Substrates	References	Component/Activity	References
Aminopyrine	(28%: 117)[a] (84, 113) (109, 120)[b]	Cytochrome P450	(28%: 117)[a] (84, 109, 118–121)
4,16-Androstadien-3-one	(145%: 122)[a]	Cytochrome P450 reductase	(109)
Aniline	(32%: 117)[a] (84, 113, 120, 123, 124)	NADPH-cytochrome c reductase	(49%: 117)[a] (84, 109, 119)
3,4-Benzpyrene	(1–3%: 113, 117)[a] (84, 112, 120, 121, 126–128) (109)[b]	Cytochrome b_5	(109)
		NADPH oxidase	(111)
Chlorpromazine	(112, 114, 128)		
Desmethylimipramine	(129, 130)		
Diazepam	(10%: 131)[a] (132)		
Ethylmorphine	(123)		
Hexobarbital	(37%: 117)[a]		
Laurate	(109)		
N-Methylaniline	(112, 126, 128)		
N,N-Dimethylaniline	(133)		
Neoprontosil	(120)		
p-Nitroanisole	(49)[b]		
p-Nitrobenzoate	(111, 112, 114, 120, 128)		
Testosterone	(109, 110)		

[a] Percentage of adult value; only studies in which comparative adult values are reported have been included.
[b] Inconsistent or negative activity.

[formation of 16 β-hydroxyepitestosterone from 4,16-androstadien-3-one expressed per mg microsomal protein (122) or aniline hydroxylation expressed per gram of liver (123)]. For most substrates, midgestational fetal liver preparations have exhibited 20–40% of adult activity. Components of the monooxygenase complex are present in comparable concentrations, with cytochrome P450 approaching one third of adult levels and NADPH cytochrome c reductase approaching one half of adult activity (117).

Consideration of changes in fractional liver weight has led Pelkonen & Kärki (104) to comment that "fetal and adult capacities to metabolize foreign compounds in vitro are at a surprisingly similar level." The question of in vivo activity of the monooxygenase complex in midgestation remains unresolved. Demonstration of metabolites of diazepam (e.g. 134) and chlorpromazine (135) in the midgestational fetus are suggestive of activity in vivo, but details of the placental transfer of many metabolites remain unexplored.

The potential significance of the presence of substantial monooxygenase activity early in human gestation with respect to teratology, carcinogenesis, and other aspects of toxicity has been emphasized (66, 67). Indeed, Rane & Gustafsson (122) have provided indirect evidence for the production of epoxides in fetal liver by documenting the formation of a 16,17-transglycolic metabolite from 4,16-androstadien-3-one. Similar preparations also catalyze the generation of potentially toxic N-oxides from N,N-dimethylaniline through a process presumably independent of cytochrome P450 (133).

Studies in the third trimester of gestation, and in the neonatal period, have been limited mainly by the difficulties inherent in sample collection. Thus far, two postmortem studies demonstrate that livers from premature and full-term newborn infants contain hepatic monooxygenase activity or possible components thereof. Soyka (136) has demonstrated the presence of cytochrome b_5 and NADPH-cytochrome c reductase in livers from two infants of 33 and 40 weeks gestation. Studies of Aranda et al with specimens from seven premature and full-term infants from 28 to 41 weeks gestation revealed the presence of cytochrome P450, NADPH-oxidase and cytochrome c reductase, aminopyrine N-demethylase, aniline p-hydroxylase (137), and microsomal lipid peroxidation (99). Considerable overlap between the highest perinatal and the lowest adult values was observed. In contrast to the midgestational plateau, a positive correlation was demonstrated between postconceptional age (gestational age + postnatal age) and the activities of aniline p-hydroxylase, NADPH-oxidase, NADPH-cytochrome c reductase, as well as cytochrome P450 content. Since the number of infants studied was limited, and the more premature infants tended to die at a younger age, it is impossible to distinguish which parameter correlates best with the increase in monooxygenase activity: gestational age, postnatal age, or postconceptional age. It is therefore difficult at this time to conclude with confidence from in vitro hepatic data whether or not there is a birth-related, significant increase in monooxygenase activity to or beyond adult values in the postnatal period. It is of considerable interest that the stumptail monkey, which, like man, exhibits appreciable midgestational hepatic monooxygenase activity (138; cf 120), experiences substantial increments in activity perinatally;

the hepatic microsomal content of cytochrome P450 increases about four-fold from 10 days before to 10 days after birth. Studies of the contents of diazepam and N-desmethyldiazepam in umbilical artery and vein have provided some evidence for in vivo function of the monooxygenase complex in term fetuses (139).

Although extrahepatic monooxygenase reactions are not reviewed herein, substantial effort has been devoted to their study in certain fetal tissues. The placental monooxygenase systems have been reviewed by Juchau (140) and Netter & Bergheim (141). It seems that human placental cytochrome P450 exhibits high selectivity in ligand binding, and that few xenobiotics are likely to be substrates for the monooxygenase complex (140). Human placental aryl hydrocarbon hydroxylase activity is well documented, especially in conjunction with maternal cigarette smoking (121, 125, 142–145). Other fetal tissues, including adrenal, kidney, gastrointestinal tract, and lung do exhibit monooxygenase activity (114, 120, 121, 126, 127, 145). Fetal adrenal, compared to liver, is reported to contain higher concentrations of cytochrome P450 (111, 120, 121) and to exhibit substantial monooxygenase activity (120, 121, 126). The perinatal development of monooxygenase activity, as well as detoxification systems, in extrahepatic tissues of animals has been studied intensively by Fouts and colleagues (e.g. 146).

DRUG OXIDATION IN THE HUMAN NEONATE

The appreciable midgestational monooxygenase activity of primate liver raises the possibility that man, unlike laboratory animals, may not experience a substantial postnatal increase in xenobiotic oxidative capacity. Since in vitro data pertaining to hepatic monooxygenase activity in perinatal man are sparse, the subsequent discussion attempts to utilize pharmacokinetic information to probe the question. Although conclusions reached about in vitro systems from pharmacokinetic data must be considered tentative, the few direct developmental comparisons that have been conducted in animals are supportive (44), as are the results of animal toxicology (147). Nonetheless, developmental aspects of distribution, hepatic uptake, storage, conjugation, and biliary and renal elimination, as well as extrahepatic oxidative metabolism (see above), are likely to contribute to the overall pharmacokinetic profile.

The disposition of diphenylhydantoin (DPH) by full-term infants has been studied in considerable detail. Metabolite patterns support applicability of such data to questions regarding oxidative metabolic capacity. Horning et al (7) have demonstrated by gas chromatographic-mass spectrometric techniques the presence of 5-phenyl-5-(4-hydroxyphenyl)-hydantoin (HPPH) and its glucuronide, as well as 5-phenyl-5-(3,4-dihydroxy-1,5-cyclohexadien-1-yl)-hydantoin, in the urine of infants who had been exposed to DPH transplacentally or postnatally. Identical metabolites have been found in adult urine. Indeed, the relative proportions of DPH, HPPH, and conjugated HPPH in urine from neonates who had acquired DPH (and perhaps, metabolites) transplacentally resemble closely those seen in urine from adult man (148, 149). Since HPPH may retard the elimination of DPH, accumulation of the unconjugated metabolite postnatally could complicate interpretation of pharmacokinetic data; accumulation did not occur, at least in the plasma of the one neonate studied (150). The binding of DPH to newborn plasma protein is decreased relative to adult values (151), and the deficiency is accentuated by hyper-bilirubinemia (152) and increased plasma concentrations of fatty acids (153). Adult-like binding is attained by the age of 3 months (154).

Pharmacokinetic investigations of DPH in infants have been conducted by Mirkin [7 newborns, transplacental acquisition (155, 156)], Rane et al [7 newborns, trans-placental acquisition (157)], Baughman & Randinitis [1 newborn, transplacental acquisition (158)], Jalling et al [steady state plasma levels in 6 infants, 5 of whom were more than 3 weeks old (159)], and Loughnan et al [15 infants from birth to 24 months, single-dose decay curves and steady state concentrations (160)]. The interpretation of events in each study and the consequent method of data analysis have influenced conclusions. Mirkin (155), although noting that elimination was "very slow on postpartum days 1 and 2, and increased markedly on postpartum day 3," elected to pool data and derived an average plasma half-life of about 60 hr. Comparative plasma half-lives in adults are much shorter: 11 to 31 hr. Rane et al (157) suggested that possibly the early slow phase of elimination reflected saturation kinetics. Analysis of the subsequent first-order decay curves omitted the events of the first few postnatal days and yielded plasma half-lives (6.6–34 hr) similar to adult values. Jalling et al (159) observed surprisingly low steady state plasma DPH concentrations after multiple intramuscular or oral doses in older infants. Loughnan et al (160) confirmed these observations, and found in single intravenous dose studies that the low steady state plasma concentrations reflected primarily a substantial diminution in half-life (5 to 7 hr) relative to the adult.

Although the question as to why apparent rates of elimination of DPH increase during the neonatal period is unresolved, we believe that the data reflect primarily a maturation of metabolic oxidative capacity. This attitude has been influenced significantly by observation (160) of a number of infants with seizures, who, after an intravenous loading dose of DPH (12 mg/kg) on the first or second postnatal day, received a maintenance (oral or intravenous) dose of 8 mg/kg per day; the plasma DPH concentrations of some infants increased to peak values (> 20 μg/ml) within a few days, only to decline to values of less than 5 μg/ml a few weeks later without alteration in dose/kg. Notably, the elimination rates of other compounds that undergo metabolic oxidation, but do not exhibit saturation kinetics at therapeutic concentrations in adults, can change similarly in the neonatal period. These agents include phenobarbital (see below), tolbutamide (161), and aminopyrine (162). Other drugs have displayed slow rates of elimination in the early postnatal period, but the time at which rates increase is less clearly defined; these include acetanilid (163), diazepam (139, 164–166), amobarbital (167), nortriptylene (168), and mepivacaine (169).

In order to probe postnatal maturation of oxidative capacity, the DPH plasma concentration versus time relationships of individual patients (155–160) have been analyzed to calculate plasma half-lives for three arbitrary age groupings (Figure 2). When half-life changed with age in an individual patient, separate estimations of half-life were made using at least 3 plasma concentration values. In some instances

DPH half-lives were estimated by calculations based on steady state plasma concentrations with assumption of an apparent volume of distribution applicable to that age (160). Such procedures have limitations, and the values generated can be regarded only as approximations. For these full-term infants, mean DPH plasma half-lives of about 80, 15, and 6 hr were derived for the age groupings 0–2, 3–14, and 14–150 days, respectively. Large interindividual variability was seen during the first few postnatal days with half-lives ranging from fewer than 10 to greater than 100 hr; the variability diminished with age. It is difficult to assess the effect of xenobiotic induction upon this maturational sequence. Many of the infants were exposed to phenobarbital along with DPH, and the barbiturate (or DPH) could accelerate maturation of oxidative (170, 171) as well as conjugative (e.g. 15, 16) processes. No dependence of DPH elimination rate on coincident exposure to phenobarbital was apparent.

Speculatively, the data presented in Figure 2 may indicate that the full-term infant is born with about 30% of the relative adult capacity to eliminate DPH. This conclusion compares favorably with in vitro measures of hepatic monooxygenase activity in second and third trimester human fetuses and the perinatal stumptail monkey (see above). The apparent rapid increase in metabolic capacity to levels about two to three fold greater than those of the adult is not without in vitro precedent in animal experiments (see above).

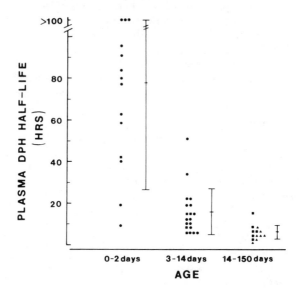

Figure 2 Plasma DPH half-lives measured in infants grouped according to postnatal age. Each infant received the drug either transplacentally (●) or as an initial therapeutic dose (■). Those half-lives calculated from steady state plasma DPH concentrations are indicated (▲). Means and standard deviations are shown. Data were obtained from several published studies (see text).

Even with the assumption that such in vivo data reflect maturation of the xenobiotic monooxygenase complex, generalization to other drugs is not possible. Four of five infants who had acquired carbamazepine transplacentally eliminated the drug in the immediate postnatal period as rapidly as adults (172). Whether or not subsequent rates of elimination would have exceeded adult values is unknown.

The elegant studies of Jalling, Boréus and colleagues (170, 171, 173–175), as well as the earlier investigations of Melchior et al (176) and Heinze & Kampffmeyer (177), permit a similar analysis of the disposition of phenobarbital by neonates and infants. In these investigations, patients acquired the barbiturate transplacentally or were treated postnatally. As seen in Figure 3, the neonates and infants exhibited mean phenobarbital plasma half-lives of greater than 200 hr, about 100 hr, and about 50 hr for the age intervals, 0–5, 5–15, and 30–900 days postnatal, respectively. Many aspects of analysis resemble closely the situation observed with DPH. The large interindividual variability seen in newborns diminished with age. The mean plasma half-life of the drug during the first five postnatal days was twice the adult value, but decreased to about half of the adult value by the age of one month.

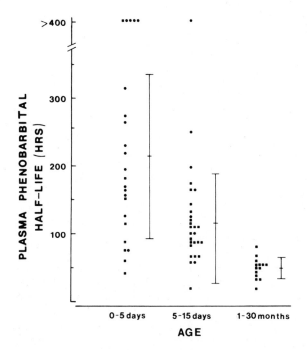

Figure 3 Plasma phenobarbital half-lives in infants grouped according to postnatal age. Some infants received the drug transplacentally (●); in others, half-lives were measured following termination of phenobarbital therapy (■). Means and standard deviations are shown. Data were obtained from several published sources (see text).

With current neonatal intensive care practices, the survival of premature infants is not negligible even when birth occurs in the late second or early third trimester of pregnancy, a circumstance not applicable to the usual animal models. An understanding of the postnatal maturation of xenobiotic oxidative capacity in prematures is of obvious clinical and biological consequence. With respect to modes of drug elimination other than oxidation, the newborn premature is deficient relative to the full-term infant although many functions improve within a few weeks of birth (178). Unfortunately, data that bear upon oxidation are sparse, and it is difficult to separate the effects of illness and nutritional status. Diazepam is eliminated more slowly by premature than full-term newborns (164, 166) but subsequent events are not clear. Unpublished studies in this laboratory indicate that two methylxanthines, caffeine and theophylline, display long plasma half-lives in premature infants (birth weight <1500 g) for at least the first 2 to 4 weeks postpartum. The plasma half-life for caffeine in such infants was greater than 2 days (compared to about 4 hr in adults) and 16 to >60 hr for theophylline [compared to 3.5 hr in children aged 1 to 4 years (179)]. Unfortunately, comparative data in full-term infants are unavailable, but Horning et al (7) have noted a decreased content of the demethylated metabolites of caffeine in urine from full-term infants.

REGULATORY MECHANISMS

The physiological factors responsible for the various developmental sequences displayed by the hepatic monoozygenase complex are not well defined, and may be multiple and/or species-specific. We have considered it appropriate in this review to view the monooxygenase complex as a functional unit that increases in capacity at certain critical periods in development. This conception is not meant to detract from the important differences in the developmental character of individual components or catalytic activities of the complex, but rather to emphasize a relationship to the problems of developmental biology. Similar control mechanisms may act also upon the development of certain other enzymes involved in xenobiotic disposition, such as UDP-glucuronyl transferase (180) and epoxide hydrase (e.g. 181). The recent finding that inducibilities of both UDP-glucuronyl transferase and monooxygenase, but not epoxide hydrase (182), are under genetic control of the "Ah locus" in mice is provocative in this recard.

It is difficult to classify the monooxygenase developmental pattern confidently within the clusters described by Greengard (36). In some species and with certain substrates, activity has increased in the late fetal period; nevertheless, the prominent increment is usually observed postnatally. In guinea pig with chlorcyclizine or benzo(a)pyrene as substrate (55), the pattern might be classified as "neonatal," whereas in the ferret with ethylmorphine as substrate (61), little increase in activity is noted until late in the suckling period. It is generally held that the event of birth per se in some way triggers the development of the monooxygenase complex, but to our knowledge direct evidence is lacking because of the difficulties inherent in the acquisition of significantly premature (or postmature) laboratory animals.

Discussions of potential physiologic control mechanisms must distinguish between direct inhibition of the monooxygenase complex, on the one hand, and agents that act at the level of transcription or translation, on the other. Applicability of one does not exclude modulation by the other. With respect to direct inhibition, the observation of reverse type I difference spectra in human fetal and neonatal animal hepatic microsomal preparations can be interpreted to indicate the presence of such potentially inhibitory endogenous ligands. Interest has focused primarily on the effects of certain steroids and phospholipids (see above). Particularly, metabolites of progesterone that are present in the plasma of pregnant women and fetuses (86) are potent inhibitors of conjugative (183) and oxidative (87–89) enzymes. Endogenous ligands have been implicated to some extent also in explanations of the perinate's decreased plasma protein binding capacity (184, 185). The action of such inhibitors of monooxygenase activity could extend into the suckling period with transmission through milk. Precocious development of coumarin 3-hydroxylase activity has been observed in rats that were weaned early, and the increase could be prevented by administration of 5 β-pregnane-5βol-20-one (89; cf 62). Other studies, however, have failed to demonstrate dependence of monooxygenase activity on the time of weaning (34, 46). It seems that most data reviewed herein indicate that the primary deficit in fetal hepatic monooxygenase activity relates more to decreased contents of the appropriate components and membrane structure than to direct enzyme inhibition.

Substantial effort has been devoted to study of fetal and perinatal induction of monooxygenase activity by xenobiotics. Most studies with nonprimate mammals have revealed that inducibility of monooxygenase activity in fetal liver by barbiturates or polycyclic hydrocarbons is negligible until near or after term (34, 45, 51, 55, 186). Experiments designed to evaluate inducibility of the hepatic monooxygenase system in midgestational human fetal liver by phenobarbital, other drugs, and cigarette smoking have yielded equivocal (128) or negative (145) results. Certain investigations in rodents have revealed some inducibility of hepatic 3, 4-benzpyrene hydroxylation as early as the end of the second trimester of pregnancy (66). After birth, inducibility by xenobiotics increases in striking fashion and has been found to exceed relative adult values later in maturation; significantly, monooxygenase activity returns to the expected basal level for age after withdrawal of the inducer (187). Oesch and colleagues (67) have explored in detail inducer specificity with respect to aryl hydrocarbon monooxygenase and epoxide hydrase activities in rat liver 1 to 3 days antepartum. The minimal responsiveness of midgestational fetal liver (including primates, above) has been hypothesized to reflect any one or a number of maturational parameters, including insufficient exposure in utero (120, 188) and absence of appropriate receptor macromolecules (188). The sequential development in responsiveness of rat liver tyrosine aminotransferase to cAMP, glucagon, hydrocortisone, dietary protein, and pyridoxine (36) offers interesting comparison. The requisite priming effect of hydrocortisone for precocious responsiveness of tryptophan oxygenase and glucokinase to inducibility by substrates may serve also as an informative analogy (36).

Investigations that involve potential physiological inducers are sparse. In liver cultures, hydrocortisone is required for glycogen storage (36), development of bile canaliculi (189), and development of tyrosine transaminase activity (36), but has no effect on aryl hydrocarbon hydroxylase activity (189a, b). The effects of thyroxine on the mixed function oxidase activity in neonatal rats have been studied (190). Conclusions are difficult to summarize because of the fluctuating effects of thyroxine with age. Finally, the possible effects of diet and arterial oxygen tension require clarification.

The presence of fetal repressors has been suggested by certain experiments. In chick embryo cultures, the precocious development of conjugative (35, 191) and oxidative enzymes (192) occurs upon removal of the embryo from the egg. The development of UDP glucuronyltransferase activity in these chick embryo cultures required protein synthesis, but not the presence of adrenal steroids; it was independent of the rate of cell proliferation (35). The potential in ovo repressor(s) has not been chemically identified. Interestingly, livers removed at an early embryonic age achieve higher levels of transferase activity on culture than those extirpated later (35). The injection of phenobarbital in ovo does provoke precocious development of the transferase in situ (35, 193).

Growth hormone has been suggested as a repressor of hepatic monooxygenase activity in the rat (42). The plasma level of growth hormone in the rat at birth is about 200 ng/ml and decreases to adult levels of about 40 ng/ml during the first 21 postnatal days. Adult rats treated with growth hormone have displayed a diminution in hepatic microsomal drug metabolism (194), and the postnatal muturation of oxidative capacity of young rats was slowed, but not prevented, by a single injection of growth hormone (195). Henderson & Kersten (46, 196) have commented that the increase in hepatic monooxygenase activity, both postnatally and during liver regeneration, in rats correlates well with the cessation of active liver growth. The asynchrony of parenchymal cell perinatal maturation with respect to content of glucose-6-phosphatase is of interest in this regard (197, 198). Provocative evidence for a repressor in rat fetal liver has been presented by Klinger et al (199) who demonstrated that the administration of supernatant fractions from fetal liver to weanling rats prevented subsequent induction of monooxygenase activity by phenobarbital, but exerted less effect on basal levels. It was noted that the effects of such manipulations were inconsistent.

Whether the low fetal hepatic monooxygenase activity relates to the lack of effective induction or the existence of repression, or a combination thereof, it should reflect decreased rates of component synthesis or increased degradation. Little data bear directly upon this question, but Short et al (34) have noted an *increase* in the rate of degradation of cytochrome P450 between the age of 5 days and 8 weeks in the pig. Relationships of perinatal maturation of oxidative capacity to membrane structure and the incorporation of heme into the apoprotein of cytochrome P450 (121) require clarification. Although δ-aminolevulinic acid synthetase is thought not to be rate limiting with respect to heme synthesis in fetal rat liver (200), Siekevitz (201) has reported evidence suggestive of the presence of the apoprotein of cytochrome P450 in hepatic microsomes from near-term fetal animals.

CONCLUSION

An attempt has been made to examine developmental aspects of the hepatic cytochrome P450 monooxygenase system as a functional unit in fetal and neonatal mammals including man. In man, monooxygenase activity is detected in liver preparations as early as the sixth week of gestation and increases to a plateau (ca 20–40% of comparative adult values) in midgestation. Aside from other primates, laboratory mammals exhibit miniscule levels of hepatic monooxygenase activity midgestationally, but experience a substantial increase more or less rapidly after birth. Pharmacokinetic and sparse in vitro studies suggest tentatively that primates, like other mammals, experience sharp increases in activity perinatally, but the temporal relationship to birth and the situation in prematures is unclear. Substantial variability is seen in both midgestational in vitro data and early postnatal pharmacokinetic data. The physiological factors involved in differentiation of the monooxygenase unit are unresolved. Indeed, the relative contributions of direct inhibition (e.g. by phospholipids or steroids) as compared to inhibition at a transcriptional or translational level are not yet defined. Certain areas wherein insufficient information is available have been emphasized; they include perinatal aspects of (a) membrane structure and composition, (b) physiological inducers and/or repressors, (c) relationship to cell division, (d) endogenous inhibitors, and (e) incorporation of heme into cytochrome P450. Continued progress in this area promises to bear significantly on the related clinical problem of drug therapy of the premature and full-term infant, as well as teratology and perinatal toxicology.

Literature Cited

1. Stern, L. 1975. *Basic and Therapeutic Aspects of Perinatal Pharmacology,* ed. P. L. Morselli, S. Garattini, F. Sereni, pp. 7–12. New York: Raven
2. Peckham, C. H., King, R. W. 1963. *Am. J. Obstet. Gynecol.* 87:609–20
3. Bleyer, W. A., Au, W. Y. W., Lange, W. A., Raisz, L. G. 1970. *J. Am. Med. Assoc.* 213:2046–48
4. Hill, R. M. 1973. *Clin. Pharmacol. Ther.* 14:654–59
5. Forfar, J. O., Nelson, M. M. 1973. *Clin. Pharmacol. Ther.* 14:632–42
6. Meschia, G., Battaglia, F. C., Bruns, P. D. 1967. *J. Appl. Physiol.* 22:1171–78
7. Horning, M. G., Butler, C. M., Nowlin, J., Hill, R. M. 1975. *Life Sci.* 16:651–71
8. Ayd, F. J., ed. 1973. *Int. Drug Ther. Newslett.* 8:33–39
9. Vorherr, H. 1974. *Postgrad. Med.* 56:97–104
10. Yeh, S. Y., Paul, R. H., Cordero, L., Hon, E. H. 1974. *Obstet. Gynecol.* 43:363–73
11. Van Petten, G. R. 1975. *Br. Med. Bull.* 31:75–79
12. Reynolds, J. W. 1974. *Clin. Obstet. Gynecol.* 17:95–114
13. Liggins, G. C., Howie, R. N. 1972. *Pediatrics* 50:515–25
14. Avery, M. E. 1975. *Br. Med. Bull.* 31:13–17
15. Wilson, J. T. 1972. *Ann. Rev. Pharmacol.* 12:423–50
16. Maurer, H. M. et al 1968. *Lancet* II:122–24
17. Aranda, J. V., Cohen, S., Neims, A. H. 1975. *Abstr. Can. Pediatr. Soc.,* Toronto, Canada
18. Pomerance, J. J., Yaffe, S. J. 1973. *Curr. Probl. Pediatr.* 4:1–60
19. Silverman, H. M. 1974. *Drug Intell. Clin. Pharm.* 8:690–93
20. Shepard, T. H. June 1974. *Dis. Mon.,* pp. 1–32
21. Herbst, A. L., Ulfelder, H., Poskanzer, D. C. 1971. *N. Engl. J. Med.* 284: 878–81
22. Silbergeld, E. K., Goldberg, A. M. 1974. *Exp. Neurol.* 42:146–57
23. Neims, A. H., Chung, L. W. K., Weimar, W. R., Hales, B. 1975. In *Clinical Pharmacology of Psychoactive Drugs,*

ed. E. M. Sellers, pp. 15–33. Toronto: Addict. Res. Found. Ontario

24. Mirkin, B. L. 1975. *Clin. Res.* 23:106–13
25. Boreus, L. O., ed. 1973. *Fetal Pharmacology.* New York: Raven
26. Dancis, J., Hwang, J. C. 1974. *Perinatal Pharmacology: Problems and Priorities.* New York: Raven
27. Morselli, P. L., Garattini, S., Sereni, F., eds. 1975. *Basic and Therapeutic Aspects of Perinatal Pharmacology.* New York: Raven
28. Ankermann, H. 1973. *Entwicklungs-Pharmakologie.* Berlin: VEB Verlag Volk Gesundheit
29. *Pediatr. Clin. North Am.* 1972. Vol. 19
30. *Clin. Pharmacol. Ther.* 1973. Vol. 14
31. *Pediatrics.* Part II. 1974. Vol. 54
32. *Clin. Perinatol.* 1975. Vol. 2
33. Yaffe, S. J., Juchau, M. R. 1974. *Ann. Rev. Pharmacol.* 14:219–38
34. Short, C. R., Kinden, D. A., Stith, R. 1975. *Drug Metab. Rev.* In press
35. Nemeth, A. M. 1973. *Enzyme* 15:286–95
36. Greengard, O. 1971. *Essays Biochem.* 7:159–205
37. Rutter, W. J., Pictet, R. L., Morris, P. W. 1973. *Ann. Rev. Biochem.* 42:601–46
38. Jondorf, W. R., Maickel, R. P., Brodie, B. B. 1958. *Biochem. Pharmacol.* 1:352–54
39. Fouts, J. R., Adamson, R. H. 1959. *Science* 129:897–98
40. Gillette, J. R., Stripp, B. 1975. *Fed. Proc.* 34:172–78
41. MacLeod, S. M., Renton, K. W., Eade, N. R. 1972. *J. Pharmacol. Exp. Ther.* 183:489–98
42. Wilson, J. T., Frohman, L. A. 1974. *J. Pharmacol. Exp. Ther.* 189:255–70
43. Sims, P., Grover, P. L. 1967. *Nature London* 216:77–78
44. Kato, R., Vassanelli, P., Frontino, G., Chiesara, E. 1964. *Biochem. Pharmacol.* 13:1037–51
45. Feuer, G., Liscio, A. 1970. *Int. J. Clin. Pharmacol.* 3:30–33
46. Henderson, P. Th. 1971. *Biochem. Pharmacol.* 20:1225–32
47. Gram, T. E., Guarino, A. M., Schroeder, D. H., Gillette, J. R. 1969. *Biochem. J.* 113:681–85
48. Basu, T. K., Dickerson, J. W. T., Parke, D. V. W. 1971. *Biochem. J.* 124:19–24
49. Pomp, H. B., Schnoor, M., Netter, K. J. 1969. *Dtsch. Med. Wochenschr.* 94:1232–40

50. Nebert, D. W., Goujon, F. M., Gielen, J. E. 1972. *Nature London New Biol.* 236:107–10
51. Pantuck, E., Conney, A.H., Kuntzman, R. 1968. *Biochem. Pharmacol.* 17:1441–47
52. Fouts, J. R., Devereux, T. R. 1972. *J. Pharmacol. Exp. Ther.* 183:458–68
53. Rane, A., Berggren, M., Yaffe, S., Ericsson, J. L. F. 1973. *Xenobiotica* 3:37–48
54. Nebert, D. W., Gelboin, H. V. 1969. *Arch. Biochem. Biophys.* 134:76–89
55. Kuenzig, W., Kamm, J. J., Boublik, M., Burns, J. J. 1975. See Ref. 27, pp. 289–300
56. Kuenzig, W. et al 1974. *J. Pharmacol. Exp. Ther.* 191:32–44
57. Wilson, J. T. 1970. *Pediatric Pharmacology, FDA Symp.,* pp. 34–37
58. Short, C. R., Davis, L. E. 1970. *J. Pharmacol. Exp. Ther.* 174:185–96
59. Short, C. R., Maines, M. D., Westfall, B. A. 1972. *Biol. Neonate* 21:54–68
60. Short, C. R., Stith, R. D. 1973. *Biochem. Pharmacol.* 22:1309–19
61. Ioannides, C., Parke, D. V. 1975. See Ref. 27, pp. 245–53
62. Yaffe, S. 1968. *Report 58th Ross Conf. Pediatr. Res.,* pp. 58–63
63. Chatterjee, I. B., Price, Z. H., McKee, R. W. 1965. *Nature London* 207:1168–70
64. Greengard, O., Federman, M., Knox, W. E. 1972. *J. Cell Biol.* 52:261–72
65. Herzfeld, A., Federman, M., Greengard, O. 1973. *J. Cell Biol.* 57:475–83
66. Robinson, J. R., Felton, J. S., Thorgeirsson, S. S., Nebert, D. W. 1975. See Ref. 27, pp. 155–69
67. Oesch, F. 1975. See Ref. 27, pp. 53–64
68. Resko, J. A. 1975. *Fed. Proc.* 34:1650–55
69. De Moor, P., Denef, C. 1968. *Endocrinology* 82:480–92
70. Denef, C. 1974. *Endocrinology* 94:1577–82
71. Einarsson, K., Gustafsson, J. A., Goldman, A. S. 1972. *Eur. J. Biochem.* 31:345–54
72. Einarsson, K., Gustaffsson, J. A., Stenberg, A. 1973. *J. Biol. Chem.* 248:4987–97
73. Chung, L. W. K., Raymond, G., Fox, S. 1975. *J. Pharmacol. Exp. Ther.* 193:621–30
74. Chung, L. W. K., Raymond, G. 1975. *Pharmacologist* 17:209
75. Levin, W., Ryan, D., Kuntzman, R., Conney, A. H. 1975. *Mol. Pharmacol.* 11:190–200

76. Dallner, G., Siekevitz, P., Palade, G. E. 1966. *J. Cell Biol.* 30:97–117
77. Uehleke, H., Reiner, O., Hellmer, K. H. 1971. *Res. Commun. Chem. Pathol. Pharmacol.* 2:793–805
78. Davies, D. S., Gigon, P. L., Gillette, J. R. 1969. *Life Sci.* 8:85–91
79. Klinger, W. et al See Ref. 27, pp. 255–64
80. Gunsalus, I. C., Pederson, T. C., Sligar, S. G. 1975. *Ann. Rev. Biochem* 44:377–407
81. Iba, M., Soyka, L. F., Schulman, M. P. 1975. *Fed. Proc.* 34:784
82. Rifkind, A., Lauersen, N., Bennett, S., New, M. 1974. *Pediatric Res.* 8:366
83. Rane, A., von Bahr, C., Orrenius, S., Sjöqvist, F. See Ref. 25, pp. 278–301
84. Pelkonen, O. 1973. *Biochem. Pharmacol.* 22:2357–64
85. Schenkman, J. B., Cinti, D. L., Orrenius, S. 1973. *Drug Metab. Dispos.* 1:111–19
86. Deshpande, G. N., Turner, A. K., Sommerville, L. F. 1960. *J. Obstet. Gynaecol. Br. Commonw.* 67:954–61
87. Soyka, L. F., Long, R. J., 1972. *J. Pharmacol. Exp. Ther.* 182:320–27
88. Soyka, L. F., Deckert, F. W. 1974. *Biochem. Pharmacol.* 23:1629–39
89. Kardish, R., Feuer, G. 1972. *Biol. Neonate* 20:58–67
90. Juchau, M. R., Lee, Q. H., Zachariah, K. 1975. *Pharmacologist* 17:208
91. Holtzman, J. L., Gram, T. E., Gigon, P. L., Gillette, J. R. 1968. *Biochem. J.* 110:407–12
92. Getz, G. S., Wentworth, J., Laiken, S. 1970. *Adv. Lipid Res.* 8:175–223
93. Lu, A. Y. H., Levin, W. 1974. *Biochim. Biophys. Acta* 344:205–40
94. Baldwin, J., Cornatzer, W. E. 1968. *Lipids* 3:361–67
95. Davison, S. C., Wills, E. D. 1974. *Biochem. J.* 140:461–68
96. Rogers, M. J., Strittmatter, P. 1974. *J. Biol. Chem.* 249:895–900
97. Kamataki, T., Kitagawa, H. 1973. *Biochem. Pharmacol.* 22:3199–3207
98. Wills, E. D. 1968. *Biochem. J.* 113:325–32
99. Renton, K. W. 1975. *Hepatic microsomal lipid peroxidation and its effects on drug metabolism.* PhD thesis. McGill Univ., Montreal, Canada. 192 pp.
100. Short, C. R. 1975. *Pharmacologist* 17:208
101. Kotake, A. N., Peloria, L. B., Abbott, V. S., Mannering, G. J. 1975. *Biochem. Biophys, Res. Commun.* 63:209–16
102. Kamataki, T., Ozawa, N., Kitada, M., Kitagawa, H. 1974. *Biochem. Pharmacol.* 23:2485–90
103. Warner, M. 1975. *Studies on the ligand-binding protein and other components of Z-fraction.* PhD thesis. McGill Univ., Montreal, Canada. 146 pp.
104. Pelkonen, O., Kärki, N. T. 1973. *Life Sci.* 13:1163–80
105. Rane, A., Sjöqvist, F., Orrenius, S. 1973. *Clin. Pharmacol. Ther.* 14:666–72
106. Netter, K. J. 1971. *Arch. Gynaekol.* 211:112–33
107. Pelkonen, O., Vorne, M., Kärki, N. T. 1969. *Acta Physiol. Scand. Suppl.* 330:69–74
108. Arvela, P., Vorne, M., Järvinen, P., Kärki, N. 1970. *Abstract, Reg. Congr. Int. Union Physiol. Sci. Brasov, Romania*
109. Yaffe, S. J., Rane, A., Sjöqvist, F., Boréus, L.-O., Orrenius, S. 1970. *Life Sci.* 9:1189–1200
110. Gustafsson, J. A., Lisboa, B. P. 1968. *Steroids* 11:555–63
111. Juchau, M. R. 1971. *Arch Int. Pharmacodyn. Ther.* 194:346–58
112. Pelkonen, O. 1973. *Arch Int. Pharmacodyn. Ther.* 202:281–87
113. Pelkonen, O., Kärki, N. T. 1973. *Biochem. Pharmacol.* 22:1538–40
114. Pelkonen, O., Vorne, M., Jouppila, P., Karki, N. T. 1971. *Acta Pharmacol. Toxicol.* 29:284–94
115. Koga, A. 1971. *Analyt. Entwickl. Gesch.* 135:156–61
116. Zamboni, L. 1965. *J. Ultrastruct. Res.* 12:509–24
117. Pelkonen, O., Kaltiala, E. H., Larmi, T. K. I., Kärki, N. T. 1973. *Clin. Pharmacol. Ther.* 14:840–46
118. Pelkonen, O., Kärki, N. T. 1971. *Acta Pharmacol. Toxicol.* 30:158–60
119. Ackermann, E., Rane, A., Ericsson, J. L. E. 1972. *Clin. Pharmacol. Ther.* 13:652–62
120. Juchau, M. R., Pedersen, M. G. 1973. *Life Sci.* 12:193–204
121. Rifkind, A. B., Bennett, S., Forster, E. S., New, M. I. 1975. *Biochem. Pharmacol.* 24:839–46
122. Rane, A., Gustafsson, J. A. 1973. *Clin. Pharmacol. Ther.* 14:833–39
123. Rane, A., Ackermann, E. 1972. *Clin. Pharmacol. Ther.* 13:663–70
124. Ackermann, E., Rane, A. 1971. *Chem. Biol. Interact.* 3:233–34
125. Juchau, M. R. 1971. *Toxicol. Appl. Pharmacol.* 18:665–75

126. Pelkonen, O., Arvela, P., Kärki, N. T. 1971. *Acta Pharmacol. Toxicol.* 30: 385–95
127. Juchau, M. R., Pedersen, M. G., Symms, K. G. 1972. *Biochem. Pharmacol.* 21:2269–72
128. Pelkonen, O., Jouppila, P., Kärki, N. T. 1973. *Arch. Int. Pharmacodyn. Ther.* 202:288–97
129. Rane, A., Ackermann, E. 1971. *Acta Pharmacol. Toxicol.* 29:Suppl. 4, 84
130. Rane, A., Sjöqvist, F., Orrenius, S. 1971. *Chem. Biol. Interact.* 3:305–6
131. Ackermann, E., Richter, K. See Ref. 27, pp. 311–18
132. Idänpään-Heikkila, J. E., Jouppila, P. I., Puslakka, J. O., Vorne, M. S. 1971. *Am. J. Obstet. Gynecol.* 109:1101–6
133. Rane, A. 1974. *Clin. Pharmacol. Ther.* 15:32–38
134. Erkkola, R., Kanto, J., Sellman, R. 1974. *Acta Obstet. Gynecol. Scand.* 53:135–38
135. Pelkonen, O., Jouppila, P., Järvinen, P., Kärki, N. T. 1973. In *Perinatal Medicine,* ed. H. Brossart, J. M. Cruz, A. Huber, L. S. Prod'hom, J. Sistek, pp. 306–7. Bern: Hans Huber
136. Soyka, L. F. 1970. *Biochem. Pharmacol.* 19:945–51
137. Aranda, J. V., MacLeod, S. M., Renton, K. W., Eade, N. R. 1974. *J. Pediatr.* 85:534–42
138. Dvorchik, B. H., Stenger, V. G., Quattropani, S. L. 1974. *Drug Metab. Dispos.* 2:539–44
139. Mandelli, M. et al 1975. *Clin. Pharmacol. Ther.* 17:564–72
140. Juchau, M. R. 1975. See Ref. 27, pp. 29–38
141. Netter, K. J., Bergheim, P. 1975. See Ref. 27, pp. 39–52
142. Nebert, D. W., Winker, J., Gelboin, H. V. 1969. *Cancer Res.* 29:1763–69
143. Welch, R. M. et al 1969. *Clin. Pharmacol. Ther.* 10:100–109
144. Juchau, M. R. et al 1974. *Drug Metab. Dispos.* 2:79
145. Pelkonen, O., Jouppila, P., Kärki, N. T. 1972. *Toxicol. Appl. Pharmacol.* 23: 399–407
146. Bend, J. R., James, M. O., Devereux, T. R., Fouts, J. R. 1975. See Ref. 27, pp. 229–43
147. Goldenthal, E. I. 1971. *Toxicol. Appl. Pharmacol.* 18:185–207
148. Rane, A. 1974. *J. Pediatr.* 85:543–45
149. Reynolds, J. W., Mirkin, B. L. 1973. *Clin. Pharmacol. Ther.* 14:891–97

150. Hoppel, C., Rane, A., Sjöqvist, F. 1975. See Ref. 27, pp. 341–45
151. Ehrnebo, M., Agurell, S., Jalling, B., Boréus, L. O. 1971. *Eur. J. Clin. Pharmacol.* 3:189–93
152. Rane, A., Lunde, P. K. M., Jalling, B., Yaffe, S. J., Sjöqvist, F. 1971. *J. Pediatr.* 78:877–82
153. Fredholm, B. B., Rane, A., Persson, B. 1975. *Pediatr. Res.* 9:26–30
154. Loughnan, P. M., Greenwald, A., Neims, A. H. 1974. *Clin. Res.* 22:726A
155. Mirkin, B. L. 1971. *J. Pediatr.* 78: 329–37
156. Mirkin, B. L. 1971. *Am. J. Obstet. Gynecol.* 109:930–33
157. Rane, A., Garle, M., Borga, O., Sjöqvist, F. 1974. *Clin. Pharmacol. Ther.* 15:39–45
158. Baughman, F. A., Randinitis, E. J. 1970. *J. Am. Med. Assoc.* 213:466
159. Jalling, B., Boréus, L. O., Rane, A., Sjöqvist, F. 1970. *Pharmacol. Clin.* 2:200–202
160. Loughnan, P. M., Watters, G., Neims, A. H. 1975. *Ped. Res.* 9:285
161. Nitowsky, H. M., Matz, L., Berzofsky, J. A. 1966. *J. Pediatr.* 69:1139–49
162. Reinicke, C., Rogner, G., Frenzel, Y., Maak, B., Klinger, W. 1970. *Pharmacol. Clin.* 2:167–72
163. Vest, M. F., Streiff, R. R. 1949. *Am. J. Dis. Child.* 98:688–93
164. Morselli, P. L. et al 1973. *J. Perinat. Med.* 1:133–41
165. Cree, J. E., Meyer, J., Hailey, D. M. 1973. *Br. Med. J.* 4:251–55
166. Morselli, P. L. et al 1974. In *Drug Interactions,* ed. P. L. Morselli, S. Garattini, S. N. Cohen, pp. 259–70. New York: Raven
167. Krauer, B. et al 1973. *Clin. Pharmacol. Ther.* 14:442–46
168. Sjöqvist, F., Bergfors, P. G., Borga, O., Lind, M., Ygge, H. 1972. *J. Pediatr.* 80:496–500
169. Meffin, P., Long, G. J., Thomas, J. 1973. *Clin. Pharmacol. Ther.* 14: 218–23
170. Boréus, L. O., Jalling, B., Kallberg, N. 1975. See Ref. 27, pp. 331–40
171. Jalling, B., Boreus, L. O., Kallberg, N., Agurell, S. 1973. *Eur. J. Clin. Pharmacol.* 6:234–38
172. Rane, A., Bertilsson, L., Palmer, L. 1975. *Eur. J. Clin. Pharmacol.* 8: 283–84
173. Jalling, B. 1976. *Acta Paediatr. Scand.* In press
174. Walling, A., Jalling, B., Boréus, L. O. 1974. *J. Pediatr.* 85:392–98

175. Jalling, B. 1974. *Dev. Med. Child. Neurol.* 16:781–93
176. Melchior, J. C., Svensmark, P., Trolle, D. 1967. *Lancet* 2:860–61
177. Heinze, E., Kampffmeyer, H. G. 1971. *Klin. Wochenschr.* 49:1146–47
178. Gladtke, E., Heimann, G. See Ref. 27, pp. 393–403
179. Loughnan, P. M. et al 1976. *J. Pediatr.* In press
180. Dutton, G. J. 1966. *Biochem. Pharmacol.* 15:947–51
181. Oesch, F., Morris, N., Daly, J. W., Gielen, J. E., Nebert, D. W. 1973. *Mol. Pharmacol.* 9:692–96
182. Owens, I. S., Nebert, D. W. 1975. *Pharmacologist* 17:217
183. Hsia, D. Y. Y., Riabov, S., Dowben, R. M. 1963. *Arch. Biochem. Biophys.* 103:181–85
184. Chignell, C. F., Vesell, E. S., Starkweather, D. K., Berlin, C. M. 1971. *Clin. Pharmacol. Ther.* 12:897–901
185. Hadjian, A. J., Chedin, M., Cochet, C., Chambaz, E. M. 1975. *Pediatr. Res.* 9:40–45
186. Welch, R. M., Gommi, B., Alvares, A. P., Conney, A. H. 1972. *Cancer Res.* 32:973–78
187. Müller, D., Forster, D., Dietze, H., Langenberg, R., Klinger, W. 1973. *Biochem. Pharmacol.* 22:905–10
188. Fouts, J. R. 1973. See Ref. 25, pp. 305–20
189. Lambiotte, M., Vorbrodt, A., Benedetti, E. L. 1972. *C.R. Acad. Sci. Ser. D.* 275:2539–42
189a. Whitlock, J. P., Miller, H., Gelboin, H. V. 1974. *J. Cell Biol.* 63:136–45
189b. Nebert, D. W., Gelboin, H. V. 1968. *J. Biol. Chem.* 243:6250–61
190. Aranda, J. V. 1975. *Thyroxin and development of hepatic microsomal drug oxidation and electron transport in man and rats.* PhD thesis. McGill Univ., Montreal. 233 pp.
191. Dutton, G. J. 1973. *Enzyme* 15:304–17
192. Poland, A., Kappas, A. 1971. *Mol. Pharmacol.* 7:697–705
193. Burchell, B., Dutton, G. J., Nemeth, A. M. 1972. *J. Cell Biol.* 55:448–56
194. Wilson, J. T. 1969. *Biochem. Pharmacol.* 18:2029–31
195. Wilson, J. T. 1970. *Nature London* 225:861–63
196. Henderson, P. Th., Kersten, K. J. 1970. *Biochem. Pharmacol.* 19:2343–51
197. Leskes, A., Siekevitz, P., Palade, G. E. 1971. *J. Cell Biol.* 49:264–87
198. Leskes, A., Siekevitz, P., Palade, G. E. 1971. *J. Cell Biol.* 49:288–302
199. Klinger, W. 1973. See Ref. 28, pp. 51–126
200. Woods, J. S., Dixon, R. L. 1972. *Biochem. Pharmacol.* 21:1735–44
201. Siekevitz, P. 1973. *J. Supramol. Struct.* 1:471–89

METHODS FOR EVALUATING THE TOXICOLOGICAL EFFECTS OF GASEOUS AND PARTICULATE CONTAMINANTS ON PULMONARY MICROBIAL DEFENSE SYSTEMS

❖6659

Elliot Goldstein, George W. Jordan, Malcolm R. MacKenzie
Department of Medicine, University of California, Davis, California 95616

John W. Osebold
Department of Veterinary Microbiology, University of California, Davis, California 95616

INTRODUCTION

Methods to evaluate the toxicity of airborne chemicals (gases and particulates) are of the utmost importance to society. Increasing numbers of potentially toxic contaminants are an invariable consequence of otherwise beneficial industrial processes. Accordingly, toxicological information is essential to assess the need for control measures to protect occupational workers and the public from contaminant-induced health injury. Ideally, these studies should be performed in man using epidemiological or volunteer methods of investigation. Unfortunately, the expense and complexity of epidemiological investigations limit these techniques to the study of selected substances that are either widely disseminated or already suspected of causing human illness. In designing volunteer studies, ethical as well as practical considerations often preclude appropriate toxicological appraisal. Because of these investigational limitations, much reliance must be placed on experiments conducted with animal or cell systems.

Traditionally, nonhuman studies have used physiological, pathological, and biochemical measurements to assess toxicity. Recognition of the association between exposure to noxious gases [ozone (1, 2), nitrogen dioxide (3–5), sulfur dioxide (1, 6)] or airborne particulates [sulfates (6), silica (7), asbestos (8)] and the development of respiratory infection has resulted in the use of microbiological and immunological parameters to evaluate toxicity. Normally, the lungs are protected from bacterial

447

and viral infection by the integrated activity of the mucociliary, phagocytic, and immune systems. Methods are available to assess components of these defense systems, the systems themselves, and their function as a unit in preventing pulmonary bacterial and viral invasion. The results of these experiments in which baseline measurements of one or more defense parameters are compared with measurements made following exposure to test compounds have provided valuable information concerning the toxicity of airborne contaminants (9–12). This article reviews the methods used to assess different microbial defense parameters, their sensitivity in detecting abnormality, the importance of the abnormality as regards susceptibility to infection, and the extent to which the method has been applied in toxicology.

TRANSPORT SYSTEMS OF THE LUNG

The mechanical removal of bacteria from the lung is a primary means of pulmonary protection against bacterial infection (13, 14). Three mechanisms of varying capabilities participate in this process: the mucociliary system, which removes bacteria from the tracheobronchial tree; the alveolar system, which is important for the removal of particulates but may also transport bacteria from alveoli; and cough reflexes, which expel secretions and bacteria from all pulmonary regions (14). The available evidence indicates that of the three, mucociliary transport is the most important. The mucociliary system extends from the nares to the terminal bronchioles (13). Ninety percent of particles that deposit on ciliated epithelium are transported out of the lungs within hours (15, 16). In contrast, the alveolar system requires days to remove intra-alveolar materials (17, 18). Because of the rapidity of bacterial proliferation, such slow rates are unlikely to prevent bacterial infection. The significance of cough mechanisms for maintaining pulmonary sterility is unknown. Cough is of undoubted importance when the lung is already diseased. Whether cough also compensates for ineffective mucociliary removal in the normal lung has not been determined. Depression of the cough reflex may ultimately be shown to be a factor in reducing pulmonary resistance to infection. However, until such data appear, the significance of alterations in cough frequency and intensity as regards infection cannot be evaluated. In accordance with these considerations, this section is confined to a discussion of the methods used to assess different components of the mucociliary transport system and the effect of airborne toxicants on these components.

Tracheobronchial Architecture

Architecturally, the nasopharynx and tracheobronchial tree may be considered as a series of bifurcating tubes of ever diminishing caliber. This configuration allows certain aerodynamic generalizations regarding sites of deposition of inhaled bacteria. Because many factors in addition to anatomic considerations interact to determine particle movement (inertia, velocity, diffusion, gravity, respiratory frequency, tidal volume), these generalizations apply only to the majority of particles of a given size. Bacteria are 0.5 to 2.0 μm in diameter and usually traverse the bronchi suspended in air by Brownian movement to settle in alveolar regions.

Agglomerations of bacteria that form larger particles, 2.0 to 10.0 μm in diameter, are influenced more by gravity than by Brownian movement. These bacterial particles often settle within the tracheobronchial tree (14). Bacterial particles greater than 10 μm in diameter tend to sediment almost immediately in the nasal or pharyngeal cavity. Because the longest diameter of most bacteria is 1.0 to 2.0 μm, single or paired bacteria are likely to reach the alveoli where they are relatively safe from mechanical removal; small groups of bacteria tend to settle on tracheobronchial surfaces where they are amenable to rapid removal, and bacterial clumps are usually too large to enter the lung.

As a consequence of these factors, experiments in which radioisotopically labeled bacterial aerosols are used to study the effect of an airborne toxicant on pulmonary defense systems are a poor means of evaluating mucociliary transport; the finely divided aerosol deposits the majority of bacteria within the alveoli (19). Calculation of mucociliary transport by measuring rates of pulmonary removal of the radioisotope for 4- or 5-hr experimental periods invariably shows unaltered mucociliary function in test animals when compared with controls (11, 19–21).

An additional point of importance pertains to differences in respiratory anatomy among rodents, canines, and primates. For example, the respiratory anatomy of rats differs from that of primates in not having interlobular septae, having fewer generations of airways, utilizing distal bronchioles for respiration rather than alveoli, and in pulmonary vasculature (22). There are also important differences among primates and rabbits, mice, pigs, and dogs (23). These distinctions in anatomy may explain why identical exposures to an airborne toxin may cause diverse mucociliary responses and make interpretation that is relevant to disease in man exceedingly difficult.

Tracheobronchial Mucosa, Mucus, and Mucociliary Movement

The celullar components of the mucociliary system are goblet, clara, ciliated epithelial cells, and apocrine glands (13, 24). The goblet and clara cells and the apocrine glands continuously produce large amounts of a sticky, viscous mucus (0.1–0.3 ml/kg body weight per 24 hr in man) (25), which serves as the backbone of the mucociliary system. This complex fluid has a surface layer with gel-like properties and an underlying layer that behaves like a sol (13). Bacteria that come into contact with mucus are trapped by its adhesiveness. Because of these physicochemical properties, mucus and attached bacteria move as a single layer upward against gravity. Ciliated epithelial cells provide the force for this purposeful movement. The cilia that line the free surface of these cells beat synchronously to propel the overlying mucus at rates of 10 to 20 mm/min (25).

Mechanisms of Injury

Although the mucociliary system is continuously exposed to the atmosphere, environmental injury is uncommon in the absence of technology. A few natural perturbations (extremely dry or cold air, dust, allergens, viruses) can inhibit mucociliary function by hardening the mucus layer, constricting bronchioles, or destroying mucosal cells (26–29). The numerous man-made insults (cigarette smoke, industrial particulates, gaseous pollutants) are considerably more important as causes of mucociliary dysfunction. Exposure to these substances damages cilia, ciliary cells, and mucus-producing cells (24, 30). Such insults result in dyssynchronous ciliary movements, the production of excessive quantities of mucus, and retarded rates of bacterial transport. Because of the relationship of bacterial transport to infection, the result is an increased susceptibility to pulmonary infection.

Measurements of Mucociliary Function

MUCUS Methods exist for determining the amount of mucus produced, its physicochemical characteristics, and its biochemical consistency. Mucus formation can be measured by collecting respiratory secretions from an anesthetized animal via an intratracheal or endotracheal cannula (31–33). The quantity of secretions collected over defined periods allows calculation of hourly or daily rates of formation. The rate in normal animals is then compared with corresponding rates for animals that have received test treatments. It is also possible for the animal receiving the treatment to be its own control. Important sources of error exist in these techniques. The need to anesthetize and to intubate the animals introduces artifacts of mucus formation (anesthesia) and extraneous substances (intubation). A more physiological method for obtaining respiratory secretions has been described by Wardell and associates (34). A 5 to 6 cm segment of the cervical trachea of a dog is separated and formed in situ into a subcutaneous pouch. The isolated system functions for months in a normal fashion. Milliliter quantities of tracheal mucus can be collected at intervals throughout this period. Studies with this experimental model have shown that exposure to sulfur dioxide interferes with mucus production (35).

The rheologic or flow properties of mucus can be measured with various types of viscometers (36–39). Considerable technical expertise is required to perform these delicate measurements. Mucus is subject to shear degradation, and only the gentlest of handling will prevent mechanical breakdown. Furthermore, the test stresses must be similar in magnitude to normal intrapulmonary forces, if the results are to be biologically applicable. When properly performed, viscoelastic measurements provide useful information, for increases in viscosity or elasticity are associated with reductions in mucociliary function (40). These kinds of tests have been used to compare the effectiveness of different mucolytic agents in reducing the viscosity of sputum (37, 41). More recently, investigations in which mucus was obtained from a canine pouch demonstrated that exposure to sulfur dioxide changed the viscosity (35). Future studies with other noxious gases or with particulate inhalants may reveal similar effects.

The concentrations of various constituents of mucus (acid polysaccharides, neutral mucopolysaccharides, sialic acid, and sulfonated compounds) can be measured biochemically (42) and histochemically (43, 44). At present the value of the biochemical measurements is uncertain because relationships between chemical concentrations and mucociliary function have not be established (45). Reid has determined by histochemical testing the percentage of bronchial cells in organ culture explants that secrete glycoproteins at 4 hr after exposure to cholinergic or anticholinergic drugs. The secretory index (percentage of cells secreting at 4 hr) increased in the presence of acetylcholine and decreased with atropine (44). These methods can be used to test the effect of noxious gases and possibly also particulate toxicants on intracellular production of mucus constituents; abnormality would be correlated with hypersecretion.

CILIARY ACTIVITY   Much more is known about ciliary activity than about mucus. Ciliastasis has been used as a bioassay for the detection and assessment of hazardous agents for years (9, 46–49). These bioassays are performed in vitro by removing a section of trachea, visually measuring changes in ciliary rate, and then comparing either changes in rate or in time to cessation of ciliary movement in control and test specimens. Numerous technical variables are inherent in the methodology. Observer error occurs in judging ciliary rate or ciliary cessation. Ciliary rates differ among animals of the same species and even in the same animal at different periods. Lastly, difficulties may occur in reproducing treatment procedures. Because of these variables, statistical evaluations using blind protocols and randomized testing are a necessary part of these experiments (50). Nevertheless, these techniques have yielded valuable information concerning the adverse effects of cigarette smoke (47, 51), chemicals (51, 52), and gaseous and particulate air pollutants (9, 26, 53) on ciliary function. Such results have improved our understanding of the pathogenesis of the toxicant-induced decrease in respiratory resistance to infection and also in some instances (cigarette smoke) allowed testing of protective devices (51).

Errors in visualization can be minimized by using objective methods for measuring ciliary rates. Ciliary activity can be continuously photographed (54, 55) or the rate of flickering can be counted photoelectrically (56, 57) or stroboscopically (58–61). Photography appears to be the most reliable of these methods. Very accurate measurements of ciliary rates can be made by means of high speed photography. Preliminary observations with photoelectric methods indicate that this method will also allow precise determination. Stroboscopy has been successful in measuring slow frequencies of ciliary activity in nonmammalian systems (57). However, attempts to use this technique to record the more rapid rates of ciliary movement in mammals have not had the same success (55). Methods are also available for observing in vivo the rate of ciliary movement (52). A microscope with a vertical light is attached to the trachea via tracheostomy. This system allows measurement of ciliary activity while the animal is exposed to noxious gases or particulates.

Nonvisualization techniques have been used to assess the effects of drugs (62, 63), cigarette smoke (64, 65), and air pollutants on cilia (65, 66). These methods have value in demonstrating beneficial as well as toxic effects of various agents. Increases in ciliary activity have been observed following treatment with several adrenergic drugs, thereby documenting the potential utility of these agents (62, 63). In contrast, exposure to realistic concentrations of cigarette smoke produced zones of ciliary inactivity similar to those observed in bronchitis (64, 65). Preliminary experiments suggest that these techniques can be used to construct dose-response curves (63).

MUCOCILIARY TRANSPORT   Mucociliary transport rates are determined by visually monitoring the rate of movement of particles placed within an excised tracheobronchial system (66), or an incised and externalized in situ system (67–71). More nearly physiological measurements may be obtained by externally monitoring the movement of inhaled radioactive particles in intact animals and humans (72–76). The visual methods that require less expertise and costly equipment have been used in most studies. In these experiments the progress of carbon particles, india ink, or graphite has been measured microscopically within murine, feline, or canine tracheas (67–71). Since all particles do not move at the same rate, arbitrary endpoints such as the fastest rate of transport are recorded. Although the evidence is sometimes inconclusive, particle transport appears to be accelerated by epinephrine (77), inhibited by numerous chemicals (acrolein, formaldehyde, acetone (51), by cigarette smoke (50), and by various noxious gases (SO_2, NO_2, NH_3) (9).

In the past, the sensitivity of mucociliary components (mucus, mucus transport, ciliary movement) to noxious inhalants was determined in an isolated fashion without concomitant measurement of overall mucociliary function. Recently, an in vivo feline model has been designed that allows the simultaneous measurement of mucus load and rheology, tracheal transport velocity, and ciliary beat frequency (71). Future studies with this model should allow assessment of the effect of noxious inhalants on each of these parameters, and on overall mucociliary function. Such data should be extremely helpful in evaluating the significance of threshold impairments to individual mucociliary components.

The intrapulmonary movement of radioactive particles (Au^{198}-Fe_2O_3, Cr^{51}-Fe_2O_3, $Mn^{54}O_2$) can be determined by externally monitoring radioactivity (72–76). A source of uniformly sized γ emitting particles and an Anger camera, or similar measuring device, is required. The human subject or the experimental animal inhales the radioactive particles from an aerosol generator. Sequential measurements of particle location are made with γ-ray–detecting cameras. Because the particles are distributed throughout the lungs, alveolar as well as tracheal clearance rates can be determined from the radioisotopic scans. These techniques have a number of potential advantages for studying airborne toxicants. The methods are physiological, nonhuman primates can be studied, the animal serves as its own control, and clearance rates are measured precisely and sequentially over prolonged periods.

The effects of inspired sulfur dioxide and carbon dust have been studied on mucociliary clearance rates using technetium-99, labeled albumin, and teflon particles. Sulfur dioxide at a concentration of 5.0 ppm had, at most, a minor effect on clearance (76), whereas carbon dust caused very rapid clearance of the radioactive spheres (78, 79). These techniques have also been used to study the deposition and clearance of 2 μm particles by individuals with a history of smoking as compared to nonsmokers (72). In the smokers, tracheobronchial clearance was delayed for periods of one to four hours.

ALVEOLAR MACROPHAGE SYSTEM

The distal alveolar regions of the lung are protected against bacterial infection by the alveolar macrophage system (14, 80). These ubiquitous pulmonary phagocytes are dispersed throughout the alveoli in a manner that allows them to intercept invading bacteria within minutes after their entry into the lung (81). The bactericidal armamentarium of the macrophage inactivates and degrades the ingested bacteria in the ensuing 2 to 4 hr (82–84). The efficiency of this phagocytic system maintains the sterility of the alveolar region under normal conditions despite the constant introduction of microorganisms (14, 85).

The extraordinary ability of the macrophage to seek out, ingest, and inactivate invading bacteria results from the integration of a number of complex biophysical reactions (86). Phagocytes are attracted to bacteria by chemotactic factors that are elaborated by the bacteria themselves, or are formed from the interaction of bacteria and host tissues (86). Simultaneously, serum opsonins attach to the bacterial cell surface rendering the microorganism susceptible to phagocyte ingestion. This opsonizing process is extremely important, because phagocytes that are surrounded by equally palatable particles will selectively ingest ones that have been opsonized (87). Once ingested, bacteria are internally isolated with phagosomes (88); microbicidal enzymes that were in inactive states (secondary lysosomes) are activated and then fuse with the phagosome, to form the phagolysosome. This process allows the delivery of highly active enzymes to the operational site without subjecting the cell's cytoplasm to potentially injurious effects (86, 88). Although the exact role of each of the many enzymes and toxic substances that participate in intracellular bacterial inactivation is not known, the available evidence suggests that lysozyme, catalase, hydrogen peroxide, and malonyldialdehyde, a catabolite of lipid peroxide with antibacterial activity, are among the more important bactericidal substances (86, 88, 89).

The complexity of the above sequence of phagocytic events provides numerous potential sites for an environmental toxin to interfere with phagocytic function. The toxin can impair chemotaxis by destroying chemotactic substances or by reducing phagocytic mobility secondary to the formation of edema. The toxin can inhibit the ingestive process by damaging the phagocytic membrane. Lastly, the toxin can damage the cell itself or the enzymatic systems involved in bacterial inactivation and degradation.

Chemotaxis

Rates of chemotaxis can be measured in vitro by removing pulmonary macrophages and then testing them in Boyden-type chambers (90–92). Highly purified macrophages are obtained by lavage techniques (93). The cells are placed in the upper compartment of the chamber and allowed to migrate through a micropore filter toward an attracting medium. After a period of incubation, the number of macrophages resting on the lower membrane is counted microscopically. Although the results are affected by many technical factors, e.g. adhesiveness of cells to the filter membrane, tortuosity and size of pore channels in the membrane, and detachment of cells into the underlying medium, the tests are sufficiently standardized to assess differences in chemotactic function (94, 95). Technical improvements such as the use of a second filter that is impermeable to cells (96) or measurement of the cell front within the filter (97) should allow better quantitation of chemotactic rates.

The few toxicological studies that have been performed with pulmonary phagocytes indicate that macrophages from otherwise healthy cigarette smokers do not have chemotactic impairments (92), and that extracts of cotton capable of causing byssinosis also do not impair chemotaxis by pulmonary macrophages (98). A wide variety of drugs have been tested with regard to their effect on the movement of polymorphonuclear leukocytes. Glucosteroids (99, 100), chloroquine (99), and colchicine (101) have been shown to suppress chemotaxis in vitro. Future tests of the effects of exposure to airborne gaseous and particulate contaminants on chemotaxis of alveolar macrophages should result in useful toxicological information. These experiments can be performed either by exposing the intact animal to the toxicant and then removing the macrophages, or by exposing macrophages that have already been removed from presumably normal animals.

Phagocytic Ingestion

A number of in vitro tests have been advised to measure rates of phagocytic ingestion (102–109). Macrophage monolayers can be prepared and tested with microbial or particulate suspensions (102–107). Alternatively, bacteria can be injected intratracheally into animals, alveolar macrophages lavaged, and the number of intracellular bacteria counted (108, 109). Different test organisms *Staphylococcus aureus* (102, 103), *S. epidermidis* (102), *Pseudomonas auriginosa* (104, 105), *Aspergillus fumigatus* (106), as well as inert particles (106, 107) have been used in these tests. Time-related visual measurements of the number of ingested microorganisms (102, 103) or particulates (106, 107), or in some instances in which radiolabeled bacteria were studied, measurements of intracellular radioactivity (104, 105) allow assessment of the ingestion rate. Visual measurements of intracellular microorganisms or particulates are sometimes complicated by an inability to differentiate intracellular from extracellular cell-associated bacteria or particulates. This technical problem can be overcome by using *S. aureus,* because this bacteria is uniquely susceptible to lysostaphin, a muralytic enzyme that does not enter phagocytes. The addition of lysostaphin to a culture dish containing macrophages and staphylococcus results in rapid lysis of extracellularly located staphylococci enabling precise determination of the number of intracellular bacteria.

The literature contains few studies of the effect of airborne toxicants on the ingestive function of alveolar macrophages (108–111). The rate of ingestion of intratracheally injected streptococci by rabbit macrophages is reduced following exposure to ozone or nitrogen dioxide (108, 109). Similar reductions in the rate of uptake of radiophosphorus labeled *S. epidermidis* were observed in cell systems in which macrophages were exposed in vitro to ozone (110). The effect of other airborne toxicants on bacterial ingestion by alveolar macrophages has received much less attention (111). Because of the importance of this parameter it is anticipated that measurement of the effects of airborne agents on ingestion rates of alveolar macrophages will be evaluated more thoroughly in future toxicologic experiments.

Bactericidal Activity of Macrophages

The techniques applied in vitro to determining bacterial ingestion rates can also be used to measure rates of intracellular bacterial killing (bactericidal activity). Instead of laborious microscopic scrutiny of phagocytes to count the number of ingested bacteria, the cell suspensions or monolayers are lysed, and the numbers of viable bacteria are determined by pour-plate techniques (103, 105, 106). Because the test results vary for different bacteria to macrophage ratios (112), fixed ratios must be present when comparing treatment and control groups or tests from different days. Much variation also exists in the ability of macrophages to kill different microorganisms (113, 114). These considerations, as well as differences due to technical factors in performing bactericidal assays, make interpretation of results exceedingly difficult.

Because alterations in the rate of bacterial killing relate directly to impairments in pulmonary resistance to infection, many studies of the effect of airborne toxicants on bactericidal function have been performed (104, 110, 115, 116). Ozone (110), nitrogen dioxide (115), cigarette smoke (116), high oxygen tensions (124), and nitrate ion (115) have been tested in phagocytic systems to determine their toxicity. With the exception of oxygen, exposure to concentrations of these agents that were much above ambient caused impairments in intracellular bacterial killing rates.

In Vivo Measurements of Pulmonary Antibacterial Activity

Methods for the evaluation in vivo of the intact pulmonary antibacterial system of rodents (mice, rats, guinea pigs) have been developed (117–120). Briefly, rodents are infected with aerosols of test bacteria. The animals are sacrificed immediately after infection and 4 hr thereafter. The lungs are excised to determine the numbers of viable bacteria by pour-plate techniques. The rate of bacterial inactivation can be determined by comparing the numbers of viable bacteria at each time period. If the bacteria are radiolabeled, precise measurements of pulmonary bacterial inactivation can be made because each animal serves as its own control (118). Histologic determination of the intra- or extracellular locations of the intrapulmonary bacteria at the two time periods reveals the rate of bacterial ingestion by pulmonary macrophages (81). The effects of exposure to ozone (11, 81, 121, 122), nitrogen dioxide (10, 21), sulfur dioxide (19, 123), cigarette smoke (124), automobile exhaust (12), silica (125), and high oxygen tensions (122, 126) have been studied by these experimental methods. According to the data obtained, exposure to above ambient levels of ozone, nitrogen dioxide, and automobile exhaust, but not sulfur dioxide, depresses bactericidal function. Tests with ozone also show that the depression in bactericidal function is due to severe impairments of intrapulmonary phagocytic killing and lesser impairments of bacterial ingestion by the alveolar macrophage (83). In addition to determining threshold levels of toxicity, these methods have also allowed the formulation of dose-response curves (11, 21), and testing of mixtures of airborne toxicants (20). Qualitatively, the results of these studies have compared favorably with other indices of respiratory disease caused by these agents (4, 127).

DEFENSE AGAINST VIRAL INFECTION

A protective function against viral infection has been proposed for the mucociliary transport system, the alveolar macrophage, the interferon system, and humoral and cellular immune mechanisms. The antiviral role of these putative host defenses has been difficult to define, partly because of a lack of the necessary ablative experiments. Studies of the effects of inhaled toxins on resistance to viral infection with concomitant monitoring of specific host defenses have begun to provide not only information on the action of these toxicants, but also information on the physiologic role of the defense mechanisms themselves.

Effect of Pollutants on Viral Respiratory Infection

Epidemiologic data have shown an association between respiratory symptoms indicative of viral infections and increased levels of air pollution (128, 129). Cigarette smoke has been shown to increase the mortality of murine influenza (124). Chronic exposure of squirrel monkeys to nitrogen dioxide renders influenza virus infection fatal, in contrast to the symptomatic, but nonfatal, infection in unexposed animals (130, 131). Mice exposed to 20 ppm of sulfur dioxide for 7 days after infection with influenza virus developed more pneumonia than control animals, although no effect was observed on the growth of influenza virus (132). Conflicting evidence on the effects of oxidants on the pathogenesis of viral infection may result from such factors as the species of animal, the concentration of the toxicant, and the intermittent or continuous nature of the exposure (133, 134). Other effects of toxic gases on the establishment of viral respiratory infection include the increased decay of infectivity of aerosolized Venezuelan equine encephalomyelitis virus in the presence of NO_2 (135) and the increased deposition of vesicular stomatitis virus in the nasal cavity of mice exposed to ozone (136). Studies illustrating detrimental effects of inhaled toxicants on respiratory tract viral infections provide models, which by further study may yield information concerning the involved host defense mechanisms.

Mucociliary Transport

The site of deposition of inhaled particles containing infectious virus may in part determine clinical manifestations. Tracheobronchitis can result from aerosolized rhinovirus type 15; however topical application to the nasal mucosa is a more efficient route for establishing infection, which then spreads down the respiratory tract. In contrast, influenza infection begins in the bronchiolar epithelium with virus swept upward by cilia to cause bronchitis and systemic disease (137, 138).

If the conjunctiva of one eye is inoculated with adenovirus type 4, the sequential development of unilateral rhinitis, tonsillitis, and pharyngitis can be observed before infection spreads to the contralateral side (138). Thus, while entrapment in mucus and physical removal by ciliary action are thought to be a primary defense of the respiratory tract, some viral infections may actually spread by this mechanism. Once viral or mycoplasmal infection of the respiratory tract is established, impaired mucociliary clearance of bacteria can be demonstrated (139, 140).

The Alveolar Macrophage

An important antiviral role for the mononuclear phagocyte has been established for infection of the peritoneum, skin, and brain—indeed, the susceptibility of newborn as opposed to weanling mice can be related to the maturation of the virucidal capacity of these cells (141, 142). Valand et al (143) have shown that lung monocytes from rabbits exposed to 25 ppm of nitrogen dioxide for 3 hr failed to produce interferon after infection with parainfluenza virus type 3 and did not develop resistance to challenge with virulent rabbitpox virus. Subsequent studies by Williams et al (144) showed that the failure of interferon production was not due to lack of attachment, penetration, or uncounting of the virus. In fact, more virus was absorbed and penetrated the macrophages from animals exposed to nitrogen dioxide. Suppression of phagocytic activity and virus-induced resistance were observed to be the most sensitive indicators of NO_2 effects on alveolar cells (145).

The establishment of a viral pulmonary infection results in enhanced susceptibility to bacterial superinfections because of the viral-induced defects in bacterial inactivation by macrophages (146, 147).

Protection of the Respiratory Tract by Interferon

A distinction should be made at the outset between a possible physiological role of interferon as a defense mechanism of the respiratory tract and the antiviral effects that have been demonstrated in vivo using high doses of locally applied interferon or interferon inducers. The cells of the respiratory tract must be exposed directly to the drug administered as an aerosol, or given as drops into the nose or trachea, before resistance to viral challenge via the respiratory route can be demonstrated (148, 149). The administration of mouse interferon intranasally or by aerosol has been shown to inhibit virus replication in the lungs of mice challenged 24 hr later with an aerosol of influenza virus (149, 150). Inducers that stimulate the local production of interferon have also been shown to be effective against intranasal challenge with influenza, mouse pneumonia, vesicular stomatitis, and Columbia SK viruses (p. 306, Table 14.2 in reference 151). These inducers have included pyran copolymer (152), statolon (153), poly I/C (152, 154), and other double-stranded RNAs (155–158). In only a few instances, however, have attempts been made to demonstrate the presence of interferon in the respiratory tract following inducer treatment (153, 154).

Human interferon has been detected in respiratory tract secretions in naturally occurring infections with influenza A_2 (159) and parainfluenza (160) viruses as well as in experimental infections with influenza A_2 (161–163) and members of the rhinovirus and Coxsackie A virus groups (164). Locally applied human interferon has been shown to suppress symptoms and decrease the virus titer during experimental rhinovirus 4 infection in a placebo-controlled double-blind trial (165). Interferon inducers have been shown to suppress symptoms (166, 167), prevent illness, and decrease viral titers in experimental rhinovirus infections (167).

In spite of numerous studies demonstrating protection of the respiratory tract by exogenous interferon or inducers, the importance of the interferon system as a physiologic mechanism is difficult to assess. Evidence that interferon plays a physiologic role in resistance to viral infection is circumstantial and is based on its presence in measurable quantities at the proper time and location to provide beneficial effects to the host. The effect of inhaled toxicants on interferon-mediated resistance has received little study. In order to study the effects of gaseous and particulate pollutants on the interferon system in the respiratory tract, several types of experiments can be envisioned. First, the response to inducers, administered by aerosol, can be determined before and after exposure to toxicants. Two types of measurable response include the level of interferon produced and the degree of protection to virus challenge obtained by the inducer following such exposure. Second, the response to virus challenge after exposure might include observations on the susceptibility to infection, the outcome of infection, and the titer of interferon and virus in respiratory secretions and in the lung.

IMMUNOLOGIC DEFENSES

A detailed presentation of the humoral and cellular immunologic reactions that protect the lung from microbial infection is beyond the scope of this review. Microorganisms that infect the lung stimulate the formation of various protective neutralizing and agglutinating antibodies. The presence of these antibodies may be assayed in respiratory secretions or in blood. Secretions are commonly obtained by pulmonary lavage through a bronchoscope in anesthetized dogs, sheep, and nonhuman primates. Variability in volume and protein concentration of the lavage fluid can be an important source of error (168, 169). Because of this difficulty in specimen collection, whole-lung lavage in terminal experiments is a preferred means for sampling secretions of the lower airways (170–172). Standardized procedures exist for measuring concentrations of neutralizing or agglutinating antibody (173–175). In these procedures the respiratory or serum specimens are serially diluted and reacted against appropriate antigens. An alternative method is to adsorb the antigen on a carrier particle, red blood cells, or latex spheres and to measure antibody-mediated agglutination. Complement fixation or gel immunodiffusion tests are additional methods of measuring antibody (175). The amount of specific antibody in a respiratory or serum sample can be measured with regard to its immunoglobulin class. A fluorescein conjugated anti IgA, IgG, or IgM antibody is added following the reaction of microbial antigen and lavage fluid or serum. If antibodies of the homologous class are bound to the antigen, the particle fluoresces (176).

The few immunologic studies of airborne toxicants indicate that prolonged exposure to carbon or sulfur dioxide can cause a progressive decrease in murine ability to form agglutinating antibodies (177). Cigarette smoke has also been shown to initially enhance and then depress murine antibody response to sheep red blood cell antigens (178). In contrast to these toxicant-induced reductions in antibody formation, continuous exposure for 21 days to nitrogen dioxide did not affect the formation of serum-neutralizing antibody or hemagglutination-inhibiting antibody to influenza virus in nonhuman primates (179). Because of the importance of antibody function in preventing bacterial or viral respiratory infections, further studies of the effect of toxicants on antibody formation are warranted. It is worth emphasizing that appropriate immunological models and test procedures are available for assessing potential toxicity.

It has recently been shown that cellular immune reactions occur locally within the lung (180, 181). These reactions involve the mononuclear population, which in lavage fluid from the normal lung is composed of 78% macrophages and 17% lymphocytes (182). Forty seven percent of the lymphocytes are identifiable as T cells by E rosette formation and 22% as B cells by surface immunoglobulin staining. The B cells are further divided in that 14.5% possess IgM, 9.3% IgG, and only 5% have IgA on their surface. There is in addition a population of cells without markers known as "null cells." Changes in cell number or composition following exposure to toxicants is unknown. Preliminary evidence indicates that in smokers the total number of mononuclear cells is increased and the proportion that are macrophages reaches 95% (182). Cigarette smoke reduces the phytohemagglutinin response of lymphocytes isolated from the peripheral blood, lymph nodes, and spleens of mice (183). The effects of cigarette smoke on pulmonary lymphocytes have not as yet been reported. Since alterations in number and type of lymphocyte can have profound effects on the production of local antibody needed for inactivating invading bacteria or viruses (184), it is likely that these changes will alter resistance to infection.

CONCLUDING REMARKS

In recent years considerable information has accumulated indicating the pathophysiological interrelationship of exposure to noxious atmospheric compounds and enhanced susceptibility to respiratory infection. Recognition of this association has resulted in many studies linking the toxicity of airborne agents to impairments in one or more parameters of pulmonary microbial defense. The development of newer methods of testing microbial resistance allows more precise evaluation of airborne toxicants. Methods are now available for (noninvasive) testing of mucociliary transport, for simultaneously measuring the component parameters of mucociliary function and overall mucociliary transport, and for testing the influence of toxicants on in vivo rates of ingestion and inactivation of bacteria by alveolar macrophages. Additionally, techniques for studying pulmonary susceptibility to viral infection and for studying the effect of toxicants on humoral and cellular immune systems can be used to obtain toxicological information. Although few studies relating exposure to a toxicant on viral susceptibility, or on immune defense have been performed, it can be anticipated that future investigations will provide data regarding these potentially significant interrelationships. Because the above studies can be performed with any inhaled contaminant, the hazard of presently unstudied agents such as pesticides, metallic vapors, and hydrocarbon-containing industrial effluents is assessable by the methods indicated in the test.

One important area for future developmental research concerns the lack of animal models corresponding to human disease states. Present evidence indicates that individuals with underlying illness, especially chronic respiratory disease, are particularly vulnerable to infection following exposure to airborne toxicants. The development and use of animal models that mimic human diseases should significantly enhance our ability to assess the hazard from exposure to man-made airborne contaminants.

460   GOLDSTEIN, JORDAN, OSEBOLD & MACKENZIE

ACKNOWLEDGMENT

This work was supported by contract F33615-73-6-4059 from the Aerospace Medi-
cal Division, Air Force Systems Command and grants from the Electric Power
Research Insitute RP-680-1, California Primate Research Center (USPHS-Grant
RROO-169), and USERDA Contract E(04-3) 472. Preparation of this review was
aided by USAF Contract F33615-76-C-5005 and by California Air Resources Board
Contract 4-611 with the Department of Community and Environmental Medicine,
California College of Medicine, University of California, Irvine, California.

Literature Cited

1. Goldsmith, J. R. 1968. In *Air Pollution,* ed. A. S. Stern, Chap. 14, 547–615. New York: Academic. 2nd ed.
2. Bates, D. V. 1972. *Am. Rev. Respir. Dis.* 105:1–13
3. Lillington, G. A. 1974. In *Environmental Problems in Medicine,* ed. W. McKee, pp. 314–24. Springfield, Ill.: Thomas
4. Goldstein, E. 1975. *Rev. Environ. Health* 2:5–37
5. Ramirez, J., Dowell, A. R. 1971. *Ann. Intern. Med.* 74:569–76
6. French, J. G. et al 1973. *Arch. Environ. Health* 27:129–33
7. Tepper, L. P., Redford, E. P. 1970. In *Harrison's Principles of Internal Medicine.* Chap. 288, 1322–27. 6th ed.
8. Selikoff, I. J., Nicholson, W. J., Langer, A. M. 1972. *Arch. Environ. Health* 25:1–13
9. Dalhamn, T., Sjöholm, J. 1963. *Acta Physiol. Scand.* 58:287–91
10. Ehrlich, R. 1966. *Bacteriol. Rev.* 30:604–14
11. Goldstein, E., Tyler, W. S., Hoeprich, P. D., Eagle, C. 1971. *Arch. Intern. Med.* 127:1099–1102
12. Coffin, D. L., Blommer, E. J. 1967. *Arch. Environ. Health* 15:36–38
13. Kilburn, K. H. 1967. *Arch. Environ. Health* 14:77–91
14. Green, G. M. 1970. *Am. Rev. Respir. Dis.* 102:691–703
15. Green, G. M. 1968. *Ann. Rev. Med.* 19:315–36
16. Morrow, P. E., Gibb, F. R., Johnson, L. 1964. *Health Phys.* 10:543–55
17. Green, G. M. 1973. *Arch. Intern. Med.* 131:109–14
18. Kilburn, K. H. 1974. *Ann. NY Acad. Sci.* 221:276–81
19. Fairchild, G. A., Kane, P., Adams, B., Coffin, D. 1975. *Arch. Environ. Health* 30:538–45
20. Goldstein, E., Warshauer, D. W., Lippert, W., Tarkington, B. 1974. *Arch. Environ. Health.* 28:85–90
21. Goldstein, E., Eagle, M. C., Hoeprich, P. D. 1973. *Arch. Environ. Health.* 26:202–4
22. Roe, F. S. C. June 1966. In *Lung Tumours in Animals,* ed. I. Severi, 111–26
23. Tyler, W. S., McLaughlin, R. F. Jr., Canada, R. O. 1967. *Arch. Environ. Health.* 14:62–69
24. Ballenger, J. J. 1960. *N. Engl. J. Med.* 263:832–35
25. Toremalm, N. G. 1960. *Acta Oto Laryngol. Suppl.* 158:43–53
26. Dalhamn, T. 1956. *Acta Physiol. Scand. Suppl.* 36:1–161
27. Kra Jina, G. Z. 1964. *Acta Oto Laryngol.* 57:342–51
28. Walsh, J. J., Dietlein, L. F., Low, F. N., Burch, G. E., Mogabgab, W. J. 1961. *Arch. Int. Med.* 108:376–88
29. Vaughan, J. H. et al 1973. In *Pathophysiology in Asthma, Physiology, Immunopharmacology, and Treatment,* ed. K. F. Austen, L. M. Lichtenstein, Chap. 1, 1–13. New York: Academic
30. Kensler, C. J., Battista, S. P. 1966. *Am. Rev. Respir. Dis.* 93:93–102
31. Perry, W. F., Boyd, E. M., 1941. *J. Pharmacol. Exp. Ther.* 73:65–77
32. Boyd, E. M., Ronan, A. 1942. *Am. J. Physiol.* 135:383–86
33. Boyd, E. M. 1954. *Pharmacol. Rev.* 6:521–42
34. Wardell, J. R. Jr., Chakrin, L. W., Payne, B. S. 1970. *Am. Rev. Respir. Dis.* 101:741–54
35. Litt, M. 1974. *Ann. NY Acad. Sci.* 221:212–13
36. Davis, S. S., Dippy, J. E. 1969. *Biorheology* 6:11–21
37. Lieberman, J. 1968. *Am. Rev. Respir. Dis.* 97:654–61, 662–72
38. Reid, L. V. 1974. *Scand. J. Respir. Dis. Suppl.* 90:27–32

39. Odeblad, E. 1974. *Scand. J. Respir. Dis. Suppl.* 90:37–39
40. Litt, M. 1970. *Arch. Intern. Med.* 126:417–23
41. Keal, E. 1974. *Scand. J. Respir. Dis. Suppl.* 90:49–53
42. Jakowska, S. 1963. *Ann. NY Acad. Sci.* 106:157–809
43. Lamb, D., Reid, L. 1969. *J. Pathol.* 98:213–29
44. Reid, L. 1974. *Scand. J. Respir. Dis. Suppl.* 90:9–15
45. Reid, L. 1970. *Arch. Environ. Med.* 126:428–34
46. Hilding, A. C. 1957. *Am. J. Physiol.* 191:404–10
47. Dalhamn, T. 1964. *Am. Rev. Respir. Dis.* 89:870–77
48. Dalhamn, T., Rosengren, A. 1968. *Arch. Environ. Health* 16:371–73
49. Cralley, L. V. 1942. *J. Ind. Hyg. Toxicol.* 24:193–98
50. Donnelly, G. M., McKean, H. E., Heird, D. S., Green, J. 1974. *Arch. Environ. Health* 28:350–355
51. Kensler, C. J., Battista, S. P. 1966. *Am. Rev. Respir. Dis.* 93:93–102
52. Gosselin, R. E. 1966. *Am. Rev. Respir. Dis.* 93:41–59
53. Dalhamn, T., Reid, L. 1967. In *Inhaled Particles and Vapours,* ed. C. N. Davies, 299–306. New York: Pergamon
54. Proetz, A. W. 1932. *Trans. Am. Laryng. Assoc.* 54:264–73
55. Dalhamn, T. 1970. *Arch. Environ. Health* 126:424–27
56. Dalhamn, T., Rylander, R. 1962. *Nature London* 196:592–93
57. Mercke, U., Hakansson, C. H., Toremalm, N. G. 1974. *Acta Oto Laryng.* 78:118–23
58. Rivera, J. 1962. *Cilia, Ciliated Epithelium, and Ciliary Activity,* 1–167. New York: Pergamon
59. Gray, J. 1930. *Proc. R. Soc. London* 107:313–32
60. Jennison, M. W., Bunker, J. W. 1934. *J. Cell. Comp. Physiol.* 5:189–97
61. Brokaw, C. S. 1966. *Am. Rev. Respir. Dis.* 93:32–40
62. Iravani, J., Melville, G. N. 1974. *Respiration* 31:350–57
63. Van As, A. 1974. *Respiration* 31:146–51
64. Iravani, J. 1972. *Respiration* 29:480–87
65. Iravani, J., Melville, G. N. 1974. *Respiration* 31:358–66
66. Barclay, A. E., Franklin, K. J. 1937. *J. Physiol.* 90:482–84
67. Lightowler, N. M., Williams, J. R. B. 1969. *Br. J. Exp. Pathol.* 50:139–49

68. Laurenzi, G. A., Yin, S., Collins, B. S. Guarneri, J. J. 1969. *Proc. 10th Aspen Emphysema Conf.,* Aspen, Colorado, June 7–10, 1967. *US Publ. Health Serv. Publ. No. 17 & 7,* p. 27
69. Laurenzi, G. A., Yin, S., Guarneri, J. J. 1968. *N. Engl. J. Med.* 279:333–39
70. Carson, J., Goldhamer, R., Carpenter, R. 1966. *Am. Rev. Respir. Dis.* 93:86–102
71. Adler, K. B., Wooten, O., Dulfano, M. J. 1973. *Arch. Environ. Health* 27:364–69
72. Lourenco, R. V., Klimek, M. E., Borowski, C. S. 1971. *J. Clin. Invest.* 50:1411–20
73. Thomson, M. L., Pavia, D., McNicol, M. W., 1973. *Thorax* 28:742–47
74. Andersen, I., Camner, P., Jensen, P. L., Philipson, K., Proctor, D. F. 1974. *Arch. Environ. Health* 29:290–93
75. Forbes, A. R. 1974. *Br. J. Anaesth.* 46:29–34
76. Sanchis, J. et al 1973. *N. Engl. J. Med.* 288:651–54
77. Kordik, P., Bulbring, E., Burn, J. H. 1952. *Br. J. Pharmacol.* 7:67–79
78. Wolf, R. K., Dolovich, M., Eng, P., Rossman, C. M., Newhouse, M. T. 1975. *Arch. Environ. Health* 30:521–27
79. Camner, P., Helström, P., Philipson, K. 1973. *Arch. Environ. Health.* 26:294–96
80. Bowden, D. H. 1971. *Curr. Top. Pathol.* 55:1–36
81. Goldstein, E., Lippert, W., Warshauer, D. 1974. *J. Clin. Invest.* 54:519–28
82. Cohn, Z. A. 1963. *J. Exp. Med.* 117:27–42
83. Gill, F. A., Cole, R. M. 1965. *J. Immunol.* 94:898–915
84. Elsbach, P., Peltis, P., Beckerdite, S., Franson, R. 1973. *J. Bacteriol.* 115:490–97
85. Kass, E. H., Green, G. M., Goldstein, E. 1966. *Bacteriol. Rev.* 30:488–97
86. Stossel, T. P. 1974. *N. Engl. J. Med.* 290:717–23, 774–80, 833–39
87. Cohn, Z. A. 1968. *Adv. Immunol.* 9:163–214
88. Weissman, G., Zurier, R. B., Hoffstein, S. 1972. *Am. J. Pathol.* 68:539–59
89. Gee, J. B. L. 1970. *Am. J. Med. Sci.* 260:195–201
90. Boyden, S. 1962. *J. Exp. Med.* 115:453–65
91. Ward, P. A. 1968. *J. Exp. Med.* 128:873–17
92. Warr, G. A., Martin, R. R. 1974. *Infect. Immun.* 9:769–71
93. Myrvik, Q. N., Leake, E. S., Fariss, B. 1961. *J. Immunol.* 86:128–32

94. Ward, P. A. 1972. *J. Lab. Clin. Med.* 79:873–77
95. Snyderman, R., Altman, L. C., Hausman, M. S., Mergenhagen, S. E. 1972. *J. Immunol.* 108:857–60
96. Keller, H. U., Borel, J. F., Wilkinson, P. C., Hess, M. W., Cottier, H. 1972. *J. Immunol. Methods* 1:165–68
97. Zigmund, S. H., Hirsh, J. G. 1973. *J. Exp. Med.* 137:387–410
98. Lynn, W. S., Muñoz, S., Campbell, J. A., Jeffs, P. W. 1974. *Ann. NY Acad. Sci.* 221:163–73
99. Ward, P. A. 1966. *J. Exp. Med.* 124:209–26
100. Perper, R. J., Sanda, M., Chinea, G., Oronsky, A. L. 1974. *J. Lab. Clin. Med.* 84:394–406
101. Phelps, P., McCarty, D. J. Jr. 1966. *J. Exp. Med.* 124:115–24
102. Mackaness, G. B. 1960. *J. Exp. Med.* 112:35–53
103. Tan, J. S., Watanakunakorn, C., Phair, J. P. 1971. *J. Lab. Clin. Med.* 78:316–22
104. Murphey, S. A., Hyams, J. S., Fisher, A. B., Root, R. K. 1975. *J. Clin. Invest.* 56:503–11
105. Reynolds, N. Y., Thompson, R. E. 1973. *J. Immunol.* 111:369–80
106. Lundborg, M., Holma, B. 1972. *Sabouraudia* 10:152–56
107. Gardner, D. E., Graham, J. A., Miller, F. J., Illing, J. W., Coffin, D. L. 1973. *Appl. Microbiol.* 25:471–75
108. Coffin, D. L., Gardner, D. E., Holzman, R. S., Wolock, F. J. 1968. *Arch. Environ. Health* 16:633–36
109. Gardner, D. E., Holzman, R. S., Coffin, D. L. 1969. *J. Bacteriol.* 98:1041–43
110. Richmond, V. L. 1974. *J. Lab. Clin. Med.* 83:757–67
111. Gee, J. B. L., Cross, C. E. 1973. In *Fundamentals of Cell Pharmacology*, ed. S. Dikstein, Chap. 14, 349–72. Springfield, Ill.: Thomas
112. Castro, O., Andriole, V. T., Finch, S. C. 1972. *J. Lab. Clin. Med.* 80:857–70
113. Steigbigel, R., Lambert, L. H. Jr., Remington, J. S. 1974. *J. Clin. Invest.* 53:131–42
114. Miller, T. E. 1971. *Infect. Immun.* 3:390–97
115. Vasallo, C. L., Domm, B. M., Poe, R. H., Duncumbe, M. L., Gee, J. B. L. 1973. *Arch. Environ. Health* 26:270–74
116. Green, G. M., Carolin, D. 1967. *N. Engl. J. Med.* 276:421–27
117. Laurenzi, G. A., Berman, L., First, M., Kass, E. H. 1964. *J. Clin. Invest.* 43:759–68

118. Green, G. M., Goldstein, E. 1966. *J. Lab. Clin. Med.* 68:669–77
119. Goldstein, E., Green, G. M., Seamans, C. 1970. *J. Lab. Clin. Med.* 75:912–23
120. Jakab, G. J., Green, G. M. 1973. *Am. Rev. Respir. Dis.* 107:776–83
121. Coffin, D. L. 1970. In *Inhalation Carcinogenesis, A.E.C. Symp. Ser.* 18, 259–69
122. Huber, G. L., Laforce, F. M. 1970. *Antimicrob. Agents Chemother.* 1:129–36
123. Rylander, R., Ohrström, M., Hellström, P. A., Bergstrom, R. 1971. In *Inhaled Particles,* ed. W. H. Walton, III: 535–41. London: Unwin Brothers
124. Spurgash, A., Ehrlich, R., Petzold, R. 1968. *Arch. Environ. Health* 16:385–91
125. Goldstein, E., Green, G. M., Seamans, C. 1969. *J. Infect. Dis.* 120:210–16
126. Shurin, P. A., Permutt, S., Riley, R. L. 1971. *Proc. Soc. Exp. Biol. Med.* 137:1202–8
127. Coffin, D. L., Gardner, D. E. 1972. *Ann. Occup. Hyg.* 15:219–34
128. Thompson, D. J. et al 1970. *Am. J. Public Health* 60:731–39
129. Ipsen, J., Deane, M., Igenito, F. E. 1969. *Arch. Environ. Health* 18:462–72
130. Henry, M. C., Findlay, J., Sprangler, J., Ehrlich, R. 1970. *Arch. Environ. Health* 20:566–70
131. Fenters, J. D., Findlay, J. C., Port, C. D., Ehrlich, R., Coffin, D. L. 1973. *Arch. Environ. Health* 27:85–89
132. Fairchild, G. A., Roan, J., McCarroll, J. 1972. *Arch. Environ. Health* 25: 174–82
133. Buckley, R. D., Loosli, C. G. 1969. *Arch. Environ. Health* 18:588–95
134. Greenburg, L. 1967. *Arch. Environ. Health* 15:167–76
135. Ehrlich, R., Miller, S. 1972. *Appl. Microbiol.* 23:481–84
136. Fairchild, G. A. 1974. *Am. Rev. Respir. Dis.* 109:446–51
137. Landahal, H. D. 1972. In *Assessment of Airborne Particles—Fundamentals, Applications, and Implications to Inhalation Toxicology,* ed. T. T. Mercer, P. E. Morrow, W. Stoler, Chap. 21, 421–28. Springfield, Ill.: Thomas
138. Ward, T. G. 1973. *Prog. Med. Virol.* 15:126–58
139. Lourenco, R. V., Stanley, E. D., Gatmaitan, B., Jackson, G. G. 1971. *J. Clin. Invest.* 50:62a
140. Jarstrand, C., Camner, P., Philipson, K. 1974. *Am. Rev. Respir. Dis.* 110:415–19
141. Allison, A. C. 1974. *Prog. Med. Virol.* 18:15–31

142. Merigan, T. C. 1974. *N. Engl. J. Med.* 290:323–29
143. Valand, S. B., Acton, J. D., Myrvik, Q. N. 1970. *Arch. Environ. Health* 20:303–9
144. Williams, R. D., Acton, J. D., Myrvik, Q. N. 1972. *J. Reticuloendothel. Soc.* 11:627–36
145. Acton, J. D., Myrvik, Q. N. 1972. *Arch. Environ. Health* 24:48–52
146. Goldstein, E., Buhles, W. L., Akers, T. G., Veedros, N. 1972. *Infect. Immun.* 6:398–402
147. Goldstein, E., Akers, T., Prato, C. 1973. *Infect. Immun.* 8:757–61
148. Finter, N. B., Ed. 1966. In *Interferons,* 232–267. Amsterdam: North-Holland
149. Finter, N. B. 1967 . In *Interferon,* ed. M. J. Wolstenholme, A. O'Connor, 204–17. London: Churchill
150. Finter, N. B. 1969. *Ann. NY Acad. Sci.* 173:131–50
151. Finter, N. B., ed. 1973. In *Interferons and Interferon Inducers,* Chap. 14, 295–361. New York: Am. Elsevier
152. DeClercq, E., Merigan, T. C. 1969. *J. Gen. Virol.* 5:359–68
153. Kleinschmidt, W. J. 1969. *Ann. NY Acad. Sci.* 173:547–56
154. Hill, D. A., Baron, S., Chanock, R. M. 1969. *Bull. WHO* 41:689–93
155. Lampson, G. P., Tytell, A. A., Field, A. K., Nemes, M. M., Hilleman, M. R. 1967. *Proc. Natl. Acad. Sci. USA* 58:782–89
156. Tytell, A. A., Lampson, G. P., Field, A. K., Hilleman, M. R. 1967. *Proc. Natl. Acad. Sci. USA* 58:1719–22
157. Nemes, M. M., Tytell, A. A., Lampson, G. P., Field, A. K., Hilleman, M. R. 1969. *Proc. Soc. Exp. Biol. Med.* 132:784–89
158. Field, A. K., Lampson, G. P., Tytell, A. A., Nemes, M. M., Hilleman, M. R. 1967. *Proc. Natl. Acad. Sci. USA* 58:2102–8
159. Gresser, I., Dull, H. B. 1964. *Proc. Soc. Exp. Biol. Med.* 115:192–95
160. Wheelock, E. F., Larke, R. P. B., Caroline, N. L. 1968. *Prog. Med. Virol.* 10:286–347
161. Jao, R. L., Wheelock, E. F., Jackson, G. G. 1965. *J. Clin. Invest.* 44:1062
162. Jao, R. L., Wheelock, E. F., Jackson, G. G. 1970. *J. Infect. Dis.* 121:419–26
163. Wheelock, E. F. 1967. *PAHO/WHO Sci. Publ. 147,* Washington, DC, p. 623

164. Cate, T. R., Douglas, G. Jr., Couch, R. B. 1969. *Proc. Soc. Exp. Biol. Med.* 131:631–36
165. Merigan, T. C., Reed, S. E., Hall, T. S., Tyrrell, D. A. 1973. *Lancet* I:563–67
166. Hill, D. A., Baron, S., Perkins, J. C., Worthington, M., Van Kirk, J. E., Mills, J., Kapikian, A. Z., Chanock, R. M. 1972. *J. Am. Med. Assoc.* 219:1179–84
167. Panusarn, C., Stanley, E. D., Dirda, V., Rubenis, M., Jackson, G. G. 1974. *N. Engl. J. Med.* 291:57–61
168. Dulfano, M. S. 1973. *Sputum: Fundamentals and Clinical Pathology.* Springfield, Ill.: Thomas
169. Muggenburg, B. A. et al 1972. *Am. Rev. Respir. Dis.* 106:219–32
170. Myrvik, Q. N., Leake, E. S., Fariss, B. 1961. *J. Immunol.* 86:128–36
171. Brain, J. D. 1970. *Arch. Intern. Med.* 126:477–87
172. Medin, N. I., Osebold, J. W., Zee, Y. C. 1976. *Am. J. Vet. Res.* In press
173. Davis, B. D., Dulbecco, R., Eisen, H. N., Ginsberg, H. S., Wood, W. B. Jr. 1973. *Microbiology,* 1198–1201. Hagerstown, Md.: Harper & Row
174. Bailey, W. R., Scott, E. G. 1974. *Diagnostic Microbiology. A Textbook for the Isolation and Identification of Pathogenic Microorganisms,* 339–46. St. Louis, Mo.: Mosby
175. Nakamura, R. M. 1974. *Immunopathology. Clinical Laboratory Concepts and Methods,* 418–58, 583–620, 620–49. Boston: Little, Brown
176. Baublis, J. V., Brown, G. C. 1968. *Proc. Soc. Exp. Biol. Med.* 128:206–10
177. Zarkower, A. 1972. *Arch. Environ. Health* 25:45–50
178. Thomas, W. R., Holt, P. G., Keast, D. 1975. *Arch. Environ. Health* 30:78–80
179. Fenters, J. D., Ehrlich, R., Findley, J., Spangler, J., Tolkacz, V. 1971. *Am. Rev. Respir. Dis.* 104:448–51
180. Mackaness, G. B. 1971. *Am. Rev. Respir. Dis.* 104:813–28
181. Truitt, G. L., Mackaness, G. B. 1971. *Am. Rev. Respir. Dis.* 104:829–43
182. Daiele, R. P., Altose, M. D., Rowlands, D. T. Jr. 1975. *J. Clin. Invest.* 56: 986–96
183. Thomas, W. G., Holt, P. G., Keast, D. 1973. *Arch. Environ. Health* 27:373–75
184. Gershon, R. K. 1973. *Contemp. Top. Immunobiol.* 3:1–74

EVALUATION OF ABNORMAL LUNG FUNCTION

◆6660

A. F. Wilson, R. D. Fairshter

California College of Medicine, Department of Medicine, University of California, Irvine, California 92668

J. R. Gillespie

School of Veterinary Medicine, Department of Physiological Sciences, University of California, Irvine, California 92668

J. Hackney

Rancho Los Amigos Hospital and Department of Medicine, University of Southern California, School of Medicine, Downey, California 90242

INTRODUCTION

Impairment of lung function is often not apparent symptomatically or by clinical examination until substantial and largely irreversible damage has occurred (1, 2). Since many substances that are toxic or potentially toxic to the lung are present in our environment (3–5) and since clinically obvious lung disease may be evident only after prolonged exposure to atmospheric contaminants, it is useful to have sensitive and noninvasive means for detection of pulmonary toxicity from inhaled substances.

Recent investigations have demonstrated that sensitive physiologic tests are capable of detecting abnormal lung function at an early, and, presumably reversible stage of development (1, 2, 6–12). These methods include such tests as maximal expiratory flow rates (6–8), single-breath and multibreath nitrogen washout (9, 10), closing volume (11), frequency dependence of compliance (1), and radioisotopic regional ventilation-perfusion studies (12). Since some of the methods are invasive and/or require expensive equipment, they are not all equally suitable as screening tests for abnormal lung function. Yet, a variety of physiologic tests are necessary since tests, such as maximal expiratory flow rates, detect airway obstruction whereas others, such as single-breath diffusing capacity for carbon monoxide (DLCO SB), are affected primarily by abnormalities of the pulmonary parenchyma or vasculature. Some methods, which are not suitable for screening purposes, are excellent confirmatory tests in specific circumstances.

465

Part I of this review describes a sequential approach to pulmonary function testing following experimental and natural exposure of humans or animals to inhalants, which includes suggestions as to screening and initial testing as well as later, more detailed investigation procedures. Approaches are suggested for differing circumstances (awake vs anesthetized) and species (large and small animals vs man). Part II, mainly presented in tabular form, offers a critical review of the limitations and applications of individual tests of pulmonary function.

I   Sequential Approach to Pulmonary Function Testing
    A.   <u>Man</u> (Unanesthetized)
                    Preexposure Testing for Control Values

                               Exposure

      1.   Screening
          a.   Closing volume (CV)
          b.   Single-breath (SB) N_2 washout
          c.   Single-breath diffusing capacity of the lung for CO (DLCO SB)
          d.   Maximum expiratory flow-volume (MEFV) curves
          e.   Spirometry
          f.   Airway resistance (R_{AW}) and thoracic gas volume (Vtg)
      2.   Follow-up testing
          a.   Arterial blood gases
          b.   Multibreath N_2 washout (7 min)
      3.   Further analysis, appropriate tests from Table 1

For screening purposes following exposure to inhalants, closing volume (11) and SB N_2 washout (9) are noninvasive, easy to perform, and both tests may be calculated from the same expiratory maneuver. The test is moderately sensitive but is quasistatic since low flow rates are employed. Dynamic methods such as MEFV curves and spirometry, particularly if flow rates are measured at low lung volumes (FEF 25–75, FEF 75–85), may be abnormal when static tests are normal (15). Both procedures are noninvasive, easy to perform, and therefore well suited for screening purposes. All measurements can be made technically from a single maneuver although the tests are usually repeated to insure "best effort." The MEFV curve is probably best utilized with the subject serving as his own control since flow rates are highly variable from person to person (16). The sensitivity of the technique may be increased by comparison of curves obtained after inhaling air and helium-oxygen mixtures (17). Airway resistance is easy to perform but is sensitive to abnormalities, primarily of large central airways (1, 18) and should not be used alone. Changes in maximal expiratory flow (particularly at low lung volumes) with no change in R_{AW} would suggest that the site of the lesion is in the small airways. DLCO SB is simple and easy to perform; this test and, possibly, SB N_2 washout might be the most sensitive detectors of early (interstitial) pulmonary edema or microatelectasis (19, 20).

Arterial blood gas analysis is a very sensitive parameter of change in respiratory status. The procedure is invasive and is best performed with local anesthesia; it therefore probably should not be considered a screening procedure. Multibreath nitrogen washout is highly sensitive to abnormalities of distribution of ventilation (10); however, not only does this procedure require more time to perform than single-breath tests, but also analysis of results is more time consuming. Multibreath nitrogen washout is best utilized in selected circumstances (i.e. to confirm borderline results, to differentiate degrees of abnormality not apparent from screening tests, and to further investigate suspected abnormalities in the presence of negative screening tests).

A variety of other tests such as radioisotopic regional ventilation and perfusion studies, static or dynamic compliance, pulmonary artery catheterization, multiple inert gas washout are detailed in Table 1. These tests will provide answers to specific questions. They are, in general, more invasive, more expensive and require greater expertise to perform.

B. Large Animals (Unanesthetized)
      Preexposure Testing for Control Values

      Exposure

1. Screening tests
    a. Spirometry—respiratory rate, tidal and minute volume
    b. Arterial blood gases—PaO_2, $PaCO_2$, pH
    c. Multibreath nitrogen washout—distribution of ventilation, functional residual capacity (FRC)
2. Confirmatory tests
    a. Dynamic compliance
    b. Dynamic resistance (airway)
    c. Total pulmonary resistance (oscillatory)
    d. Steady state diffusing capacity for carbon monoxide (DLCO SS)
    e. Other appropriate tests from Table 1

C. Large Animals (Sedated or Anesthetized)
      Preexposure Testing for Control Values

      Exposure

1. Screening tests
   a. Spirometry—respiratory rate, tidal and minute volume
   b. Lung volumes—total lung capacity (TLC), vital capacity (VC), functional residual capacity (FRC), residual volume (RV)
   c. Arterial blood gases—PaO_2, $PaCO_2$, pH
   d. Multibreath nitrogen washout—distribution of ventilation, FRC
   e. Lung compliance—static (Cst), dynamic (Cdyn) including measurements at different respiratory rates (frequency dependence of compliance)
   f. Dynamic resistance (airway)
   g. Total pulmonary resistance (oscillatory)
2. Confirmatory tests
   a. Closing volumes
   b. DLCO SS
   c. DLCO SB
   d. Maximal expiratory flow-volume (MEFV) curves
   e. Radioisotopic regional ventilation-perfusion ($\dot{V}/\dot{Q}$) studies
   f. Other appropriate tests from Table 1

Unanesthetized large animals may be tested using either a face mask (21) or chronic tracheostomy (22). These techniques are used most frequently in relatively cooperative, trainable animals such as dogs. Alternatively, any animal may be tested using general anesthesia, although this method seems less desirable since the effects of anesthesia must also be assessed. Recently, however, Muggenburg & Mauderly have shown that general anesthesia, using triflupromazine HC1, is associated with minimal respiratory side effects (23).

Screening procedures, such as spirometry or multibreath nitrogen washout, are usually easy to perform, noninvasive, and require relatively little equipment or training of animals (see Table 1). Arterial blood gases, although invasive, also require relatively little time and equipment. They probably are best obtained from an indwelling catheter in a femoral or exteriorized carotid artery. Multiple samples can be obtained without causing pain and agitation, which are often associated with reflex changes in respiration.

The confirmatory tests either require intubation and are, therefore, invasive (dynamic compliance, dynamic resistance, radioisotopic regional ventilation studies, MEFV curves), require expensive equipment (DLCO, dynamic compliance, dynamic resistance, radioisotopic regional ventilation-perfusion studies, MEFV curves), or are time consuming (dynamic compliance, dynamic resistance, radioisotopic regional ventilation-perfusion studies) and, therefore, are poorly suited for screening purposes except in anesthetized animals. However, many of these latter methods are also the most sensitive and yield the most information. MEFV curves, for example, have recently been used successfully in monkeys to evaluate the effects of coal dust upon the small airways (24). Although relatively elaborate equipment was required, individual subjects (monkeys) could be completely tested within 10–12 min following induction of anesthesia (24).

D. Small Animals

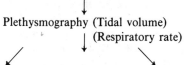

Preexposure Testing for Control Values

↓

Exposure

↓

Plethysmography (Tidal volume)

↓ (Respiratory rate)

Postmortem studies

a. Total respiratory resistance (Amdur-Mead technique	a. Histology	¹³³Xe washout
	b. Pressure volume curves	
b. Maximum expiratory flow-volume curves	c. Lung lavage for surface active material	
	d. Pulmonary edema analysis (wet/dry weight ratios)	

The most suitable technique for in vivo screening for response to inhalants is plethysmography. The plethysmograph is relatively easy to construct, and small animals such as rats may be monitored even (with difficulty) without anesthesia. The technique is sensitive and tidal volume and respiratory rate can be measured. Postmortem studies may be sensitive but are both time consuming and tedious and therefore poorly suited for screening purposes in large numbers of small animals. Pulmonary resistance as measured by the technique of Amdur & Mead (25) requires placement of an intrapleural catheter; a plethysmograph and physiologic recorder are also required. The procedure has merit for in vivo testing of small animals but probably should not be considered a screening procedure. ^{133}Xe washout requires expensive equipment as well as use of radioisotopes. As yet, this procedure has not been widely used in small animals. Its utility is not definitely established and therefore is currently under evaluation.

II Specific Types of Tests

The following is a description of pulmonary function methods, their sensitivity and limitations, physiologic interpretation, and the equipment needed for their performance. The material is presented in tabular form as a convenient reference for the inhalation toxicologist (Table 1). This description of methods is divided into the following categories: 1. Ventilatory exchange, measurement of volumes of gases exchanged during (usually quiet) breathing. These tests are ordinarily not very useful. 2. Static lung volumes. These tests are simple and provide useful information about the strength and elasticity of the respiratory system. They are usually combined with other types of tests since they, by themselves, do not provide definitive information. 3. Tests of respiratory mechanics, analysis of the forces that provide resistance to airflow and inflation or deflation of the lung. Tests of respiratory mechanics vary from the simple to the complex. They are important for the detection and analysis of most types of exposure. 4. Tests of distribution of ventilation, description of the degree of uniformity of alveolar ventilation. Maldistribution of the inspired gas is often associated with early lung disease even though total ventilation is normal or increased. Methods of detecting airway closure are also considered in this section of the table. 5. Tests describing the pulmonary circulation including measurement of vascular pressures, right to left shunting, and distribution of perfusion. Since these measurements are relatively insensitive and require special equipment, they are usually reserved for particular circumstances. 6. Tests describing regional ventilation/perfusion matching ($\dot{V}/\dot{Q}$). This includes direct evaluation of regional ventilation and perfusion as well as several different tests. These measurements are more important to understanding the mechanism of pulmonary function abnormalities than early detection. 7. Tests of diffusion. Although impaired diffusion of oxygen across the alveolar-capillary membrane is not a common cause of hypoxemia (13, 14), diffusing capacity is affected by a wide variety of lung diseases and therefore is a good screening test. 8. Blood gas measurement. These important parameters are affected by abnormalities, single or combined, including altered respiratory mechanics, right to left shunting, altered $\dot{V}/\dot{Q}$ relationships, control of respiration, and acid-base balance. Although not specific for any one type of abnormality, arterial hypoxemia is a sensitive indicator of impaired pulmonary function from a multitude of causes, while mixed venous oxygen tension is more indicative of tissue oxygenation and more often reflects the state of cardiac rather than pulmonary function.

DISCUSSION

Pathologic studies indicate that a surprisingly high percentage of autopsied nonsmoking adults have pulmonary emphysema (135, 136), while a higher incidence of emphysema in both smokers and nonsmokers has been found in areas with high atmospheric concentrations of sulfur oxides, nitrogen oxides, hydrocarbons, and particulates (136). Clinical chronic bronchitis is more common in urban areas (137), and children from urban environments have maximal expiratory flow rates lower than predicted (138). Though much of this data can be explained by high atmospheric levels of common pollutants, viral respiratory infections and cigarette smoking probably have additive deleterious effects upon lung function (136, 138).

The toxicity of all potential atmospheric contaminants, alone or in combination, as well as safe exposure limits, needs to be defined. One approach to this problem is exposure of humans or animals, under strictly controlled experimental conditions, to varying concentrations, durations, and combinations of inhalants. The results of such investigations must be objective and reproducible, and the methods must be sensitive and capable of large-scale utilization. The use of the pulmonary

Table 1 Characteristics and limitations of pulmonary function tests

	Name of test	Physiological interpretation	Animal species	Experimental conditions	Sensitivity	Limitations	Equipment needed	References
Ventilatory exchange	Respiratory rate.	Frequency of breathing.	Any.	Many.	Low, large animals; moderate, small animals.	Very few.	Spirometer, face mask for large animals or plethysmograph, pressure transducer, recorder for small animals. Pneumograph and transthoracic impedance are noninvasive.	26
	Tidal volume.	Depth (volume of breathing).	Any.	Many.	Low, large animals; moderate, small animals.	Very few.	Spirometer, face mask for large animals or plethysmograph, pressure transducer, recorder for small animals. Pneumograph and transthoracic impedance are noninvasive.	26
	Minute ventilation.	Total volume of breathing in one minute (may measure inspiration or expiration). Equals the product of respiratory rate multiplied by tidal volume.	Any.	Many.	Low, large animals; moderate, small animals.	Very few.	Spirometer, face mask for large animals or plethysmograph, pressure transducer, recorder for small animals. Pneumograph and transthoracic impedance are noninvasive.	26
Static lung volumes[a]	Total lung capacity.	Elasticity of lungs and thorax, muscle strength.	Any (see experimental conditions).	Only man without external forces; animals (30 cm H_2O) distending pressure.	Good.	Requires maximal effort or external distending and/or withdrawing pressures.	Spirometer plus helium catharometer, nitrogen meter, or other inert gas measuring device or body plethysmograph.	27–30
	Vital capacity.	Elasticity of lungs and thorax, muscle strength.	Any (see experimental conditions).	Only man without external forces; animals (30 cm H_2O) distending pressure.	Good.	Requires maximal effort or external distending and/or withdrawing pressures.	Spirometer.	30, 31

Table 1 *(Continued)*

Name of test	Physiological interpretation	Animal species	Experimental conditions	Sensitivity	Limitations	Equipment needed	References
Static lung volumes[a] *(continued)*							
Residual volume.	Elasticity of lungs and thorax, muscle strength.	Any (see experimental conditions).	Only man without external forces; animals (30 cm H_2O distending pressure.	Good.	Requires maximal effort or external distending and/or withdrawing pressures.	Spirometer plus inert gas measuring device of body plethysmograph.	30, 31
Expiratory reserve volume.	Expiratory force, diaphragm position.	Any (see experimental conditions).	Only man without external forces; animals (30 cm H_2O distending pressure.	Good.	Requires maximal effort or external distending and/or withdrawing pressures.	Spirometer	31
Functional residual capacity.	Elasticity of lungs and thorax.	Any (see experimental conditions).	Resting.	Good.	Almost none.	Spirometer (body plethysmograph, with cooperation).	30, 32, 33
Inspiratory capacity.	Inspiratory force, diaphragm position.	Any (see experimental conditions).	Only man without external forces.	Good.	See TLC.	Spirometer (body plethysmograph, with cooperation).	31
Respiratory mechanics **Compliance**							
Static lung and thoracic cage compliance (C total).	Stiffness of respiratory system. $$\frac{1}{C_{total}} = \frac{1}{C_{stat}(\ell)} + \frac{1}{C_{stat}(W)}$$ (liter/cm H_2O)	Any (see experimental conditions).	Results uncertain without anesthesia and paralysis of respiratory muscles.	Moderate or less.	Requires cooperation or relaxing anesthesia plus external forcing.	Pressure and volume transducers, amplifiers and recorders. One method requires head-out body chamber.	34, 35
Static lung compliance. (Static volume pressure curves) [$C_{st}(\ell)$]	Stiffness of the lungs quasistatic. A measure of distensibility, reciprocal of elastance. (liter/cm H_2O)	Mammals, any (see experimental conditions).	Only in man without relaxing anesthesia, for full curves. Animals: for $C_{st}(\ell)$ in tidal volume range in unanesthetized or full range with relaxing anesthesia.	Moderate.	Requires cooperation or relaxing anesthesia plus external forcing (see experimental conditions).	Pleural (animals only) or esophageal balloon, pressure and volume transducers, amplifiers, recorder, or CRT, or X-Y plotter, or tape.	36

Table 1 *(Continued)*

Respiratory mechanics
Compliance *(continued)*

Static thoracic cage compliance [C_{stat} (w)].	Stiffness of chest wall. (liter/cm H_2O)	See Cst and C total.	See Cst and C total.	See Cst and C total.	See Cst and C total.	See Cst and C total.	37
"Specific" compliance.	Cst/V_{tg} where V_{tg} is usually at functional residual capacity. (liter/cm H_2O per liter)	Mammals, any (see experimental conditions).	For Cst (ℓ) in tidal volume range. Relaxing anesthesia may not be required.	Moderate or less.	See Cst (ℓ), requires measurement of FRC.	See Cst (ℓ) and FRC.	37
Dynamic lung compliance [Cdyn (ℓ)].	Stiffness of lung at specified frequency. Frequency dependent if Cdyn is a function of frequency. (liter/cm H_2O)	Mammals, any (see experimental conditions).	Usually only man without relaxing anesthesia for studies at a full range of frequencies.	Moderate or less.	Usually requires co-operation or relaxing anesthesia plus external forcing.	Same as for static volume pressure curves plus a pneumotachograph measure flow.	1, 38, 39
Static volume pressure curves of saline-filled excised lungs.	Tissue (quasistatic) distensibility. (liter/cm H_2O)	Mammals, any (at necropsy).	Saline-filled excised lungs.	Moderate.	Leakage and lack of uniform filling can create problems. Excised lungs.	Pressure and volume transducers, amplifiers, and recording devices.	40
Airflow	Spirometry-forced expired volume vs time.	Overall mechanical function of lungs and thoracic wall including flow rates at various parts of the expiratory curve (e.g. maximum midexpiratory flow in liters/sec) and FEV in liters at various times (e.g. 0.75, 1, 2, 3 sec).	Any (see experimental conditions).	Usually only man without relaxing anesthesia with external forcing.	Good to moderate.	Usually requires co-operation, a relaxing anesthesia plus external forcing.	Low resistance spirometer or pneumotachograph with integrator.	41

474   WILSON, FAIRSHTER, GILLESPIE & HACKNEY

Table 1 *(Continued)*

Name of test	Physiological interpretation	Animal species	Experimental conditions	Sensitivity	Limitations	Equipment needed	References
Respiratory mechanics **Airflow** *(continued)*							
Flow-volume maximum expiratory flow-volume curves (MEF).	Overall mechanical function of lung and thoracic wall including Peak Flow Rates (PEFR) and flow rates at various volumes (e.g. MEF_{50} at 50% of vital capacity).	Mammals, any (see experimental conditions).	Usually only man without relaxing anesthesia. Measurements with gases of different physical properties can be done (e.g. He or SF_6).	Good to moderate.	Usually requires cooperation or relaxing anesthesia plus external forcing.	Storage oscilloscope or a photographic X-Y recorder or tape. Low resistance spirometer or pneumotachograph with integrator.	42
Flow-volume inspiratory maximum inspiratory flow-volume curves (MIF).	Overall mechanical function of lung and thoracic wall including Peak Flow Rates (PIFR) and flow rates at various volumes (e.g. MIF_{50} at 50% of vital capacity).	Mammals, any (see experimental conditions).	Usually only man without relaxing anesthesia. Measurements with gases of different physical properties can be done (e.g. He or SF_6).	Good to moderate.	Usually requires cooperation or relaxing anesthesia plus external forcing.	Storage oscilloscope or a photographic X-Y recorder or tape. Low resistance spirometer or pneumotachograph with integrator.	42
Lung and thoracic cage flow resistance (total resistance) (Rrs).	Changes in total respiratory system. (cm H_2O/liter per sec)	Mammals, any.	Can use several frequencies (e.g. 3, 6, 12, 24 Hz).	Good to moderate.	Specificity of interpretation limited.	Oscillatory equipment, transducers for flow, pressure, amplifiers, recorders: stripchart, tape.	43, 44
Total lung flow-resistance (Rℓ).	Flow-resistance of airways and lung tissue $Rℓ = Raw + Rℓt$. (cm H_2O/liter per sec)	Mammals, any; (see Cst (ℓ)).	See Cst (ℓ).	Moderate.	See Cst (ℓ).	Pleural (animals only) or esophageal balloon, pressure and flow transducers, amplifiers, recorder or CRT or X-Y plotter, or tape.	45, 46

Table 1 *(Continued)*

Respiratory mechanics Airflow *(continued)*							
Airway flow-resistance (Raw).	Flow-resistance of airways. $Raw = R_{peripheral} + R_{central}$ ($cm\ H_2O$/liter per sec)	Mammals, usually only man.	(Method #1, body plethysmograph) Usually only man.	Moderate or less.	Requires panting.	Body plethysmograph.	47
Small airways flow-resistance (R_p).	Partition of flow-resistance to airways usually of < 2-3 mm diameter. ($cm\ H_2O$/liter per sec).	Difficult with small animals.	Only animals or excised human lungs.	Good to moderate.	Requires invasive procedure.	Retrograde catheter, transducers for flow pressure, amplifiers, recorders (see $R\ell$).	48
Specific airway resistance [SR (aw)].	$1/SG$ (aw).	See SG (aw).	See SG (aw).	See SG (aw).	See SG (aw).	See SG (aw).	49
Frictional resistance lung tissue ($R\ell$).	Subtraction of Raw from total lung flow-resistance. $R\ell t = R\ell - Raw$. ($cm\ H_2O$/liter per sec).	See Raw and total lung flow-resistance.	See Raw and total lung flow-resistance.	See Raw and total lung flow-resistance.	See Raw and total lung flow-resistance.	See Raw and total lung flow resistance.	50
Airway conductance (Gaw).	$Gaw = 1/Raw$. (liter/sec per $cm\ H_2O$)	See Raw.	See Raw.	See Raw.	See Raw.	See Raw.	28, 51, 52
Specific airway conductance [SG (aw)].	$(1/Raw)/V_{tg}$ where V_{tg} usually = FRC airway conductance per unit lung volume.	See Raw and V_{tg}; see V_{tg}.	See Raw; see V_{tg}.	Moderate.	Need measure of V_{tg}.	See Raw and V_{tg}.	28, 51, 52

Table 1 *(Continued)*

	Name of test	Physiological interpretation	Animal species	Experimental conditions	Sensitivity	Limitations	Equipment needed	References
Respiratory mechanics								
Work of breathing	Work of breathing, lungs and thoracic wall.	Work of moving lungs and thoracic wall (kgM/min).	Any (see experimental conditions).	Results uncertain without anesthesia and paralysis of respiratory muscles. Work of inspiration and expiration can be separated.	Moderate or less.	Combined measure.	See C total pressure, flow volume (recorder), body respirator.	35, 53, 54
	Work of breathing, lungs.	Work of moving lungs. (kgM/min).	Any.	See Cst and total lung flow-resistance. Work of inspiration can be separated.	Moderate.	See Cst and total lung flow-resistance.	See Cst and total lung flow-resistance.	35, 53, 54
	Work of breathing, thoracic wall.	Work of moving thoracic wall. (kgM/min).	Any.	Results uncertain without anesthesia and paralysis of respiratory muscles. Work of inspiration and expiration can be separated.	Moderate or less.	See experimental conditions.	See C total pressure, flow volume (recorder), body respirator.	35, 53, 54
Distribution of ventilation[b]	Closing volume ^{133}Xe (bolus distribution).	Closure of dependent airways.	Man, rabbit probably minimal size; larger animals better.	Requires cooperation. Only man without anesthesia. May be done in large animals with anesthesia, positive and negative pressure breathing.	Moderate; most sensitive if measured as closing capacity/TLC (Closing capacity = CV + RV).	See experimental conditions.	Spirometer; flow meter; scintillation counter; digital rate meters, physiologic recorder.	55, 56
	Closing volume (helium bolus distribution).	Closure of dependent airways.	Man, rabbit probably minimal size; larger animals better.	Requires cooperation. Only man without anesthesia. May be done in large animals with anesthesia, positive and negative pressure breathing.	Moderate; most sensitive if measured as closing capacity/TLC (Closing capacity = CV + RV).	See experimental conditions.	Spirometer; flow meter; critical orifice helium analyzer; physiologic recorder.	57

Table 1 *(Continued)*

Distribution of ventilation *(continued)*							
Closing volume (argon bolus distribution).	Closure of dependent airways.	Man, rabbit probably minimal size; larger animals better.	Requires cooperation. Only man without anesthesia. May be done in large animals with anesthesia, positive and negative pressure breathing.	Moderate; most sensitive if measured as closing capacity/TLC (Closing capacity = CV + RV).	See experimental conditions.	Spirometer; flow meter; mass spectrometer, physiologic recorder.	11
Closing volume (nitrogen dilution).	Closure of dependent airways.	Man, rabbit probably minimal size; larger animals better.	Requires cooperation. Only man without anesthesia. May be done in large animals with anesthesia, positive and negative pressure breathing.	Moderate; may be slightly less sensitive than bolus techniques. Measure as CC/TLC.	See experimental conditions.	Spirometer, flow meter, nitrogen analyzer, physiologic recorder.	58
Nitrogen washout, single breath.	Distribution of ventilation.	Man, rabbit probably minimal size; larger animals better.	Requires cooperation. Only man without anesthesia. May be done in large animals with anesthesia, positive and negative pressure breathing.	Moderate; may be normal when dynamic measurements are abnormal.	See experimental conditions.	Spirometer, flow meter, nitrogen analyzer, physiologic recorder.	9, 59
Nitrogen washout, multi-breath.	Distribution of ventilation.	Man, large animal, beagle dog, Shetland pony, monkey, baboon.	Only man and beagle without anesthesia; animals require tight-fitting face mask; restraints.	High; sensitivity increased by washout at high respiratory rates and poor collateral ventilation.	See experimental conditions.	Spirometer or pneumotachograph; nitrogen analyzer; physiologic recorder.	60-62
Regional pulmonary function, 133Xe technique.	Topographical distribution of ventilation.	Man, baboon, monkey.	Only man without E-T tube; anesthesia, controlled ventilation.	High; man: low, animals (due to limited experience).	See experimental conditions.	Spirometer; multiple scintillation counters or Anger camera; computer or strip charts, physiologic recorder, ventilator, air pump (animals).	12, 63
133Xe washout multi-breath.	Distribution of ventilation.	Man, baboon.	Only man without E-T tube; anesthesia, controlled ventilation.	High; man: low, animals; not yet well quantitated or subjected to compartmental analysis in animals.	See experimental conditions.	Spirometer; multiple scintillation counters or Anger camera; computer or strip charts, physiologic recorder, ventilator, air pump (animals).	63-65

Table 1 *(Continued)*

	Name of test	Physiological interpretation	Animal species	Experimental conditions	Sensitivity	Limitations	Equipment needed	References
Pulmonary circulation	Cardiovascular pressures.	Intravascular diastolic, systolic, and/or mean pressures. Detects hyper- or hypotension in vascular system. Necessary for calculations of vascular resistances and ventricular work.	Any (see conditions). Difficult in small rodents.	Awake animals following preparation of indwelling catheters. Anesthetized animals usual.	Can be done with good accuracy and reproducibility. Moderate to low sensitivity for pulmonary disease.	Few limitations if one has adequate training and equipment. Frequency-response of equipment and proper application essential. Animals should be studied under similar conditions and levels of activity.	Cardiac catheters, strain gauges, and recorder. Surgical equipment. Fluids, drugs, and variety of stopcocks.	65–75
	Cardiovascular volumes, flows, resistance, and work.	Cardiovascular performance.	Any (see conditions). Difficult in small rodents.	All can be done on reasonably tractable awake animal *except* pulmonary capillary blood volume and pulmonary capillary blood flow.	Can be done with good accuracy and reproducibility. Moderate to low sensitivity for pulmonary disease.	Calculated (derived) values. Each value depends upon several variables. Otherwise limitations as listed above.	As above. Dye dilution equipment, body plethysmograph, and appropriate strain gauges. Appropriate drugs and test gases.	65–81
	Distribution of perfusion ^{133}Xe technique.	Regional distribution of pulmonary blood in the lung.	Meaningful only in animals the size of cats *or larger.*	Animals usually anesthetized and positioned with limited movement.	Moderate to low.	Expensive equipment. Useful only on larger animals. Requires use of radioactive material.	Four scintillation detectors and cylindrical collimetors. Magnetic tape recorder. Rate meter.	82–84
	^{135}I-macroaggregated albumin technique.	Regional distribution of pulmonary blood in the lung.	Meaningful only in animals the size of cats *or larger.*	Animals usually anesthetized and positioned with limited movement.	Moderate to low.	Expensive equipment. Useful only on larger animals. Requires use of radioactive material.	Scanner. Radiological equipment.	82–84
	Right to left pulmonary vascular shunt during O_2 breathing.	Percentage of the cardiac output that is bypassing ventilated exchange area in the lung.	More conveniently done in animals at least the size of cats.	Animal must breathe 100% O_2 without rebreathing. Animals usually anesthetized. Must measure O_2 concentration in inspired air, expired air, arterial and mixed venous blood.	Depends upon how rigorously each measurement is made for the shunt calculation. Moderate to good for advanced, chronic lung disease.	Accuracy of measure of O_2 content in mixed venous blood and alveolar O_2.	Blood gas analysis equipment; blood gas pressure analysis, Scholander and perhaps Van Slyke or gas chromatograph with gas extractor.	85, 86

Table 1 *(Continued)*

Pulmonary circulation *(continued)*	Matching of ventilation and perfusion.	Regional distribution of ventilation relative to perfusion in the lungs.	Meaningful only in animals the size of cats *or larger*.	Animals usually anesthetized and positioned with limited movement.	Moderate to low.		Expensive equipment. Useful only on larger animals. Requires use of radioactive material.	55, 87-93
	Reflexes Pulmonary vascular effects of breathing O_2.	Measurement of effect of high O_2 concentrations upon pulmonary vascular resistance (see Cardiovascular resistance, and work, above) and and distribution of perfusion (see Distribution of perfusion, above, and Matching of ventilation and perfusion, above).	All experimental animals.	Awake animals following preparation of indwelling catheters. Anesthetized animals usual.	Moderate to low.	Few limitations if one has adequate training and equipment. Frequency-response of equipment and proper application essential. Animals should be studied under similar conditions and levels of activity.	As in Cardiovascular pressures, above, and breathing equipment for giving O_2.	94-102
	Histamine, fibrinopeptide B, bradykinin analysis.	Chemical and/or biological analysis for concentration of pulmonary vasoactive agents.	All experimental animals.	Chemical and/or biological analyses of concentrations in plasma, blood or tissue.	Low.	Availability of techniques.	Cardiac catheters, strain gauges, and recorder. Surgical equipment, fluids, drugs, and variety of stopcocks. Breathing equipment for giving O_2.	103, 104
	Diffusion perfusion ratio studies.	Measure of the distribution of pulmonary diffusion relative to pulmonary perfusion.	Animals at least the size of cats.	Animals anesthetized and usually terminal preparation. Requires special gas handling equipment.	Moderate to unknown.	Requires excellent experimental control and measurement of pulmonary and cardiovascular variables.	Respiratory gas chromatograph. Ability to handle and analyze labeled O_2. Breathing equipment.	105-107
	Edema evaluation. In vivo, 112 indium-transferrin.	Estimate of extravascular fluid accumulation in the lung.	Animals at least the size of cats. Technique confirmed only on sheep.	Animal must be restrained by counters.	Moderate to unknown.	New technique must be confirmed on species other than sheep.	Four scintillation detectors and cylindrical collimeters. Magnetic tape recorder. Rate meter.	108-111

Table 1 *(Continued)*

Name of test	Physiological interpretation	Animal species	Experimental conditions	Sensitivity	Limitations	Equipment needed	References
Pulmonary circulation *(continued)*							
Edema evaluation. *(continued)*							
In vitro wet/dry weight ratios.	Measurement of total lung H_2O.	All experimental species.	Study of lung tissue after death.	Moderate to good.	Animals must be sacrificed.	Laboratory balance and desiccating oven.	108–111
In vivo pulmonary tissue volume.	Estimate of tissue volume exposed to and in equilibrium with gas in airways.	Meaningful only in animals the size of cats *or larger.*	Anethetized controlled airways in animals.	Moderate.	Indirect measurement.	Gas analysis gas-volume measurement.	76
Postmortem pulmonary arterial and bronchial arterial casts.	Relative distribution of pulmonary and bronchial circulations.	All experimental species and postmortem material from human beings.	Postmortem material.	Moderate to low.	Access to material. Tedious work requiring long man hours.	Vascular canula, latex, or other appropriate injection material.	112
Regional ventilation/ perfusion matching ($\dot{V}/\dot{Q}$)							
Arterial PO_2.	See Blood gases.						
$AaDO_2$.	$\dot{V}/\dot{Q}$ or shunt.	Any but larger better.	Good.	Good.	Requires arterial blood and measurement of alveolar gas (Scholander, gas chromatograph, mass spectrometer).		86, 113
$AaDN_2$.	$\dot{V}/\dot{Q}$.	← Similar to $AaDO_2$.	Good.		Requires arterial blood and measurement of alveolar gas (blood gas extractor, gas chromotograph, recorder).		114
Radioisotopes.	Regional $\dot{V}/\dot{Q}$.	Rabbit probably minimal size.	Any.	Fair.	Restraint, cooperation or anesthesia required.	Multiple probes or scintillation camera.	83
Radioisotopes.	Regional ventilation.	Rabbit probably minimal size.	May be measured during breath holding or during breathing.	Fair.		Deposited aerosols do not measure ventilation; 133Xe most convenient isotope.	115
Radioisotopes.	Regional perfusion.	Rabbit probably minimal size.	May be measured during breath holding or during breathing.	Fair.		113In, 131I, or 99mTc, combined with albumin or other 30 μ particles most widely used; 133Xe dissolved in saline useful when studies need to be repeated rapidly.	115

Table 1 *(Continued)*

Regional ventilation/ perfusion matching (V̇/Q̇) *(continued)*							
Single expiration PCO_2 and R.	V̇/Q̇	Any, but larger better.	Slow, complete expiration.	Fair	Cannot quantitate.	CO_2, O_2 meters of mass spectrometer.	5, 116
V_D/V_t:	V̇/Q̇ particularly high ratios.	Any, but larger better.	Need constant breathing pattern.	Fair.	Hard to quantitate.	Analysis of CO_2 in mixed expired gas and arterial blood.	113
Lobar gas sampling.	Regional V̇/Q̇.	Large.	Requires lobar catheters.	Fair.	Invasive, anesthesia.	Catheter, gas analyzers.	117
Multiple inert gas washout.	Distribution of V̇/Q̇.	Any, but larger better.	Collection of expired gas, venous infusion, cardiac output measurement.	Good.	Somewhat complicated.	Gas chromatography mass spectography; dye dilution or Fick cardiac output.	118
Diffusion							
D_LCO (SB).	D_M, V_C, Hgb (see below).	Larger better.	Timed breath holding at TLC.	Good.	Cooperation or anesthesia.	Co and He meters or gas chromatograph.	119, 120
D_LCO (SS).	Above plus V̇/Q̇.	Larger better.	Regular breathing.	Good.	Cooperation or anesthesia.	Same plus measurement of V_D (physiol).	121–123
DM.	Thickness and quantity of membrane.	Larger better.	Timed breath holding at TLC.	Good.	Cooperation or anesthesia.	CO, O_2, and He measurement.	124
V_C.	Pulmonary capillary blood volume.	Larger better.	Timed breath holding at TLC.	Good.	Cooperation or anesthesia.	CO, O_2, and He measurement.	124
D_LO_2.	D_LO_2.	Larger better.	Regular breathing.	Good.	Computation of mean capillary PO_2 difficult.	Measurement of VO_2, V_{CO_2} at 2 levels of oxygenation.	107, 125
D_LCO (RB).	Less affected by V̇/Q̇.	Larger better.	Breath by breath analysis.	Good.	Complex method and computation.	Rapidly responding analyzers.	126, 127

Table 1 *(Continued)*

	Name of test	Physiological interpretation	Animal species	Experimental conditions	Sensitivity	Limitations	Equipment needed	References
Blood gases	Arterial PCO$_2$.	Total alveolar ventilation.	Any, but larger better.	Any.	Good.	Requires accessibility of artery.	Anaerobic blood collection, anticoagulant (blood gas analyzer).	128–130
	Mixed venous PCO$_2$.	Total alveolar ventilation.	Any, but larger better.	Any.	Good.	Requires mixed venous blood.	Anaerobic blood collection, anticoagulant (blood gas analyzer).	131
	Arterial pH.	HCO$_3$/PCO$_2$.	Any, but larger better.	Any.	Good.	Arterial blood.	Anaerobic blood collection, anticoagulant (blood gas analyzer).	129, 130 132, 133
	Mixed venous pH.	HCO$_3$/PCO$_2$.	Any, but larger better.	Any.	Good.	Mixed venous blood.	Anaerobic blood collection, anticoagulant (blood gas analyzer).	132–134
	Arterial PO$_2$.	Regional $\dot{V}/\dot{Q}$ R → L shunt, alveolar ventilation.	Any, but larger better.	Any.	Good.	Arterial blood.	Anaerobic blood collection, anticoagulant (blood gas analyzer).	128, 129
	Mixed venous PO$_2$.	Above plus cardiac output and $\dot{V}O_2$.	Any, but larger better.	Any.	Good.	Mixed venous blood.	Anaerobic blood collection, anticoagulant (blood gas analyzer).	128, 129

[a] In general, FRC is measured by inert gas dilution, nitrogen washout, or body plethysmography; VC, ERV, and IC by spirometry; TLC and RV are usually calculated.
[b] Distribution of ventilation may be defined as a description of the uniformity of distribution of inspired gas. In a hypothetical lung with perfectly uniform distribution of ventilation, the ratio regional tidal volume per regional lung volume is equal for all alveoli.

function tests described in this manuscript would seem satisfactory for these purposes.

Similar considerations apply to the pulmonary toxicology of a variety of other inhaled (and, in some cases, ingested) substances. If a potentially toxic inhalant is to be investigated, certain tests are more valuable than others. While the factors of reproducibility, sensitivity, and specificity are important, the choice of specific pulmonary function tests also depends upon other factors such as anatomic characteristics of the species to be tested. For example, in dogs, multibreath nitrogen washout might be expected to be a relatively insensitive detector of mild physiologic abnormality since the dog lung has a highly developed collateral ventilation system, a factor known to decrease the sensitivity of tests measuring distribution of ventilation. On the other hand, since the pig lung has poorly developed collateral pathways, multibreath nitrogen washout should be an effective means of detecting maldistribution of ventilation. Multibreath nitrogen washout would be expected to be a reasonably sensitive technique in man, whose lung has collateral pathway development intermediate between that of the dog and the pig. Hence, effective selection of pulmonary function methods will depend not only on the scientific information sought but also the nature of the subject, the test itself, and the experimental conditions. These factors should all be considered in designing inhalation toxicology protocols.

ACKNOWLEDGMENT

Preparation of this review was aided by USAF Contract F33615-76-C-5005 and by California Air Resources Board Contract 4–611 with the Departments of Medicine and of Community and Environmental Medicine, California College of Medicine, University of California, Irvine, California.

Literature Cited

1. Woolcock, A. J., Vincent, N. J., Macklem, P. T. 1969. *J. Clin. Invest.* 48:1097–1105
2. Macklem, P. T. 1972. *Am. J. Med.* 52:721–24
3. Lundgren, D. A. 1970. *J. Pure Air Pollut. Control Assoc.* 20:603–8
4. Gorden, R. J., Bryan, R. J. 1973. *Environ. Sci. Technol.* 7:645–47
5. Bates, D., Hazucha, M. 1973. In *Proc. Conf. Health Eff. Air Pollut., Nat. Acad. Sci.,* 507–40
6. McFadden, E. R. Jr., Lincoln, D. A. 1972. *Am. J. Med.* 52:725–37
7. Morris, J. F., Koski, A., Breese, J. D. 1975. *Am. Rev. Respir. Dis.* III:755–62
8. Gelb, A. F., Zamel, N. 1973. *N. Engl. J. Med.* 268:395–98
9. Buist, A. S., Ross, B. B. 1973. *Am. Rev. Respir. Dis.* 108:1078–87
10. Wanner, A., Zarzeck, S., Atkins, N., Zapata, A., Sackner, M. A. 1974. *J. Clin. Invest.* 54:1200–1213
11. McCarthy, D. S., Spencer, R., Greene, R., Milic-Emili, J. 1972. *Am. J. Med.* 52:747–53
12. Milic-Emili, J., Henderson, J. A. M., Dolovich, M. B., Trop, D., Kaneko, K. 1966. *J. Appl. Physiol.* 21:749–59
13. Bates, D. V., Macklem, P. T., Christie, R. V. 1971. *Respiratory Function in Disease,* p. 71. Philadelphia: Saunders
14. Cole, R. B., Bishop, J. M. 1963. *J. Appl. Physiol.* 18:1043–48
15. McFadden, E. R. Jr., Kiker, R., Holmes, B., De Groot, W. J. 1975. *Am. J. Med.* 57:171–81
16. Black, L. F., Offord, K., Hyatt, R. E. 1975. *Am. Rev. Respir. Dis.* 110:282–92
17. Hutcheon, M., Griffin, P., Lewison, H., Zamel, N. 1974. *Am. Rev. Respir. Dis.* 110:458–65

18. Hogg, J. C., Macklem, P. T., Thurlbeck, W. 1968. *N. Engl. J. Med.* 278:1355–60
19. Arndt, H., King, T. K. C., Briscoe, W. A. 1970. *J. Clin. Invest.* 49:408–22
20. Bouhys, A. 1974. *Breathing*, p. 102. New York: Grune & Stratton
21. Mauderly, J. L. 1972. *Am. J. Vet. Res.* 33:1485–91
22. Thelenius, O. C. 1963. *J. Appl. Physiol.* 18:439–40
23. Muggenburg, B. A., Mauderly, J. L. 1974. *J. Appl. Physiol.* 37:152–57
24. Moorman, W. J., Lewis, T. R., Wagner, A. D. 1975. *J. Appl. Physiol.* 39:444–48
25. Amdur, M. O., Mead, J. 1958. *Am. J. Physiol.* 192:364–68
26. Comroe, J. H. Jr., Forster, R. E. II, Dubois, A. B., Briscoe, W. A., Carlsen, E. 1962. *The Lung: Clinical Physiology and Pulmonary Function Tests*, pp. 27–51. Chicago Yearb. Med.
27. Gilson, J. C., Hugh-Jones, P. 1949. *Clin. Sci.* 7:185–216
28. DuBois, A. B., Botelho, S. Y., Bedell, G. N., Marshall, R., Comroe, J. H. Jr. 1956. *J. Clin. Invest.* 35:322–26
29. Baldwin, E. de F., Cournand, A., Richards, D. W. Jr. 1948. *Medicine* 27:248–78
30. Robinson, N. E., Gillespie, J. R. 1973. *J. Appl. Physiol.* 35:317–21
31. Kory, R. C., Callahan, R., Boren, H. G., Syner, J. C. 1961. *Am. J. Med.* 30:243–58
32. Tierney, D. F., Nadel, J. A. 1962. *J. Appl. Physiol.* 17:871–73
33. Darling, R. C., Cournand, A., Richards, D. W. Jr. 1940. *J. Clin. Invest.* 19:609–18
34. Rohrer, F. 1916. *Arch. Gesch. Physiol.* 165:419–44
35. Rahn, H. et al 1946. *Am. J. Physiol.* 146:161–78
36. Fry, D. L. 1954. *Am. J. Med.* 16:80–97
37. Comroe, J. H., Forster, R. E. II, Dubois, A. B., Briscoe, W. A., Carlsen, E. 1968. See Ref. 26, pp. 172–73
38. Neergaard, K., Wirz, K. 1927. *Z. Tschr. Klin. Med.* 105:35–51
39. Otis, A. B., McKerrow, C. B., Bartlett, R. A., et al. 1956. *J. Appl. Physiol.* 8:427–443
40. Neergaard, K. 1929. *Z. Gesamte Exp. Med.* 66:373–94
41. Gaensler, E. A. 1961. *Ann. Rev. Med.* 12:385–408
42. Hyatt, R. E., Schilder, D. P., Fry, D. L. 1958. *J. Appl. Physiol.* 13:331–36
43. DuBois, A. B. et al 1956. *J. Appl. Physiol.* 8:587–94
44. Goldman, M. et al 1970. *J. Appl. Physiol.* 28:113–16
45. Mead, J., Whittenberger, J. L. 1953. *J. Appl. Physiol.* 5:779–96
46. Milic-Emili, J. et al 1964. *J. Appl. Physiol.* 19:207–11
47. Mead, J., Whittenberger, J. L. 1954. *J. Appl. Physiol.* 6:408–16
48. Macklem, P. T., Mead, J. 1967. *J. Appl. Physiol.* 22:395–401
49. Bates, D. V., Macklem, P. T., Christie, R. V. 1971. See Ref. 13, pp. 27–28
50. Marshall, R., DuBois, A. B. 1956. *Clin. Sci.* 15:161–70
51. DuBois, A. B., Botelho, S. Y., Comroe, J. H. 1956. *J. Clin. Invest.* 35:327–35
52. DuBois, A. B., van de Woestijne, K. P., eds. 1969. *Int. Symp. Body Plethysmography*, Nijmegen, 1968, *Prog. Respir. Res.*, Vol. 4. Basel & New York: Karger
53. Otis, A. B. 1954. *Physiol. Rev.* 34:449–59
54. Otis, A. B. 1964. *Handb. Physiol.* 1:463–76
55. Dolfuss, R. E., Milic-Emili, J., Bates, D. V. 1967. *Respir. Physiol.* 2:234–46
56. Leblanc, P., Ruff, F., Milic-Emili, J. 1970. *J. Appl. Physiol.* 28:448–51
57. Green, M., Travis, D. M., Mead, J. 1972. *J. Appl. Physiol.* 33:827 (Abstr.)
58. Anthonisen, N. R., Danson, J., Robertson, P. C., Ross, W. R. D. 1969. *Respir. Physiol.* 8:58–65
59. Fowler, W. S. 1949. *J. Appl. Physiol.* 2:283–99
60. Fowler, W. S., Cornish, E. R., Kety, S. S. 1952. *J. Clin. Invest.* 31:40–50
61. Mauderly, J. L., Pickrell, J. A. 1972. *Proc. Nat. Conf. Lab. Animals Med.*, NIH, Washington DC
62. Dubin, S. E., Westcott, R. J. 1969. *Am. J. Vet. Res.* 30:2027–30
63. Tsai, S. A., Loken, M. K., Ponto, R., Griswa, P. 1969. *Minn. Med.* 52:1893–97
64. Heidendal, G. K., Fontana, R. S., Tauxe, W. N. 1972. *Cancer* 30:1358–67
65. Deland, F. H., Wagner, H. N. Jr. 1970. *Atlas of Nuclear Medicine*, Vol. 2, *Lung and Heart.* Philadelphia: Saunders
66. Bergofsky, E. H. 1974. *Am. J. Med.* 57:378–94
67. Roos, A., Thomas, L. I., Nagel, E. L. 1961. *J. Appl. Physiol.* 16:77–84
68. Duke, H. N., Lee, G. 1963. *Br. Med. Bull.* 19:71–75
69. Comroe, J. H. Jr. 1966. *Circulation* 33:146–58
70. Caro, C. G. 1963. *Br. Med. Bull.* 19:66–70

71. Eberly, V. E., Gillespie, J. R., Tyler, W. S. 1964. *Am. J. Vet. Res.* 25:1712–15
72. Eberly, V. E., Tyler, W. S., Gillespie, J. R. 1966. *J. Appl. Physiol.* 21:883–89
73. Steffey, E. P., Gillespie, J. R., Berry, J. D., Eger, E. I., Rhode, E. A. 1974. *Am. J. Vet. Res.* 35:1315–19
74. Steffey, E. P., Gillespie, J. R., Berry, J. D., Eger, E. I., Rhode, E. A. 1974. *Am. J. Vet. Res.* 35:1289–93
75. Brody, J. S., Stemmler, E. J., DuBois, A. B. 1968. *J. Clin. Invest.* 47:783–99
76. Cander, L., Forster, R. E. 1959. *J. Appl. Physiol.* 14:541–51
77. Becklake, M. R., Varvis, C. J., Pengelly, L. D., Kenning, S., McGregor, M., Bates, D. V. 1962. *J. Appl. Physiol.* 17:579–86
78. Feisal, K. A., DuBois, A. B. 1962. *J. Clin. Invest.* 41:390–400
79. Lee, G. D. Van de Woestijne, K. P., eds. 1969. See Ref. 52, pp. 140–63
80. Lee, G. D., DuBois, A. B. 1955. *J. Clin. Invest.* 34:1380–90
81. Sackner, M. A., DuBois, A. B. 1965. *7th Conf. Res. Emphysema,* Aspen, 1964; *Med. Thorac.* 22:146–57
82. Anthonisen, N. R., Milic-Emili, J. 1966. *J. Appl. Physiol.* 21:760–66
83. Bell, W. C. Jr., Stewart, P. B., Newsham, L. G. S., Bates, D. V. 1962. *J. Clin. Invest.* 41:519–31
84. Hoppin, F. G. Jr., York, E., Kuhl, D. E., Hyde, R. W. 1967. *J. Appl. Physiol.* 22:469–74
85. Riley, R. L. 1951. *Am. J. Med.* 10: 210–20
86. Riley, R. L., Cournand, A. 1949. *J. Appl. Physiol.* 1:825–47
87. Dollery, C. T., Hugh-Jones, P. 1963. *Br. Med. Bull.* 19:59–65
88. Kaneko, K., Milic-Emili, J., Dolovich, M. B., Dawson, A., Bates, D. V. 1966. *J. Appl. Physiol.* 21:767–77
89. Maloney, J. E. 1967. *Phys. Med. Biol.* 12:161–72
90. Markello, R. A., Olszowka, A., Winter, P., Farhi, L. 1973. *Respir. Physiol.* 19:221–32
91. West, J. B. 1963. *Br. Med. Bull.* 19:53–58
92. Yokoyama, T., Farhi, L. E. 1967. *Respir. Physiol.* 3:166–76
93. West, J. B., Dollery, C. T. 1960. *J. Appl. Physiol.* 15:405–10
94. Dawson, A. 1969. *J. Clin. Invest.* 48:301–10
95. Cotes, J. E., Pisa, Z., Thomas, A. J. 1963. *Clin. Sci.* 25:305–10
96. Arborelius, M. Jr. 1969. *J. Appl. Physiol.* 26:101–4

97. Dugard, A., Naimark, A. 1967. *J. Appl. Physiol.* 23:663–71
98. Thilenius, O. G., Hoffer, P. B., Fitzgerald, R. S., Perkins, J. F. Jr. 1964. *Am. J. Physiol.* 206:867–74
99. Harris, P., Segel, N., Green, I., Housley, E. 1968. *Cardiovasc. Res.* 2:84–92
100. Said, S. I. 1974. *Science* 185:1181–83
101. Vane, J. R. 1969. *Br. J. Pharmacol.* 35:209–42
102. Piper, P., Vane, J. 1971. *Ann. NY Acad. Sci.* 180:363–85
103. Hauge, A. 1968. *Circ. Res.* 22:371–83
104. Hauge, A., Melmon, K. L. 1968. *Circ. Res.* 22:385–92
105. Staub, N. C. 1963. *J. Appl. Physiol.* 18:673–80
106. Piper, J. 1961. *J. Appl. Physiol.* 16:507–16
107. Hyde, R. W., Rynes, R., Power, G. G., Nairn, J. 1967. *J. Clin. Invest.* 46: 463–74
108. Liebow, A. A. 1969. In *The Pulmonary Circulation and Interstitial Space,* ed. A. P. Fishman. Chicago: Univ. Chicago Press
109. Gump, F. E., Mashima, Y., Ferenczy, A., Kinney, J. M. 1971. *J. Trauma* 11:474–82
110. Staub, N. C. 1970. *Hum. Pathol.* 1:419–32
111. Robin, E. D., Cross, C. E., Zelis, R. 1973. *N. Engl. J. Med.* 288:239–45, 292–304
112. Phelan, R. F., Yeh, H. C., Raabe, O. G., Velasquez, D. J. 1973. *Anat. Rec.* 177:255–63
113. Raino, J. M., Bishop, J. M. 1963. *J. Appl. Physiol.* 18:284–89
114. Groom, A. C., Morin, R., Farhi, L. E. 1967. *J. Appl. Physiol.* 23:706–12
115. Wilson, A. F. 1969. *Ann. Int. Med.* 71:155–76
116. West, J. B., Hugh-Jones, P. 1959. *Clin. Sci.* 18:553–59
117. Young, A. C., Martin, C. J., Pace, W. R. 1963. *J. Appl. Physiol.* 18:47–50
118. Wagner, P. D., Laravuso, R. B., Uhl, R. R., West, J. B. 1974. *J. Clin. Invest.* 54:54–68
119. Ogilvie, C. M., Forster, R. E., Blakemore, W. S., Morton, J. W. 1957. *J. Clin. Invest.* 36:1–7
120. Meade, F., Saunders, M. J., Hyett, F., Reynolds, J. A., Pearl, N., Cotes, J. E. 1965. *Lancet* 2:573–75
121. Krogh, A., Krogh, M. 1910. *Skand. Arch. Physiol* 22:236–47
122. Filley, G. F., MacIntosh, D. J., Wright, G. W. 1954. *J. Clin. Invest.* 33:530–39

123. Marshall, R. 1958. *J. Clin. Invest.* 37:394–408
124. Roughton, F. J. W., Forster, R. E. 1957. *J. Appl. Physiol.* 11:290–302
125. Farhi, L., Riley, R. L. 1957. *J. Appl. Physiol.* 10:179–85
126. Lewis, B. M., Lin, T. H., Noe, F. E., Hayford-Welsing, E. J. 1959. *J. Clin. Invest.* 38:2073–86
127. Mittman, C. 1967. *J. Appl. Physiol.* 23:131–38
128. Severinghaus, J. W., Bradley, A. F. 1958. *J. Appl. Physiol.* 13:515–20
129. Severinghaus, J. W., Stupfel, M., Bradley, A. F. 1956. *J. Appl. Physiol.* 9:189–96
130. Astrup, P. 1956. *Scand. J. Clin. Lab. Invest.* 8:33–43
131. Hackney, J. D., Sears, C. H., Collier, C. R. 1958. *J. Appl. Physiol.* 12:425–30

132. Bates, R. C. 1964. *Determination of pH: Theory and Practice,* pp. 379–80. New York: Wiley
133. Wilson, A. F., Simmons, D. H. 1970. *Clin. Sci.* 39:731–45
134. Denison, D., Edwards, R. H. T., Jones, G., Pope, H. 1969. *Respir. Physiol.* 7:326–34
135. Anderson, A. E. Jr., Hernandez, J. A., Holmes, W. L., Foraker, A. G. 1966. *Arch. Environ. Health* 12:569–77
136. Ishikawa, S., Bowden, D. H., Fisher, V., Wyatt, J. P. 1969. *Arch. Environ. Health* 18:660–66
137. Lambert, P. M., Reid, D. D. 1970. *Lancet* I:853–57
138. Zapletal, A., Jech, J., Paul, T., Samanek, M. 1973. *Am. Rev. Respir. Dis.* 107:400–409

HISTORY AND HIGHLIGHTS ❖6661
OF PHARMACOLOGY IN HUNGARY

J. Knoll

Department of Pharmacology, Semmelweis University of Medicine, Budapest, Hungary

In the Middle Ages universities were already established in Hungary. The first record of the teaching of medicine in Hungary is to be found in the papal bull of Boniface IX (1399), which referred to the medical course at the high school of Esztergom, a town in northern Hungary. The occupation of Hungary by the Turks (1526–1676), however, devastated the country and paralyzed its universities.

In 1635 Péter Pázmány, the famous polemist of the Hungarian Counter-Reformation, a professor at the University of Graz for ten years, and archbishop of Esztergom from 1616, founded a new university in Nagyszombat (now Trnava in Czechoslovakia). This university, which was named after its founder, was completed with a medical faculty in 1769. In 1777 it was moved to Buda and then in 1789 to Pest (the two cities united in 1872). In 1951 the medical faculty had been divided into faculties of general medicine, dentistry, and pharmacy and became the independent University of Medicine of Budapest. In 1969 at the bicentennial of the founding of the faculty of medicine it was named Semmelweis University of Medicine.

I. P. Semmelweis (1818–1865), whose research activity belongs to the history of pharmacology, was professor of gynecology at this university. He was one of the most outstanding personalities of the history of general medicine and has been called the "Savior of mothers" (1). In his work at the first obstetrical clinic of Vienna following his graduation he noticed the high incidence of puerperal fever in the obstetrical ward, which was visited by medical students. In 1847 he analyzed this problem and concluded that "... das Kindbettfieber ist eine von einer kranken Wöchnerin auf eine gesunde Wöchnerin übertragbare Krankheit durch Vermittlung eines zersetzten thierisch-organischen Stoffes" (2, p. 108). He realized that the mothers were infected by medical students coming from the autopsy room to the labor ward who after dissecting corpses had their hands contaminated with cadaveric toxins ("disintegrative bioorganic material"). He suggested that pus might also cause infection and performed animal experiments to prove this hypothesis. In May 1847 in order to inactivate the "disintegrative bioorganic material" he initiated the use of "chlorina liquida." He decreased the incidence of puerperal fever in the obstetrical ward of the Allgemeines Krankenhaus of Vienna from 11.4 to 1.27% by having the medical students wash their hands thoroughly in chlorinated lime before examining patients. This discovery of Semmelweiss was first mentioned in a paper by Hebra (one of the founders of dermatology) in April 1848, and then in 1849 by the famous Skoda in his report to the Academy of Sciences in Vienna

> Ich glaube, dass ich der sehr geehrten Abteilung eine der wichtigsten Entdeckungen auf dem Gebiet der medizinischen Wissenschaft zu kenntniss bringe, wenn ich die Entdeckung von Doctor Semmelweis, dem früheren Assistenten der hiesigen Geburtshilflichen Klinik, mitteile, die sich auf die Ursache der in diesem Institut mit ungewöhnlicher Häufigkeit auftretenden Kindesbetterkrankungen und auf das Mittel bezieht, mit dem diese Krankheit auf das normale Mass herabgedrückt werden kann (cf 1).

Semmelweis was a modest man. At the beginning of his career he wrote letters to professors of gynecology and published his discovery first in 1858 in Hungarian, while at the University of Pest. In 1861 his famous book was edited in German in Pest under the title *Die Aetiologie, der Begriff und die Prophylaxis des Kindbettfibers* (2). According to the data and conclusions of this monograph Semmelweis can be regarded as the discoverer of the principles of asepsis and antisepsis.

In 1872 the first edition of *Pharmacopoea Hungarica* was published. Before that the *Pharmacopoea Austriaca* (Editions IV and V) were used in Hungary. The second edition followed in 1888, the third in 1909, the fourth in 1933, the fifth in 1954, and the sixth (three volumes, 1564 pages) in 1967.

In 1872 the first independent department of pharmacology in Hungary was established in Budapest, headed by K. Balogh. Balogh was followed in 1890 by Bókay, whose successor was Vámossy in 1920; Issekutz took the chair in 1939 and was succeeded in 1962 by Knoll.

Hungary has four medical universities: Budapest, Szeged, Debrecen, and Pécs. The Universities of Szeged and Debrecen were founded in 1921, and the one at Pécs in 1923. Their medical faculties became independent universities of medicine in 1951.

Besides the university departments of pharmacology, the Drug Research Institute, the Medical Research Institute of the Hungarian Academy of Sciences, and pharmaceutical firms (Chinoin, Gedeon Richter, and EGYT) have important divisions of experimental pharmacology.

A network devoted to clinical pharmacological research was established in 1967. At present 21 units of this network, distributed mainly in different clinical departments of the medical universities, work in close collaboration with the pharmacological research laboratories.

As in other countries, pharmacologists of Hungary are members of their national physiological society. The Hungarian Pharmacological Society (HPS) was founded in 1962. It supported the activities of the Section of Pharmacology (SEPHAR) of the International Physiological Society and as one of the members participated in the foundation of the International Union of Pharmacology (IUPHAR).

The 289 members of the HPS work in five areas: experimental pharmacology, clinical pharmacology, biochemical pharmacology, medicinal chemistry, and chemotherapy. The society organizes congresses with international participation triannually in Budapest. The first was held in 1971 with 313 Hungarian participants and 187 guests from 25 countries. Pharmacological agents and biogenic amines in the central nervous system (3), drugs and heart metabolism (4), pharmacology of analgetics (5), pharmacology of learning and retention (6), drug-induced metabolic changes (7), and the pharmacology of gastrin and its antagonists (8) were the selected topics for the symposia. The second congress in 1974 had 510 active participants (192 guests from 24 countries) presenting 301 papers. Again six symposia were organized; the six volumes are now in press.

The HPS collaborates with other pharmacological societies. Reciprocal joint symposia were organized with the pharmacological societies of the Soviet Union, Czechoslovakia, and Italy. According to a recent agreement between the Hungarian and Polish pharmacological societies, starting in 1976 joint symposia will be organized biannually. In 1974 a joint meeting of the German, Hungarian, Portuguese, and Yugoslav pharmacological societies, organized by Professor F. Lembeck, was held in Graz, Austria. Hungarian pharmacologists (9) presented 51 papers at the meeting.

Pharmacological research in Hungary produced its first results by the end of the 19th century. In 1886 Jendrassik (10, 11) analyzed the diuretic effect of calomel and demonstrated its high efficiency when combined with opium. In 1885 Bókay demonstrated the antagonism between picrotoxin and paraldehyde (cf 1), and the studies of Kossa (12) and Köppen (13) in 1892 revealed the analeptic effect of picrotoxin. In 1897 Vámossy described the local anesthetic effect of trichloroisobutyl alcohol (14). In 1902 he analyzed the toxicity of phenolphthalein in animals for the Hungarian government in order to determine the safety of this compound, which was to be used as a means of identifying artificial wines. When he learned that it was nontoxic in animals he took one gram and discovered its strong cathartic effect (15). Tablets (Purgo) were soon marketed by a small pharmaceutical enterprise in Hungary, and because of its lack of untoward systemic effects in children, phenolphthalein is still widely employed as a cathartic all over the world.

Issekutz demonstrated in 1917 that the quaternary ammonium bases of atropine and homatropine are strong parasympatholytics with low central effects and proposed their combination with papaverine (16, 17). Homatropine methylbromide (novatropine) is still used in Hungary. Issekutz's structure-activity relationship studies led to the synthesis of useful spasmolytics at Chinoin (Perparin®, 18; No-Spa®, 19) and different curare-like tropeine-derivatives (20). As founder and head of the pharmacology laboratory of the Medical Research Institute of the Hungarian Academy of Sciences Issekutz catalyzed detailed studies in the field of central and peripheral cholinolytics. Between 1955 and 1960 Nádor, his pupil, synthesized a series of new tropeine derivatives, whose pharmacology in relation to their steric structure was studied by Gyermek (21), leading to the introduction of xentropinium-bromid (Gastripon®) into therapy. Further structure-activity relationship studies by György et al (22) resulted in the use of tropinium-xanthene-9-carboniacidmethylbromide (Gastrixon®), and potent central cholinolytics were found among tertiary tropanes (23, 24). It has been shown recently in this laboratory that the chloroethylamino derivative of oxotremorine is irreversibly bound to central M-cholinoreceptors (25).

Using the isolated perfused liver Issekutz found in 1924 that glycogenolysis is inhibited by insulin (26) and in 1937 analyzed the effects of thyroxin on the central nervous system (27).

Between 1927 and 1932 Jancsó, a pupil of Issekutz, developed new histochemical methods (28) for research in chemotherapy, demonstrated that trypaflavine and Solganal® find entrance into trypanosomes and *Borrelia recurrentis* (29), and also discovered the storage of Neo-Salvarsan® in the reticuloendothelial system (28).

Issekutz (30) and Jancsó (31–33) proved in 1933–1935 that suramin acts on specific enzyme systems of the trypanosomes by lowering their oxygen and glucose consumption. From these experiments Jancsó thought that hypoglycemic compounds that deprive the protozoons of their main nutriment might be potent trypanocides. In 1935 he and his wife succeeded in demonstrating that Synthalin®, a guanidine derivative with hypoglycemic effect, is a potent trypanocidal agent (34). It was soon demonstrated by Yorke (35) that Synthalin was actively trypanocidal in vitro, i.e. this action proved to be entirely unrelated to the hypoglycemic effect. The discovery of the trypanocidal effect of Synthalin, however, became of practical importance initiating the structure-activity relationship studies of King et al (36) which led to the development of useful protoacidal guanidine derivatives.

Jancsó, a professor of pharmacology in Szeged from 1940 until his death in 1966, was a splendid scientist, rich in new ideas. He described histamine in 1947 as a physiological activator of the reticuloendothelial system (37) and using new techniques with Jancsó-Gábor analyzed the storage mechanism in the organism (38–42). He summarized his results and ideas in his important monograph "Speicherung. Stoffanreicherung im Retikuloendothel und in der Niere" in 1955 (43). In his last research period he became involved in the mechanism of neurogenic inflammatory responses (44) and with his co-workers analyzed the pharmacology of capsaicin (45–47). He demonstrated that capsaicin selectively and irreversibly inactivates the receptors of chemical pain as well as the peripheral and hypothalamic thermodetectors (44, 48). He concluded that chemical and physical pain are mediated by different receptors and that stimulation of the receptors of chemical pain leads to the release of a mediator that increases permeability ("neurogenic inflammation") (49).

Szent-Györgyi, one of the founders of biochemistry, was professor of this subject in Szeged. It was for his work at Szeged that he won his Nobel prize in 1937. Many of his works can be regarded as highly important contributions to pharmacology. Through his study of the oxidizing mechanism of the adrenal cortex in 1928 he isolated from the adrenals a powerful reducing agent in crystalline form, believing it to be hexuronic acid. In 1932 King & Waugh isolated a crystalline compound from lemon juice, identified it as hexuronic acid, and demonstrated its potent antiscorbutic effect (50). At the same time Svirbely and Szent-Györgyi announced the isolation of hexuronic acid from adrenal glands, cabbages, and oranges (51, 52). In 1932 Szent-Györgyi discovered the presence of the substance in the paprika that was cultivated extensively near Szeged and soon extracted a few kilograms of the substance in his department. The Hungarian pharmaceutical firm, Chinoin, became the first en masse producer of vitamin C from paprika. Chemists soon identified vitamin C as ascorbic acid and revealed it as an endogenous oxidation-reduction system, as proposed by Szent-Györgyi.

In 1929 Drury & Szent-Györgyi noted the coronary artery dilating effect of adenosine and adenylic acid (53).

Szent-Györgyi & Rusznyák (professor of medicine in Szeged and later in Budapest and president of the Hungarian Academy of Sciences between 1949 and 1970) noticed that crude preparations of ascorbic acid obtained from natural sources were more effective in alleviating the capillary lesions and prolonging the life of scorbutic animals than was purified vitamin C. In 1936 they isolated an unknown substance from lemon, called *citrin* or *vitamin P* (Permeability vitamin), which protected the capillaries (54–56). Bruckner & Szent-Györgyi demonstrated in 1936 that eriodictyol and hesperidin are the joint components of citrin (57). It became evident that a variety of naturally occurring flavone derivatives possess vitamin P activity. The chemical structure of sophorabioside, an isoflavine glycoside isolated from the fruits of *Sophora japonica* L., was described by Zemplén & Bognár in 1942 (58). Zemplén et al (59) clarified the precise structure also of sophoricoside, whose capillary resistance–elevating and estrogenic effects were demonstrated by Gábor and Kiss in 1953 (cf 60).

Hungary received international recognition for the work of Kabay who developed a method still used throughout the world for obtaining industrial quantities of opium alkaloids from the poppy head and straw (cf 1).

After World War II many young, mainly medical, students worked in the Department of Pharmacology headed by Issekutz. Many of them were to become professors of pharmacology, physiology, biochemistry, or medicinal chemistry in Hungary and abroad (e.g. K. Nádor, J. Knoll, I. Horváth, K. Kelemen in Budapest; J. Pórszász in Pécs; J. Szegi in Debrecen; J. Szerb in Halifax, Canada; I. Bonta in Rotterdam) and leaders of research laboratories (e.g. E. Komlós, F. Herr, G. Wix, I. Pataki, K. Pfeifer, L. Gyermek, G. Fekete, L. Tardos, L. György, J. Borsy, B. Knoll). Between 1946 and 1960 structure-activity relationship studies and methodological problems were the main interest of this department. Komlós, Pórszász & Knoll studied the mechanism of the potentiation of the effects of narcotic analgesics by parasympathomimetics (61–67). Pataki, Pfeifer, and co-workers analyzed (68–70) the creatine-creatinine metabolism of the central nervous system and described the early inhibitory effects of thyroxine on convulsive thresholds as a consequence of a shift in this metabolism; later Pfeifer studied the role of catecholamines in the regulation of convulsive threshold (71). J. Knoll & B. Knoll developed new methods in psychopharmacology (72–78) and they studied with Kelemen drive-motivated behavior (79–87) and J. Knoll proposed a new psychophysiological theory in his monograph "Theory of Active Reflexes" (88). These works initiated structure-activity relationship studies in the field of psychopharmacology.

In 1961 new aminoketones with a major tranquilizing effect synthesized by Nádor, were described (89). After the finding of Knoll (cf 3, pp 13–36) that amphetamine and in smaller doses methamphetamine enhance performance of rats in behavioral tests by increasing the catcholaminergic tone and that higher doses are inhibitory because of activation of the 5-hydroxytryptamine (5-HT) system, the goal of synthesizing new phenylalkylamines with only stimulatory or only inhibitory effects in the tests was set. Methamphetamine was the starting substance. At Chinoin Ecsery synthesized a series of new derivatives and the goal was reached by appropriate substitutions at the para position. Parabromomethamphetamine (V-111) was found to be a derivative which in small and large doses exerted only inhibitory effects, while N_1-O-carboxyphenyl-N_2 2,2-methylaminopropyl-1-phenylacetamidine (I-1703) exerted only stimulatory effects. In contrast to the acute central effects of V-111 the chronic administration of the compound was found to facilitate the learning performance of the rats because it diminished the 5-HT content of the brain and exerted a long-lasting inhibitory effect on the intraneuronal uptake of 5-HT and dopamine (90–105).

One of the practical fruits resulting from the structure-activity relationship studies with the newly synthesized metamphetamine derivatives was the discovery of the first and up to now the only selective B-type monoamine oxidase (MAO) inhibitor, 1-deprenyl. The pharmacology of deprenyl (under the code name E-250) was described by Knoll et al in 1965 as a new spectrum psychic energizer, which in contrast to other MAO inhibitors did not potentiate the effect of tyramine. Its high selectivity in inhibiting the oxidation of benzylamine (a substrate of the B-type of MAO) was demonstrated by Knoll and Magyar in 1971. The pharmacology of selective MAO inhibitors was summarized in 1975 (106–110). The antidepressant effect of deprenyl in man was demonstrated by Varga et al (111) in 1967 and 1-deprenyl was recently described as an excellent drug for preventing the potentiation of the anti-akinetic effect after L-dopa treatment and for the off-phenomena in parkinsonian patients (112).

Knoll et al developed a new family of non-narcotic analgesics containing the 1,5-diazanaphthalene ring system (113–116) synthesized by Mészáros et al at Chinoin (117). Probon®, the first marketed drug of this family, which potentiates the analgesic and antagonizes the respiratory depressant effect of narcotic analgesics, proved to be a useful analgesic in man (118).

Knoll et al (119–127) demonstrated the peculiar spectrum of activity of the 6-azido-7,8-dihydroisomorphine (azidomorphine) derivatives synthesized by Bognár & Makleit (128). They proved to be the most potent of all semisynthetic analgesics and antitussives containing the morphine structure. Azidomorphine showed an unusually great dissociation between analgesic activity and tolerance and dependence capacity in both animals (119–127) and man (129–131), and in combination with Probon® it proved to exert much less untoward central and peripheral effects in man than either morphine or pentazocine (129–131).

Knoll observed in 1951 the existence of an unknown cardiotonic substance in the perfusate of the frog liver. This substance was described in 1952 and 1955 (132–136). He discovered in 1956 that the isolated frog heart arrested by 16- to 45-fold potassium excess that cannot be antagonized by known cardiotonics, like β-receptor stimulants, cardiac glycosides, or calcium, starts beating again in the course of time. The auricle proved to be the determinant in the adaptation of the frog heart to the high potassium milieu. Ventricles isolated from their auricles were found to be unable to adapt themselves, but when an isolated ventricle was in touch with the bathing fluid of an intact heart it regularly gained, sometimes even earlier than the intact heart, the ability to work in presence of the high potassium concentration. This showed that an unknown substance is produced by the auricle that enables the frog heart to work under unfavorable circumstances. This endogeneous substance was named *celluline* by Knoll, who soon demonstrated that different organ extracts exert celluline-like activity. To rule out the effect of known substances with cardiotonic effect the biological titration of celluline-like activity was based on the observation that it is unique in making the frog or mammalian heart contract in the presence of the combination of high potassium concentrations, tetrodotoxin and propranolol. Celluline-A, prepared from frog skin, was purified by gel chromatographic procedure. The unknown structure seems to be an organic Ca complex in which "salt" is produced by fatty acids and phenylalkylcarbonic acids which is surrounded by phenylalkylamines (phenylethylamine and tyramine) as ligands. Celluline-A was also found to antagonize the effect of tetrodotoxin in the guinea pig vas deferens (137–142).

Kelemen, Kecskeméti & Knoll demonstrated that celluline—A is the only substance that markedly increases at an unchanged resting potential the overshoot and rate of depolarization of the transmembrane action potential of heart cells and that under voltage clamp conditions it increases the inward sodium current. Analysis of the electrophysiological effects of PGE_1 and PGE_2 suggested the possibility of the release or activation of celluline by prostaglandins in the heart (143–148).

Vizi & Knoll presented evidence that in Auerbach's plexus the acetylcholine output per stimulus depends on the frequency and length of stimulation applied and demonstrated that the inhibition of the release of acetylcholine by the adrenergic transmitter is mediated via α-adrenoceptors situated presynaptically. It was found that the release of acetylcholine by gastrointestinal hormones can be inhibited by the stimulation of opiates and α-adrenoceptors of Auerbach's plexus. It has also been shown that the inhibitory effect of the presynaptic α-adrenoceptor stimulation on the noradrenergic transmission depends on the frequency of stimulation (149–154). Similar interaction was found for PGE_1 on guinea pig vas deferens, and it was further demonstrated that PGE_2 markedly retards the onset and depresses the velocity of mechanical responses to continous sympathetic stimulation in the guinea pig vas deferens (155). PGE_1 was found to reduce vagal bradycardia by antagonizing the effect of acetylcholine on the atrial cells (156). Vizi demonstrated (157) the stimulation by inhibition of $(Na^+\text{-}K^+\text{-}Mg^{2+})$-activated adenosine triphosphatase (ATPase) of acetylcholine release in cortical slices from rat brain. Fürst (158) proved that the intraventricular administration of naloxone increased the output of acetylcholine into perfused lateral cerebral ventricle in cats.

Szekeres, who first worked in the Department of Pharmacology in Pécs and who in 1967 succeeded Jancsó at Szeged, concentrated with his group on problems of the cardiovascular system, in particular on the pathomechanism and drug therapy of cardiac arrhythmias. The results of this work were summarized by Szekeres in 1966 (159) and by Szekeres & Papp in 1968 (160) and 1971 (161). Their studies revealed that increased excitation of the autonomic nervous centers makes the heart more susceptible to external arrhythmogenic stimuli in the initial, moderately severe phase of hypoxia and hypothermia (162–165). Stimulation of the adrenergic β-receptors was found to promote the appearance of arrhythmias. Failure of mainly the α-receptor stimulators (phenylephrine, synephrine, and methoxamine) to decrease electrical fibrilloflutter threshold has been demonstrated, as well as the biphasic action of epinephrine and norepinephrine, which stimulates both α- and β-receptors. In dopamine- and L-dopa-induced arrhythmia, shortening of repolarization can be prevented by β-blockade. Analysis of the role of hormones and metabolites in the pathomechanism of cardiac arrhythmias has revealed that arrhythmia-producing and cardiotoxic effects of ouabain increased in experimental hyperthyroidism. In other experiments increased susceptibility of the failing heart to the arrhythmogenic action of acute stretch by sudden overloading has been observed (166–168).

Studies of the role of local myocardial ischemia in the genesis of early arrhythmias appearing after coronary occlusion revealed that appearance of arrhythmias depends on (a) the extent of inhomogeneity of the electrophysiological parameters between the noninfarcted myocardium and the ischemic area and (b) the asynchrony of conduction and inequality of repolarization within the ischemic area and the noninfarcted myocardium, respectively. Also transient metabolic alterations appeared after coronary occlusion in the noninfarcted myocardium. Pharmacological interventions protecting against early postocclusion arrhythmias such as infusion of nitroglycerine or lidocaine and especially chemical denervation (atropine with practolol or pindolol) prevented shortening of the refractory period and reduced asynchrony in recovery of excitability at nearby sites in the nonischemic myocardium.

A rational screening program for the assay of antiarrhythmic and antianginal drugs was recommended (169–171). A new type of electrode for continuous recording of monophasic action potentials from the heart in situ has been introduced (172). Alkylamine-substituted phthalimide derivatives with antiarrhythmic activity and new isoquinoline derivatives possessing marked and long-lasting antianginal action were described (173).

At Szeged Minker & Koltai studied the modulation of the receptor function of the synapses and smooth muscle under the influence of transmitters, enzymes, hormones, and peptides (174–178). It has been shown on rats that some nucleic acid and protein synthesis inhibitors inhibit the inflammatory response induced by dextran (179) and that the insulin-induced sensitization of anaphylactoid reaction is due to a release of a factor derived from lymphocytes (180). The effects of various irritants were prevented by agents producing hyperlipemia and by interferon inducers (181–183).

In the Department of Pharmacology of the Medical University of Pécs the late J. Pórszász, who was head of the department, and his group studied physiological problems of pharmacological interest, such as the effects of blood pressure changes on single-unit activity in the bulbar reticular formation, the physiological properties of tonic exspiratory vagal afferent fibers from the pulmonary stretch receptors, and the dynamics of the somatic and visceral sympathoinhibitory reflexes (184–186).

Pórszász was earlier engaged in structure-activity relationship studies mainly with aminoketones of nicotinic and antinicotinic activity, synthesized by Nádor, which led to the introduction of spiractin, a new respiratory stimulant compound, and mydetone, a new interneurone-blocking compound possessing potent peripherial vasodilator activity (187–195). In the same department Varga, who became chairman after the death of Pórszász, by studying the intestinal absorption of chloroquine presented an interesting example of an effect of a drug on the body, which in turn modifies the pharmacokinetics of the drug itself (196). Decsi studied the biochemical effects of psychopharmacological agents (197–199) and the subcortical organization of the chemically evoked rage reaction on the freely moving cat (200, 201).

The Department of Pharmacology at the University of Debrecen became independent in 1948. The late Vályi-Nagy, who was head of the department, and his co-workers isolated primycin, a new antibacterial antibiotic (202), and flavofungin and desertomycin, new antifungal antibiotics (203, 204). Between 1963 and 1971 he and his co-workers studied the mode of antitumor action of cytotoxic hexits. These compounds, in contrast to the biological alkylating agents, do not affect thermodenaturation of DNA. According to these studies the indicator of the anticarcinogenic effect is the increased RNA synthesis in the sensitive tumor cells. Based on the observations that under the effect of Dibrombulcit® cytotoxic hexits inhibited the development of the nucleohistone complex, it was suggested that by the abolishment of histone function a depression of DNA occurs and results in an increased RNA synthesis. It has not been settled whether increased RNA synthesis is only a side product of the impairment of chromatic substance or whether the increasing synthesis of RNA has a decisive role in the proliferation of tumor cells (205–211).

In the Department of Pharmacology at Debrecen, Hernádi et al analyzed the mechanism of the metabolic radioprotective effect of cysteine on *Escherichia coli* and on primordial hemopoietic germ cells of the mouse. Inhibition of the biosynthesis of amino acids, primarily the blockade of the homoserindehydrogenase and hydroxyacetic acid synthetase, was thought to be responsible for the reversible inhibition of the division of *E. coli* cells. Cysteine was found to inhibit cell division also in the primordial hemopoietic germ cell population of the mice (212–219). Kelentey et al studied the passage of drugs into and out of the central nervous system (220, 221). Hepatoendocrine regulations and sex differences in the sensitivity for different drugs were studied by Kulcsár & Kulcsár-Gergely (222–229). Szegi et al analyzed the isoproterenol-induced myocardial necrosis. (230).

In 1950 the nationalized pharmaceutical firms of the country decided to promote and intensify drug research and started a far-reaching program with a goal toward the development of their own firm base for experimental research. In the spirit of these decisions the biggest firms (Chinoin, Gedeon Richter, EGYT) successfully established new laboratories, and the Drug Research Institute, which numbers 170 research workers, was founded in Budapest in 1950. One of its departments, headed by J. Borsy, is engaged in experimental pharmacology and toxicology.

The Drug Research Institute developed a number of therapeutically useful cytostatics. The first of these, mannomustine (Degranol,® 1,6-bis (2-chloroethylamino)-1,6-dideoxy-D-mannitol) synthesized by Vargha in 1955 (231), was found more potent and less toxic than nitrogen mustard (232). Degranol was followed by a number of new cytostatics. Mitobronitol (Myleobromol®, 1,6-dibromo-1,6-dideoxy-mannitol) was found to be effective in several forms of hemopoietic diseases and tumors (233–235a). Mannosulfan, (Zitostop®, D-mannitol-1,2,5,6-tetrabis-methanesulphonate), a new compound with a better safety margin proved to produce some delay in the development of pulmonary tumors (236), while licurim [1,4-di(2-methylsulphonooxyethylamino)-1,4-dideoxy-*m*-eritritdimethylsulphonate] is useful in lymphopoietic disorders (237, 238).

In the field of chemotherapy, the Institute solved practical problems. In collaboration with the pharmaceutical firms, workers at the institute developed procedures for producing known antibacterial and antifungal antibiotics. Penicillin, streptomycin, oxytetracycline, 6-aminopenicillanic acid, neomycin, paromomycin, gentamycin C, erythromycin, viomycin, polymyxin B and D, actinomycin D, mitramycin, nigericin, antimycin, nystatin, candicydin, nyfimycin, and mykoheptin were produced by fermentation, and among others, chloramphenicol, cycloserine, and trimethoprim were synthesized. They also worked out an efficient method for the isolation of soil actinomycetes (239) and isolated in pure form 60 antibiotics of which 50 were identified as earlier known ones; oleficin (240), desoxinigericin (241), mannoside-hydroxystreptomycin, citotetrin, cinerubin C, griseofagin, new macrolids (10-desoximetimicin and 12-desoxi-4-dehydropicromycin), parvulin, krotocin (242), heptafungin A (243), and pentafungin (244) proved to be new. Pirazocillin [1-(2,6-dihydrophenyl)-4-methyl-5-pyrazolilpenicillin Na], a new semisynthetic penicillin derivative (245), was found to be of practical value.

In the domain of steroid research Krámli & Horváth (246) and Wix et al (247–249) made important observations regarding the microbiological transformation of steroids.

Structure-activity relationship studies by Borsy in the field of psychopharmacology led to the introduction of trimetozine (Trioxazin®) a useful antianxiety agent (250,251) and metofenazate (Frenolon®) a potent neuroleptic drug, synthesized by Toldy (252, 253).

In 1966 a research group of the Institute led by Bajusz in collaboration with Medzihradszky working in the Department of Organic Chemistry of the Eötvös Lóránd University in Budapest (headed by Professor Bruckner) synthesized human corticotropin according to sequences described in the literature (254, 255). This synthetic human ACTH showed an activity of 120–130 unit/mg, and clinical studies revealed that it was tolerated also in patients hypersensitive to highly purified pig corticotropin (256). Analytic studies in the institute in 1971 by Gráf et al (257, 258) revealed that the structure of pig and human corticotropins given in the literature are incorrect, because they contain at position 25–27 aspartic acid-alanine-glycine instead of the described asparagine-glycine-alanine, and at position 30, glutaminic acid instead of glutamine. The synthesis of the human ACTH with the correct structure was performed in collaboration with Gedeon Richter Co. and described by Kisfaludy et al (259).

Headed by G. Fekete the research laboratories of Gedeon Richter have made detailed studies into the effects of glucocorticoids on the adrenal cortex (260–268), a pharmacological analysis of newly synthesized ACTH fragments of different sequences (269), and studies into the testing problem and mechanism of inflammation (270–275).

As fruits of drug research, a water-soluble glucocorticoid preparation (275), a new neuromuscular blocking agent among nitrogen-containing steroids (276), and coronary and peripheric vasodilators (277) were produced. Economical methods for the isolation of the natural alkaloids of Vinca minor L and series of half synthetic and synthetic derivatives of vincamine were developed and detailed pharmacological studies with the alkaloids were performed (278–282).

Drug research is now one of the very few fields which, in recognition of scientific accomplishments, enjoy special governmental care and support in Hungary. The history of pharmacology in this country which dates back more than a century makes, I hope, this honorable distinction understandable.

Literature Cited

1. Issekutz, B. 1971. *Die Geschichte der Arzneimittel forschung.* Budapest: Akad. Kiadó. 651 pp.
2. Semmelweis, I. P. 1861. *Die Aetiologie, der Begriff und die Prophilaxis des Kindbettfibers.* Pest, Wien & Leipzig: Hartleben's Verlags-Expedition. 543 pp.
3. Knoll, J., Magyar, K., eds. 1973. *Symp. Pharmacol. Agents Biogenic Amines Central Nervous System.* Budapest: Akad. Kiadó. 274 pp.
4. Knoll, J., Szekeres, L., Papp, J. Gy., eds. 1973. *Symp. Drugs Heart Metab.* Budapest: Akad. Kiadó. 369 pp.
5. Knoll, J., Vizi, E. S., eds. 1974. *Symp. Curr. Probl. Pharmacol. Analgetics.* Budapest: Akad. Kiadó. 183 pp.
6. Knoll, J., Knoll, B. eds. 1974. *Symp. Pharmacol. Learn. Retention.* Budapest: Akad. Kiadó. 103 pp.
7. Knoll, J., Jávor, T., Gógl, A., eds. 1974. *Symp. Drug-Induced Metabolic Changes.* Budapest: Akad. Kiadó. 253 pp.
8. Knoll, J., Borsy, J., Mózsik, Gy. eds. 1973. *Symp. Gastrin and its Antagonists.* Budapest: Akad. Kiadó. 153 pp.
9. Abstr. Pharmacol. Meet. Graz. Sept. 2–5, 1974. *Arch. Pharmacol,* Suppl. to Vol 285
10. Jendrassik, E. 1886. *Dtsch. Arch. Klin Med.* 38:499–524
11. Jendrassik, E. 1891. *Dtsch. Arch. Klin. Med.* 47:226–88
12. Kossa, Gy. 1892. *Magy. Orv. Arch.* 1:469–91
13. Köppen, L. 1892. *Arch. Exp. Pathol. Pharmakol.* 29:327–52

14. Vámossy, Z. 1897. *Dtsch. Med. Wochenschr. Ther. Beil.* 23:457–61
15. Vámossy, Z. 1902. *Ther. Ggw.* 43:201
16. Issekutz, B. 1916. *Orv. Hetil.* 60:485–87
17. Issekutz, B. 1917. *Z. Exp. Pathol. Ther.* 19:99
18. Issekutz, B., Leinzinger, M., Dirner, Z. 1932. *Arch. Exp. Pathol. Pharmakol.* 164:158–72
19. Issekutz, B. 1964. *Ther. Hung.* 12:3–9
20. Issekutz, B. 1952. *Arch. Exp. Pathol. Pharmakol.* 215:283–98
21. Gyermek, L., Nádor, K. 1957. *J. Pharm. Pharmacol.* 9:209–29
22. György, L., Dóda, M., Nádor, K. 1961. *Arzneim. Forsch.* 11:444–50
23. György, L. et al 1968. *Arzneim. Forsch.* 18:517–24
24. György, L. et al 1970. *Acta Physiol. Acad. Sci. Hung.* 37:313–18
25. György, L. et al 1971. *Acta Physiol. Acad. Sci. Hung.* 40:373–79
26. Issekutz, B. 1924. *Biochem. Z.* 147:264–74
27. Issekutz, B. et al 1937. *Arch. Exp. Pathol. Pharmakol.* 185:673–84
28. Jancsó, N. 1928–1929. *Z. Exp. Med.* 61:63, 64:256, 65:98
29. Jancsó, N. 1931–1932. *Zentralb. Bacteriol.* 122:388, 393; 123:129; 124:167
30. Issekutz, B. 1933. *Arch. Exp. Pathol. Pharmakol.* 173:479–98
31. Jancsó, N., Jancsó, H. 1934. *Ann. Trop. Med. Parasitol.* 28:419–38
32. Jancsó, N., Jancsó, H. 1935. *Ann. Trop. Med. Parasitol.* 29:95–109
33. Jancsó, N., Jancsó, H. 1935. *Z. Immunitaetsforsch.* 84:471–504
34. Jancsó, N., Jancsó, H. 1935. *Z. Immunitaetsforsch.* 86:1–30

35. Yorke, W. 1940. *Trans. R. Soc. Trop. Med. Hyg.* 33:463–82
36. King, H., Lourie, E. M., Yorke, W. 1938. *Ann. Trop. Med. Parasitol.* 32:177–92
37. Jancsó, N. 1947. *Nature London* 160:227–28
38. Jancsó, N., Jancsó-Gábor, A. 1952. *Experientia* 8:465–67
39. Jancsó, N., Jancsó-Gábor, A. 1952. *Nature London* 170:567–68, 568–69
40. Jancsó, N., Jancsó-Gábor, A. 1952. *Acta Physiol. Acad. Sci. Hung.* 3:537–554, 555–62
41. Jancsó, N., Jancsó-Gábor, A. 1954. *Experientia* 10:256–57
42. Jancsó, N. 1955. *Acta Med. Acad. Sci. Hung.* 7:173–210
43. Jancsó, N. 1955. *Speicherung. Stoffanreicherung im Retikuloendothel und in der Niere.* Budapest. Akad. Kiadó. 468 pp.
44. Jancsó, N. 1962. *J. Pharm. Pharmacol.* 13:577–94
45. Jancsó, N. et al 1967. *Br. J. Pharmacol. Chemother.* 31:138–51
46. Jancsó, N. et al 1968. *Br. J. Pharmacol. Chemother.* 33:32–41
47. Pórszász, J., Jancsó, N. 1959. *Acta Physiol. Acad. Sci. Hung.* 16:299–306
48. Jancsó, N., Jancsó-Gábor, A. 1965. *Arch. Exp. Pathol. Pharmakol.* 251:136–37
49. Jancsó, N. 1965. *Orv. Hetil.* 106:289–96
50. King, C. G., Waugh, W. A. 1932. *Science* 75:357–58
51. Svirbely, J. L., Szent-Györgyi, A. 1932. *Biochem. J.* 26:865–70
52. Svirbely, J. L., Szent-Györgyi, A. 1932. *Nature London* 129:576
53. Drury, A. N., Szent-Györgyi, A. 1929. *J. Physiol.* 68:213–37
54. Rusznyák, I. Szent-Györgyi, A. 1936. *Nature London* 138:27
55. Armentano, L. et al 1936. *Dtsch. Med. Wochenschr.* 62:1325–28
56. Bentsáth, A., Rusznyák, I., Szent-Györgyi, A. 1936. *Nature London* 138:798
57. Bruckner, V., Szent-Györgyi, A. 1936. *Nature London* 138:1057
58. Zemplén, G., Bognár, R., Farkas, L., 1943. *Ber. Dtsch. Chem. Ges.* 76:267
59. Zemplén, G., Bognár, R., Farkas, L. 1943. *Ber. Dtsch. Chem. Ges.* 76:267
60. Gábor, M. 1974. *Pathophysiology and Pharmacology of Capillary Resistance.* Budapest: Akad. Kiadó. 235 pp.
61. Komlós, E., Pórszász, J., Knoll J. 1950. *Acta Physiol. Acad. Sci. Hung.* 1:77–90

62. Knoll, J., Komlós, E. 1951. *Acta Physiol. Acad. Sci. Hung.* 2:57–69
63. Pórszász, J., Knoll, J., Komlós, E. 1951. *Acta Physiol. Acad. Sci. Hung.* 2:469–77
64. Knoll, J., Komlós, E. Pórszász, J. 1951. *Acta Physiol. Acad. Sci. Hung.* 2:479–91
65. Komlós, E., Knoll J. 1952. *Acta Physiol. Acad. Sci. Hung.* 3:123–26
66. Knoll, J., Komlós, E. 1952. *Acta Physiol. Acad. Sci. Hung.* 3:127–36
67. Knoll, J., Komlós, E., Tardos, L. 1953. *Acta Physiol. Acad. Sci. Hung.* 4:131–40
68. Pataki, I. et al 1948. *Arch. Int. Pharmacodyn. Ther.* 77:17–22, 204–11
69. Pataki, I. et al 1951. *Acta Physiol. Acad. Sci. Hung.* 2:71–76, 199–205
70. Pfeifer, A. K. et al 1952. *Acta Physiol. Acad. Sci. Hung.* 3:153–64
71. Pfeifer, A. K. et al 1967. *Arch. Int. Pharmacodyn. Ther.* 165:201–11, *J. Pharm. Pharmacol.* 19:400–402
72. Knoll, J., Knoll, B. 1958. *Arzneim. Forsch.* 8:330–33
73. Knoll, J., Knoll, B. 1959. *Arzneim. Forsch.* 9:633–36
74. Knoll, J. 1961. *Arch. Int. Pharmacodyn. Ther.* 130:141–54
75. Knoll, J., Knoll, B. 1961. *Arch. Int. Pharmacodyn. Ther.* 133:310–26
76. Knoll, J., Knoll, B. 1964. *Arch. Int. Pharmacodyn. Ther.* 148:200–216
77. Knoll, J. 1961. *Acta Biol. Med. Ger. Suppl.* 1:9–45
78. Knoll, J. 1959. In *Neuropsychopharmacology,* ed. P. B. Bradley, 1:334–37. Amsterdam:Elsevier
79. Knoll, J., Kelemen, K., Knoll, B. 1955. *Acta Physiol. Acad. Sci. Hung.* 8:327–45
80. Knoll, J., Kelemen, K., Knoll, B. 1955. *Acta Physiol. Acad. Sci. Hung.* 8:347–67
81. Knoll, J., Kelemen, K., Knoll, B. 1955. *Acta Physiol. Acad. Sci. Hung* 8:369–88
82. Knoll, J., Kelemen, K., Knoll, B. 1956. *Acta Physiol. Acad. Sci. Hung.* 9:99–109
83. Knoll, J. 1956. *Acta Physiol. Acad. Sci. Hung.* 10:89–100
84. Knoll, J. 1957. *Acta Physiol. Acad. Sci. Hung.* 12:65–92
85. Kelemen, K., Bovet, D. 1961. *Acta Physiol. Acad. Sci. Hung.* 19:143–54
86. Kelemen, K. et al 1961. *Electroencephalogr. Clin. Neurophysiol.* 13:745–51
87. Knoll, B. 1961. *Acta Physiol. Acad. Sci. Hung.* 20:265–75
88. Knoll, J. 1969. *The Theory of Active Reflexes. An Analysis of Some Fundamental Mechanisms of Higher Nervous Activity.* Budapest: Akad. Kiadó. 131 pp.

89. Knoll, J. et al 1961. *Arch. Int. Pharmacodyn. Ther.* 130:155–69
90. Knoll, J., Vizi, E. S., Ecseri, Z. 1964. *Magy. Tud. Akad. V. Oszt. Közl.* 15:413–20
91. Knoll, J. 1965. In *Pharmacology of Conditioning, Learning and Retention,* ed. M. J. Michelson, 221–30. London: Pergamon
92. Knoll, J., Vizi, E. S., Ecseri, Z. 1966. *Arch. Int. Pharmacodyn. Ther.* 159: 442–51
93. Knoll, J. 1967. In *Recent Developments of Neurobiology in Hungary,* ed. K. Lissák, 72–97. Budapest: Akad. Kiadó
94. Knoll, J. 1967. In *Animal and Clinical Pharmacologic Techniques in Drug Evaluation,* ed. P. E. Siegler, 305–21. Chicago: Yearb. Med.
95. Vizi, E. S., Knoll, B., Knoll, J. 1968. *Int. J. Neuropharmacol.* 7:503–50
96. Knoll, J. 1970. In *Amphetamines and Related Compounds,* ed. E. Costa, S. Garattini, 761–80. New York: Raven
97. Knoll, J., Vizi, E. S. 1970. *Pharmacol. Res. Commun.* 2:67–70
98. Knoll, J., Vizi, E. S. 1970. *Pharmacology* 4:278–86
99. Knoll, J., Vizi, E. S., Knoll, B. 1970. *Acta Physiol. Acad. Sci. Hung.* 37: 151–70
100. Knoll, J., Vizi, E. S., Knoll, B. 1970. *Excerpta Med. Int. Congr. Ser.* 220: 50–55
101. Knoll, B., Held, K., Knoll, J. 1971. In *Symp. Pharmacol. Learn. and Retention,* ed. J. Knoll, B. Knoll, pp. 43–47. Budapest: Akad. Kiadó
102. Knoll, J., Kelemen, K., Knoll, B. 1971. In *Biology of Memory,* ed. G. Ádám, 247–53. Budapest: Akad. Kiadó
103. Knoll, J. 1973. In *Proc. 5th Int. Congr. Pharmacol.* ed. F. E. Bloom, G. H. Acheson, 4:55–68. Basel: Karger
104. Magyar, K. et al 1972. *Acta Physiol. Acad. Sci. Hung.* 41:356
105. Knoll, J., Knoll, B. 1975. *Int. J. Neurol.* 10:198–221
106. Knoll, J. et al 1965. *Arch. Int. Pharmacodyn. Ther.* 155:154–64
107. Magyar, K. et al 1967. *Acta Physiol. Acad. Sci. Hung.* 32:377–87
108. Knoll, J. et al 1968. *Arzneim. Forsch.* 18:109–12
109. Knoll, J., Magyar, K. 1972. *Adv. Biochem. Psychopharmacol.* 5:393–408
110. Knoll, J. 1976. *CIBA Symp.* In press
111. Varga, E., Tringer, L. 1967. *Acta Med. Acad. Sci. Hung.* 23:289–95
112. Birkmayer, W. et al 1975. *J. Neural Transm.* 36:303–26

113. Knoll, J. et al 1971. *Arzneim. Forsch.* 21:717–19
114. Knoll, J., Fürst, Zs., Mészáros, Z. 1971. *Arzneim. Forsch.* 21:719–27
115. Knoll, J., Fürst, Zs., Mészáros, Z. 1971. *Arzneim. Forsch.* 21:727–33
116. Knoll, J., Magyar, K., Bánfi, D. 1971. *Arzneim. Forsch.* 21:733–38
117. Mészáros, Z. et al 1972. *Arzneim. Forsch.* 22:815–29
118. Gráber, H. 1972. *Int. J. Clin. Pharmacol.* 6:354–57
119. Knoll, J., Fürst, Zs., Kelemen, K. 1971. *Orvostudomány* 22:265–84
120. Knoll, J. et al 1975. *Orvostudomány* 26:89–95; 96–102; 103–10; 111–27
121. Knoll, J., Fürst, Zs., Vizi, E. S. 1973. *Pharmacology* 10:354–62
122. Knoll, J. et al 1974. *Pharmacology* 12:283–89
123. Knoll, J. 1973. *Pharmacol. Res. Commun.* 5:175–91
124. Knoll, J., Fürst, Zs., Kelemen, K. 1973. *J. Pharm. Pharmacol.* 25:929–39
125. Knoll, J., Fürst, Zs., Makleit, S. 1975. *J. Pharm. Pharmacol.* 27:99–105
126. Knoll, J. et al 1974. *Arch. Int. Pharmacodyn.* 210:241–49
127. Knoll, J., Zsilla, G. 1974. *Biochem. Pharmacol.* 23:745–50
128. Bognár, R., Makleit, S. 1968. *Acta Chim. Acad. Sci. Hung.* 58:203–5
129. Rétsági, Gy., Schwarzmann, É. 1973. *Orvostudomány* 24:359–69
130. Rétsági, Gy. et al 1973. *Orvostudomány* 24:371–78
131. Rétsági, Gy. et al 1974. *Orvostudomány* 25:83–90
132. Knoll, J., Komlós, E., Tardos, L. 1952. *Orv. Hetil.* 93:757–58
133. Knoll, J. et al 1955. *Acta Physiol. Acad. Sci. Hung.* 8:173–86
134. Knoll, J. et al 1955. *Acta Physiol. Acad. Sci. Hung.* 8:187–208
135. Knoll, J. et al 1957. *Acta Physiol. Acad. Sci. Hung.* 12:183–87
136. Knoll, J. 1958. *Klin, Wochenschr.* 36:141
137. Knoll, J. 1956. *Experientia* 12:262
138. Knoll, J., Kelemen, K., Knoll, B. 1958. *Pfluegers Arch. Gesamte Physiol. Menschen Tiere* 267:150–57
139. Knoll, J. 1965. *Magy. Tud. Akad. V. Oszt. Közl.* 16:311–26
140. Knoll, J., Kelemen, K., Knoll, B. 1965 *Magy. Tud. Akad. V. Oszt. Közl.* 16:327–38
141. Knoll, J. et al 1965. *Magy. Tud. Akad. V. Oszt. Közl.* 16:339–49
142. Knoll, J. 1970. *Orvostudomány* 21:271–324

143. Kelemen, K., Kecskeméti, V., Knoll, J. 1965. *Magy. Tud. Akad. V. Oszt. Közl.* 16:351–58

144. Kelemen, K. 1967. *Magy. Tud. Akad. V. Oszt. Közl.* 18:305–22

145. Kelemen, K. et al 1968. *Acta Physiol. Acad. Sci. Hung.* 33:269–84

146. Kelemen, K., Kecskeméti, V., Knoll. J. 1972. *Orvostudomány* 23:231–41

147. Kelemen, K., Skolnik, J., Knoll, J. 1972. *Orvostudomány* 23:391–402

148. Kecskeméti, V., Kelemen, K., Knoll, J. 1973. *Eur. J. Pharmacol.* 24:289–95

149. Vizi, E. S., Knoll, J. 1971. *J. Pharm. Pharmacol.* 23:918–25

150. Knoll, J., Vizi, E. S. 1971. *Br. J. Pharmacol.* 41:263–72

151. Vizi, E. S. 1973. *Br. J. Pharmacol.* 47:765–77

152. Vizi, E. S. et al 1972. *Eur. J. Pharmacol.* 17:175–78

153. Vizi, E. S. et al 1973. *Gastroenterology* 64:286–97

154. Vizi, E. S. et al 1973. *Arch. Pharmakol.* 280:79–91

155. Illés, P. et al 1973. *Eur. J. Pharmacol.* 24:29–36

155a. Knoll, J., Illés, P., Torma, Z. 1975. *Neuropharmacology* 14:317–24

156. Hadházy, P., Illés, P., Knoll, J. 1973. *Eur. J. Pharmacol.* 23:251–55

157. Vizi, E. S. 1973. *J. Physiol. London* 226:95–117

158. Fürst, Zs. et al 1975. *Sixth Int. Congr. Pharmacol.*, p. 179 (Abstr.)

159. Szekeres, L. 1966. *Actual. Pharmacol.* XIX:149–86

160. Szekeres, L., Papp, J. Gy. 1968. *Fortschr. Arzneimittelforsch.* 12:292–369

161. Szekeres, L., Papp, J. Gy. 1971. *Experimental Cardiac Arrhythmias and Anti-Arrhythmic Drugs.* Budapest: Akad. Kiadó. 374 pp.

162. Szekeres, L., Méhes, J., Papp, J. Gy. 1961. *Br. J. Pharmacol.* 17:167–75

163. Szekeres, L., Papp, J. Gy., Förster, W. 1965. *Experientia* 21:720–22

164. Szekeres, L., Papp, J. Gy. 1965. *Acta Physiol. Acad. Sci. Hung.* 26:277–86

165. Szekeres, L., Papp, J. Gy. 1967. *Acta Physiol. Acad. Sci. Hung.* 32:143–62

166. Papp, J. Gy., Szekeres, L. 1968. *Eur. J. Pharmacol.* 3:4–14

167. Papp, J. Gy., Szekeres, L. 1968. *Eur. J. Pharmacol.* 3:15–26

168. Papp, J. Gy., Szekeres, L. 1967. *Acta Physiol. Acad. Sci. Hung.* 32:163–74

169. Szekeres, L. 1971. *Methods Pharmacol.* I: 151–82

170. Szekeres, L., Papp, J. Gy. 1973. *Herzrhythmusstörungen. 2nd Wiener Symp.*, ed. H. Antoni. Stuttgart & New York: Schattauer Verlag

171. Szekeres, L., Papp, J. Gy. 1976. In *Handbuch für Experimentelle Pharmakologie.* Berlin:Springer. In press

172. Szekeres, L., Szurgent, J. 1974. *Cardiovasc. Res.* 8:132–37

173. Szekeres, L. et al 1965. *Acta Physiol. Acad. Sci. Hung.* 26:287–95

174. Minker, E., Koltai, M. 1962. *Acta Physiol. Acad. Sci. Hung.* 22:99–109

175. Minker, E., Koltai, M. 1964. *Acta Physiol. Acad. Sci. Hung.* 24:365–71

176. Koltai, M., Minker, E. 1966. *Acta Physiol. Acad. Sci. Hung.* 29:410

177. Minker, E., Koltai, M. 1967. *Acta Physiol. Acad. Sci. Hung.* 31:167–76

178. Minker, E., Koltai, M. 1965. *Naturwissenschaften* 52:189

179. Koltai, M., Minker, E. 1969. *Eur. J. Pharmacol.* 6:175

180. Koltai, M., Minker, E., Ottlecz, A. 1971. *Life Sci.* 10:315–20

181. Koltai, M., Minker, E., Ottlecz, A. 1972. *Experientia* 28:302–3

182. Ottlecz, A. et al 1974. *Pharmacology* 11:346–49

183. Koltai, M., Mécs, E. 1973. *Nature London* 242:525–26

184. Pórszász, J., Barankay, T., Pórszász-Gibiszer. 1965. *Acta Physiol. Acad. Sci. Hung.* 27:119–24

185. Pórszász, J., Pórszász-Gibiszer, K. 1968. *Acta Physiol. Acad. Sci. Hung* 34:249–58

186. Pórszász, J., Such, G., Pórszász-Gibiszer, K. 1972. *Acta Physiol. Acad. Sci. Hung.* 42:387–402

187. Herr, F., Pórszász, J. 1951. *Acta Physiol. Acad. Sci. Hung.* 2:17

188. Pórszász, J., Nádor, K., Pórszász-Gibiszer, K., Bacsó, I. 1957. *Acta Physiol. Acad. Sci. Hung.* 11:95–108

189. Pórszász, J. et al 1975. *Acta Physiol. Acad. Sci. Hung.* 11:211–24

190. Pórszász, J. 1958. *Acta Physiol. Acad. Sci. Hung.* 14:375–90

191. Pórszász, J., Nádor, K., Pórszász-Gibiszer, K. 1958. *Acta Physiol. Acad. Sci. Hung.* 14:403–9

192. Pórszász, J. et al 1960. *Acta Physiol. Acad. Sci. Hung.* 18:149–70

193. Nádor, K., Pórszász, J. 1956. *Arzneim. Forsch.* 6:696–98

194. Pórszász, K., Pórszász, J. 1958. *Arzneim. Forsch.* 8:313–15

195. Pórszász, J. et al 1961. *Arzneim. Forsch.* 11:257–60

196. Varga, F. 1966. *Arch. Int. Pharmacodyn. Ther.* 163:38–46
197. Decsi, L. 1960. *Arzneim. Forsch.* 10:432–34
198. Decsi, L. 1961. *Psychopharmacologia* 2:224–42
199. Decsi, L. 1964. *Fortschr. Arzneimittelforsch.* 8:53–194
200. Decsi, L. 1974. *Pharmacol. Biochem. Behav.* 2:141–43
201. Decsi, L., Nagy, J. 1974. *Neuropharmacology* 13:1153–62
202. Vályi-Nagy, T., Uri, J., Szilágyi, I. 1954. *Nature London* 1974:1105
203. Uri, J., Békési, I. 1958. *Nature London* 181:908
204. Uri, J. et al 1958. *Nature London* 182:401
205. Jeney, A. et al 1968. *Neoplasma* 15:237–40
206. Jeney, A., Szabó, J., Vályi-Nagy, T. 1968. *Neoplasma* 15:231–36
207. Jeney, A. et al 1969. *Neoplasma* 16:151–60
208. Zsindely, A. et al 1972. *Neoplasma* 19:89–94
209. Szabó, J. et al 1973. *Neoplasma* 20:13–25
210. Vályi-Nagy, T. et al 1969. *Eur. J. Cancer* 5:403
211. Jeney, A., Szabó, I., Vályi-Nagy, T. 1970. *Eur. J. Cancer* 6:297
212. Hernádi, F. et al 1962. *Radiat. Res.* 16:464
213. Nagy, Zs. et al 1968. *Radiat. Res.* 35:652–60
214. Kovács, P. et al 1968. *Radiat. Res.* 36:217–24
215. Nagy, Zs. et al 1968. *Biochem. Pharmacol.* 17:861–66
216. Kari, Cs., Nagy, Zs., Hernádi, F. 1971. *Biochem. Pharmacol.* 20:975–78
217. Kovács, P., Daróczy, A., Hernádi, F. 1971. *Stud. Biophys.* 26:13
218. Kovács, P., Hernádi, F. 1971. *Stud. Biophys.* 27:149
219. Hernádi, F., Kari, Cs. 1972. *Experientia* 28:155
220. Kelentey, B. et al 1961. *Acta Physiol. Acad. Sci. Hung.* 20:81–88
221. Kelentey, B. et al 1964. *Arch. Int. Pharmacodyn. Ther.* 150:363–72
222. Kulcsár-Gergely, J., Kulcsár, A. 1960. *J. Pharm. Pharmacol.* 12:313–16
223. Kulcsár, A., Kulcsár-Gergely, J. 1960. *Naturwissenschaften* 47:183
224. Kulcsár, A., Kulcsár-Gergely, J. 1966. *Tohoku J. Exp. Med.* 89:315–20
225. Kulcsár-Gergely, J., Kulcsár, A. 1964. *Naturwissenschaften* 51:390–91
226. Kulcsár, A., Kulcsár-Gergely, J. 1970. *Tohoku J. Exp. Med.* 101:251–56
227. Kulcsár, A. et al 1969. *Rev. Int. Hepatol.* 19:359–64
228. Kulcsár-Gergely, J., Kulcsár, A. 1973. *Toxicology* 288:125–30
229. Kulcsár-Gergely, J., Kulcsár, A. 1974. *Arzneim. Forsch.* 24:1772–74
230. Csáky, L., Szabó, J., Szegi, J. 1974. *Experientia* 30:428
231. Vargha, L. 1955. *Naturwissenschaften* 42:582
232. Kellner, B., Németh, L., Sellei, C. 1955. *Naturwissenschaften* 42:582–83
233. Institoris, L., Horváth, I. P. 1964. *Arzneim. Forsch.* 14:668–70
234. Csányi, E., Horváth, P., Institoris, L. 1964. *Arzneim. Forsch.* 14:670–73
235. Csányi, E. 1965. *Arzneim. Forsch.* 15:198
235a. Institoris, L., Horváth, I. P., Csányi, E. 1967. *Arzneim. Forsch.* 17:145–49
236. Szentkláray, I., Sellei, C. 1967. *Neoplasma* 14:83–90
237. Csányi, E., Elekes, I. 1972. *Neoplasma* 19:189–95
238. Börzsönyi, M. et al 1967. *Arzneim. Forsch.* 17:1596–98
239. Horváth, I., Lovrekovich, I., Magyar, K. 1964. *Z. Allg. Mikrobiol.* 4:225
240. Gyimesi, J. et al 1971. *J. Antibiot.* 24:217
241. Gyimesi, J., Horváth, I., Szentirmai, A. 1964. *Z. Allg. Mikrobiol.* 4:269
242. Gláz, E. T. et al 1959. *Nature London* 184:908
243. Kalász, H. et al 1972. *Acta Microbiol. Acad. Sci. Hung.* 19:111–20
244. Bérdy, I., Horváth, I. 1965. *Z. Allg. Mikrobiol.* 5:345
245. Gadó, I. et al 1961. *Acta Microbiol. Acad. Sci. Hung.* 8:291–302
246. Krámli, A., Horváth, J. 1948. *Nature London* 162:619
247. Wix, Gy. et al 1959. *Nature London* 183:1279
248. Wix, Gy. et al 1961. *Acta Microbiol. Acad. Sci. Hung.* 8:339
249. Wix, Gy. et al 1968. *Steroids* 11:401
250. Borsy, J. et al 1959. *Acta Physiol. Acad. Sci. Hung.* 15:107–17
251. Vargha, L. et al 1962. *Biochem. Pharmacol.* 11:639–49
252. Toldy, L. et al 1964. *Acta Chim. Acad. Sci. Hung.* 42:351–58
253. Borsy, J., Toldy, L., Dumbovics, B. 1965. *Acta Physiol. Acad. Sci. Hung.* 27:65–80
254. Bajusz, S. et al 1967. *Acta Chim. Acad. Sci. Hung.* 52:335

502   KNOLL

255. Bajusz, S. et al 1968. In *Peptides,* ed. E. Brices, p. 237. Amsterdam: North-Holland
256. Kovács, K. et al 1968. *Lancet.* 1:698
257. Gráf, L. et al 1971. *Acta Biochim. Biophys. Hung.* 6:415
258. Gráf, L. et al 1972. *Acta Biochim. Biophys. Hung.* 7:293
259. Kisfaludy, L. et al 1972. In *Chemistry and Biology of Peptides,* ed. J. Meienhofer, p. 299. Ann Arbor, Mich.: Ann Arbor Sci.
260. Fekete, Gy. 1962. *Acta Physiol. Acad. Sci. Hung.* 21:77–82
261. Fekete, G., Görög, P. 1962. *Acta Physiol. Acad. Sci. Hung.* 21:83–86
262. Fekete, Gy., Görög, P. 1963. *J. Endocrinol.* 27:123
263. Fekete, Gy. et al 1964. *Steroids* 3:163
263a. Fekete, Gy. et al 1966. *Steroids* 6:159
264. Fekete, Gy., Szeberényi, Sz. 1965. *Endokrinologie* 49:23
265. Fekete, Gy., Szeberenyi, Sz. 1968. *Arzneim. Forsch.* 18:451–52
266. Szeberényi, Sz. et al 1964. *Steroids* 4:587
267. Szeberényi, Sz. et al 1966. *Acta Physiol. Acad. Sci. Hung.* 30:328
268. Szeberényi, Sz. et al 1966. *J. Endocrinol.* 35:323
269. Szporny, L. et al 1968. *Nature London* 218:1169
270. Szporny, L., Fekete, Gy. 1960. *Arch. Exp. Pathol. Pharmakol.* 238:233–34
271. Tóth, E., Szporny, L., Görög, P. 1965. *Arch. Exp. Pathol. Pharmakol.* 250:265–66
272. Görög P. et al 1968. *Arzneim. Forsch.* 18:227–30
273. Görög P. et al 1962. *Arch. Int. Pharmacodyn.* 136:165
274. Görög, P., Szporny, L. 1965. *Biochem. Pharmacol.* 14:1673–77
275. Görög, P., Szporny, L. 1965. *J. Pharm. Pharmacol.* 7:250–51
276. Szporny, L., Biro, H. K., Kárpáti, E. 1974. *Arch. Exp. Pathol. Pharmacol.* 285:80
277. Kárpáti, E. et al 1968. *J. Pharm. Pharmacol.* 20:735–36
278. Kárpáti, E., Dömök, L., Szporny, L. 1969. *Arzneim. Forsch.* 19:1011–1115
279. Szporny, L. et al 1958. *Acta Physiol. Acad. Sci. Hung.* 14:46
280. Molnár, J., Szporny, L. 1962. *Acta Physiol. Acad. Sci. Hung.* 21:169–75
281. Szporny, L., Görög, P. 1962. *Arch. Int. Pharmacodyn. Ther.* 138:451–61
282. Szporny, L. et al 1962. *Biochem. Pharmacol.* 8:259–62

REVIEW OF REVIEWS[1]   ♦6662

Chauncey D. Leake
University of California, San Francisco, California 94143

A few years ago I gave a short report on the questionable progress and present problems of primary journals (*J. Chem. Doc.* 10:27–29, 1970). My purpose was to propose a study of ways to get rid of the burden of primary journals by developing current technology on an international scale by the recording, storage, and retrieval of bit-by-bit scientific information, quite as is done so well in airline reservations. Further, my purpose was to promote the use of reviews, either periodically or in monographs. I advocated the specific training of library scientists for the writing of reviews on items of current interest.

Eugene Garfield, the keen documentalist who founded the very successful Institute for Scientific Information (ISI), has long been interested in these matters. The services offered by ISI are indicative of what can be done. The financial success of ISI testifies to satisfaction with its services. Reviewing has now become such an important part of the science enterprise that ISI is offering an annual index of scientific reviews. It is a huge compilation!

In the nearly half a century of *Annual Reviews,* scientists generally have become fully aware of the significance of reviews, both in orienting novices in a field, and in keeping scientific workers abreast of progress in their respective areas. *Annual Reviews* has set a high standard of reviewing excellence, and its various editorial boards deserve much praise for their achievement. Special thanks and honors are always due Murray Luck and his devoted staff for initiating *Annual Reviews* and for maintaining them so well for so long.

GENERAL

In a recent survey of about 2000 acknowledged pharmacologists, 91% were found to have doctoral degrees; 92% are males; 7% are from various minorities; about half hold positions in medical schools; and about a fourth are in the drug industry. I would say that about 15% are in schools of pharmacy.

---

[1]This review was completed July 1, 1975, for material available at that time. References are cited by author, without numbering. Names are arranged alphabetically for convenience.

Drug-transport processes were reviewed in 23 contributions to a London conference edited by Callingham. The role of nutrition in drug-metabolizing enzyme systems was surveyed by Campbell & Hayes in regard both to macro and micro nutrient deficiencies. Some 27 reviews on endocrine aspects of malnutrition were edited by Gardner & Amacher.

A useful review of bibliography on foreign drug identification was given by Closson. Dancis & Hwang edited 18 discussions on problems and priorities in perinatal pharmacology. A more comprehensive survey of basic and therapeutic aspects of perinatal pharmacology was edited by Morselli, Garattini & Sereni. Farnsworth and associates reviewed the potential value of plants as sources of new antifertility agents. With 43 references, Silverman surveyed fetal and newborn adverse drug reactions. Susman edited many case reports dealing with various aspects of drug use and social policy.

A series of 19 discussions on insolubilized enzymes was edited by Salmona, Saronio & Garattini. These dealt with fiber entrapment, artificial membranes, and drug-release devices. Schmitt, Schneider & Crothers edited 16 discussions on functional linkage in biomolecular systems, with much on transductive coupling.

Popular is sophisticated methodology for approaching pharmacological problems. Frigerio & Castagnoli edit 34 descriptions of mass spectrometric methods involving many types of drugs, and usually including gas chromotography. Industrial aspects of enzymes and drug actions are discussed at length in 48 reports edited by Spencer.

PHARMACOKINETICS AND DRUG INTERACTIONS

In discussing drug interactions, Cohen & Armstrong advise adjusting dosage and mode of administration to reduce interactive potential. They offer much tabular data and consider mechanisms. Morselli, Garattini & Cohen edit 37 essays on drug interactions, from absorption to microsomal enzymes and protein binding. With 72 references, Suffness & Rose discuss adverse effects related to aspirin, from ulcerogenic to ion imbalance.

Csaky edits 20 reviews on intestinal absorption and malabsorption, ranging from membrane-bound enzymes to the "brush border" and the influence of bacterial enterotoxins. Lauterbach reviews absorption and secretion of drugs by mucosal epithelium of the gastroenteric tract. Saunders offers an outline review of the absorption and distribution of drugs, with special reference to anionic drugs and to uncharged drugs.

Metabolism of tobacco alkaloids is reviewed by Gorrod & Jenner. Age and exposure factors in drug metabolism are surveyed by Hanninen. With 109 references, Jerina & Daly reveal that many aromatic organic compounds metabolize to potentially carcinogenic arene oxides. With appropriate dedication to the memory of Wallace O. Fenn (1893–1971), Nahas & Schaefer edit 31 essays on carbon dioxide in relation to metabolic regulation. Using 95 references, O'Brien gives tabulated data on excretion of drugs in milk. The rectal administration of drugs is reviewed by Senior.

CHEMOTHERAPY

Chemotherapeutic interest seems to be centering on cancer control. Clark introduces a Houston symposium on the pharmacological basis of cancer chemotherapy. This includes discussions on drug design by Ariens, with 73 references, and by Cheng with 261 references. Toxicity aspects are well covered by Sieber & Adamson with 297 references. Mechanisms of action of antimicrobial and antitumor agents are analyzed by Corcoran & Hahn in regard to interference with nucleic acid, protein, and enzyme biosynthesis. A series of 33 contributions on differentiation and control of malignancy of tumor cells is well edited by Nakahara, Sugimura, Ono & Sugano. With much on alkylating agents and cell kinetics, Sartorelli & Johns edit discussions on antineoplastic and immunosuppressive agents. A series of 31 full reports on adenine arabinoside as an antiviral agent is edited by Pavon-Langston, Buchanan & Alford.

AUTONOMIC NERVOUS SYSTEM

Ablad and associates edit a comprehensive symposium on "metoprolol," another new adrenergic β-1-receptor antagonist. Magnani edits 15 reports on β-adrenergic blocking agents in the management of hypertension and angina pectoris, with much on "timolol maleate," another new one. With 423 references, Paul, Miller & Trendelenberg review molecular geometry in relation to adrenergic drug activity, emphasizing stereo selectivity at receptors, as well as enzyme selectivity. They conclude that for β-adreno-receptor antagonists, the stereochemical explanation still holds.

Brimblecombe reviews drug actions on cholinergic systems for both peripheral and central muscarinic and nicotinic sites, and with much on anticholinesterase agents. A comprehensive survey, with 51 reviews on cholinergic mechanisms is well edited by Waser. This included morphology of cholinergic synapses, estimation of cholines, their pharmacokinetics, enzymes in synthesis and degradation, transmitter action on receptors, anticholinesterase poisoning, and pharmacological and behavioral aspects.

CENTRAL NERVOUS SYSTEM

Social aspects of the medical use of psychotropic drugs were reviewed in a volume edited by Cooperstock. A full survey of benzodiazepines was edited by Garattini, Mussini & Randall. Dealing mostly with chlordiazepoxide and diazepam, it includes biochemorphology, pharmacokinetics, antianxiety actions, muscle-relaxing effects, sleep, and antiaggressive action. Triazolo derivatives are described in relation to central nervous system depression, and interactions with other drugs are discussed. With 128 references (1974), Hartshorn reviews drug interactions with monamine oxidase, and with 78 references (1975) he surveys anti-anxiety drug interactions. Tolerance among these drugs seems to be induced by microsomal enzyme reactions. With 34 essays, Usdin edits an important volume on the neuropsychopharmacology of monoamines and their regulatory enzymes. This includes much on dopamine.

Mandell edits 16 important surveys of neurobiological mechanisms of adaptation and behavior in relation to psychotropic drugs.

Gibbins and colleagues at the Toronto Addiction Research Foundation begin a series of volumes on research advances in alcohol and drug problems. The first includes reviews of methods, of marihuana, of narcotic addiction, and survey data on alcohol use. Gross edits proceedings of 30th congress on alcoholism, dealing with alcohol intoxication and withdrawal, with mechanisms of tolerance, and with human experimentation.

With 394 references, Kostrzewa & Jacobowitz review pharmacological actions of 6-hydroxydopamine, finding that in high doses it induces peroxides and destroys neurons. In an unusual volume of 39 essays, Sandler & Gessa edit much material on the pharmacology of sexual behavior, especially with humoral, endocrine, serotonin, and aminergic mechanisms. Zimmermann & George edit 18 surveys regarding narcotics and the hypothalamus, including mechanisms of action of narcotics on the diencephalon, effects of morphine on neuroendocrine regulation, and effects of blood-brain barriers on narcotic action. Munkvad surveys mechanisms of action of psychopharmacological agents on behavior.

Siva Sankar edits a comprehensive review on LSD. With 84 references, Hoskins reviews the current status of anti-epilepsy drugs. In surveying the use of lithium salts in psychiatry, Shopsin & Gershon advise. Vernadakis & Weiner edit 28 contributions to our knowledge of the action of drugs on developing brains.

ANESTHESIA

A new serial publication, *Progress in Anesthesiology,* is inaugurated by a volume of 46 contributions on molecular mechanisms of anesthesia edited by Fink. These are grouped by neuronal systems, physicochemical models, high pressure, biochemical studies, cellular systems, and cardiac muscle studies. With 78 references, Aviado reviews the regulation of bronchomotor tone during anesthesia. Brunner, Cheng & Berman review the effects of anesthesia on intermediate metabolism. Gyermek & Soyka, in surveying steroid anesthetics, using 92 references, conclude that dione steroids have advantages in low toxicity with little cardiac or respiratory depression. Ketamine anesthesia is reviewed by Lanning & Harmel. Larson and associates survey anesthetic effects on cerebral, renal, and splanchnic circulations. With 185 references, Rowe analyzes the response of the coronary circulation to various drugs used in anesthesia, finding increases with ketamine, barbitals, atropine, epinephrine, dopamine, guanethidine, and papaverine. Ueda, Shieh & Eyring note that anesthetics expand membrane areas. In reviewing local anesthetic effects on vascular smooth muscle, using 180 references, the Alturas find that local anesthetics stabilize cell membranes.

CARDIOVASCULAR-RENAL

Anderson & Kepler, with 96 references, review thiazide diuretics. With 472 references, Bennett, Singer & Coggins offer a guide to drug therapy in renal failure.

Davies & Wilson survey mechanisms of action and clinical applications of various diuretics. Murray & Goldberg warn about renal disease from analgesic abuse.

Doherty & Kane survey the clinical pharmacology of digitalis glycosides. Donoso edits a two-part review of the many drugs used in cardiology. Øye reviews the status of cyclic AMP in cardiovascular pharmacology. With 86 references, Porter reports on digitalis toxicity.

Appropriately, Page & Bumpus edit a comprehensive survey on angiotensin. Regoli, Park & Rioux use 354 references in reviewing the pharmacology of angiotensin, with comments on the biochemorphology of three-dimensional structures in receptor theory. With 729 references, Schwartz, Lindenmayer & Allen review the pharmacological aspects of Na^+–K^+ adenosine triphosphatase, raising the question as to whether or not it may be a receptor for digitalis, and showing the wide range of drugs modifying its action from mercurial diuretics to dimethylsulfoxide (DMSO). The Meisels question whether or not adenosine may be a mediator for coronary circulation regulation and for efficiency of coronary dilators.

TOXICOLOGY

An important comprehensive account of uranium, plutonium, and transplutonic elements has been carefully edited by Hodge, Stannard & Hursh. This gives full details on toxicity, protective criteria, monitoring, body burdens, excretion, biomedical properties, and assays. The toxicology of nonradioactive heavy metals and their salts is described by Venugopal & Luckey.

Toxicological analysis of drugs in biological specimens is reviewed by Goldbaum & Dominguez, while Koles surveys microcrystal tests for drugs. Bastos & Mule describe uses of fluorescence in toxicological analysis while Feldstein does likewise for polarography.

Ciegler reviews occurrence, chemistry, and activity of mycotoxins. Wolfe & Devries survey oxygen toxicity.

CLINICAL

With 134 references, Duhme, Greenblatt & Miller review the pharmacology of essential hypertension, while Fozard reviews the pharmacology of drugs used in treating migraine. Glenn edits 24 reviews on the use of steroids in shock, including discussions on cardiovascular actions of corticosteroids and their use in circulatory shock. Lithium therapy is reviewed by Greene. With 126 references, Holloway considers drug problems in geriatric patients. Parratt reviews pharmacological approaches to angina therapy. Pories, Strain, Hsu & Woosley edit reports on clinical applications of zinc metabolism, with much on zinc sulfate therapy.

MISCELLANEOUS

Gastric antisecretory and anti-ulcer drugs are reviewed by Bass, and Bennett reviews prostaglandin antagonists. Robinson & Vane edit 28 reviews on prostaglandin synthetase inhibitors, especially aspirin, antipyretics, and indomethacin. Bennett & Aberg edit a symposium on hormonal and antifertility action of silicon derivatives, such as 2,6,cis-diphenylhexamethyl-cyclotetra siloxane. The effect is antigonadotrophic.

Carter edits discussions on inhibitors of viral functions, with much on interferon and amantadine, while Parkes gives a full review of amantadine which blocks entry of virus into cells. With 212 references, Coburn, Hartenbower & Norman review the metabolism and calcium homeostatic action of hormone vitamin D. Hellon surveys monoamines, pyrogens, and cations with regard to their effects on the central control of body temperature. Lomax, Schönbaum & Jacob edit Paris symposium on temperature regulation and drug action, covering 46 reports.

Scherrer & Whitehouse edit 11 reports on anti-inflammatory agents, including aryl-carboxylic, alkanoic and enolic acids, sulfonamides, gold compounds, steroids, colchicine, and allopurinol. They then edited 10 surveys on the evaluation, kinetic metabolism, and toxicity of such agents.

Howe reviews hypolipodaemic agents. Jacob & Herschler edit an important symposium on the biological actions of DMSO. This includes reports on its mechanisms of action, toxicity, metabolism, effects on tumor systems, use in agriculture and in radiation and cold protection, effects on the central nervous system, and its clinical potential. Rando, with 34 references, reviews the enzymology of "k_{cat}" inhibitors. This is a catalytic constant reflecting the probability that substrate molecules once bound may be converted into a product. He notes that an acetylene moiety, as in pargyline and its derivatives, irreversibly inhibits monamine oxidases. Vogt reviews the activation of pharmacologically active products of complement. With 38 references, he notes 9 components acting sequentially in a properdin system activating lipopolysaccharides.

LOOKING AHEAD

Reviews of pharmacological information will continue to increase in number and importance. Fortunately, the annual *Index to Scientific Reviews* issued by the Institute for Scientific Information in Philadelphia will help greatly in locating and using them.

Literature Cited

Ablad, B. et al 1975. *Acta Pharmacol. Toxicol.* 36: Suppl. 5. 142 pp.
Altura, B. M., Altura, B. T. 1974. *Anesthesiology* 41:197–214
Anderson, P. O., Kepler, J. A. 1975. *Am. J. Hosp. Pharm.* 32:473–80
Ariens, E. J. 1975. See Clark & Cumler 1975, pp. 127–52
Aviado, D. M. 1975. *Anesthesiology* 42:68–80
Bass, P. 1974. *Adv. Drug Res.* 8:205–330
Bastos, M. L., Mule, S. K. 1974. *Pharmacokinetics of Poisons and Their Metabolites,* 187–272. New York: Academic

Bennett, A. 1974. *Adv. Drug Res.* 8:83–118
Bennett, D. R., Aberg, B. 1975. *Acta Pharmacol. Toxicol.* 36:Suppl. 3. 145 pp.
Bennett, W. M., Singer, I., Coggins, C. J. 1974. *J. Am. Med. Assoc.* 230:1544–53
Brimblecombe, R. W. 1974. *Drug Actions on Cholinergic Systems.* Baltimore: Univ. Park Press. 256 pp.
Brunner, E. A., Cheng, S. C., Berman, M. L. 1975. *Ann. Rev. Med.* 26:391–401
Callingham, B. A., ed. 1974. *Drugs and Transport Processes.* Baltimore: Univ. Park Press. 356 pp.

Campbell, T. C., Hayes, J. R. 1974. *Pharmacol. Rev.* 26:171–98

Carter, W. A., ed. 1973. *Selective Inhibitors of Viral Functions.* Cleveland: Chem. Rubber. 388 pp.

Cheng, C. C. 1975. See Clark & Cumler, pp. 165–95

Ciegler, A. 1975. *Lloydia* 38:21–36

Clark, R. L., Cumler, R., eds. 1975. *Pharmacological Basis of Cancer Chemotherapy.* Baltimore: Williams & Wilkins. 737 pp.

Closson, R. 1974. *Drug Intell. Clin. Pharm.* 8:437–43

Coburn, J. W., Hartenbower, P. L., Norman, A. W. 1974. *West. J. Med.* 121:22–44

Cohen, S. N., Armstrong, M. F. 1974. *Drug Interactions.* Baltimore: Williams & Wilkins. 385 pp.

Cooperstock, R. 1974. *Social Aspects of Medical Use of Psychotropic Drugs.* Toronto: Addict. Res. Found. 179 pp.

Corcoran, J. W., Hahn, F. E. 1975. *Mechanism of Action of Antimicrobial and Antitumor Agents.* New York: Springer. 750 pp.

Csaky, T. C., ed. 1975. *Intestinal Absorption and Malabsorption.* New York: Raven. 320 pp.

Dancis, J., Hwang, J. C., eds. 1974. *Perinatal Pharmacology.* New York: Raven. 310 pp.

Davies, D. L., Wilson, G. M. 1975. *Drugs* 9:178–226

Doherty, J. E., Kane, J. J. 1975. *Ann. Rev. Med.* 26:159–72

Donoso, E., ed. 1975. *Drugs in Cardiology.* New York: Stratton. Vol. 1, Pt. 1, 239 pp.; Vol. 1, Pt. 2, 194 pp.

Duhme, D. W., Greenblatt, D. J., Miller, R. R. 1975. *Am. J. Hosp. Pharm.* 32:508–16

Farnsworth, N. R., Bingel, A. S., Cordell, G. A., Crane, F. A., Fong, H. H. 1975. *J. Pharmaceut. Sci.* 64:535–98

Feldstein, M. 1974. *Pharmacokinetics of Poisons and Their Metabolites,* 369–89. New York: Academic

Fink, B. R., ed. 1975. *Molecular Mechanisms of Anesthesia.* New York: Raven. 685 pp.

Fozard, J. R. 1975. *J. Pharm. Pharmacol.* 27:297–321

Frigerio, A., Castagnoli, N., eds. 1974. *Mass Spectrometry in Biochemistry and Medicine.* New York: Raven. 532 pp.

Garattini, S., Mussini, E., Randall, L. O., eds. 1973. *The Benzodiazepines.* New York: Raven. 685 pp.

Gardner, L. I., Amacher, P., eds. 1973. *Endocrine Aspects of Malnutrition.* New York: Raven. 520 pp.

Gibbins, R. J., Israel, Y., Kalani, H., Popham, R. E., Schnidt, W., Smart, R. G., eds. 1974. *Research Advances in Alcohol and Drug Problems.* New York: Wiley. 384 pp.

Glenn, T. M., ed. 1974. *Steroids and Shock.* Baltimore: Univ. Park Press. 470 pp.

Goldbaum, L. R., Dominguez, A. M. 1974. *Pharmacokinetics of Poisons and Their Metabolites,* 101–50. New York: Academic

Gorrod, J. W., Jenner, P. 1975. *Essays Toxicol.* 6:35–79

Greene, R. J. 1975. *Drug Intell. Clin. Pharm.* 9:17–25

Gross, M. M., ed. 1973. *Alcohol Intoxication and Withdrawal.* New York: Plenum. 422 pp.

Gyermek, L., Soyka, L. F. 1975. *Anesthesiology* 42:331–44

Hanninen, O. 1975. *Acta Pharmacol. Toxicol.* 36:Suppl. 2, 3–21

Hartshorn, E. A. 1974. *Drug Intell. Clin. Pharm.* 8:591–606

Hartshorn, E. A. 1975. *Drug Intell. Clin. Pharm.* 9:26–35

Hellon, R. F. 1974. *Pharmacol. Rev.* 26:289–322

Hodge, H. C., Stannard, J. N., Hursh, J. B., eds. *Uranium, Plutonium and Transplutonic Elements.* New York: Springer. 1017 pp.

Holloway, D. A. 1974. *Drug Intell. Clin. Pharm.* 8:632–42

Hoskins, N. M. 1974. *Am. J. Hosp. Pharm.* 31:1170–78

Howe, R. 1974. *Adv. Drug Res.* 9:7–40

Jacob, S. W., Herschler, R., eds. 1975. *Biological Actions of Dimethyl Sulfoxide,* 243:1–508. New York: Ann. NY Acad. Sci.

Jerina, D. M., Daly, J. W. 1974. *Science* 185:573–81

Koles, J. E. 1974. *Pharmacokinetics of Poisons and Their Metabolites,* 293–368. New York: Academic

Kostrzewa, R. M., Jacobowitz, D. M. 1974. *Pharmacol. Rev.* 26:199–288

Lanning, C. F., Harmel, M. H. 1975. *Ann. Rev. Med.* 26:137–42

Larson, C. P., Mazze, R. I., Cooperman, L. H., Wollman, H. 1974. *Anesthesiology* 41:169–81

Lauterbach, F. 1975. *Arzneim. Forsch.* 25:479–88

Lomax, P., Schönbaum, E., Jacob, J., eds. 1975. *Temperature Regulation and Drug Action.* Basel: Karger. 405 pp.

Magnani, B., ed. 1974. *Beta-Adrenergic Blocking Agents in the Management of Hypertension and Angina Pectoris.* New York: Raven. 220 pp.

Mandell, A. J., ed. 1975. *Neurobiological Mechanisms of Adaptation and Behavior.* New York: Raven. 344 pp.

Meisel, M., Meisel, P. 1974. *Pharmacie* 29:561–68

Morselli, P. L., Garattini, S., Cohen, S. N., eds. 1974. *Drug Interactions.* New York: Raven. 406 pp.

Morselli, P. L., Garattini, S., Sereni, F., eds. 1975. *Basic and Therapeutic Aspects of Perinatal Pharmacology.* New York: Raven. 452 pp.

Munkvad, I. 1975. *Acta Pharmacol. Toxicol.* 36:21–30

Murray, T., Goldberg, M. 1975. *Ann. Rev. Med.* 26:537–50

Nahas, G., Schaefer, K. E., eds. 1974. *Carbon-Dioxide and Metabolic Regulation.* New York: Springer. 387 pp.

Nakahara, W., Sugimura, T., Ono, T., Sugano, H., eds. 1975. *Differentiation and Control of Malignancy of Tumor Cells.* Baltimore: Univ. Park Press. 556 pp.

O'Brien, T. E. 1974. *Am. J. Hosp. Pharm.* 31:844–54

Øye, I. 1975. *Acta Pharmacol. Toxicol.* 36:Suppl. 2, pp. 31–40

Page, I. H., Bumpus, F. M., eds. 1974. *Angiotensin.* New York: Springer. 610 pp.

Parkes, D. 1974. *Adv. Drug Res.* 8:11–82

Parratt, J. R. 1974. *Adv. Drug Res.* 9:103–30

Paul, P. N., Miller, D. D., Trendelenberg, V. 1974. *Pharmacol. Rev.* 26:323–92

Pavon-Langston, D., Buchanan, R. A., Alford, C. A., eds. 1975. *Adenine Arabinoside: An Antiviral Agent.* New York: Raven. 448 pp.

Pories, W. J., Strain, W. H., Hsu, J. M., Woosley, R. L., eds. 1975. *Clinical Application of Zinc Metabolism.* Springfield, Ill: Thomas. 320 pp.

Porter, L. K. 1974. *Drug Intell. Clin. Pharm.* 8:700–708

Rando, R. R. 1974. *Science* 185:320–24

Regoli, D., Park, W. K., Rioux, F. 1974. *Pharmacol. Rev.* 26:69–123

Robinson, H. J., Vane, J. R., eds. 1974. *Prostaglandin Synthestase Inhibitors.* New York: Raven. 416 pp.

Rowe, G. G. 1974. *Anesthesiology* 41:182–96

Salmona, M., Saronio, C., Garattini, S., eds.

1974. *Insolubilized Enzymes.* New York: Raven. 275 pp.

Sandler, M., Gessa, G. L., eds. 1975. *Sexual Behavior: Pharmacology and Biochemistry.* New York: Raven. 368 pp.

Sartorelli, A. C., Johns, D. G., eds. 1974. *Antineoplastic and Immunosuppressive Agents.* New York: Springer. 762 pp.

Saunders, L. 1974. *The Absorption and Distribution of Drugs.* Baltimore: Williams & Wilkins. 272 pp.

Scherrer, R. A., Whitehouse, M. W., eds. 1974. *Antiinflammatory Agents.* New York: Academic. Vol. 1, 432 pp.; Vol. 2, 400 pp.

Schmitt, F. O., Schneider, D. M., Crothers, D. M., eds. 1975. *Functional Linkage in Biomolecular Systems.* New York: Raven. 387 pp.

Schwartz, A., Lindenmayer, G. E., Allen, J. C. 1975. *Pharmacol. Rev.* 27:3–134

Senior, N. 1974. *Adv. Pharm. Sci.* 4:363–410

Shopsin, B., Gershon, S. 1974. *Am. J. Med. Sci.* 268:306–25

Sieber, S. M., Adamson, R. H. 1975. See Clark 1975, pp. 401–68

Silverman, H. M. 1974. *Drug Intell. Clin. Pharm.* 8:690–93

Siva Sankar, D. V., ed. 1975. *LSD: A Total Study.* Westbury, NY: PJD Publ. 960 pp.

Spencer, B., ed. 1974. *Industrial Aspects of Biochemistry.* New York: Elsevier. 980 pp.

Suffness, M., Rose, B. S. 1974. *Drug Intell. Clin. Pharm.* 8:694–99

Susman, J., ed. 1975. *Drug Use and Social Policy.* New York: AMS. Vol. 1, 616 pp.; Vol. 2, 500 pp.

Ueda, I., Shieh, D. D., Eyring, H. 1974. *Anesthesiology* 41:217–25

Usdin, E., ed. 1974. *Neuropsychopharmacology of Monoamines and Their Regulatory Enzymes.* New York: Raven. 530 pp.

Venugopal, B., Luckey, T. D. 1975. *Heavy Metal Toxicity,* 4–73. Stuttgart: Thieme

Vernadakis, A., Weiner, N., eds. 1974. *Drugs and the Developing Brain.* New York: Plenum. 537 pp.

Vogt, W. 1974. *Pharmacol. Rev.* 26:125–69

Waser, P. G., ed. 1975. *Cholinergic Mechanisms.* New York: Raven. 465 pp.

Wolfe, W. G., Devries, W. C. 1975. *Ann. Rev. Med.* 26:203–18

Zimmermann, E., George, R., eds. 1974. *Narcotics and the Hypothalamus.* New York: Raven. 290 pp.

AUTHOR INDEX

A

Aach, R. D., 369
Aaron, R. K., 181
Abbanat, R. A., 192, 193
Abbatiello, E. R., 353
Abbott, V. S., 431
Abboud, F. M., 290
Abelwann, W. H., 62
Aberg, B., 508
Aberg, H., 296
Abiko, Y., 183
Ablad, B., 291, 505
Abrahamsson, H., 21
Abramow, M., 209
Acheson, G. H., 195
Ackermann, E., 432, 433
Ackers, R. P., 180
Ackrill, P., 224
Acton, J. D., 457
Adachi, K., 406
Adam, N., 76
Adams, B., 449, 455
Adams, D. R., 387
Adams, P. R., 167, 171
Adams, W. C., 37
Adamson, I. Y. R., 395
Adamson, R. H., 428, 505
Adamson, W., 293, 298
Addison, G. M., 238
Adelman, L. S., 216
Adesso, V. J., 353
Adler, K. B., 452
Adlin, E. V., 297-99, 302
Agranoff, B. W., 149
Agurell, S., 435-37
Agus, Z. S., 202, 205
Ahlenius, S., 352
Ahlquist, R. P., 296
Airaksinen, M. M., 67, 68, 72, 73, 345
Akers, T. G., 457
Akers, W., 402, 409
Al-Baker, A., 354
Albinus, M., 17, 20
Albuquerque, E. X., 144, 154, 166, 167, 169, 171
Alcaraz, M., 414-17, 424
Aldo, M. A., 218
Alegnani, W. C., 56
Alexander, E. A., 204
Alexander, J. O'D., 56
Aleyassine, H., 273, 274
Alford, C. A., 505
Alguire, P. C., 208
Al-Hachim, G. M., 254
Ali, B., 240
Allen, A. C., 59, 223
Allen, A. S., 194
Allen, F. M., 275

Allen, J. C., 507
Allen, R., 143, 146, 147
Allen, R. D., 144
Allison, A. C., 152, 457
Allison, D. J., 296
Allison, P. S., 368, 369
Allott, P. R., 71
Almirante, L., 295
Almon, R. R., 156, 220
Alper, M. H., 293
Alpers, H. S., 182, 329
Alter, H., 68
Altman, G.E., 92
Altman, K., 219
Altman, L. C., 454
Altmann, K. P., 118
Altose, M. D., 459
Altschule, M. D., 33, 34
Altura, B. M., 506
Altura, B. T., 506
Alumot, E., 135
Alvares, A. P., 407, 439
Amacher, P., 504
Amdisen, A., 233-36, 238
Amdur, M. O., 469
Amery, A., 296, 297
Amery, A. K. P. C., 299
Ametani, T., 146
Amiel, C., 202
Aminoff, M. J., 236
Amit, Z., 340, 350
Ammon, J., 318, 319
Amorico, L., 334, 354
Amposta, B., 340
Amsel, A., 341
An, R., 345
Anden, N. E., 117
Andersen, I., 452
Anderson, A. E. Jr., 396, 470
Anderson, C. R., 165, 168, 170
Anderson, F. G., 296
Anderson, G. H., 297, 303
Anderson, G. W., 324, 325
Anderson, J., 290
Anderson, J. R., 278
Anderson, K. E., 155
Anderson, M. L., 59
Anderson, M. W., 68
Anderson, P. O., 506
Anderson, S., 18
Anderson, T. F., 388
André-Bougaran, J., 396
Andreoli, T. E., 203
Andreoli, V. M., 237
Andrew, A., 271
Andrew, C. G., 220
Andriole, V. T., 455
Angel, C., 335

Ankermann, H., 428
Ankerst, J., 377
Annau, Z., 355
Anslow, W. P., 204
Anthonisen, N. R., 477, 478
Anton, S., 38, 39
Anton-Tay, F., 35, 36, 38-40
Anwyl, R., 262
Aoki, M., 317
Apajalahti, A., 62
Appel, J. B., 345, 351
Appel, S. H., 220
Aprison, M. H., 246, 252, 253, 258
ARANDA, J. V., 427-45; 427, 433, 440
Araujo, P. E., 354
Araujo-Silva, M. T., 341
Arbit, J., 76
Arborelius, M. Jr., 479
Archer, J. A., 281
Archer, M. C., 33, 39
Arefos, K. E., 181
Ariens, E. J., 169, 505
Arimura, A., 20
Armentano, L., 491
Armstrong, C. M., 165, 166
Armstrong, M. F., 504
Arndorfer, R. C., 19
Arndt, H., 467
Arnold, A., 296
Aron, C., 338
Aronow, L., 68
Arp, D. J., 340
Arroyave, R., 185
Arstila, A. U., 127, 395
Arth, C., 130
Arutyunyan, G. J., 40
Arvela, P., 431, 432, 434
Asbornsen, M. T., 406
Ascher, P., 257, 259-61
Aschkenase, L. J., 76
Asherson, G. L., 375
Ashmore, J., 275
Askenase, P. W., 375
Assaykeen, T. A., 296
Assem, E.-L. K., 17
Astrada, C. A., 352
Astrup, P., 482
Astwood, E. B., 324, 325
Atallah, M. M., 67, 68
Athanassopoulos, S., 127, 128
Atkins, L. L., 290
Atkins, N., 465, 467
Atkins, T., 38
Atkinson, D. J., 354

511

SUBJECT INDEX

2-Bromlysergic acid diethyl-
    amide
  behavioral pharmacology of,
    345
BS 100/141
  see N-Amidino-2-(2-6-di-
    ' chlorophenyl)acetamide
    HC1
Bufotenidine
  on gastrointestinal motility,
    25
Bulbogastrone
  on gastric secretion, 19
Bumetanide
  site and mechanism of action
    of, 208
  structure-activity of, 320,
    323
α-Bungarotoxin
  on invertebrate neural trans-
    mission, 257, 261
  at postjunctional membrane,
    162-63
Burinamide
  on gastric secretion, 16-
    17
Butanetrioltrinitrate (BTTN)
  metabolism of, 83
N-Butanol
  at postjunctional membrane,
    167, 172
Butylated hydroxyanisole
  behavioral effects of, 354
Butylated hydroxytoluene
  behavioral effects of, 354
1-Butyl-3-sulfanylurea carbut-
    amide
  structure-activity of, 324
Butyrophenones
  behavioral pharmacology of,
    339, 352

C

Caerulein
  on gastric motility. 23-25
  on gastric secretion, 20
Caffeine
  developmental metabolism
    of, 438
  in myopathies, 222
Calcium
  and insulin secretion, 281
  and lithium, 237-38
  in myopathies, 222, 224
    hypercalcemia, 224
    hypocalcemia, 224
  at postjunctional membrane,
    161, 163, 171
Calcium gluconate
  in mypathies, 221
Calomel
  diuretic effects of, 489
Cancer
  cell-mediated immunity to,
    376-77
  chemotherapy, reviews of,

    505
  and melatonin, 40
Cancer (crab genus)
  transmitter neurochemistry
    in, 254
Cannabis derivatives
  behavioral toxicology of,
    350
Carbacholine
  at postjunctional membrane,
    164
Carbamates
  behavioral toxicology of,
    353
Carbamazepine
  developmental metabolism
    of, 437
Carbohydrate metabolism
  lithium effect on, 239-40
Carbon dioxide
  review of, 504
Carbon dust
  on respiratory defense sys-
    tem, 452
Carbonic anhydrase inhibitors
  sites and mechanisms of
    action of, 205-6
  structure-activity of, 313-
    17, 321
Carbon tetrachloride (CCl_4)
  and lipid peroxidation,
    132-34, 137
N_1-O-Carboxyphenyl-N_2-2,2-
    methylaminopropyl-1-
    phenylacetamide
  as stimulant, 492
Carcinoembryonic antigen
    (CEA)
  in immunosuppression,
    369
Carcinogens
  in manufacture of arsenicals,
    95-100
  reviews of, 504
Carcinus
  transmitter neurochemistry
    in, 254
Cardiac glycosides
  bioavailability of, 62
Cardiovascular disease
  renin as prognostic factor
    for, 299-300
Cardiovascular system
  reviews of, 506-7
Castor oil
  mode of action of, 28
Catecholamines
  colchicine effect on, 149
  on convulsive threshold,
    491
  effects of neurotoxic indole-
    amines on, 101-9
  on gastrointestinal motility,
    22
  in hypertension, 288
  on pancreatic islet, 277-78,
    280-82

  and thrombogenesis, 183
Catechol-O-methyltransferase
    (COMT)
  in pancreatic islets, 273
Catharanthine
  on intracellular movement,
    151
Cathartics
  mode of action of, 27
Catron
  see Pheniprazine
Celluline
  discovery and activity of,
    493
Central control of blood pres-
    sure, 113-25
  central β-adrenergic recep-
    tors, 120-21
  central cardiovascular
    effects of α-adrenergic
    agonists, 115-20
  clonidine, 117-19
  desipramine-clonidine
    interaction, 120
  drugs related to clonidine,
    119
  methyldopa, 116-17
  norepinephrine and related
    substances, 115-16
  conclusions, 121
  distribution, 113-14
  noradrenergic neurons in
    experimental hyperten-
    sion, 114-15
Central nervous system (CNS)
  anesthetic effects on brain
    electrical activity, 413-
    26
    classical schema of CNS
    excitation and depression,
    414
    continuum of states, 416-
    17
    control mechanism for
    sensory input and arousal,
    diagram of, 422
  effects of chronic anesthetics
    on, 76
  effects of melatonin on, 38-
    40
  effects of neurotoxic amines
    on, 101-9
    morphological effects,
    106
    regeneration, 107
  reviews of, 505-6
Cephalin
  and thrombogenesis, 182
Chemotaxis
  measurement of, 453-54
Chemotherapy
  bioavailability as factor in,
    54-58
  Hungarian work on,
    496
  reviews of, 505
Chistrionicotoxin

review of, 505
Tyramine
  on pancreatic islet, 277
  pineal effects of, 43, 45-46
  and thrombogenesis, 183
Tyrode solution
  in skin perfusion, 407-8
Tyrosine
  and immunity, 368
Tyrosine aminotransferase
  developmental studies of, 439
Tyrosine transaminase
  developmental studies of, 440

U

Ultraviolet irradiation
  cutaneous effects of, 408
Uranium
  toxicology of, 507
Urethane
  and thrombogenesis, 181
Urine flow
  lithium effect on, 238
Urogastrone
  on gastric secretion, 19

V

Valine
  and immunity, 368
Vasoactive intestinal peptide
  (VIP)
  on gastric secretion, 19-20
Vasoconstriction
  invertebrate
    acetylcholine in, 261
  and thrombogenesis, 184
Vasodilators
  on hypertension, 291-92
Vasopressin

and lithium, 240
and thrombogenesis, 182
Ventilatory exchange
  tests of, 471, 476-77, 480
Villikinin
  on gastric secretion, 19
Vinblastine
  on intracellular movement, 149, 151-52
  and platelet formation, 179
Vinca alkaloids
  intracellular transport role of, 147, 149-52
Vincamine
  synthetic derivatives of, 497
Vincristine
  on intracellular movement, 149, 151
  and platelet formation, 179
Vindoline
  on intracellular movement, 151
Virus infection
  inhibitors of, reviewed, 508
  respiratory defense against, 456-58
    alveolar macrophage, 457
    effects of pollutants on, 456
    mucociliary transport, 457
    protection by interferon, 457-58
Vital capacity
  and lung function, 471
Vitamin A (retinol)
  cutaneous effects of, 409
Vitamin C
  discovery of, 490-91
Vitamin D
  review of, 508
Vitamin E

and lipid peroxidation, 129-30, 133
  myopathy from, 226
Vitamin P
  discovery of, 491
Vitamins
  bioavailability of, 63

W

Warfarin sodium
  bioavailability of, 63
Water
  normal renal physiology of, 202-4
Water, heavy
  on intracellular movement, 155-56
Withdrawal
  physical and psychic aspects of, 349

X

Xenobiotics
  and hepatic monooxygenase system development, 427-45
Xentropiniumbromid (gastripon)
  cholinolytic action of, 489
X irradiaton
  in immunosuppression, 368-69
Xylazine (Bayer 1470)
  central cardiovascular effects of, 119

Z

Zinc
  metabolism of, 507
Zinc sulfate
  review of, 507
Zoxazolamine
  and lipid peroxidation, 128

CUMULATIVE INDEXES

CONTRIBUTING AUTHORS VOLUMES 12-16

CHAPTER TITLES VOLUMES 12-16